Neurosurgery's Frontline Role in Gliomas Treatment

Daniele Armocida • Diego Garbossa
Maurizio Salvati
Editors

Neurosurgery's Frontline Role in Gliomas Treatment

Trends, Technologies and Treatments

Springer

Editors
Daniele Armocida
Neurosurgery Unit, Dept. Neuroscience
"Rita Levi Montalcini"
Università degli studi di Torino
Torino, TO, Italy

Diego Garbossa
Neurosurgery Unit, Dept. Neuroscience
"Rita Levi Montalcini"
Università degli studi di Torino
Torino, TO, Italy

Maurizio Salvati
Neurosurgery Unit
University di Roma "Tor Vergata"
Roma, Italy

ISBN 978-3-031-81852-3 ISBN 978-3-031-81850-9 (eBook)
https://doi.org/10.1007/978-3-031-81850-9

This Springer imprint is published by the registered company Springer Nature Switzerland AG
The registered company address is: Gewerbestrasse 11, 6330 Cham, Switzerland

Preface

Gliomas are known to be one of the most challenging tumors to treat and have a relatively poor prognosis with the current standard of care. To address this, treatment paradigms depend on a multidisciplinary clinical effort that incorporates the expertise of dedicated neurosurgeons, neuro-oncologists, radiation oncologists, neuropathologists, and radiologists. This comprehensive clinical focus from several specialties underscores the significance of the combined effort of each discipline in providing patients with the most advanced care options available.

The fields of medicine, research, and technology are currently undergoing significant changes, and this is also evident in the most recent studies concerning the brain tumors. The newly established World Health Organization (WHO) classification system has introduced novel concepts for understanding gliomas by emphasizing the importance of molecular profiling over traditional histology-based methods. These developments have not only altered the way brain tumors are classified but also affected their treatment, from initial care to recurrence.

Neuro-oncology, a critical area in the study and treatment of gliomas, encompasses numerous areas of expertise. However, it is essential to recognize that surgery for diagnostic and therapeutic purposes remains the primary and often the most critical step in treating patients affected by gliomas. Therefore, a comprehensive overview of the current state-of-the-art treatments for gliomas, organized by subspecialized disciplines, will provide physicians with updated information on new therapeutic paradigms and future advancements.

The primary objective of this research is to delve into every facet of patient assessment and care, with a particular emphasis on the skills and challenges associated with surgical interventions. It is not to say that neurosurgeons are more important than other medical professionals, but rather that surgical procedures often serve as a critical juncture in a patient's care and are typically their most stressful and uncomfortable moments. This book is designed for medical or nonmedical professionals who are eager to confront the challenging and intriguing obstacles posed by complex conditions such as gliomas.

Torino, Italy — Daniele Armocida
Torino, Italy — Diego Garbossa
Rome, Italy — Maurizio Salvati

Contents

Part I

Part I

1 Neurosurgery at the Frontline of Glioma Care: What do We Really Mean?

Daniele Armocida, Alessandro Pesce, Diego Garbossa, Maurizio Salvati, and Alessandro Frati

1.1 Still a Long Search

At the time of writing this book, the number of results obtained from a search on PubMed for the keyword "glioma" was over 125,000 papers, which includes studies, reviews, book chapters, and case series. While this appears to be a large quantity of research, it is actually quite small compared to the more than 450,000 results obtained from a search, for example, "lung cancer" as a keyword. Gliomas are relatively uncommon compared to other types of cancers [1]. However, research in the field of neuro-oncology has accelerated significantly in recent decades, with numerous studies providing a better understanding of glioma pathogenesis [2]. When looking at the distribution of publications over the years, it is evident that most of them have been produced in the last two decades (Fig. 1.1). This increase in publications is not surprising, given the significant rise in the number of annual publications and the emergence of new journals, editorials, books, and publishers in all fields of research. It is also worth noting that despite this significant increase in publications and studies, there has not been a corresponding improvement in patient outcomes from a purely clinical-prognostic perspective for those suffering from gliomas, which is a concerning issue.

For glioblastoma, which remains the most prevalent histotype among adults, survival rates typically range between 16 and 18 months under optimal care [3]. Although several prognostic markers and subcategories have been identified to distinguish the most aggressive forms, the general population's disease progression has not significantly improved. Notably, the most frequently cited paper in the literature on gliomas is a 2005 study by Stupp et al. [4], which reported the outcomes of the eponymous treatment protocol for glioblastomas. Upon closer examination of recent research, it becomes evident that there is a significant focus on preclinical studies. Out of the approximately 125,000 initial results, only about 35,000 involve neurosurgical studies or incorporate the surgical procedure component in some way.

D. Armocida (✉) · D. Garbossa
Neurosurgery Unit, Dept. Neuroscience "Rita Levi Montalcini", Università degli studi di Torino, Torino, TO, Italy
e-mail: danielearmocida@yahoo.it

A. Pesce
Policlinico Tor Vergata (PTV), Neurosurgery Unit, Università degli studi di Roma (Tor Vergata), Rome, Italy

M. Salvati
Neurosurgery Unit, University di Roma "Tor Vergata", Rome, Italy

A. Frati
IRCCS "Neuromed", Pozzilli, IS, Italy

Neurosurgery Division, Human Neurosciences Department, "La Sapienza" University, Rome, Italy

D. Armocida et al. (eds.), *Neurosurgery's Frontline Role in Gliomas Treatment*,
https://doi.org/10.1007/978-3-031-81850-9_1

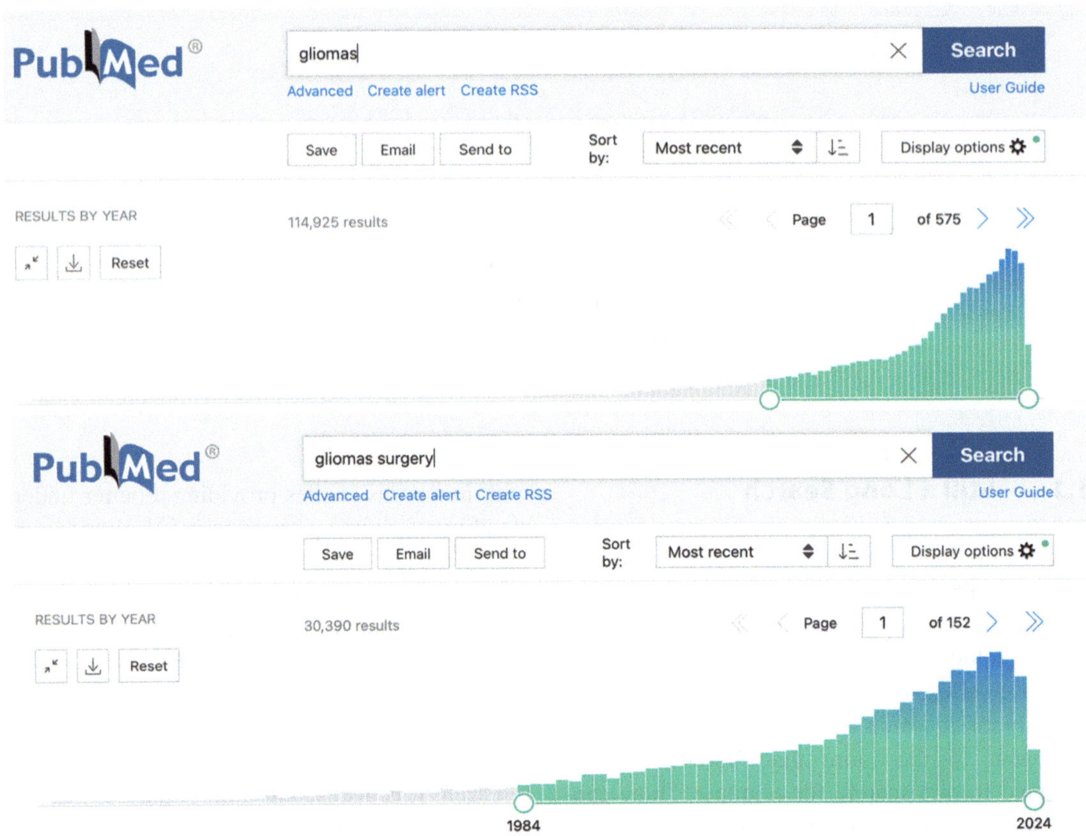

Fig. 1.1 Searching on pubmed, generically for the term "glioma" yields over 110,000 results, the majority of which refer to papers published in the last 20 years. It is also observed that entering "surgery" as the keyword MESH the results are around 30,000 papers denoting the strong imbalance between pre-clinical and surgical research

In a recent bibliometric study from 2020 [5], it was reported that gliomas, as primary topic in oncology, also extend into fields such as neurosurgery, neurology, radiation therapy, basic sciences, and general medicine, which accounts for the diverse range of journals in which the most highly cited articles were published. Only 12% of articles were published in neuroscience-specific journals, while the majority were published in oncology, basic sciences, and general medicine journals. A significant portion of the studies conducted were concentrated in a few national centers, mainly in the United States and a few European countries, such as France and Switzerland. This differs from bibliometric findings in other fields, like cardiology and thrombolytic therapy, where most of the pioneering articles are widely distributed across countries and originate from specialty journals, considering that advancements in these fields are primarily of interest to researchers and clinicians in those specialties. This observation seems counterintuitive because surgical intervention is generally considered a key aspect of glioma patient management, and it often serves as the initial step in the management process, whether for diagnostic or therapeutic purposes.

Why is there a difference in research priorities between neurosurgical and biological-molecular interests? The answer to this question is multifaceted and not straightforward. The primary limitation of oncologic neurosurgery is that surgery alone is usually insufficient to ensure a complete cure, even for the least aggressive forms of the disease. Oncologic neurosurgery, as specialized field of neurosurgery, faces significant challenges in its procedures, including the need for complete tumor resection, which often requires sacrificing important sensory-motor and neuro-cognitive functions. The limitations of the surgical approach become even more substantial for deep-seated tumors. From a technical standpoint, the lack of a proper tumor capsule, the similarity in appearance between the tumor and healthy tissue, and the absence of macroscopic landmarks make the surgical procedure complex and do not guarantee complete resection [6]. Recent advancements in resection methods have been made possible by the integration of new technologies including neuronavigation, immunofluorescence, and augmented reality. These innovations have revolutionized the approach to tumor resection and overall survival, which were previously the only parameters used to measure treatment success and quality of care for patients with glioma over several decades. However, with the emergence of new systemic therapeutic approaches and imaging technologies as well as a deeper understanding of brain connectivity and molecular mechanisms of glioma, individualized patient-centered therapy for glioma is a promising standard of care [7].

The use of new biological drugs in chemotherapy for gliomas has become increasingly popular as a viable option for adjuvant treatment in most cases. There is a growing interest in immunotherapy, including immune checkpoint molecules, tumor-associated macrophages, dendritic cell vaccines, and CAR-T, as well as the tumor microenvironment and the combination of different effective methods [8]. The emergence of many targeted therapy options has also led to a focus on biomarkers that guide the prescription of a specific targeted therapy [9]. To develop successful treatments for gliomas, faithful in vivo disease modeling and rigorous preclinical testing are necessary. Murine models, including xenograft, syngeneic, and genetically engineered models, are used to study glioma-genesis, identify methods of tumor progression, and test novel treatment strategies. Improvements in preclinical models that capture the phenotypic and molecular heterogeneity of gliomas are crucial for the development of new effective therapies [10]. It is also important to consider new disciplines introduced in recent years, such as computer analysis, machine and deep learning, radiomics, and applications of artificial intelligence [11, 12].

Despite numerous advancements in surgical and oncologic techniques, precise methods for enhancing glioma patient outcomes remain unclear. Neuro-oncology is a field that demands a cooperative strategy, with no particular individual dominating the others. All clinical decisions ranging from diagnosis to neurorehabilitation and follow-up plans should be made jointly. Furthermore, it is not reasonable to assume that a molecular biologist could carry out a study on brain gliomas without first interacting with medical professionals who specialize in the clinical aspects of the disease, such as neurooncologists or neurosurgeons. As you read the following chapters, you will observe how each functional clinical moment determines the story of the disease, from in-depth neuroradiology to surgical planning, procedure, and rehabilitation.

The optimal management of glioma patients involves a multidisciplinary approach that includes specialists from neurosurgery, neuro-oncology, and radiation oncology. The initial management should focus on addressing urgent clinical symptoms and conducting a comprehensive molecular diagnosis. Although surgery is a crucial aspect of glioma management, the infiltrative nature of these tumors means that even complete surgical resection is typically not curative (Fig. 1.2). Therefore, adjuvant therapy is essential for extending progression-free survival (PFS) and overall survival (OS) [13]. The text will provide an overview of the entire management process for patients with cerebral glioma, acknowledging that surgery is often unavoidable in most cases. The initial part of the text will cover the current state of knowledge on the topic, while the latter part will discuss future perspectives. The book begins with an overview of general epidemiological knowledge, coherently to all traditional medical-scientific texts.

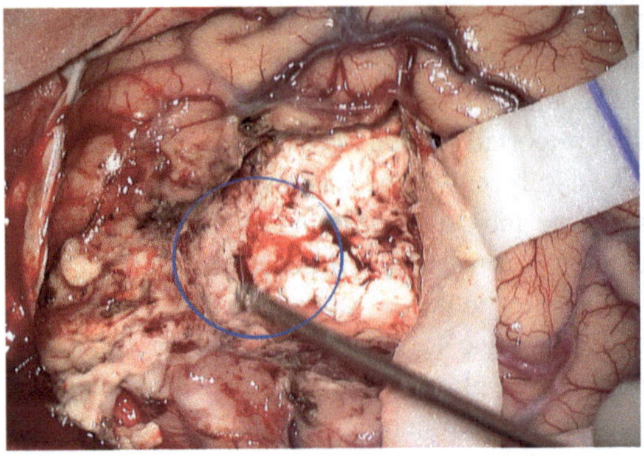

Fig. 1.2 From the present surgical image, it is possible to observe the great difficulty of removing a glioblastoma, as it is challenging to define the margin and boundaries around healthy tissue

1.2 Glioma's Definition and Epidemiology

Gliomas are the most common primary neoplasms of the central nervous system (CNS) in adults [14, 15]. They are typically distinct for their astrocytic or oligodendrocytic origin and are categorized according to the World Health Organization (WHO) grade [16]. Approximately, 85,000 individuals in the United States and 5/100000 in Europe are diagnosed with a primary brain tumor each year [17], of which approximately 80–85% of these are gliomas, which diffusely infiltrate the brain parenchyma. The incidence of glioblastoma (GB), the most common malignant primary brain tumor in adults, increases after the age of 40 and peaks in adults aged 75–84 years. Lower-grade diffuse gliomas usually affect patients younger than 50 years old and are further subclassified into astrocytomas and oligodendrogliomas [15].

Less than 5% of adults with a malignant brain tumor report a family history of brain tumors or have a cancer predisposition syndrome [18]. However, the contribution of heritability to brain tumor formation is likely higher, based on germline sequencing and analysis using Genome-wide Complex Trait Analysis (GCTA). Prior exposure to ionizing radiation to the CNS, usually during treatment for another cancer, such as childhood leukemia, is considered a risk factor for brain tumors. Exposure to low-frequency electromagnetic fields is not an established risk factor. No high-quality evidence demonstrates an association between cellular telephone use and brain tumor formation. Furthermore, a large and recent multicenter study involving five different nations and more than 1 million participants, no relationship was found between intensive cellular phone use and the occurrence of brain tumors [19].

In an international case-control study of 4533 glioma patients and 4171 controls, a history of respiratory allergies, asthma, or eczema was associated with a statistically significant lower risk of glioma. Those with glioma (229 patients) are also less likely than controls (289 patients) to report a history of varicella virus (adjusted OR, 0.59 [95% CI, 0.40–0.86]) and have lower levels of immunoglobulin G to varicella virus [20].

Since identifying key molecular alterations that provided a definitive prognosis and led to the 2021 WHO classification of CNS tumors, understanding of glioma behavior has rapidly evolved [21]. The mutations in isocitrate dehydrogenase (IDH) 1 and 2 are present in all of the adult grade 2 and 3 gliomas, and the use of 1p/19q codeletion for classification is now limited to the oligodendroglioma distinction. Furthermore, new molecular key factors were discovered to improve distinction and to better predict the prognosis (Fig. 1.3). As such, low-grade glioma (LGG) encompasses all grade 2 and 3 tumors, while high-grade gliomas (HGG, grade 4) are definitely identified with the IDH-wild type mutation or the new additional molecular characterization. With this definitive shift in the understanding of lower-grade gliomas, disease management is being redefined in the setting of emerging molecular-genetic biomarkers rather than historical pathological findings (Fig. 1.4, [22]).

Comprehensive molecular profiling has dramatically mutated the diagnostic neuropathology of brain tumors. Diffuse gliomas are now classified by highly recurrent biomarkers instead of histo-morphological characteristics. The advent of molecular profiling technology has altered neoplastic disease classification, delineating more biologically and clinically uniform entities that often transcend conventional histopathologi-

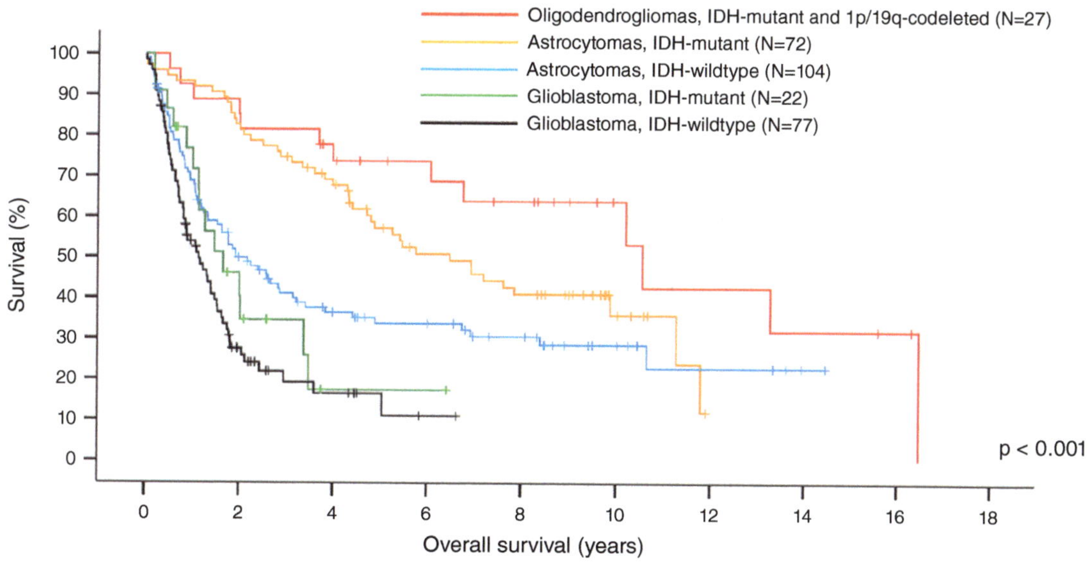

Fig. 1.3 This Keplen-Meier chart shows how the distinction between oligodendroglioma, astrocytoma and glioblastoma with IDH mutation alone is capable of determining important prognostic stratification

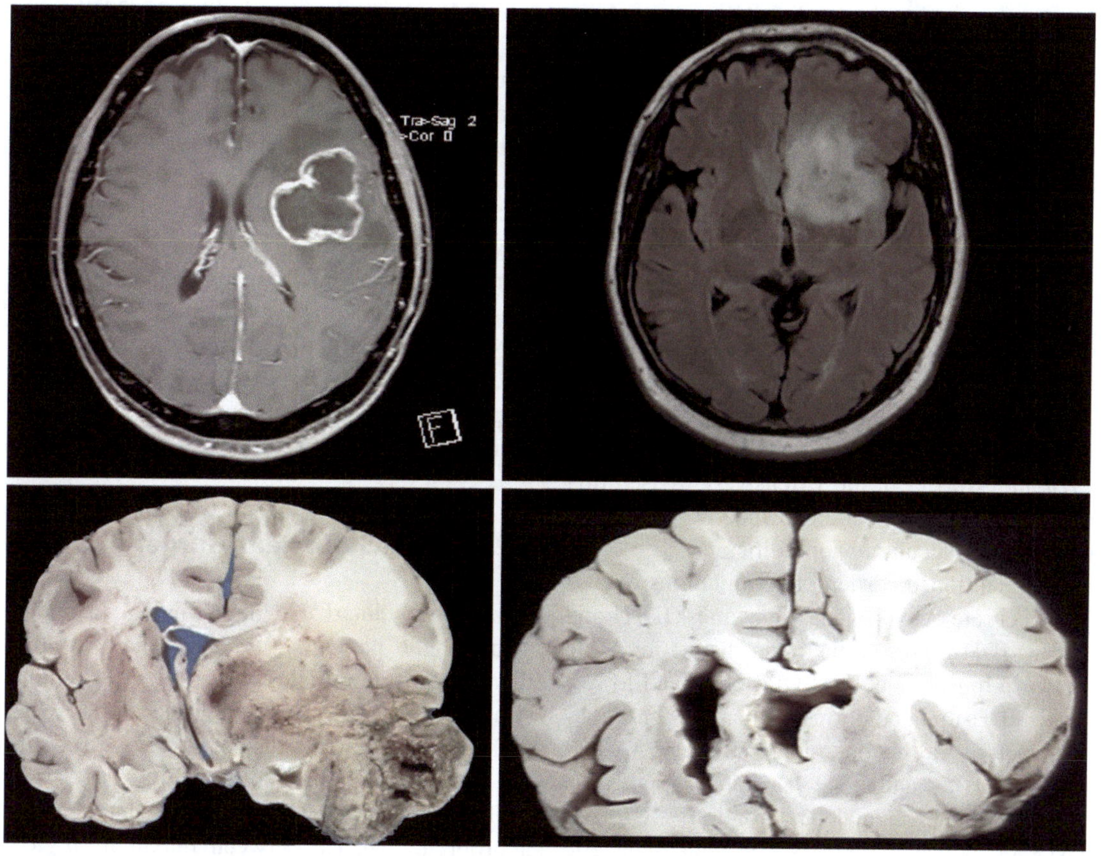

Fig. 1.4 The image shows the pathological counterpart of high- and low-grade gliomas, respectively, compared with imaging according to historical and traditional classification criteria

cal categorization [23]. This is particularly evident in brain tumor taxonomy, where this fundamental shift in approach has led to both the refinement of existing diagnostic categories and the creation of several novel tumor types.

Neoplastic categories based on the histopathological features of astrocytes and oligodendrocytes have been revised and optimized with the integration of disease-defining molecular markers, stratifying biologically, clinically, and prognostically distinct entities in adult and pediatric populations. Moreover, above and beyond tumor classification, these developments have revealed novel pathogenic mechanisms involving epigenetic regulator genes not previously been implicated in oncogenesis.

Historically, diffuse gliomas have been classified solely based on histological characteristics into HGG, lower-grade astrocytomas, or oligodendrogliomas, with a portion of lower-grade tumors expressing both glial phenotypes (oligoastrocytomas). Histological diagnosis of HGG was performed based on central pseudopallisading necrosis and microvascular proliferation. In contrast, diffuse astrocytomas and oligodendrogliomas were typically characterized by moderately increased cellularity, small nuclear atypia, low mitotic activity, absence of necrosis, and microvascular proliferation [24].

Morphology alone does not sufficiently predict clinical behavior, with tumor progression varying notably across each histological subtype. More recently, the WHO, informed by large genomic profiling studies like the Cancer Genome Atlas [25], has extensively revised diffuse glioma classification to incorporate highly penetrant molecular abnormalities.

As mentioned earlier, gene mutations encoding isocitrate dehydrogenase enzymes (IDH1 and IDH2) IDH represent the main distinction node between high-grade (IDH wild-type) and lower-grade IDH-mutated forms. Other key biomarkers, such as H3 histone monomers (H3F3A and HIST1H3B), and the histone chaperone α-thalassemia mental retardation X-linked (ATRX), induce disruptions in normal epigenetic functionality, revealing previously unappreciated oncogenic mechanisms [26].

IDH mutations, as codified in the WHO 2021 [16], designate predominantly lower-grade (WHO grade 2 and 3) diffuse gliomas distinct from IDH-wildtype GB, the archetypical WHO grade 4 primary brain tumors. IDH-wildtype GBM almost invariably arises de novo in a fully malignant state characterized by the aggressive histopathological features of microvascular proliferation and necrosis, and although exclusively low-grade morphology is occasionally encountered, rapid clinical progression is the rule. GB and WHO grade 4, with histologically LGG, possess highly infiltrative patterns, such as gliomatosis cerebri growth patterns with widespread involvement [24].

IDH-mutant gliomas, while ultimately deadly, typically progress at a more measured pace through repeated cycles of treatment and recurrence before emerging as high-grade lesions [27]. The prognosis of the glioma patient is influenced mostly by the molecular profile [27–29], extent of surgical resection, age, and initial and postoperative performance status [30]. Survival varies significantly by grade across all glioma subtypes and expression of key biomarkers [31]. GB has the poorest overall survival (OS), with only 0.05–4.7% of patients surviving 5 years past diagnosis and a median survival of approximately 15 months [32], while gliomas with an oligodendroglial component have increased survival, as opposed to those with an astrocytic component. Age is significantly associated with survival after diagnosis for all glioma, but the effect is most pronounced for GB [33].

1.2.1 First Step: Neurosurgery

Despite the remarkable improvement in understanding the pathogenesis of gliomas, the first therapeutic step remains surgery. It was demonstrated in population-based parallel cohorts that early surgical resection is associated with better OS than biopsy and watchful waiting [15].

Therefore, it is necessary to maintain an appropriate balance between maximal surgical resection and the risk of neurological damage contributed to the patient [34]. The goals of surgery are maximal tumor removal associated with minimal postoperative morbidity and maximal patient functional preservation [35]. Surgery is important since it relieves symptoms and provides accurate histological and molecular diagnosis. Extent of resection (EOR) remains a critical determinant of oncologic outcomes for patients with high- and low-grade glioma [36]. Realizing the true benefit of neurosurgical resection requires a balance between surgical cytoreduction and preservation of neurological function. This surgical concept is defined as "Maximal safe resection" and "Neuro-oncological balance" [14].

But while there is the issue of a balance between surgical radicality and preservation of function, fully understanding what it means to perform a total resection and understanding whether all functions, including higher cognitive functions, have been preserved has not yet been achieved [37].

At first, it is known that the carcinogenic process and mutations leading to the tumor-disease phenotype are already initiated by surrounding cells beyond the contrast-enhancing tumor visible on MRI [38]. Supratotal resection is the emerging concept within GB-surgery, which aims to achieve a more extensive resection of the tumor than is possible with conventional techniques [39]. The technique involves the removal of more than 100% of the visible tumor tissue, which means that the surgeon removes not only the tumor itself but also some surrounding healthy brain tissue [40]. This may be accomplished with 5-aminolaevulinic acid (5-ALA)-guided tumor tissue elimination, using intraoperative MRI for non-enhancing residual tumors, or resection until improvement in clinical outcome is achieved [41].

Neuronavigation using 5-ALA fluorescence and microsurgical techniques have been developed to enable maximal safe neurosurgical tumor resection and minimize the neurological consequences of glioma surgery [42]. Furthermore, in glioma radiotherapy treatment planning, a margin of 15–25 mm is typically applied to the edge of the gross tumor to create the CTV, and a further 5 mm is added to generate a safety margin [43]. This raises the probability of progression-free recession and survival while lowering the likelihood of recurrence, but on the other side can notably increment the risk of functional damage [44] and treatment-related cerebral necrosis.

Second, within the neurosurgical planning, the definition of what brain tissue must be considered "eloquent" is still mostly based on a classic localizationist model, which assumes that cortical areas are specialized for specific aspects of neurological functions. On the other hand, this model is now outdated, and cognitive neuroscience research suggests that every cognitive and motor function depends on complex neuroplastic networks connecting many cortical areas by means of long- and short-association white-matter (WM) fibers [45]. According to this connectionist model, cortical and subcortical functional interplay may be highly variable among human beings and can reorganize in response to brain damage, such as a relatively slow-growing tumor mass [46, 47]. These neuroplastic properties might explain why, despite bearing an extensive mass located close or within brain tissue considered to be critical according to the classic localizationist model, patients with brain tumors usually display very mild or even no neurological deficit at presentation and can maintain this status even after surgery with extensive tumoral and peritumoral tissue resection [48]. Preserving cortical and subcortical function is important for better postoperative outcomes and improved quality of life; thus, the concept of neuroplasticity should be considered for accurate presurgical planning, but the full translation of this factor from basic to clinical neuroscience is still lacking because of an incomplete understanding of its mechanisms [49]. Currently, it is still impossible to predict its impact on the post-surgical outcome based on an objective measure of how much the brain of the patient has already reorganized in response to the tumor and may still reorganize after surgery. From this point of view, cortical and subcortical structures show different plastic potential. The cortex seems to have great neuroplastic potential, and it can reorganize effectively in the case of brain tumors, while white-matter bundles seem to have low plastic potential, and extensive surgical resections might depend mainly on white-matter boundaries rather than on the cortical extension of the tumor [50]. Although the goal of maximal safe resection is clear, it is often difficult in clinical practice to identify the correct planning because the limit of a maximum EOR is unclear, and the preservation of neurological function is undefined.

As discussed in the opening section of this chapter, surgery is the primary therapeutic option for patients with cerebral glioma. However, achieving balanced function while ensuring complete resection is challenging. Without the support of adjuvant chemotherapy, radiation therapy, appropriate clinical-radiological follow-up, and rehabilitation, the chances of a cure are reduced. It is important to note that each of these areas alone is insufficient, and a long search is still necessary.

References

1. Bello L, Gambini A, Castellano A, Carrabba G, Acerbi F, Fava E, Giussani C, Cadioli M, Blasi V, Casarotti A, Papagno C, Gupta AK, Gaini S, Scotti G, Falini A. Motor and language DTI fiber tracking combined with intraoperative subcortical mapping for surgical removal of gliomas. NeuroImage. 2008;39(1):369–82. https://doi.org/10.1016/j.neuroimage.2007.08.031.
2. Ostrom QT, Gittleman H, Farah P, Ondracek A, Chen Y, Wolinsky Y, Stroup NE, Kruchko C, Barnholtz-Sloan JS. CBTRUS statistical report: Primary brain and central nervous system tumors diagnosed in the United States in 2006–2010. Neuro Oncol. 2013;15(Suppl 2):ii1–56. https://doi.org/10.1093/neuonc/not151. Erratum in: Neuro Oncol. 2014 May;16(5):760.
3. Louis DN, et al. The 2021 WHO classification of tumors of the central nervous system: a summary. Neuro-Oncology. 2021;23:1231–51.
4. Leece R, Xu J, Ostrom QT, Chen Y, Kruchko C, Barnholtz-Sloan JS. Global incidence of malignant brain and other central nervous system tumors by histology, 2003-2007. Neuro-Oncology. 2017;19(11):1553–64. https://doi.org/10.1093/neuonc/nox091.
5. Schaff LR, Mellinghoff IK. Glioblastoma and other primary brain malignancies in adults: a review. JAMA. 2023;329(7):574–87. https://doi.org/10.1001/jama.2023.0023.
6. Armocida D, Pesce A, Santoro A, Salvati M, Frati A. Letter to the editor: "the neurosurgical perspective for the 2021 WHO classification of tumors of the central nervous system: a missed opportunity?". World Neurosurg. 2021;155:203–4. https://doi.org/10.1016/j.wneu.2021.07.149.
7. Tom MC, Cahill DP, Buckner JC, Dietrich J, Parsons MW, Yu JS. Management for different glioma subtypes: are all low-grade gliomas created equal? Am Soc Clin Oncol Educ Book. 2019;39:133–45. https://doi.org/10.1200/EDBK_238353.
8. Yan H, Parsons DW, Jin G, McLendon R, Rasheed BA, Yuan W, Kos I, Batinic-Haberle I, Jones S, Riggins GJ, Friedman H, Friedman A, Reardon D, Herndon J, Kinzler KW, Velculescu VE, Vogelstein B, Bigner DD. IDH1 and IDH2 mutations in gliomas. N Engl J Med. 2009;360(8):765–73. https://doi.org/10.1056/NEJMoa0808710.
9. Motomura K, Kibe Y, Ohka F, Aoki K, Yamaguchi J, Saito R. Clinical characteristics and radiological features of glioblastoma, IDH-wildtype, grade 4 with histologically lower-grade gliomas. Brain Tumor Pathol. 2023;40(2):48–55. https://doi.org/10.1007/s10014-023-00458-5. Epub 2023 Mar 29.
10. Berger MF, Mardis ER. The emerging clinical relevance of genomics in cancer medicine. Nat Rev Clin Oncol. 2018;15(6):353–65. https://doi.org/10.1038/s41571-018-0002-6.
11. Liu XY, Gerges N, Korshunov A, Sabha N, Khuong-Quang DA, Fontebasso AM, Fleming A, Hadjadj D, Schwartzentruber J, Majewski J, Dong Z, Siegel P, Albrecht S, Croul S, Jones DT, Kool M, Tonjes M, Reifenberger G, Faury D, Zadeh G, Pfister S, Jabado N. Frequent ATRX mutations and loss of expression in adult diffuse astrocytic tumors carrying IDH1/IDH2 and TP53 mutations. Acta Neuropathol. 2012;124(5):615–25. https://doi.org/10.1007/s00401-012-1031-3.
12. Kurokawa R, Kurokawa M, Baba A, Ota Y, Pinarbasi E, Camelo-Piragua S, Capizzano AA, Liao E, Srinivasan A, Moritani T. Major changes in 2021 World Health Organization classification of central nervous system tumors. Radiographics. 2022;42(5):1474–93. https://doi.org/10.1148/rg.210236. Epub 2022 Jul 8.
13. Shirahata M, Ono T, Stichel D, et al. Novel, improved grading system(s) for IDH-mutant astrocytic gliomas. Acta Neuropathol. 2018;136(1):153–66. https://doi.org/10.1007/s00401-018-1849-4. Epub 2018 Apr 23.
14. Armocida D, Pesce A, Di Giammarco F, Frati A, Santoro A, Salvati M. Long term survival in patients suffering from Glio-blastoma multiforme: a single-center observational cohort study. Diagnostics (Basel). 2019;9(4):209. https://doi.org/10.3390/diagnostics9040209.
15. Yoshikawa MH, Rabelo NN, Telles JPM, Figueiredo EG. Modifiable risk factors for glioblastoma: a systematic review and meta-analysis. Neurosurg Rev. 2023;46(1):143. https://doi.org/10.1007/s10143-023-02051-y.
16. Creighton H, Beach B, Bamford S-M. Rethinking cancer, 2015. Available: www.ilcuk.org.uk.
17. Armocida D, Pesce A, Palmieri M, Cofano F, Palmieri G, Cassoni P, Busceti CL, Biagioni F, Garbossa D,

Fornai F, Santoro A, Frati A. EGFR-driven mutation in non-small-cell lung cancer (NSCLC) influences the features and outcome of brain metastases. J Clin Med. 2023;12(10):3372. https://doi.org/10.3390/jcm12103372.
18. van den Bent MJ, Geurts M, French PJ, Smits M, Capper D, Bromberg JEC, Chang SM. Primary brain tumours in adults. Lancet. 2023;402(10412):1564–79. https://doi.org/10.1016/S0140-6736(23)01054-1.
19. Brown TJ, Brennan MC, Li M, Church EW, Brandmeir NJ, Rakszawski KL, et al. Association of the extent of resection with survival in glioblastoma: a systematic review and meta- analysis. JAMA Oncol. 2016;2:1460–9.
20. de Leeuw CN, Vogelbaum MA. Supratotal resection in glioma: a systematic review. Neuro-Oncology. 2019;21(2):179–88. https://doi.org/10.1093/neuonc/noy166.
21. Incekara F, Koene S, Vincent AJ, van den Bent MJ, Smits M. Association between supratotal glioblastoma resection and patient survival: a systematic review and meta-analysis. World Neurosurg. 2019;127:617–24.
22. Suero Molina E, Schipmann S, Stummer W. Maximizing safe resections: the roles of 5- aminolevulinic acid and intraoperative MR imaging in glioma surgery-review of the literature. Neurosurg Rev. 2019;42(2):197–208. https://doi.org/10.1007/s10143-017-0907-z.
23. Castellano A, Bailo M, Cicone F, Carideo L, Quartuccio N, Mortini P, Falini A, Cascini GL, Minniti G. Advanced imaging techniques for radiotherapy planning of gliomas. Cancers (Basel). 2021;13(5):1063. https://doi.org/10.3390/cancers13051063.
24. Aziz PA, Memon SF, Hussain M, Memon AR, Abbas K, Qazi SU, Memon RAR, Qambrani KA, Taj O, Ghazanfar S, Ellahi A, Ahmed M. Supratotal resection: an emerging concept of glioblastoma Multiforme surgery-systematic review and meta-analysis. World Neurosurg. 2023;179:e46–55. https://doi.org/10.1016/j.wneu.2023.07.020.
25. Armocida D, Pesce A, Palmieri M, D'Andrea G, Salvati M, Santoro A, Frati A. Periventricular zone involvement as a predictor of survival in glioblastoma patients: a single centre cohort-comparison investigation concerning a distinct clinical entity. Interdiscip Neurosurg. 2021;25:101185. https://doi.org/10.1016/j.inat.2021.101185.
26. Di Cristofori A, Basso G, de Laurentis C, Mauri I, Sirtori MA, Ferrarese C, Isella V, Giussani C. Perspectives on (a)symmetry of arcuate fasciculus. A short review about anatomy, tractography and TMS for arcuate fasciculus reconstruction in planning surgery for gliomas in language areas. Front Neurol. 2021;10(12):639822. https://doi.org/10.3389/fneur.2021.639822.
27. Julkunen P, Karhu J. Brain plasticity in neurosurgery. In: Krieg SM, editor. Navigated transcranial magnetic stimulation in neurosurgery. Cham: Springer; 2017. p. 267–85. https://doi.org/10.1007/978-3-319-54918-7_16.
28. Sanai N, Berger MS. Extent of resection influences outcomes for patients with gliomas. Rev Neurol. 2011;167:648–54. https://doi.org/10.1016/j.neurol.2011.07.004.
29. Hicks WH, Bird CE, Traylor JI, Shi DD, El Ahmadieh TY, Richardson TE, McBrayer SK, Abdullah KG. Contemporary mouse models in glioma research. Cells. 2021;10(3):712. https://doi.org/10.3390/cells10030712.
30. Mitchell D, Shireman JM, Dey M. Surgical neuro-oncology: management of glioma. Neurol Clin. 2022;40(2):437–53. https://doi.org/10.1016/j.ncl.2021.11.003. Epub 2022 Mar 31.
31. Akmal M, Hasnain N, Rehan A, Iqbal U, Hashmi S, Fatima K, Farooq MZ, Khosa F, Siddiqi J, Khan MK. Glioblastome multiforme: a bibliometric analysis. World Neurosurg. 2020;136:270–82. https://doi.org/10.1016/j.wneu.2020.01.027.
32. Stupp R, Mason WP, Van Den Bent MJ, Weller M, Fisher B, Taphoorn MJ, Belanger K, Brandes AA, Marosi C, Bogdahn U, Curschmann J. Radiotherapy plus concomitant and adjuvant temozolomide for glioblastoma. N Engl J Med. 2005;352:987–96.
33. Hossain R, Ibrahim RB, Hashim HB. Automated brain tumor detection using machine learning: a bibliometric review. World Neurosurg. 2023;175:57–68. https://doi.org/10.1016/j.wneu.2023.03.115.
34. Yang X, Man D, Zhao P, Li X. Quantitative study of bioinformatics analysis on glioma: a bibliometric analysis. Front Oncol. 2023;13:1222797. https://doi.org/10.3389/fonc.2023.1222797.
35. Du X, Chen C, Yang L, Cui Y, Tan B. Bibliometric and visualized analysis of the application of nanotechnology in glioma. Front Pharmacol. 2022;13:995512. https://doi.org/10.3389/fphar.2022.995512.
36. Yang K, Wu Z, Zhang H, Zhang N, Wu W, Wang Z, Dai Z, Zhang X, Zhang L, Peng Y, Ye W, Zeng W, Liu Z, Cheng Q. Glioma targeted therapy: insight into future of molecular approaches. Mol Cancer. 2022;21(1):39. https://doi.org/10.1186/s12943-022-01513-z.
37. Ghiaseddin AP, Shin D, Melnick K, Tran DD. Tumor treating fields in the management of patients with malignant gliomas. Curr Treat Options in Oncol. 2020;21(9):76. https://doi.org/10.1007/s11864-020-00773-5.
38. Finch A, Solomou G, Wykes V, Pohl U, Bardella C, Watts C. Advances in research of adult gliomas. Int J Mol Sci. 2021;22(2):924. https://doi.org/10.3390/ijms22020924.
39. Feychting M, Schüz J, Toledano MB, Vermeulen R, Auvinen A, Harbo Poulsen A, Deltour I, Smith RB, Heller J, Kromhout H, Huss A, Johansen C, Tettamanti G, Elliott P. Mobile phone use and brain tumour risk - COSMOS, a prospective cohort study. Environ Int. 2024;185:108552. https://doi.org/10.1016/j.envint.2024.108552.
40. Dadey DYA, Medress ZA, Sharma M, Ugiliweneza B, Wang D, Rodrigues A, Parker J, Burton E, Williams B, Han SS, Boakye M, Skirboll S. Risk of developing glioblastoma following non-CNS primary cancer:

a SEER analysis between 2000 and 2018. J Neuro-Oncol. 2023;164(3):655–62. https://doi.org/10.1007/s11060-023-04460-x.
41. Forster MT, De Witt HP, Hervey-Jumper SL, Renovanz M. Editorial: Quality of care of glioma patients. Front Neurol. 2022;13:1041388. https://doi.org/10.3389/fneur.2022.1041388. Erratum in: Front Neurol. 2022 Dec 01;13:1084412.
42. Dharmaiah S, Huse JT. The epigenetic dysfunction underlying malignant glioma pathogenesis. Lab Investig. 2022;102(7):682–90. https://doi.org/10.1038/s41374-022-00741-7.
43. Dadario NB, Brahimaj B, Yeung J, Sughrue ME. Reducing the cognitive footprint of brain tumor surgery. Front Neurol. 2021;12:711646. https://doi.org/10.3389/fneur.2021.711646.
44. Skrap M, Marin D, Ius T, Fabbro F, Tomasino B. Brain mapping: a novel intraoperative neuropsychological approach. J Neurosurg. 2016;125(4):877–87. https://doi.org/10.3171/2015.10.JNS15740.
45. Kciuk M, Yahya EB, Mohamed Ibrahim Mohamed M, Rashid S, Iqbal MO, Kontek R, Abdulsamad MA, Allaq AA. Recent advances in molecular mechanisms of cancer immunotherapy. Cancers (Basel). 2023;15(10):2721. https://doi.org/10.3390/cancers15102721.
46. Lugano R, Ramachandran M, Dimberg A. Tumor angiogenesis: causes, consequences, challenges and opportunities. Cell Mol Life Sci. 2020;77(9):1745–70. https://doi.org/10.1007/s00018-019-03351-7.
47. Ostrom QT, Francis SS, Barnholtz-Sloan JS. Epidemiology of brain and other CNS tumors. Curr Neurol Neurosci Rep. 2021;21(12):68. https://doi.org/10.1007/s11910-021-01152-9.
48. Ius T, Sabatino G, Panciani PP, Fontanella MM, Rudà R, Castellano A, Barbagallo GMV, Belotti F, Boccaletti R, Catapano G, Costantino G, Della Puppa A, Di Meco F, Gagliardi F, Garbossa D, Germanò AF, Iacoangeli M, Mortini P, Olivi A, Pessina F, Pignotti F, Pinna G, Raco A, Sala F, Signorelli F, Sarubbo S, Skrap M, Spena G, Somma T, Sturiale C, Angileri FF, Esposito V. Surgical management of glioma grade 4: technical update from the neuro-oncology section of the Italian Society of Neurosurgery (SINch®): a systematic review. J Neuro-Oncol. 2023;162(2):267–93. https://doi.org/10.1007/s11060-023-04274-x.
49. Baik SH, Kim SY, Na YC, Cho JM. Supratotal resection of glioblastoma: better survival outcome than gross total resection. J Pers Med. 2023;13(3):383. https://doi.org/10.3390/jpm13030383. PMID: 36983564; PMCID: PMC10053695.
50. Maizey L, Evans CJ, Muhlert N, Verbruggen F, Chambers CD, Allen CPG. Cortical and subcortical functional specificity associated with response inhibition. NeuroImage. 2020;15(220):117110. https://doi.org/10.1016/j.neuroimage.2020.117110. Epub 2020 Jun 30. PMID: 32619711; PMCID: PMC7573537.

The Current State of Gliomagenesis Knowledge in Light of New Classifications

2

Lorenzo Sgarbanti, Daniele Armocida, and Francesco Paglia

2.1 Introduction

Gliomas are a large group of tumors that originate from glial cells, which are responsible for supporting the function of brain nerve cells. The central nervous system (CNS) and brain microenvironment are naturally equipped to control proliferative cells and prevent cancer development [1, 2]. However, due to an imbalance between proto-oncogenic and oncosuppressive genetic factors, cancerous foci can develop and escape immune control, leading to a process known as "gliomagenesis" [3]. Glioma cells possess fundamental characteristics of growth and survival beyond a normal homeostatic or favorable environment, and their growth, survival, oncogenic proliferation, and apoptosis are regulated by signaling pathways [4]. To date, three core signaling pathways have been identified for gliomas: the receptor tyrosine kinase (RTK)/phosphatidylinositol 3-kinase (PI3K)/protein kinase AKT pathway, the TP53 pathway, and the RB1 pathway [3, 5]. These pathways are highly dependent on various epigenetic modifications and the molecular microenvironment. This chapter will provide a comprehensive summary of the key findings on the pathogenesis of gliomas, starting with the conventional phenotypic classification and moving on to describe the primary genetic pathways, the role of epigenetic mutations, and finally the significance of the tumor growth environment within the stem foci present in the brain's periventricular zone.

2.2 Biomolecular Classification

The new classification system for glioma tumors by integrating both tumor morphology and biomolecular features [6]. The classification evaluated the correlation between microarray expression profiling of gliomas and tumor grades, progression, malignancy, and prognosis to identify the molecular subtypes [7]. The substantial cellular and genetic heterogeneity of the tumor activates different pathological pathways leading to increased difficulty in treatment. Consequently, gliomas are classified into four transcriptional phenotypes: proneural, neural, mesenchymal, and classical. These classes differ according to genetic mutations, response to therapies, and consequently also prognosis (Fig. 2.1).

L. Sgarbanti
Department of Neurosurgery, University Hospital S. Anna of Ferrara, Ferrara, Italy

D. Armocida
Neurosurgery Unit, Dept. Neuroscience "Rita Levi Montalcini", Università degli studi di Torino, Torino, TO, Italy

F. Paglia (✉)
Rome Human Neurosciences Department, AUO "Policlinico Umberto I", Neurosurgery Division, Sapienza University, Rome, Italy
e-mail: Francesco.paglia@hotmail.it

D. Armocida et al. (eds.), *Neurosurgery's Frontline Role in Gliomas Treatment*,
https://doi.org/10.1007/978-3-031-81850-9_2

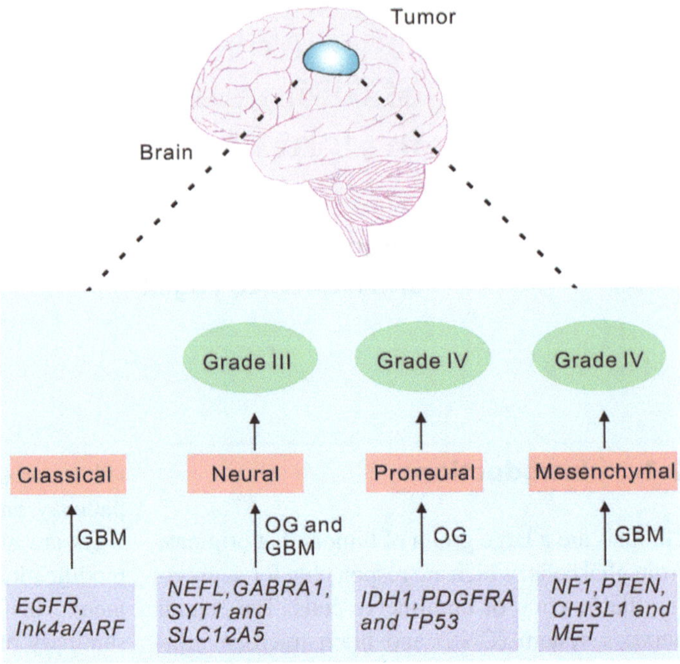

Fig. 2.1 The resumed characteristics of the molecular classification of gliomas [8]

2.2.1 Proneural Subtype

The proneural subtype is characterized by specific alterations such as PDGFRA focal amplifications at the 4q12 locus, high levels of PDGFRA gene expression, and point mutations in IDH1. PDGFRA mutations can be found in the Ig-domain, potentially affecting ligand interaction. Although PDGFRA amplification is present in all subtypes of glioblastoma (GBM), it is more prevalent in the proneural subtype [9]. However, the proneural subtype's characteristic signature for PDGFRA includes focal amplification and high expression of the PDGFRA gene [10]. Ten out of sixteen PIK3CA/PIK3R1 mutations and 11 out of 12 IDH1 mutations were observed in the proneural subtype, with no PDGFRA abnormalities. PT53 mutations were also frequently detected in this subtype. In contrast, the classical GBM event of amplifying Chr 7 and losing Chr 10 occurred less frequently and only in 54% of proneural subtype samples. The proneural subtype expresses highly the oligodendrocyte development genes PDGFRA, NKX2-2, and OLIG2, as well as several proneural development genes like SOX, DCX, DLL3, ASCL1, and TCF4. TP53 mutations and loss of heterozygosity are also common. Finally, high OLIG2 expression can promote proliferation and induce tumorigenesis by downregulating CDKN1A expression [11].

2.2.2 Neural Subtype

The neural subtype is especially characterized by expression of neuron markers, such as NEFL, GABRA1, SYT1, and SLC12A5, which were involved in the processes of neuron projection and axon and synaptic transmission. In addition, extensive pathological analysis confirmed the diagnosis of high-grade glioma (HGG) events in samples of this subtype. This classification offers a markedly better prognosis and includes the expression of certain genes, which were involved in the process of neurogenesis in the normal brain [5, 12].

2.2.3 Classical Subtype

The classic phenotype is defined by the presence of chromosome 7 amplification and the loss of chromosome 10 in all cases. A common feature of this subtype is the alteration of EGFR, which is often accompanied by a lack of TP53 mutations. Although chromosome 7 amplification was also observed in other subtypes of glioma, the high expression of EGFR was infrequently detected in other subtypes. It is well known that TP53 mutations are one of the most common events in GBM patients. However, compared to the high frequency of EGFR mutations, TP53 mutations are rarely observed in the classical subtype. Additionally, homozygous deletion of 9p21.3, which targets CDKN2A, is a frequent and significantly associated event in the classical subtype and is usually accompanied by EGFR amplification in most classical subtype samples. Moreover, previous reports have shown that the neural precursor and stem cell marker NES as well as the regulators of Notch and Sonic hedgehog (SH) signaling pathways, including NOTCH3, JAG1, LFNG, SMO, GAS1, and GLI2, are frequently amplified in the classical subtype [5].

2.2.4 Mesenchymal Subtype

The mesenchymal subtype primarily demonstrates increased expression of markers such as CHI3L1 and MET [12]. It is characterized by focal hemizygous deletions of a region at 17q11.2, which contains the NF1 gene, leading to low levels of NF1 expression. Approximately, 53% of cases of this subtype exhibit this alteration, which is also associated with PTEN mutations. Tumor markers for the mesenchymal histotype include CHI3L1 (also known as YKL40), MET, CD44, and MERTK (which are mesenchymal and astrocytic markers). This subtype highly expresses genes such as TRADD, RELB, and TNFRSF1A, which are probably related to the high necrotic and inflammatory component of the mesenchymal histotype. Verhaak et al. reported that 70% of samples were classified as the mesenchymal subtype in NF1-mutated samples. Furthermore, most of the mesenchymal subtype samples were detected as having NF1 and PTEN dual mutations, which play an essential role in the RTK/PI3K pathway [5].

2.3 Specific Genetic Alterations in Gliomagenesis

The majority of tumors were successfully divided into classical, proneural, and mesenchymal phenotypes using five immunohistochemical markers. However, in some cohorts classified according to the WHO-2021 system, protein signatures did not correlate with patient survival. At the time of recurrence, IDH-mutated tumors mainly retained proneural signatures, while IDH-wild type tumors mostly retained or gained mesenchymal signatures. It appears that these phenotypic shifts, which are associated with increased aggressiveness in GBM, did not affect survival when compared to other specific mutations [13]. In 2009, The Cancer Genome Atlas Network (TCGA) used gene sequencing to analyze variations in 601 tumor-associated genes in more than 200 glioma samples [14]. TCGA's analysis of DNA methylation, DNA copy number, and other genetic mutations in glioma patients identified core glioma pathways, and the regulatory functions of these pathways were mainly summarized in the RTK/PI3K/AKT, TP53, and RB1 signaling pathways [15].

In the RTK/Ras/PI3K pathway, receptor tyrosine kinases (RTKs) mediate many growth signals through diffusive growth factors. Several RTK ligands, such as PDGFR, EGFR, and VEGFR, are frequently overexpressed in glioma specimens. EGFR, the most common RTK target mutation, is often amplified in HGGs together with intra-genic deletion, resulting in a constitutively activated form that induces primary GBMs. VEGF and its receptors are critical regulators of glioma angiogenesis. Additionally, local degradation of the vascular basement membrane and extracellular matrix promotes the phosphorylation of focal adhesion kinase (FAK) [16]. EGFR amplification is also associated with Ink4a and TP53 mutations in primary GBMs [17], and the overexpression of dual EGFR, Ink4a-Arf mutations leads to the development of glioma-like lesions [18]. As a major effector of the RTK/PI3K pathway, RAS is responsible for activating downstream cascades and regulating cellular proliferation and differentiation in various cell types

[19]. The RTK/RAS/PI3K pathway promotes cell survival, and its activation can occur through the loss of negative regulators such as NF1 and PTEN. NF1 is a tumor suppressor gene that, when inactive, can lead to the formation of malignant tumors like gliomas [20–23]. In glial cells and gliomas, NF1 inactivation enhances the activation potential of RAS and its downstream effectors [24]. Additionally, NF1 mutations have been linked to sporadic astrocytoma and activations of RAF/MEK/MAPK and PI3K/AKT signaling pathways in glioma patients [25]. PTEN, another regulator, acts as a dual-specificity protein phosphatase and may also contribute to glioma pathogenesis. Mutated PTEN can activate the AKT signaling pathway, which regulates multiple downstream AKT substrates, including FOXO and mTOR [26]. These substrates are often downregulated in different types of cancers, including GBMs [27].

2.4 Epigenetics

For many years, the study of gliomagenesis has primarily focused on genetic mutations. However, with the advancement of sequencing technologies and high-throughput gene editing, it is now possible to analyze both genetic and epigenetic changes in tumors [28].

Following the advancement of research and knowledge in the field of epigenetic biology, important scientific evidence on their role in the evolution of tumor progression has emerged [29]. Alteration of epigenetic mechanisms such as chromatin remodeling and post-translational DNA/histone mutations can cause a change in cell behavior and an initial drive to tumor formation [24]. Understanding these phenomena can lead to better knowledge of this type of cancer and consequently more specific targeted treatments.

2.4.1 Nucleosome and Histone Modification

DNA is normally packaged into chromatin, whose basic units are nucleosomes. These structures are formed by 146 base pairs surrounding 1.7 times the center of the nucleosome, formed by two pairs of four types of specialized proteins called histones, such as H2A, H2B, H3, and H4. Subtypes of histones, such as H3.1, H3.2, H3.3, and CENPA, have been found in humans, which exhibit structural dissimilarities [30]. Each histone has an amino acid "tail" that protrudes from the nucleosome center, which is critical for the regulation of DNA transcription [31, 32]. In the process of regulating DNA transcription, certain enzymes, the so-called writers or erasers, are recruited that have the power to change the state of chromatin and make genes, respectively, accessible or not [33].

2.4.2 Histone Acetylation

Acetylation of the amino acid tail of histones adds a negative charge to these proteins. Thus, this process creates more repulsion with the enveloped DNA which is negatively charged, detaching a bit and exposing itself more to the arrival of transcriptional enzymes. In the gliomagenesis, acetylation of histones promotes the insertion and acceleration of the action of RNA Polymerase II (RNAP II) with the initiation of transcription [32–34].

2.4.3 DNA Methylation

Another factor that regulates gene transcription is DNA methylation, where a methyl group is attached to cytosine of the CpG dinucleotide, causing gene silencing. There are clusters or "islands" in the genome where this phenomenon occurs more frequently, but it varies greatly from tissue to tissue [32].

2.4.4 Histone Methylation

Methylation, on the other hand, does not change the charge and interaction between histones and the DNA chain but goes to modulate the interaction of proteins that have specific methyl histone-binding domains by favoring or blocking binding. Histone lysine residues can be mono-, di-, or trimethylated, whereas arginines can be monomethylated or symmetrically/asymmetrically dimethylated, with each modification having a specific biologic effect. Methylation of H3K4, H3K36, and H3K79 leads to increased glioma's transcription activity; in contrast, methylation of H3K9, H3K27, and H4K20 promotes chromatin silencing [8, 9] (Fig. 2.2).

2.5 Epigenetic Dysregulation in Brain Tumor

Advances in epigenetic biology research have demonstrated that aberrant epigenetic modifications play a crucial role in almost every stage of tumor development and progression [35]. Recent findings in glioma biology have uncovered a

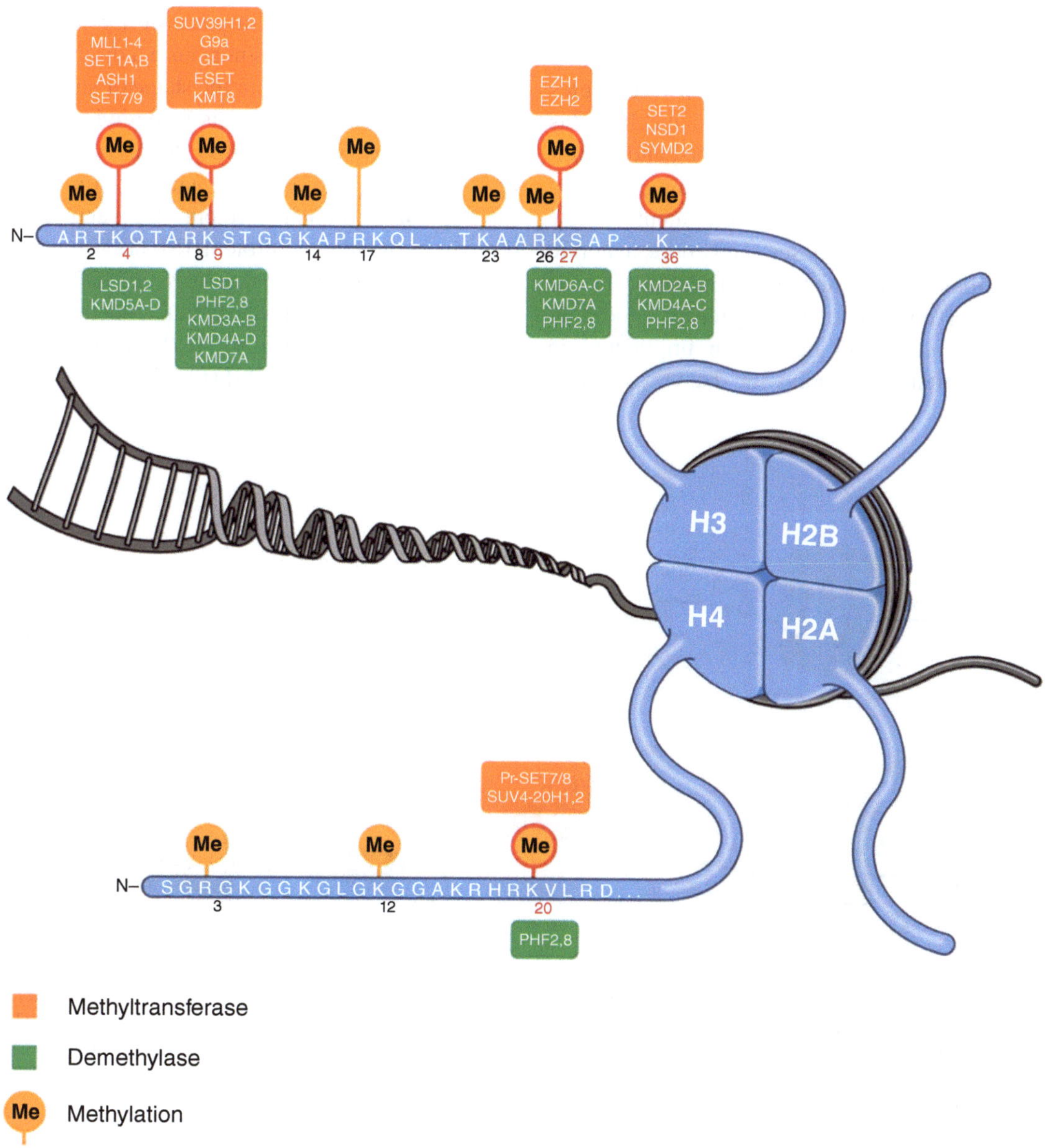

Fig. 2.2 Maury et al. in this image go to depict sites with lysine residues of histone tails where methyl groups may be deposited. Circled in red are the sites investigated in tumorigenesis [32]

strong relationship between epigenetic dysregulation and the formation of high-grade gliomas (HGGs). Several studies have explored the genetic and epigenetic mechanisms underlying the development of pediatric and adult HGGs [32]. Dysregulation of epigenetic mechanisms, such as chromatin remodeling and post-translational DNA/histone modifications, can lead to altered gene expression, ultimately resulting in tumor formation [24]. Understanding these alterations is critical for improving prognosis, developing novel drugs, and enhancing current tumor-specific therapeutic strategies [32]. Dysregulation of epigenetic mechanisms can initiate the onset of brain tumors, and a comprehensive and in-depth understanding of these processes can lead to the development of new therapies, better prognoses, and more accurate predictions of treatment response [35]. In the context of epigenetic tumorigenesis, modifications to histone H3 have been implicated in tumor formation, earning the name "oncohistones." In particular, pediatric and adult HGGs have been found to have two missense mutations in histone variant H3.3, such as G34V7R and K27M, with only one amino acid substitution [35, 36].

2.5.1 H3.3G34R/V Mutation

The H3.3G34R/V mutation has the substitution of an arginine or valine in place of a glycine at position 34 [5]. This does not cause a direct post-transcriptional alteration in the shape or structure of the protein, but it prevents trimethylation on the lysine residue at position 36, thus altering epigenetic regulation. The nuclear receptor-binding SET domain protein 1–3 and SET domain containing 2 protein (SETD2) are the major H3K36 methyltransferases. SETD2 is the only enzyme that can carry out trimethylation and upon mutation H3.3G34R/V undergoes a loss of function [32, 37, 38] (Fig. 2.3).

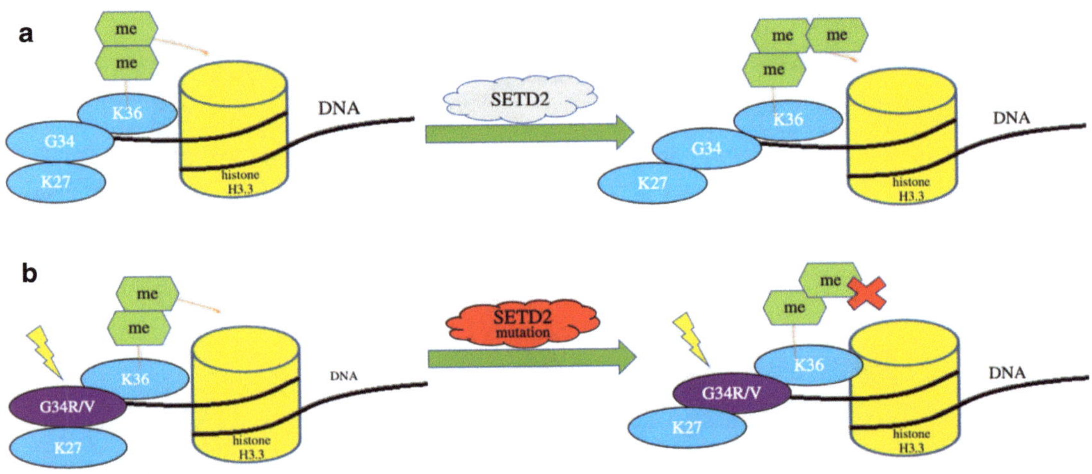

Fig. 2.3 Phasaludeen et al. have described with this picture how H3.3G34R/V mutation or directly SETD2 mutation prevent trimethylation on H3K36, altering its regulation. (**a**) Normal epigenetic regulation. (**b**) Block of trimethylation due to G34R7V mutation or SETD2 mutation [4]. This alteration occurs principally in hemispheric high-grade gliomas (HHG) of children (15% of tumors) compared with those of older adults (8% of tumors). The median age of onset of HHG with G34V/R mutation is 15 years with an overall survival of 2 years [13]

2.5.2 SETD2 Mutation

SETD2 is a histone-modifying enzyme whose function is to catalyze trimethylation on the lysine residue at position 36 of histone H3. Trimethylation can be impaired either as a result of G34R/V mutation or, instead, as a result of a mutation that leads to loss of function of SETD2, silencing it [36, 39]. With reduced trimethylation, there is an increase in spontaneous mutations and chromosomal instability, in fact, it is seen in several types of cancer including pediatric and adult HHG, but also, rarely, in low-grade glioma [40, 41].

2.5.3 K27 Mutation

Another mutation that can alter the epigenetic control of chromatin is that which occurs at the lysine site at position 27 in histones H3.1 and H3.3. This amino acid is substituted with a methionine and this causes altered binding to histone N-methyltransferase, enhancer of zeste homologue 2 (EZH2), which catalyzes the di- and trimethylation reaction, mutating the gene. In the case of mutation, there is a decrease in H3K27me2/3 mark and this DNA hypomethylation induces gene activation and cell proliferation [42, 43]. The mutation was only oncogenic in a specific cell type, neural progenitors derived from embryonic stem cells, and not in undifferentiated embryonic stem cells or astrocytes derived from these cells [32]. Has been documented, moreover, the association between H3K27M mutation, loss-of-function mutation of TP53, and gain-of-function mutations or amplification of platelet- derived growth factor receptor alpha (PDGFRA) [36, 39] (Fig. 2.4).

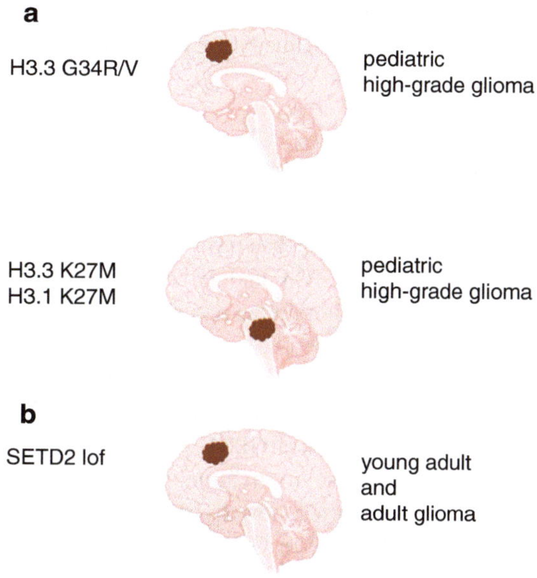

Fig. 2.4 Phasaludeen et al. have described how specific mutations, such as H3.3G34R/V, H3.1K27M, H3.3K27M, and SET2 lost-of-function, occur more frequently with high- or low-grade gliomas in distinct brain regions

2.5.4 ATRX/DAXX Mutations

The ATRX protein is a component of the SWItch/sucrose non-fermentable family of chromatin remodeling proteins, and when it collaborates with the transcription cofactor DAXX (death domain-associated protein), it helps preserve genomic stability by depositing the replication-independent histone variant H3.3 at telomeres, pericentromeric heterochromatin, and other DNA repeat regions [31]. In gliomas, ATRX loss has been demonstrated to promote alternative lengthening of telomeres (ALT), a mechanism that allows cancer cells to extend telomere length without the action of telomerase reverse transcriptase. This leads to the avoidance of cell death by telomere loss, allowing cells to continue proliferating and the tumor to progress. Additionally, ATRX inactivation has been strongly linked to DNA damage and replicative stress [44, 45]. ATRX loss within gliomas can result from mutations, deletions, gene fusions, or a combination of these causes and has been observed more commonly in primary glioblastoma and anaplastic glioma, where it serves as a marker of malignancy [46]. PDGFRA amplification, K27M has been associated with this type of mutation and the ALT phenotype [46]. Ikemura et al. demonstrated that ATRX loss mainly occurred in young subjects in non-hemispheric locations [47].

2.5.5 Alteration of DNA Methylation

DNA methylation patterns have been extensively studied in adult GBM and have helped guide clinical trials, predicting the recurrence of tumors and resistance to radiotherapy [48]. Indeed, CpG island methylator phenotype (G–CIMP) helped subdivide GBMs into glioma, G–CIMP-positive and G–CIMP-negative GBM subsets, partially predicting response to treatment [49]. Several studies have reported how hypermethylation of some particular loci in GBM frequently affects the expression of genes with known tumor suppressor functions and/or involved in cell proliferation or radiation sensitivity. Thereby, it alters the normal regulatory functions of the cell [43].

2.6 The Influence Between Epigenetic and Metabolic Dysregulation

Altered cellular metabolism is a distinctive feature of tumors. Like all other types of cancer, gliomas upregulate metabolism to increase cell proliferation, growth, and survival tasks, including macromolecule synthesis, ATP generation, and antioxidant regeneration. Metabolic abnormalities in cancer play an important role in the regulation of gene expression. Although metabolic effects may have some impact at the genetic level, they show a key role in epigenomic regulation. Epigenetics, which mainly involves DNA and histone modification, is an intrinsic process that connects nutrient supply to cellular function. Therefore, metabolic wiring can induce the epigenetic mechanism of cancer cells to transmit a mitogenic gene expression profile. At the same time, altered expression of genes involved in cellular metabolism is mediated by epigenetic dysregulation in cancer, suggesting a complex cross-talk between metabolome and epigenome during tumorigenesis [50].

The impact of metabolism on epigenetic regulation in gliomas can be seen in the role of isocitrate dehydrogenase (IDH). This group of enzymes plays a crucial role in the Krebs cycle by catalyzing the oxidative decarboxylation reaction of isocitrate, converting it into α-ketoglutarate. When these enzymes undergo loss-of-function mutations, they no longer carry out their physiological function, instead producing the (R) enantiomer of 2-hydroxyglutarate, (R)-2HG (also known as D-2HG). Accumulation of this metabolite leads to changes in the methylation pattern of DNA and histones, promoting the development of cancer [51]. On the other hand, an example of the influence of epigenetic regulation on metabolism control in gliomas is the effect of loss of SETD2. This mutated enzyme is involved in the regulation of glucose, mitochondrial, and fatty acid metabolism, including the upregulation of peroxisome proliferator gamma coactivator 1 (PGC1α), which could induce oxidative phosphorylation and TCA cycle gene expression [52].

2.7 Micro-tumor Environment

In recent times, there has been growing recognition of the shared mechanisms underlying gliomagenesis and nervous system development. Numerous experimental studies have suggested that neural stem cells (NSCs) residing in the subventricular zone (SVZ) play a crucial role in both processes [53, 54]. Furthermore, recent evidence indicates that gliomas contain a small number of cells with NSC properties, including the ability to self-renew, proliferate, and differentiate in vitro. Identifying the cell-of-origin of gliomas could help create more relevant animal models to study the biology of these tumors. Additionally, it could explain the high recurrence rate of gliomas despite adequate cytoreduction, leading to the development of more effective therapies. Understanding the biology of the SVZ, which is the largest NSC depot, is critical to achieving this goal.

It is now widely acknowledged that adult human brains contain self-renewing and multipotent NSCs capable of generating neurons, astrocytes, and oligodendrocytes. Researchers have isolated NSCs from various regions of the brain, such as the dentate gyrus, subcortical white matter, and SVZ. These cells have been found to proliferate in living organisms and behave as multipotent progenitor cells, giving rise to neurons, astrocytes, and oligodendrocytes in laboratory settings. The cellular composition and cytoarchitecture of the adult human SVZ, which contains a unique periventricular astrocyte "ribbon," have been thoroughly characterized [55]. The lateral wall of the lateral ventricles in the adult human brain is reported to exhibit varying thicknesses and cell densities and is comprised of four layers: the innermost layer, a monolayer of ependymal cells that lines the ventricular cavity (layer I); a hypocellular gap (layer II) abutting the ependymal layer; a ribbon of cells consisting of astrocytes (layer III); and a transitional zone (layer IV) into the brain parenchyma. Electron microscopy has revealed that the hypocellular gap (layer II) contains an extensive network of interconnected glial fibrillary acid protein (GFAP)-positive astrocytic processes linked by junctional complexes [56]. This layer appears to be a region of interaction between astrocytes and ependymal cells, possibly exchanging signals. Layer III contains GFAP-positive astrocytes, corresponding to the multipotent progenitor cells previously described. Electron microscopy has also revealed three distinct astrocytic subtypes within layer III. Oligodendrocytes have been observed in this layer. However, the astrocyte ribbon (layer III) has not been observed along the third ventricle, fourth ventricle, or the medial (septal) wall of the lateral ventricles. Myelinated axons delineate the transition between layer III and the underlying brain parenchyma (layer IV) [57]. Glass et al. have demonstrated that endogenous precursor cells are attracted to gliomas and mediate anti-tumorigenic effects, as shown by their study [58]. In their experiment, GBM cells were implanted into the basal ganglia of adult mice, and subsequently, endogenous SVZ neural precursor cells migrated toward the tumors, enveloping and inducing apoptosis of tumor cells. This resulted in decreased tumor size and improved survival of the animals. Another study inoculated the brain of adult rats with glioma cells, which triggered neuropoietic activity. Nestin and GFAP-positive cells then streamed from the ipsilateral SVZ, encompassing and infiltrating the tumor. Overall, these studies suggest that SVZ stem cells have the potential to both give rise to gliomas after undergoing malignant transformation and to be attracted to gliomas, contributing to their overall mass effect or exhibiting anti-tumor effects [57]. The SVZ lies at the intersection of two biological processes, namely brain development and gliomagenesis. Further studies are needed to prove the hypothesis that NSCs of the SVZ give rise to gliomas.

2.8 Limitations: The "Model Problem"

Gliomas exhibit considerable variations based on genetic, histological, and physiological characteristics, which ultimately contribute to their different malignancies, prognoses, and invasive phenotypes [59]. However, despite advances in understanding of the molecular pathogenesis of glioma, outcomes remain dismal. Developing successful treatments requires faithful in vivo disease modeling and rigorous preclinical testing. Murine models, including xenograft, syngeneic, and genetically engineered models, are used to study gliomagenesis, identify methods of tumor progression, and test novel treatment strategies. Since the discovery of highly recurrent IDH mutations in lower-grade gliomas, there has been a growing emphasis on effectively modeling IDH mutant brain tumors. To develop effective new therapies, it is critical to improve preclinical models that capture the phenotypic and molecular heterogeneity of gliomas. Glioma animal models offer several advantages over in vitro two-dimensional glioma cell cultures, as they better replicate the genetic, morphologic, and immunologic characteristics of human tumors.

Over the past 70 years, there have been numerous advances in glioma animal models, including the creation of PDXs and GEMMs [60]. These developments have enabled the creation of faithful glioma models to study the genetic and molecular changes driving gliomagenesis, immunologic tumor recognition, and therapeutic response. A suitable animal model can be a valuable tool for studying the mechanisms and potential treatments of glioma. The utility of animal models allows for the systematic identification of molecular features that contribute to the initiation and progression pathways in glioma, potentially improving therapeutic strategies for the treatment of glioma. Although the molecular mechanisms of gliomagenesis have been widely investigated in cultured cells, limitations for modeling invasion, angiogenesis, and metastasis still exist. An ideal glioma animal model should possess several features, including genetic similarity to human glioma, invasive and angiogenic-like growth, and the imitation of therapeutic response, to allow for more accurate prediction of clinical outcomes [61].

References

1. Altieri R, Barbagallo D, Certo F, Broggi G, Ragusa M, Di Pietro C, Caltabiano R, Magro G, Peschillo S, Purrello M, Barbagallo G. Peritumoral microenvironment in high-grade gliomas: from FLAIRectomy to microglia-glioma cross-talk. Brain Sci. 2021;11(2):200. https://doi.org/10.3390/brainsci11020200.
2. De Luca C, Virtuoso A, Papa M, Certo F, Barbagallo GMV, Altieri R. Regional development of glioblastoma: the anatomical conundrum of cancer biology and its surgical implication. Cells. 2022;11(8):1349. https://doi.org/10.3390/cells11081349.
3. Johnson BE, Mazor T, Hong C, Barnes M, Aihara K, McLean CY, Fouse SD, Yamamoto S, Ueda H, Tatsuno K, Asthana S, Jalbert LE, Nelson SJ, Bollen AW, Gustafson WC, Charron E, Weiss WA, Smirnov IV, Song JS, Olshen AB, Cha S, Zhao Y, Moore RA, Mungall AJ, Jones SJM, Hirst M, Marra MA, Saito N, Aburatani H, Mukasa A, Berger MS, Chang SM, Taylor BS, Costello JF. Mutational analysis reveals the origin and therapy-driven evolution of recurrent glioma. Science. 2014;343(6167):189–93. https://doi.org/10.1126/science.1239947.
4. Luo J, Junaid M, Hamid N, Duan JJ, Yang X, Pei DS. Current understanding of gliomagenesis: from model to mechanism. Int J Med Sci. 2022;19(14):2071–9. https://doi.org/10.7150/ijms.77287.
5. Verhaak RGW, Hoadley KA, Purdom E, et al. Integrated genomic analysis identifies clinically relevant subtypes of glioblastoma characterized by abnormalities in PDGFRA, IDH1, EGFR, and NF1. Cancer Cell. 2010;17(1):98–110. https://doi.org/10.1016/j.ccr.2009.12.020.
6. Kane JR, Miska J, Young JS, Kanojia D, Kim JW, Lesniak MS. Sui generis: gene therapy and delivery systems for the treatment of glioblastoma. Neuro-Oncology. 2015;17(Suppl 2):ii24–36. https://doi.org/10.1093/neuonc/nou355.
7. Wong ML, Kaye AH, Hovens CM. Targeting malignant glioma survival signalling to improve clinical outcomes. J Clin Neurosci. 2007;14(4):301–8. https://doi.org/10.1016/j.jocn.2006.11.005.
8. Mackay A, Burford A, Carvalho D, et al. Integrated molecular meta-analysis of 1000 pediatric high-grade and diffuse intrinsic pontine glioma. Cancer Cell. 2017;32(4):520–37. https://doi.org/10.1016/j.ccell.2017.08.017.
9. Barski A, Cuddapah S, Cui K, et al. High-resolution profiling of histone methylations in the human genome. Cell. 2007;129(4):823–37. https://doi.org/10.1016/j.cell.2007.05.009.
10. Noble M, Pröschel C, Mayer-Pröschel M. Getting a GR(i)P on oligodendrocyte development. Dev Biol. 2004;265(1):33–52. https://doi.org/10.1016/j.ydbio.2003.06.002.
11. Ligon KL, Huillard E, Mehta S, Kesari S, Liu H, Alberta JA, Bachoo RM, Kane M, Louis DN, Depinho RA, Anderson DJ, Stiles CD, Rowitch DH. Olig2-regulated lineage-restricted pathway controls replication competence in neural stem cells and malignant glioma. Neuron. 2007;53(4):503–17. https://doi.org/10.1016/j.neuron.2007.01.009.
12. Phillips HS, Kharbanda S, Chen R, Forrest WF, Soriano RH, Wu TD, Misra A, Nigro JM, Colman H, Soroceanu L, Williams PM, Modrusan Z, Feuerstein BG, Aldape K. Molecular subclasses of high-grade glioma predict prognosis, delineate a pattern of disease progression, and resemble stages in neurogenesis. Cancer Cell. 2006;9(3):157–73. https://doi.org/10.1016/j.ccr.2006.02.019.
13. Dénes A, Bontell TO, Barchéus H, Vega SF, Carén H, Lindskog C, Jakola AS, Smits A. The clinical value of proneural, classical and mesenchymal protein signatures in WHO 2021 adult-type diffuse lower-grade gliomas. PLoS One. 2023;18(5):e0285732. https://doi.org/10.1371/journal.pone.0285732.
14. Cancer Genome Atlas Research Network. Comprehensive genomic characterization defines human glioblastoma genes and core pathways. Nature. 2008;455(7216):1061–8. https://doi.org/10.1038/nature07385.

15. Chow LM, Endersby R, Zhu X, Rankin S, Qu C, Zhang J, Broniscer A, Ellison DW, Baker SJ. Cooperativity within and among Pten, p53, and Rb pathways induces high-grade astrocytoma in adult brain. Cancer Cell. 2011;19(3):305–16. https://doi.org/10.1016/j.ccr.2011.01.039.
16. Ahir BK, Engelhard HH, Lakka SS. Tumor development and angiogenesis in adult brain tumor: glioblastoma. Mol Neurobiol. 2020;57(5):2461–78. https://doi.org/10.1007/s12035-020-01892-8.
17. Zheng H, Ying H, Yan H, Kimmelman AC, Hiller DJ, Chen AJ, Perry SR, Tonon G, Chu GC, Ding Z, Stommel JM, Dunn KL, Wiedemeyer R, You MJ, Brennan C, Wang YA, Ligon KL, Wong WH, Chin L, DePinho RA. p53 and Pten control neural and glioma stem/progenitor cell renewal and differentiation. Nature. 2008;455(7216):1129–33. https://doi.org/10.1038/nature07443.
18. Saadeh FS, Mahfouz R, Assi HI. EGFR as a clinical marker in glioblastomas and other gliomas. Int J Biol Markers. 2018;33(1):22–32. https://doi.org/10.5301/ijbm.5000301.
19. Hobbs GA, Der CJ, Rossman KL. RAS isoforms and mutations in cancer at a glance. J Cell Sci. 2016;129:1287–92.
20. Ngeow J, Sesock K, Eng C. Breast cancer risk and clinical implications for germline PTEN mutation carriers. Breast Cancer Res Treat. 2017;165(1):1–8. https://doi.org/10.1007/s10549-015-3665-z.
21. Rosenbaum T, Wimmer K. Neurofibromatosis type 1 (NF1) and associated tumors. Klin Padiatr. 2014;226:309–15.
22. Kaul A, Toonen JA, Cimino PJ, et al. Akt- or MEK-mediated mTOR inhibition suppresses Nf1 optic glioma growth. Neuro-Oncology. 2015;17:843–53.
23. Abounader R. Interactions between PTEN and receptor tyrosine kinase pathways and their implications for glioma therapy. Exp Rev Anticancer. 2009;9:235–45.
24. Delcuve GP, Rastegar M, Davie JR. Epigenetic control. J Cell Physiol. 2009;219(2):243–50. https://doi.org/10.1002/jcp.21678.
25. Vogt PK, Hart JR, Gymnopoulos M, Jiang H, Kang S, Bader AG, Zhao L, Denley A. Phosphatidylinositol 3-kinase: the oncoprotein. Curr Top Microbiol Immunol. 2010;347:79–104. https://doi.org/10.1007/82_2010_80.
26. Armocida D, Busceti CL, Biagioni F, Fornai F, Frati A. The role of cellular prion protein in glioma tumorigenesis could be through the autophagic mechanisms: a narrative review. Int J Mol Sci. 2023;24(2):1405. https://doi.org/10.3390/ijms24021405.
27. Pérez-Ramírez C, Cañadas-Garre M, Molina MÁ, Faus-Dáder MJ, Calleja-Hernández MÁ. PTEN and PI3K/AKT in non-small-cell lung cancer. Pharmacogenomics. 2015;16(16):1843–62. https://doi.org/10.2217/pgs.15.122.
28. Weiss WA, Burns MJ, Hackett C, Aldape K, Hill JR, Kuriyama H, Kuriyama N, Milshteyn N, Roberts T, Wendland MF, DePinho R, Israel MA. Genetic determinants of malignancy in a mouse model for oligodendroglioma. Cancer Res. 2003;63(7):1589–95.
29. Timp W, Feinberg AP. Cancer as a dysregulated epigenome allowing cellular growth advantage at the expense of the host. Nat Rev Cancer. 2013;13(7):497–510. https://doi.org/10.1038/nrc3486. Epub 2013 Jun 13.
30. Hake SB, Allis CD. Histone H3 variants and their potential role in indexing mammalian genomes: the "H3 barcode hypothesis". Proc Natl Acad Sci USA. 2006;103(17):6428–35. https://doi.org/10.1073/pnas.0600803103.
31. Phasaludeen B, Emerald BS, Ansari SA. The epigenetic–metabolic interplay in gliomagenesis. Open Biol. 2022;12(4):210350. https://doi.org/10.1098/rsob.210350.
32. Maury E, Hashizume R. Epigenetic modification in chromatin machinery and its deregulation in pediatric brain tumors: insight into epigenetic therapies. Epigenetics. 2017;12(5):353–69. https://doi.org/10.1080/15592294.2016.1278095.
33. Furey TS, Sethupathy P. Genetics. Genetics driving epigenetics. Science. 2013;342(6159):705–6. https://doi.org/10.1126/science.1246755.
34. Stasevich TJ, Hayashi-Takanaka Y, Sato Y, et al. Regulation of RNA polymerase II activation by histone acetylation in single living cells. Nature. 2014;516(7530):272–5. https://doi.org/10.1038/nature13714.
35. Weinberg DN, Allis CD, Lu C. Oncogenic mechanisms of histone H3 mutations. Cold Spring Harb Perspect Med. 2017;7(1):a026443. https://doi.org/10.1101/cshperspect.a026443.
36. Schwartzentruber J, Korshunov A, Liu XY, et al. Driver mutations in histone H3.3 and chromatin remodelling genes in paediatric glioblastoma. Nature. 2012;482(7384):226–31. https://doi.org/10.1038/nature10833.
37. Panditharatna E, Yaeger K, Kilburn LB, Packer RJ, Nazarian J. Clinicopathology of diffuse intrinsic pontine glioma and its redefined genomic and epigenomic landscape. Cancer Genet. 2015;208(7-8):367–73. https://doi.org/10.1016/j.cancergen.2015.04.008.
38. St. Jude Children's Research Hospital–Washington University Pediatric Cancer Genome Project. Somatic histone H3 alterations in pediatric diffuse intrinsic pontine gliomas and non-brainstem glioblastomas. Nat Genet. 2012;44(3):251–3. https://doi.org/10.1038/ng.1102.
39. Fontebasso AM, Schwartzentruber J, Khuong-Quang DA, et al. Mutations in SETD2 and genes affecting histone H3K36 methylation target hemispheric high-grade gliomas. Acta Neuropathol. 2013;125(5):659–69. https://doi.org/10.1007/s00401-013-1095-8.
40. Wang Q, Hu B, Hu X, et al. Tumor evolution of glioma-intrinsic gene expression subtypes associates with immunological changes in the microenviron-

ment. Cancer Cell. 2017;32(1):42–56. https://doi.org/10.1016/j.ccell.2017.06.003.
41. Edmunds JW, Mahadevan LC, Clayton AL. Dynamic histone H3 methylation during gene induction: HYPB/Setd2 mediates all H3K36 trimethylation. EMBO J. 2008;27(2):406–20. https://doi.org/10.1038/sj.emboj.7601967.
42. Harutyunyan AS, Chen H, Lu T, et al. H3K27M in gliomas causes a one-step decrease in H3K27 methylation and reduced spreading within the constraints of H3K36 methylation. Cell Rep. 2020;33(7):108390. https://doi.org/10.1016/j.celrep.2020.108390.
43. Sturm D, Bender S, Jones DTW, et al. Paediatric and adult glioblastoma: multiform (epi)genomic culprits emerge. Nat Rev Cancer. 2014;14(2):92–107. https://doi.org/10.1038/nrc3655.
44. Haase S, Garcia-Fabiani MB, Carney S, et al. Mutant ATRX: uncovering a new therapeutic target for glioma. Expert Opin Ther Targets. 2018;22(7):599–613. https://doi.org/10.1080/14728222.2018.1487953.
45. Ramamoorthy M, Smith S. Loss of ATRX suppresses resolution of telomere cohesion to control recombination in ALT cancer cells. Cancer Cell. 2015;28(3):357–69. https://doi.org/10.1016/j.ccell.2015.08.003.
46. Nandakumar P, Mansouri A, Das S. The role of ATRX in glioma biology. Front Oncol. 2017;7:236. https://doi.org/10.3389/fonc.2017.00236.
47. Ikemura M, Shibahara J, Mukasa A, et al. Utility of ATRX immunohistochemistry in diagnosis of adult diffuse gliomas. Histopathology. 2016;69(2):260–7. https://doi.org/10.1111/his.12927.
48. Nervi C, De Marinis E, Codacci-Pisanelli G. Epigenetic treatment of solid tumours: a review of clinical trials. Clin Epigenetics. 2015;7:127. https://doi.org/10.1186/s13148-015-0157-2.
49. Hashizume R, Andor N, Ihara Y, et al. Pharmacologic inhibition of histone demethylation as a therapy for pediatric brainstem glioma. Nat Med. 2014;20(12):1394–6. https://doi.org/10.1038/nm.3716.
50. Johnson C, Warmoes MO, Shen X, Locasale JW. Epigenetics and cancer metabolism. Cancer Lett. 2015;356(2):309–14. https://doi.org/10.1016/j.canlet.2013.09.043.
51. Gagné L, Boulay K, Topisirovic I, Huot MÉ, Mallette FA. Oncogenic activities of IDH1/2 mutations: from epigenetics to cellular signaling. Trends Cell Biol. 2017;27(10):738–52. https://doi.org/10.1016/j.tcb.2017.06.002.
52. Austin S, St-Pierre J. PGC1α and mitochondrial metabolism–emerging concepts and relevance in ageing and neurodegenerative disorders. J Cell Sci. 2012;125(Pt 21):4963–71. https://doi.org/10.1242/jcs.113662.
53. Armocida D, Pesce A, Palmieri M, D'Andrea G, Salvati M, Santoro A, Frati A. Periventricular zone involvement as a predictor of survival in glioblastoma patients: a single centre cohort-comparison investigation concerning a distinct clinical entity. Interdiscip Neurosurg. 2021;25:101185. https://doi.org/10.1016/j.inat.2021.101185.
54. Sanai N, Alvarez-Buylla A, Berger MS. Neural stem cells and the origin of gliomas. N Engl J Med. 2005;353(8):811–22. https://doi.org/10.1056/NEJMra043666.
55. Rhoton AL. Lateral and third ventricles. Neurosurgery. 2002;51:207–71.
56. Quiñones-Hinojosa A, Sanai N, Soriano-Navarro M, Gonzalez-Perez O, Mirzadeh Z, Gil-Perotin S, Romero-Rodriguez R, Berger MS, Garcia-Verdugo JM, Alvarez-Buylla A. Cellular composition and cytoarchitecture of the adult human subventricular zone: a niche of neural stem cells. J Comp Neurol. 2006;494(3):415–34. https://doi.org/10.1002/cne.20798.
57. Barami K. Biology of the subventricular zone in relation to gliomagenesis. J Clin Neurosci. 2007;14(12):1143–9. https://doi.org/10.1016/j.jocn.2007.04.009.
58. Glass R, Synowitz M, Kronenberg G, Walzlein JH, Markovic DS, Wang LP, Gast D, Kiwit J, Kempermann G, Kettenmann H. Glioblastoma-induced attraction of endogenous neural precursor cells is associated with improved survival. J Neurosci. 2005;25(10):2637–46. https://doi.org/10.1523/JNEUROSCI.5118-04.2005.
59. Hicks WH, Bird CE, Traylor JI, Shi DD, El Ahmadieh TY, Richardson TE, McBrayer SK, Abdullah KG. Contemporary mouse models in glioma research. Cells. 2021;10(3):712. https://doi.org/10.3390/cells10030712.
60. Tomaszewski W, Sanchez-Perez L, Gajewski TF, Sampson JH. Brain tumor microenvironment and host state: implications for immunotherapy. Clin Cancer Res. 2019;25(14):4202–10. https://doi.org/10.1158/1078-0432.CCR-18-1627.
61. Lah TT, Novak M, Breznik B. Brain malignancies: glioblastoma and brain metastases. Semin Cancer Biol. 2020;60:262–73. https://doi.org/10.1016/j.semcancer.2019.10.010.

Brief Insight Into Central Nervous System Tumors: An Update on Current Status in Glioma Classification

3

Francesca Rizzo, Alberto Morello, Roberta Rudà, Diego Garbossa, and Fabio Cofano

3.1 Introduction

The ongoing updating of central nervous system (CNS) tumor biology and advances in diagnostic technologies have led to the integration of ancient histopathological models with a new molecular diagnostic approach to classify them. The synthesis of this process is represented in the fifth classification of the World Health Organization (WHO) published in 2021, redefining the diagnostic and therapeutic aspects of several tumor types and providing important insights into this complex field. Radiogenomics may become a new frontier in neuro-oncology by combining imaging features with specific molecular pathways. In doing so, the discovery of new biomarkers, development of novel treatment strategies, and introduction of therapeutic targets may open up access to personalized treatment strategies, offering better care. In this review, we summarize the main changes from the old editions and the most relevant aspects of the new classification of glioma tumors, emphasizing the need for continuous innovation.

F. Rizzo (✉) · A. Morello · F. Cofano
Neuroscience Department "Rita Levi Montalcini", Neurosurgery Unit, Università degli Studi di Torino, Turin, Italy
e-mail: fr.rizzo@unito.it

R. Rudà
Neuroscience Department "Rita Levi Montalcini", Neuro-oncology Unit, Università degli Studi di Torino, Turin, Italy

D. Garbossa
Neurosurgery Unit, Dept. Neuroscience "Rita Levi Montalcini", Università degli studi di Torino, Torino, TO, Italy

3.2 Historical Background

Historically, tumors of the central nervous system have been classified according to histopathological criteria, which date back to the work of Virchow [1] and later, Bailey and Cushing, who believed that tumors originate from immature precursors of normal cells [2]. Kernohan and Ringertz then focused on cytological and immunohistochemical criteria, leading to the creation of an international classification system by the WHO [3, 4]. The first edition of this classification system was published in 1979 and has undergone numerous revisions since then (1993, 2000, 2007, 2016, 2021), reflecting the rapid advancements in tumor biology and diagnostic technologies [5]. The fourth edition of 2007 identified genes involved in gliomagenesis, such as IDH1/2 for gliomas in adults and H3F3A and HIST1H3B/C for midline tumors. In 2016, the concept of molecular markers was introduced to define certain entities, particularly the main changes associated with diffuse astrocytic and oligodendroglial gliomas and embryonic tumors [6–8]. The development of cIMPACT-NOW (the Consortium to

D. Armocida et al. (eds.), *Neurosurgery's Frontline Role in Gliomas Treatment*,
https://doi.org/10.1007/978-3-031-81850-9_3

Inform Molecular and Practical Approaches to CNS Tumor Taxonomy—Not Official WHO) was a significant step, with seven updates, the most recent in 2019 in Utrecht. cIMPACT-NOW aimed to implement the 2016 classification in light of rapid discoveries in the field of genomics and proposed the introduction of new entities while laying the foundations for subsequent classification. In particular, the grading of non-mutated IDH gliomas is now better understood, with molecular criteria (amplification of the EGFR gene, mutation of the TERT promoter, loss of chromosome 10, and acquisition of chromosome 7) being used to classify grade II–III gliomas as grade IV. The role of the deletion in homozygosity of the CDK2A gene in mutated IDH gliomas, the histomolecular importance of MYB genes, MYBL1 or FGFR1 in diffuse low-grade tumors, and the BRAF V600E mutation are also now recognized [9, 10]. The fifth edition of the WHO, published in 2021, thus establishes a new approach to the nomenclature of central nervous system tumors, integrating histopathology, grading, and molecular information [5], to improve diagnostic classification and make treatment choices more targeted [11, 12].

3.2.1 Limitations of the WHO 2016 Classification

Focusing on the category of gliomas, the following variants are described in the fourth edition: mutated IDH gliomas, which in turn are subdivided into mutated IDH astrocytomas and mutated IDH 1p/19q codeletes oligodendrogliomas, and non-mutated IDH gliomas. In the category of diffuse astrocytic and oligodendroglial gliomas, a new molecular entity is identified, namely diffuse midline gliomas with the H3K27M mutation. In cases where a molecular diagnosis is not possible, the term "NOS" is used for "not otherwise specified." This categorization, however, is limiting; in particular, it does not allow a clear distinction of tumors according to the age of the patient and especially the grading of mutated IDH gliomas is not very satisfactory [6].

3.3 Fifth Edition of the WHO Classification (2021)

The first major change from the previous editions is the possibility to associate a different grade with the same entity. The histopathological criteria remain unchanged, with the difference that the grade is indicated by an Arabic numeral and the number of mitosis is indicated in mm^2 and no longer by ten magnification fields (HPF). In terms of nomenclature, in the new edition, the term "entity" is replaced by "type" and the term "variant" is replaced by "subtype." In the fifth edition, 22 new tumor types are included, mainly in the pediatric and adult neoplasms. Tumors that in the previous classifications included the entities of diffuse astrocytic and oligodendroglial gliomas, other astrocytic tumors, other gliomas, neuronal and glioneuronal tumors, ependymomas, are now grouped in the category of "gliomas, neuronal, and glioneuronal tumors" [5, 13, 14].

3.3.1 Gliomas, Neuronal, and Glioneuronal Tumors

Considering the great limitation of the previous classifications in not taking into account the age of the patient, in the new edition gliomas are subdivided according to the age of onset, extension characteristics, and aggressiveness. The first important categorization concerns diffuse gliomas and circumscribed astrocytic gliomas; the former are subdivided into adult and pediatric gliomas, the latter comprise tumors with well-defined margins and lesser tendency to infiltrative growth [5, 15] (Fig. 3.1).

3.3.2 Circumscribed Astrocytic Gliomas

Formerly recognized as "other astrocytic tumors," this category includes gliomas with more defined margins separated from surrounding tissue. They are characterized by a solid rather than an infiltrative growth pattern, most frequently affecting children, adolescents and young adults, and

World Health Organization Classification of Tumors of the Central Nervous System, fifth edition
Gliomas, glioneuronal tumors, and neuronal tumors
Adult-type diffuse gliomas
Astrocytoma, IDH-mutant
Oligodendroglioma, IDH-mutant, and 1p/19q-codeleted
Glioblastoma IDH-wildtype
Pediatric-type diffuse low-grade gliomas
Diffuse astrocytoma, *MYB- or MYBL1*-altered
Angiocentric glioma
Polymorphous low-grade neuroepithelial tumor of the young
Diffuse low-grade glioma, MAPK pathway-altered
Pediatric-type diffuse high-grade gliomas
Diffuse midline glioma, H3 K27-altered
Diffuse hemispheric glioma, H3 G34-mutant
Diffuse pediatric-type high-grade glioma, H3-wildtype and IDH-wildtype
Infant type hemispheric glioma
Circumscribed astrocytic gliomas
Pilocytic astrocytoma
High-grade astrocytoma with piloid features
Pleomorphic xanthoastrocytoma
Subependymal giant cell astrocytoma
Chordoid glioma
Astroblastoma, *MN1*-altered
Glioneuronal and neuronal tumors
Ganglioglioma
Desmoplastic infantile ganglioglioma / desmoplastic infantile astrocytoma
Dysembryoplastic neuroepithelial tumor
Diffuse glioneuronal tumor with oligodendroglioma-like features and nuclear clusters
Papillary glioneuronal tumor
Rosette-forming glioneuronal tumor
Myxoid glioneuronal tumor
Diffuse leptomeningeal glioneuronal tumor
Gangliocytoma
Multinodular and vacuolating neuronal tumor
Dysplastic cerebellar gangliocytoma (Lhermitte-Duclos disease)
Central neurocytoma
Extraventricular neurocytoma
Cerebellar liponeurocytoma

Fig. 3.1 According to Louis et al. in the WHO 2021 Glioma, Glioneuronal Tumors, and Neuronal tumors are divided into six different types: adult-type diffuse gliomas, pediatric-type diffuse low-grade gliomas, pediatric-type diffuse high-grade gliomas, circumscribed astrocytic gliomas, glioneuronal and neuronal tumors, ependymomas (the latter not reported in the figure above). Each of these is subdivided into several subtypes

rarely the elderly. For this type of gliomas, the EANO-EURACAN-SNO Task Force recognizes specific molecular mutations, again emphasizing their prognostic and predictive importance. Among the main molecular alterations recognized in the pathway of these tumors, those with therapeutic relevance are the BRAF and MEK mutations in pilocytic astrocytoma and pleomorphic xanthoastrocytoma, the mTOR pathway in subependymal giant cell astrocytoma [16, 17].

- *Pilocytic astrocytoma (PA)*: CNS grade 1, usually characterized by alteration in the MAPK pathway (most frequently KIAA1549-BRAF fusion). It usually presents radiologically as a cystic lesion with a contrast-enhancing nodule, in the cerebellum in children, while in adults, it can also be found supratentorially. If there is brainstem involvement, there is typically extension to the fourth ventricle due to its exophytic appearance (Fig. 3.2).

- *Pleomorphic Xanthroastrocytoma (PXA)*: CNS grade 2 or 3 based on mitotic count, typically featured with mutations in BRAF V600E. It may radiologically present the appearance of a diffuse glioma, with cystic components, intense contrast grip, and perilesional edema.
- *Subependymal large cell astrocytoma (SEGA)*: Strongly associated with tuberous sclerosis (TS). The mTOR pathway is typically involved. Pathognomonic is the localization at the level of the foramen of Monro.
- *Chordoid glioma*: Typically involves the anterior portion of the third ventricle, often expressing TTF1.
- *High-grade astrocytoma with piloid features (HGAP)*: Loss of expression of ATRX can be characteristic and the diagnosis is based on methyloma.
- *Astroblastoma, MN1 altered:* They need molecular confirmation to distinguish them from other entities with astoblastoma-like rosettes.

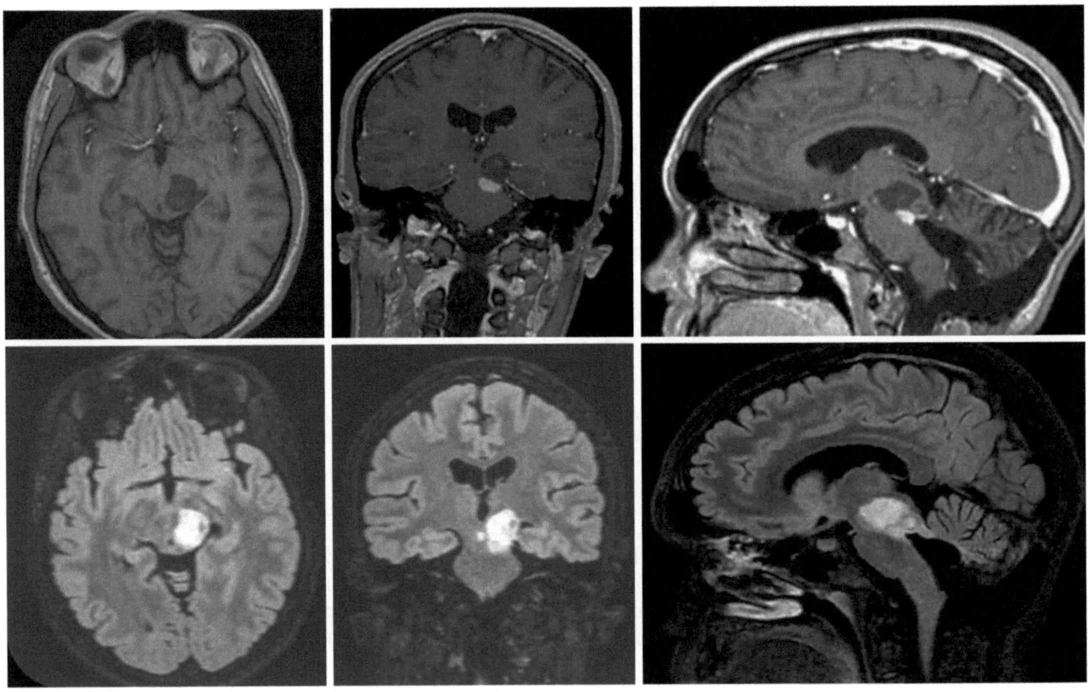

Fig. 3.2 Pediatric patient with history pilocytic astrocytoma localized in cerebral peduncle and inferior part of left thalamus. Molecular analysis revealed non-canonical BRAF mutation BRAFV600insT [c.1796_1797insTAC, p.T599_V600insT]

3.3.3 Diffuse Gliomas

As noted above, among the most significant changes in the new edition, there is the division of diffuse gliomas into those found primarily in children (pediatric type) and those found primarily in adults (adult type), as they are characterized by different molecular drivers and different prognostic impact. The term primarily emphasizes that pediatric ones may rarely be found in adults and vice versa [4]. Previously, the division into histopathological categories was based on the presumed cell of origin. Today, genomics is known to have the greatest impact on clinical behavior. In particular, the use of techniques in the field of genomics and epigenomics has made it possible to identify a complex biological landscape, especially in pediatric forms [3, 11].

3.3.4 Pediatric-Type Diffuse High-Grade Glioma (PDHGG)

In this group, we identify the following four types:

- *Diffuse H3K27 midline gliomas altered.* The new nomenclature implies the term "altered" and not "mutated," to emphasize that other mutations are also included, in addition to those previously identified in H3K27. They are grade 4. It is a perfect example of how localization, histology, and genetics define a specific type that also differs from the altered H3K27 form of adults. In the pediatric population, they generally involve the brainstem, usually the pons (DIPG), but often also bi-thalamic. The characteristic alteration is the loss of nuclear expression of H3K27me3, which determines both the mutation of H3K27 and the mutation of EGFR (bi-thalamic localization is common here), or even an overexpression of EZHIP. This allows a division into four clinically and biologically distinct subtypes: *H3.3 p.K27-mutant*, often co-occurring with TP53/PPM1D mutation and PDGFRA; *H3.1 and H3.2 p.K27M-mutant* often co-occurring with PIK3CA, PIK3R1, or PTEN mutations, and ACVR1 mutation; *H3-wild-type with EZHIP overexpression* are quite rare; the EGFR-mutant subgroup often co-occurring with TP53 mutation [18].
  Although they are more frequent in the pediatric population, this type of tumor is currently found in different age groups. In particular, unilateral thalamic or spinal involvement is more frequent in the adult population [19] (Fig. 3.3).
- *Diffuse hemispheric glioma H3 G34-mutant.* It generally affects adolescents and young adults. There is no expression of OLIG2, but there is loss of nuclear expression of ATRX and overexpression of p53 (Fig. 3.4).
- *Diffuse pediatric-type high-grade glioma H3-wildtype and IDH-wildtype.* It is characterized by histological high-grade features, absence of histone H3 and IDH mutations, and aggressive biological behavior (CNS WHO grade 4).
- *Infant-type hemispheric glioma.* It appears as a large intra-axial tumor with a solid and a cystic component, often with a marked mass effect and often with intratumoral hemorrhage.

3.3.5 Pediatric Low-Grade Gliomas

In this group, we disclose:

- *Diffuse astrocytoma with alteration of MYB or MYBL1.* A diffusely infiltrative astroglial neoplasm, typically assigned to CNS WHO grade 1 and indolent [20].
- *Angiocentric glioma.* This tumor has an indolent behavior and is assigned to CNS WHO grade 1.
- *Polymorphous low-grade neuroepithelial tumor of the young (PLNTY).* CNS WHO grade 1, characterized by indolent behavior, diffuse growth pattern, oligodendroglioma-like elements, calcifications, CD34 expres-

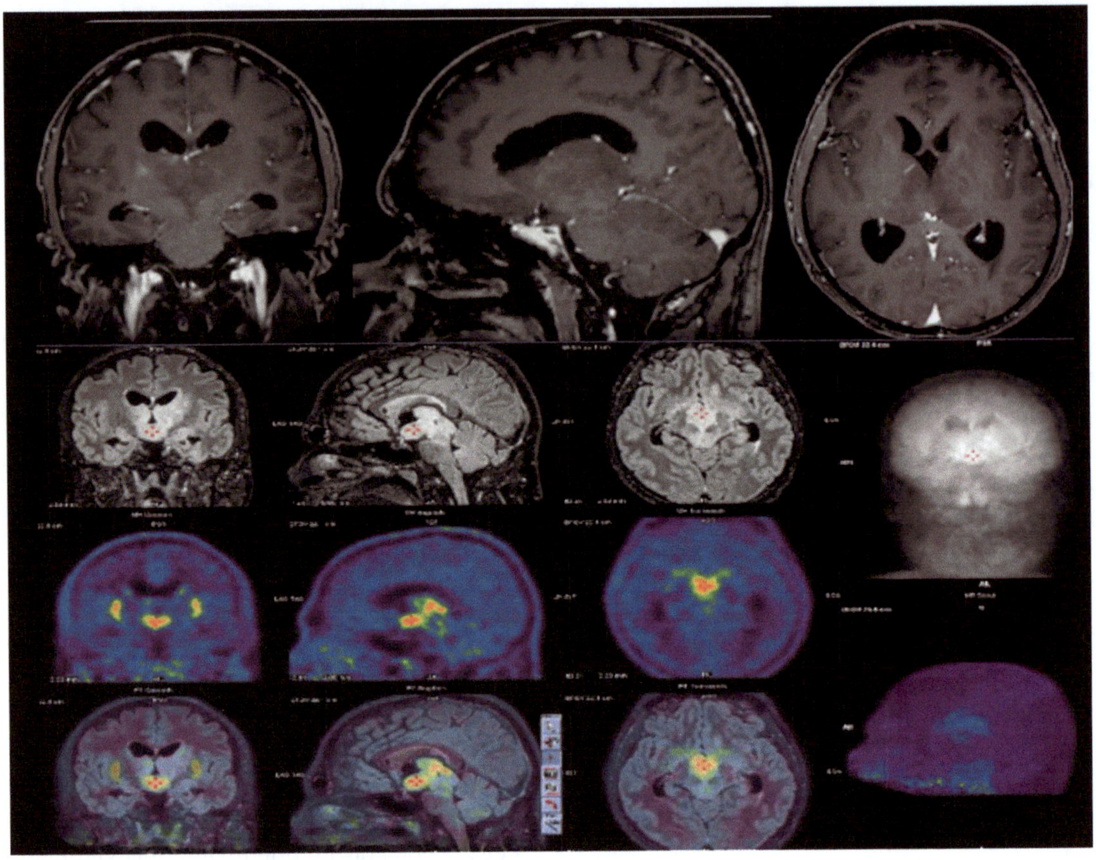

Fig. 3.3 Patient with thymic deflection with ideo-motor slowing; imaging on MRI with evidence of widespread signal alteration of interest the anterior and posterior thalamic nuclei, with also hypothalamic, and mesencephalic involvement; heterogeneous anomalous accumulation of 18F-DOPA at the note lesion involving the structures of the midline, suggestive of diffuse midline glioma. After stereotactic biopsy diagnosis was made: H3K27M-ALTERED DIFFUSE MIDLINE GLIOMAS, GRADE 4 (CNS WHO 2021)

sion, and genetic alterations activating MAPK signaling.

- *Diffuse low-grade glioma, MAPK pathway-altered.* The presence of a single gene alteration (usually BRAF or FGFR) allowed the treatment to be rapidly transferred to a target therapy.

3.3.6 Adult-Type Diffuse Gliomas

The classification of adult diffuse gliomas is summarized into three main types [21], unlike the 15 entities described in the previous edition:

- *Astrocytoma IDH mutant.* Several studies have shown that this type of tumor may originate from the precursors of the central nervous system cells. They are classified as grade 2, 3, or 4. The presence of the homozygous deletion of CDKN2A and/or CDKN2B (CDKN2A/B) is important, as it causes it to be classified as a grade 4 glioma regardless of histopathological criteria [8, 22, 23] (Fig. 3.5). The methylation status of the MGMT promoter is also relevant from a prognostic point of view. Most IDH-mutated tumors are found at a supratentorial level, mainly in the frontal lobe, while spinal or infratentorial rarely

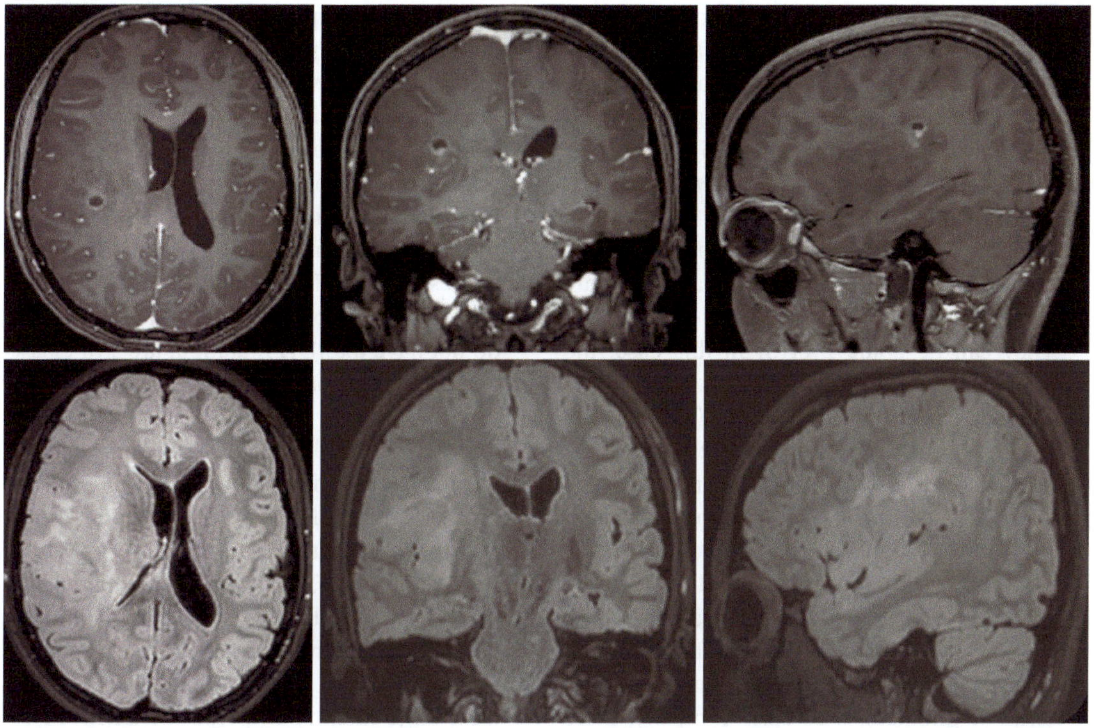

Fig. 3.4 Patient with partial motor seizure and finding on MRI of a diffuse glioma with extension to insula and corpus callosum. After biopsy diagnosis was made: DIFFUSE HEMISFERIC GLIOMA H3 G34-MUTANT, anti-OLIG2 negative, GRADE 4

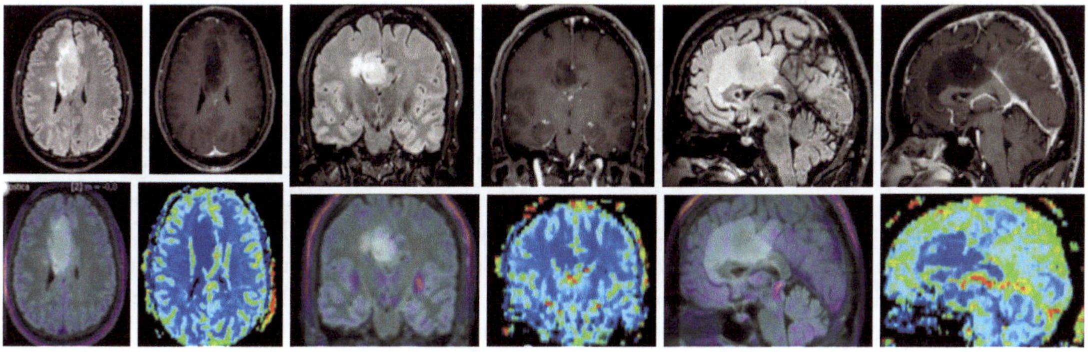

Fig. 3.5 Patient with generalized seizure; imaging on MRI show an extensive alteration signal at the right parasagittal frontal level characterized by a nuance hyperintensity on FLAIR and T2, hypointense on T1, without diffusion restriction; after contrast not significant enrichment; the perfusion study shows no increase in rCBV; not significant accumulation of 18F-DOPA. After surgery diagnosis was made: ASTROCYTOMA, IDH-MUTATED, MGMT METHYLATED, HOMOZYGUS DELETION OF CDKN2A, GRADE 4

occur. Latter localizations are frequently associated with IDH1/2 mutations variants other than the canonical IDH1 R132H and with lack of ATRX mutations, configuring a mutated IDH astrocytoma subtype [24, 25].

- *Oligodendroglioma, IDH-Mutant, and 1p/19q-Codeleted.* Some studies suggest that these tumors arise from oligodendrocyte precursors while others believe that they may arise from astrocytes and neural progenitors. They can be grade 2 or 3. In this case, the homozygous deletion of CDKN2A is not considered for grading, despite the fact that in a french study, its greater aggressiveness is described [26]. This implies that there is no grade 4. Also in this type, the most frequent localization is at the frontal level, but often also at the temporal and parietal level, more rarely at the occipital level; very rarely we find them in posterior cranial fossa, brainstem or with bilateral multiple involvement with patterns of gliomatosis cerebri. Typically, there may be leptomeningeal or intraventricular spread in the case of recurrence. Characteristic mutations, in addition to the IDH and the 1p/19q mutations, are the clear loss of ATRX expression and/or diffuse expression of TP53, TERT mutations are also typical.
- *Glioblastoma, IDH wild type.* The pathogenesis is currently unclear. Some studies suggest that it may derive from various progenitors, including neuronal, astrocytic, and oligodendroglial ones; in particular, several studies suggest that it can arise from neuronal progenitors at the level of the subventricular zones. It is classified as grade 4. They are typically subcortical, involving the white matter without a predilection for lobes. In the previous classification, the diagnosis of glioblastoma was based on histopathological features such as central pseudopalisate necrosis and microvascular proliferation, regardless of the presence or absence of certain mutations. Different studies, however, have shown that the presence of the IDH mutation determined a different biological behavior and a different response to therapy. The first major difference compared to the previous classification is that the term glioblastoma is no longer used for mutated IDH gliomas, which means that if histologically they configure grade 4, the current correct nomenclature is astrocytoma IDH-mutated grade 4, emphasizing once again the impact of molecular biology on tumor aggressiveness. This implies that tumors with low-grade histopathological features, if they do not have the IDH mutation, are still classified as glioblastoma, underlining the prognostic role of this molecular marker. In fact, glioblastoma is defined as a diffuse astrocytic glioma IDH wild type and H3 wild type with one or more of the following conditions: microvascular proliferation, necrosis, mutation of the TERT promoter, epidermal growth factor receptor (EGFR) gene amplification, a concomitant gain of chromosome 7 and loss of chromosome 10 (+7/−10) [27, 28]. This allowed to identify two types of GBM: histological glioblastoma (hist-GBM) characterized by the histopathological aspects of grade 4, and molecular glioblastoma (mol-GBM), i.e., tumors with histopathological aspects of grade 2 or 3 but the aforementioned mutations, generally classified as relatively low-grade [29, 30]. If none of these criteria are identified, they are classified as diffuse gliomas "non-elsewhere classified" (NEC) or pediatric-type diffuse glioma, including MYB- or MYBL1-altered low-grade diffuse astrocytoma and H3-wildtype and IDH wild type pediatric-type high-grade diffuse glioma. Several studies have shown that mol-GBM has specific clinical features, such as diffuse infiltration patterns (gliomatosis), multicentric loci or gyriform spread, so they are often only biopsied instead of gross total resection. In most cases, mol-GBM lack contrast enhancement in MRI defining a "low-grade" appearance in imaging (non-CE glioblastoma, when $\leq 1\ cm^3$ contrast enhancement is identified in preoperative imaging) and also from a prognostic point of view they have a better overall

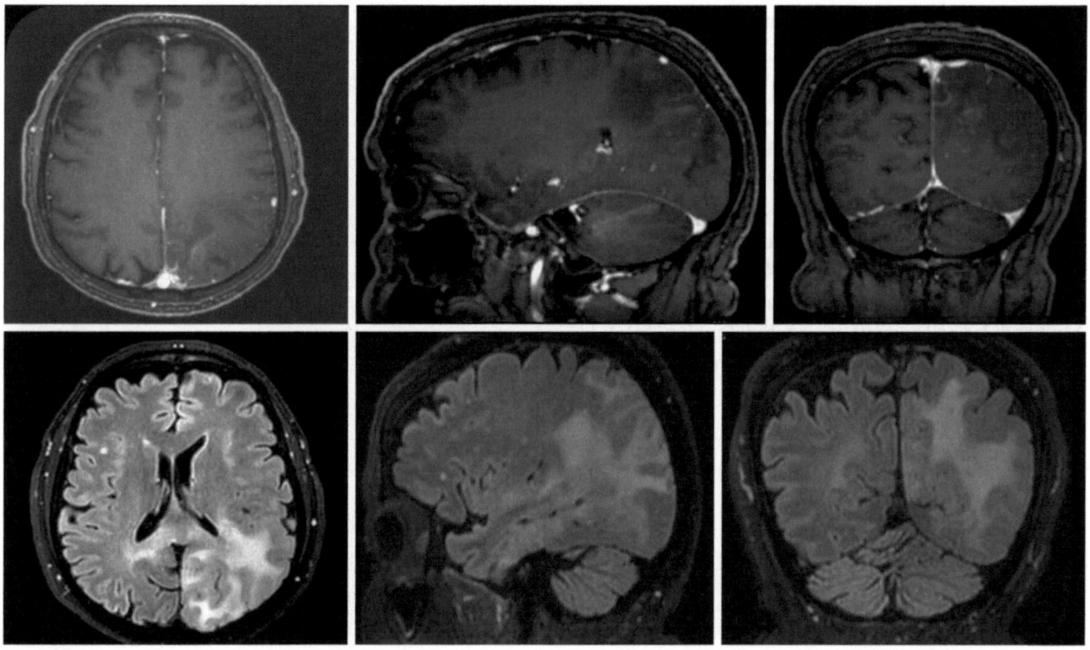

Fig. 3.6 Patient with nominum aphasia and visual field deficit. At MRI alteration on FLAIR at the left temporo-parietooccipital level with extension through the splenium of the corpus callosum to the contralateral white matter with two focal and thin contrast enhancement. After biopsy, diagnosis was made: GLIOBLASTOMA, IDH WILD TYPE, MGMT METHYLATED, TP53 MUTATED, GRADE 4

survival than histological GBM [31, 32] (Fig. 3.6). Many studies also incorporate the mRNA expression of 840 genes, proposed by Verhaak in 2010, into the molecular classification, distinguishing four-subtypes: proneural—PN, classical—CL, mesenchymal—ME, and neural—NE, demonstrating that that mesenchymal transition of glioblastomas is associated with a more aggressive course of disease and therapy resistance[33–35]. Gliosarcoma, giant cell glioblastoma, and epithelioid cell glioblastoma are still registered as histological subtypes of glioblastomas.

3.3.7 Neuronal and Glioneuronal Tumors

Briefly, glioneuronal tumors are rare tumors with several neuronal and glial components. In this category, compared to the previous classification, we recognize three new types: diffuse glioneuronal tumor with oligodendroglioma like features and nuclear clusters (DGONC), multinodular and vacuolating neuronal tumor (MVNT), and myxoid glioneuronal tumor (MGNT) (Table 3.1). Although histopathologically ganglioglioma and neurocytoma have more aggressive features, they are nowadays recognized as grade 1 and 2, respectively [16].

3.3.8 Ependymal Tumors

Ependymal tumors are a heterogeneous group of neuroepithelial tumors that originate from ependymal cells. Within this category, the new classification identifies 10 types, divided into three groups: supratentorial, posterior cranial fossa (PF), and spinal. They are typically viewed as a unique cancer entity, possessing specific qualities, and are not the primary focus of this book.

Table 3.1 Glioneuronal and neuronal tumors

Ganglioglioma
Gangliocytoma
Desmoplastic infantile ganglioglioma (DIG)/desmoplastic infantile astrocytoma (DIA)
Dysembryoplastic neuroepithelial tumor (DNT)
Diffuse glioneuronal tumor with oligodendroglioma-like features and nuclear clusters (DGONC)
Papillary glioneuronal tumor (PGNT)
Rosette-forming glioneuronal tumor (RGNT)
Myxoid glioneuronal tumor (MGNT)
Diffuse leptomeningeal glioneuronal tumor (DLGNT)
Multinodular and vacuolating neuronal tumor (MVNT)
Dysplastic cerebellar gangliocytoma (Lhermitte-Duclos disease)
Central neurocytoma
Extraventricular neurocytoma
Cerebellar liponeurocytoma

3.4 Insight Into Imaging Diagnosis

An emerging field in the diagnosis and management of CNS tumors is radiogenomics or genomic imaging, which allows molecular aspects to be correlated with radiological features [36–38]. In diffuse IDH-mutant astrocytomas of grade 2–3, the T2-FLAIR mismatch sign (T2 homogeneity of the mass with relatively hypointense signal throughout most of the lesion on FLAIR compared with T2 sequences except for a peripheral rim of hyperintense signal) has a high predictive value and is the most specific of the radiogenomic features. Elevated maximum relative CBV MRI value might be useful for differentiating grade 2 from grade 3. They are generally poorly contrast enhanced, have well-defined margins, a high apparent diffusion coefficient (ADC) value, increased level of oncometabolite 2-hydroxyglutarate (2HG) on 2HG MRI spectroscopy [15, 39]. Typical imaging features of oligodendroglioma, IDH-mutant and 1p/19q-codeleted, include localization in the frontal lobe, T1/T2 heterogeneity signal, and calcification with variable enhancement. In oligodendroglioma, calcifications and cystic changes are evident in 90% of cases; another characteristic is represented by the infiltration of the tumor in the cortex, which is evidenced in FLAIR MRI; the heterogeneous mild-to-moderate enhancement on contrast-enhanced MRI appears to be related to the histological appearance of "chicken-wire vasculature." Diffuse midline gliomas, H3 K27-altered, typically occur in the brainstem, pons, or bi-thalamic regions in children, while in adolescents and adults, they are more commonly found involving a single thalamus or spinal cord. Within the category of glioblastomas, multifocal or multicentric forms (m-GBM) are found in approximately 34% of patients, which have a worse outcome than single localization. Specifically, multifocal GBM is defined if there are several foci with contrasting plugs connected to each other, while multicentric GBM is defined if the foci are unconnected. Genomic analysis concluded that generally the majority of multiple foci taking contrast are wild type IDHs and generally expressing the mesenchymal molecular signature and therefore with a worse prognosis. From a molecular point of view, m-GBMs often show higher frequencies of epidermal growth factor receptor (EGFR) amplifications and concurrent alterations of EGFR with phosphatase and tensin homolog/mutated in multiple advanced cancers (PTEN/MMAC) gene, as well as the reverse transcriptase (TERT) promoter, which radiologically correlates with a larger volume of contrast enhancement and T2 FLAIR hyperintensity compared to EGFR non-amplified tumors. The term gliomatosis cerebri GC refers to an infiltrative growth pattern, involving three or more lobes, but since there is no distinctive histopathological or molecular criterion for such a pattern, it no longer falls under the WHO classification as a separate tumor. It is possible to identify three subtypes recognizable in MRI: subtype 1 (diffuse infiltrative) which less frequently presents contrast sockets and often does not present the histopathological aspects of GBM but presents its molecular structure; type 2 (multifocal); Type 3 (large) [40].

3.5 Future Perspectives

To date, the treatment of these tumors, in particular diffuse ones, still remains challenging, underlining the need to better identify diagnostic and therapeutic strategies. In the field of neuro-oncology, the rapid development of genomics and sequencing techniques allows to easily identify new tumor biomarkers useful in clinical practice as diagnostic, prognostic and predictive factors (The Cancer Genome Atlas project TCGA glioma database) [41]. Several authors have attempted to identify new specific molecular pathways. Wang et al. [42] in a sample of 98 elderly patients with GBM, identified KRAS and PPM1D as negative prognostic factors, but to date molecular profile of GBM in elderly patients is not completely understood, but several genetic factors can negatively affect the prognosis [43]; Chen et al. [44] analyzed 20 adult patients with pediatric-type gliomas, identifying KMT5B and MET as factors influencing survival and potentially therapeutic targets; Ge et al. [45] and Zhang et al. [46] studied brain structural and functional variations particularly in frontal and temporal gliomas; Song et al. [47] identified ARSD as a promoter of tumorigenesis, influencing the tumor microenvironment, and regulating the JAK2/STAT3 pathway, providing potential therapeutic targets for glioma treatment. Focusing on the tumor microenvironment, more and more importance is given to the immune system and its interaction with tumor cells (e.g., extracellular vesicles that contain various signaling molecules, including miRNAs that regulate the tumor microenvironment and promote tumorigenesis) encouraging the search for these diagnostic, prognostic, and predictive biomarkers [48, 49].

3.6 Conclusions

Although the current WHO classification is a valuable tool for integrating histomolecular diagnosis and clinical-prognostic trends, there are still several aspects to be improved. The classification is attributed on the basis of estimated clinical data obtained from epidemiological studies, without always taking into account the individuality of the patient. This underlines the need to evolve the current classification toward a patient-oriented type of precision medicine and to further stratify this type of neoplasms.

References

1. Walter E, Scott M. The life and work of Rudolf Virchow 1821–1902: "cell theory, thrombosis and the sausage duel". J Intensive Care Soc. 2017;18(3):234–5. https://doi.org/10.1177/1751143716663967.
2. Eastman FC. A classification of the tumors of the Glioma Group on a histogenetic basis with a correlated study of prognosis. Ann Surg. 1926. https://doi.org/10.1097/00000658-192607000-00018.
3. Whitfield BT, Huse JT. Classification of adult-type diffuse gliomas: Impact of the World Health Organization 2021 update. Brain Pathol. 2022. https://doi.org/10.1111/bpa.13062.
4. Torp SH, Solheim O, Skjulsvik AJ. The WHO 2021 classification of central nervous system tumours: a practical update on what neurosurgeons need to know—a mini review. Acta Neurochir. 2022. https://doi.org/10.1007/s00701-022-05301-y.
5. Louis DN, Perry A, Wesseling P, et al. The 2021 WHO classification of tumors of the central nervous system: a summary. Neuro-Oncology. 2021. https://doi.org/10.1093/neuonc/noab106.
6. Figarella-Branger D, Appay R, Metais A, Tauziède-Espariat A, Colin C, Rousseau A, Varlet P. La classification de l'OMS 2021 des tumeurs du système nerveux central. Ann Pathol. 2022. https://doi.org/10.1016/j.annpat.2021.11.005.
7. Weller M, van den Bent M, Preusser M, et al. EANO guidelines on the diagnosis and treatment of diffuse gliomas of adulthood. Nat Rev Clin Oncol. 2021. https://doi.org/10.1038/s41571-020-00447-z.
8. Chen W, Guo S, Wang Y, et al. Novel insight into histological and molecular astrocytoma, IDH-mutant, grade 4 by the updated WHO classification of central nervous system tumors. Cancer Med. 2023. https://doi.org/10.1002/cam4.6476.
9. Louis DN, Ellison DW, Brat DJ, et al (2019) cIMPACT-NOW: a practical summary of diagnostic points from Round 1 updates. Brain Pathol 29(4): 469-472

10. Louis DN, Wesseling P, Aldape K, et al. cIMPACT-NOW update 6: new entity and diagnostic principle recommendations of the cIMPACT-Utrecht meeting on future CNS tumor classification and grading. Brain Pathol. 2020;30:844–56.
11. Thomas DL. 2021 updates to the World Health Organization classification of adult-type and pediatric-type diffuse gliomas: a clinical practice review. Chin Clin Oncol. 2023. https://doi.org/10.21037/cco-22-120.
12. Sahm F, Brandner S, Bertero L, et al. Molecular diagnostic tools for the World Health Organization (WHO) 2021 classification of gliomas, glioneuronal and neuronal tumors; an EANO guideline. Neuro-Oncology. 2023. https://doi.org/10.1093/neuonc/noad100.
13. Kurokawa R, Kurokawa M, Baba A, Ota Y, Pinarbasi E, Camelo-Piragua S, Capizzano AA, Liao E, Srinivasan A, Moritani T. Major changes in 2021 World Health Organization classification of central nervous system tumors. Radiographics. 2022. https://doi.org/10.1148/rg.210236.
14. Horbinski C, Berger T, Packer RJ, Wen PY. Clinical implications of the 2021 edition of the WHO classification of central nervous system tumours. Nat Rev Neurol. 2022. https://doi.org/10.1038/s41582-022-00679-w.
15. Park YW, Vollmuth P, Foltyn-Dumitru M, Sahm F, Ahn SS, Chang JH, Kim SH. The 2021 WHO classification for gliomas and implications on imaging diagnosis: part 1—key points of the fifth edition and summary of imaging findings on adult-type diffuse gliomas. J Magn Reson Imaging. 2023. https://doi.org/10.1002/jmri.28743.
16. Rudà R, Capper D, Waldman AD, et al. EANO - EURACAN - SNO guidelines on circumscribed astrocytic gliomas, glioneuronal, and neuronal tumors. Neuro-Oncology. 2022. https://doi.org/10.1093/neuonc/noac188.
17. d'Amati A, Bargiacchi L, Rossi S, et al. Pediatric CNS tumors and 2021 WHO classification: what do oncologists need from pathologists? Front Mol Neurosci. 2024. https://doi.org/10.3389/fnmol.2024.1268038.
18. Vallero SG, Bertero L, Morana G, Sciortino P, Bertin D, Mussano A, Ricci FS, Peretta P, Fagioli F. Pediatric diffuse midline glioma H3K27- altered: a complex clinical and biological landscape behind a neatly defined tumor type. Front Oncol. 2023. https://doi.org/10.3389/fonc.2022.1082062.
19. Bin-Alamer O, Jimenez AE, Azad TD, Bettegowda C, Mukherjee D. H3K27M-altered diffuse midline gliomas among adult patients: a systematic review of clinical features and survival analysis. World Neurosurg. 2022. https://doi.org/10.1016/j.wneu.2022.06.020.
20. Bale TA, Rosenblum MK. The 2021 WHO classification of tumors of the central nervous system: an update on pediatric low-grade gliomas and glioneuronal tumors. Brain Pathol. 2022. https://doi.org/10.1111/bpa.13060.
21. Antonelli M, Poliani PL. Adult type diffuse gliomas in the new 2021 WHO classification. Pathologica. 2022. https://doi.org/10.32074/1591-951X-823.
22. Gritsch S, Batchelor TT, Gonzalez Castro LN. Diagnostic, therapeutic, and prognostic implications of the 2021 World Health Organization classification of tumors of the central nervous system. Cancer. 2022. https://doi.org/10.1002/cncr.33918.
23. Komori T. Grading of adult diffuse gliomas according to the 2021 WHO classification of tumors of the central nervous system. Lab Investig. 2022. https://doi.org/10.1038/s41374-021-00667-6.
24. Martin KC, Ma C, Yip S. From theory to practice: implementing the WHO 2021 classification of adult diffuse gliomas in neuropathology diagnosis. Brain Sci. 2023. https://doi.org/10.3390/brainsci13050817.
25. Śledzińska P, Bebyn MG, Furtak J, Kowalewski J, Lewandowska MA. Prognostic and predictive biomarkers in gliomas. Int J Mol Sci. 2021. https://doi.org/10.3390/ijms221910373.
26. Appay R, Dehais C, Maurage CA, et al. CDKN2A homozygous deletion is a strong adverse prognosis factor in diffuse malignant IDH-mutant gliomas. Neuro-Oncology. 2019. https://doi.org/10.1093/neuonc/noz124.
27. Guo X, Wang Y, Ma W. Editorial: Impacts of 2021 WHO classification on the precise diagnosis and management of gliomas. Front Neurosci. 2024. https://doi.org/10.3389/fnins.2024.1366523.
28. Muench A, Teichmann D, Spille D, et al. A novel type of IDH-wildtype glioma characterized by gliomatosis cerebri-like growth pattern, TERT promoter mutation, and distinct epigenetic profile. Am J Surg Pathol. 2023. https://doi.org/10.1097/PAS.0000000000002118.
29. Rudà R, Bruno F, Ius T, et al. IDH wild-type grade 2 diffuse astrocytomas: prognostic factors and impact of treatments within molecular subgroups. Neuro-Oncology. 2022. https://doi.org/10.1093/neuonc/noab239.
30. Guo X, Gu L, Li Y, et al. Histological and molecular glioblastoma, IDH-wildtype: a real-world landscape using the 2021 WHO classification of central nervous system tumors. Front Oncol. 2023. https://doi.org/10.3389/fonc.2023.1200815.
31. Karschnia P, Dietrich J, Bruno F, et al. Surgical management and outcome of newly diagnosed glioblastoma without contrast enhancement (low-grade appearance): a report of the RANO resect group. Neuro-Oncology. 2024. https://doi.org/10.1093/neuonc/noad160.
32. Nakasu S, Deguchi S, Nakasu Y. IDH wild-type lower-grade gliomas with glioblastoma molecular features: a systematic review and meta-analysis. Brain Tumor Pathol. 2023. https://doi.org/10.1007/s10014-023-00463-8.
33. Steponaitis G, Kucinskas V, Golubickaite I, Skauminas K, Saudargiene A. Glioblastoma molecular classification tool based on mRNA analysis: from

wet-lab to subtype. Int J Mol Sci. 2022. https://doi.org/10.3390/ijms232415875.
34. Dénes A, Bontell TO, Barchéus H, Vega SF, Carén H, Lindskog C, Jakola AS, Smits A. The clinical value of proneural, classical and mesenchymal protein signatures in WHO 2021 adult-type diffuse lower-grade gliomas. PLoS One. 2023. https://doi.org/10.1371/journal.pone.0285732.
35. Verhaak RGW, Hoadley KA, Purdom E, et al. Integrated genomic analysis identifies clinically relevant subtypes of glioblastoma characterized by abnormalities in PDGFRA, IDH1, EGFR, and NF1. Cancer Cell. 2010. https://doi.org/10.1016/j.ccr.2009.12.020.
36. Lasocki A, Roberts-Thomson SJ, Gaillard F. Radiogenomics of adult intracranial gliomas after the 2021 World Health Organisation classification: a review of changes, challenges and opportunities. Quant Imaging Med Surg. 2023. https://doi.org/10.21037/qims-22-1365.
37. Lee SJ, Park JE, Park SY, Kim YH, Hong CK, Kim JH, Kim HS. Imaging-based versus pathologic survival stratifications of diffuse glioma according to the 2021 WHO classification system. Korean J Radiol. 2023. https://doi.org/10.3348/kjr.2022.0919.
38. Osborn AG, Louis DN, Poussaint TY, Linscott LL, Salzman KL. The 2021 World Health Organization classification of tumors of the central nervous system: what neuroradiologists need to know. Am J Neuroradiol. 2022. https://doi.org/10.3174/ajnr.A7462.
39. Park YW, Vollmuth P, Foltyn-Dumitru M, Sahm F, Ahn SS, Chang JH, Kim SH. The 2021 WHO classification for gliomas and implications on imaging diagnosis: part 2—summary of imaging findings on pediatric-type diffuse high-grade gliomas, pediatric-type diffuse low-grade gliomas, and circumscribed astrocytic gliomas. J Magn Reson Imaging. 2023. https://doi.org/10.1002/jmri.28740.
40. Divé I, Weber KJ, Hartung TI, et al. Gliomatosis cerebri (GC) growth pattern: a single-center analysis of clinical, histological, and molecular characteristics of GC and non-GC glioblastoma. Neuro-Oncol Adv. 2023. https://doi.org/10.1093/noajnl/vdad131.
41. Zakharova G, Efimov V, Raevskiy M, Rumiantsev P, Gudkov A, Belogurova-Ovchinnikova O, Sorokin M, Buzdin A. Reclassification of TCGA diffuse glioma profiles linked to transcriptomic, epigenetic, genomic and clinical data, according to the 2021 WHO CNS tumor classification. Int J Mol Sci. 2023. https://doi.org/10.3390/ijms24010157.
42. Wang Y, Li J, Cao Y, et al. Characteristic analysis and identification of novel molecular biomarkers in elderly glioblastoma patients using the 2021 WHO classification of central nervous system tumors. Front Neurosci. 2023. https://doi.org/10.3389/fnins.2023.1165823.
43. Bruno F, Pellerino A, Palmiero R, Bertero L, Mantovani C, Garbossa D, Soffietti R, Rudà R. Glioblastoma in the elderly: review of molecular and therapeutic aspects. Biomedicine. 2022. https://doi.org/10.3390/biomedicines10030644.
44. Chen W, Jin S, Liu Q, et al. Spotlights on adult patients with pediatric-type diffuse gliomas in accordance with the 2021 WHO classification of CNS tumors. Front Neurosci. 2023. https://doi.org/10.3389/fnins.2023.1144559.
45. Ge H, Yan Z, Liu D, et al. Synergetic reorganization of the contralateral structure and function in patients with unilateral frontal glioma. Front Neurosci. 2022. https://doi.org/10.3389/fnins.2022.1016693.
46. Zhang Y, Xu H, Liu Y, Yang K, Zou Y, Liu H. Stable functional compensation within hippocampal-subregion networks in patients with temporal glioma before and after surgery. Front Neurosci. 2022. https://doi.org/10.3389/fnins.2022.991406.
47. Song Z, Zhao Z, Zhu S, Jin Q, Zhang S, Wang Z, Shen B, Wang Z, Zhao Z. Arylsulfatase D is a prognostic biomarker that promotes glioma cells progression through JAK2/STAT3 pathway and M2 macrophage infiltration. Front Oncol. 2023. https://doi.org/10.3389/fonc.2023.1228426.
48. Bianconi A, Aruta G, Rizzo F, Salvati LF, Zeppa P, Garbossa D, Cofano F. Systematic review on tumor microenvironment in glial neoplasm: from understanding pathogenesis to future therapeutic perspectives. Int J Mol Sci. 2022. https://doi.org/10.3390/ijms23084166.
49. Nikolova E, Laleva L, Milev M, Spiriev T, Stoyanov S, Ferdinandov D, Mitev V, Todorova A. miRNAs and related genetic biomarkers according to the WHO glioma classification: from diagnosis to future therapeutic targets. Non-coding RNA Res. 2024. https://doi.org/10.1016/j.ncrna.2023.10.003.

Clinical Onset of Gliomas and Its Impact on Prognosis

4

Giovanni Paternò, Barbara Buccilli, Fabio Grassia, Riccardo Boccaletti, and Fulvio Tartara

4.1 Introduction

Clinical manifestations of gliomas can range from mass effects due to tumor invasion, to symptoms of obstructive hydrocephalus, presenting diverse clinical signs. The initial symptoms, from headaches to debilitating seizures, are not only critical for early detection but also significantly influence prognosis and treatment strategies [1]. The clinical onset of gliomas—particularly the nature and timing of initial symptoms—can inform predictions about disease progression and patient outcomes. By understanding the relationship between initial symptoms and tumor behavior, healthcare professionals can better tailor treatment strategies, thereby improving patient care and enhancing quality of life. This discussion aims to provide a nuanced perspective on the prognostic value of the clinical onset in gliomas, refining our approach to managing this complex disease.

G. Paternò (✉)
Humanitas Pio X, Spine and Robotic Surgery, Milan, Italy
e-mail: giovannipaterno@yahoo.com

B. Buccilli
Department of Neurosurgery, Icahn School of Medicine at Mount Sinai, New York, NY, USA

Global Neurosurgical Alliance, Phoenix, AZ, USA

F. Grassia
University of Colorado School of Medicina, Aurora, CO, USA

R. Boccaletti · F. Tartara
Neurosurgical Department, Ospedale Maggiore University of Parma, Parma, Italy

4.2 Pre-diagnostic Symptoms

The challenge of identifying pre-diagnostic symptoms of glioma highlights a critical gap in the early detection of this serious condition. Typically, the symptoms associated with glioma are common and nonspecific, making it difficult for general practitioners to distinguish these patients from those suffering from more benign conditions. Additionally, many individuals may not seek medical advice for symptoms that are perceived as mild or do not drastically impact daily life, further complicating early diagnosis efforts. The year before the diagnosis fatigue (58%), mental exhaustion (51%), sleeping difficulty and sleep disorders (41%), headache (39%), and stress (34%), were the five symptoms most commonly identified [2]. These findings illustrate the prevalence and variety of symptoms that can be associated with gliomas, yet each of these symptoms is also commonly found in a wide range of less serious health issues. This overlap of symptoms with non-malignant conditions poses a significant challenge for healthcare providers, especially in primary care settings where such symptoms are often treated as routine ailments. The similarity and ubiquity of these symptoms can delay refer-

D. Armocida et al. (eds.), *Neurosurgery's Frontline Role in Gliomas Treatment*,
https://doi.org/10.1007/978-3-031-81850-9_4

rals and more comprehensive neurological evaluations, critical steps in diagnosing gliomas earlier. Understanding this pattern and the commonality of symptoms in the year leading up to a glioma diagnosis can aid healthcare professionals in developing a more refined index of suspicion, particularly in patients who present multiple nonspecific symptoms concurrently over an extended period. It also underscores the need for more detailed patient histories and possibly the development of screening guidelines or tools that can better flag these cases for further neurological assessment. This could potentially lead to earlier diagnosis and improved outcomes for glioma patients, emphasizing the importance of integrating such insights into clinical practice.

4.3 Symptomatology at Onset

Glioma symptoms are diverse and depend on the tumor's location, size, growth rate, and the presence of peritumoral edema. Common symptoms include headaches, seizures, cognitive and personality changes, motor deficits, sensory abnormalities, and language disturbances. The symptomatology can provide insight into the affected brain regions and may correlate with the tumor's grade (Fig. 4.1).

Headaches are often vague and worse in the morning, and typically stem from increased intracranial pressure caused by the tumor's mass effect or associated hydrocephalus. Although headaches are a common complaint, they seldom occur as the sole initial symptom and are usually accompanied by other symptoms, indicating broader neurological impact [3, 4].

Seizures are a common symptom and are especially prevalent in patients with low-grade gliomas (LGGs). Seizures often result from irritation of the cerebral cortex by the tumor or its related edema, disrupting normal neural activity [5, 6]. About 25% of glioma patients experience a seizure at diagnosis, and another 20% develop seizures later [7].

In high-grade gliomas (HGGs), rapid growth can lead to focal peritumoral ischemia and deafferentation of cortical areas due to mass effect, contributing further to seizure activity [6, 8]. Seizures can present years before diagnosis and they can be the only symptom for months or years in the non-progressing phase; a large number of patients develop refractory seizures [6, 8, 9]. Tumors located near the primary motor cortex or within the limbic and perilimbic cortical areas, supratentorial or motor cortex, and leptomeningeal involvement are more likely to cause seizures [6, 10]. Seizures seem to be a more common presentation in younger patients with LGGs [11].

Cognitive and personality changes, including memory deficits and executive dysfunction, may reflect involvement of the frontal lobes or diffuse infiltration of the tumor [12, 13]. With their relatively lengthy longevity and (often) younger age, LGG-patients are seen to be the most affected group when it comes to neurocognitive impairment, but cognitive disorders are actually more common in older patients with HGGs [11, 14]. Numerous processes, including local mechanical impacts of the tumor mass and ischemia changes resulting from it, as well as excitotoxins generated by the tumor that cause cell death and disruptions in synaptic transmission, can cause neurocognitive deficiencies [15, 16].

Glioma patients need a neuropsychological examination employing sensitive and comprehensive tests in order to identify neurocognitive abnormalities. Since they lack sensitivity and domain-specific information, standard screening tests for cognitive decline, such the Folstein Mini Mental State Examination (MMSE) and the Montreal Cognitive Assessment (MoCA), can fail to yield accurate findings [14]. Motor deficits, such as weakness or paralysis, typically indicate involvement of the motor cortex or its descending pathways, while sensory abnormalities suggest involvement of the sensory cortex or thalamic pathways [5, 17]. Language disturbances, including aphasia, are associated with tumors in the dominant hemisphere's language areas, such as Broca's or Wernicke's areas. Visual field deficits, such as hemianopia, can occur with tumors affecting the optic pathways or occipital lobe [10].

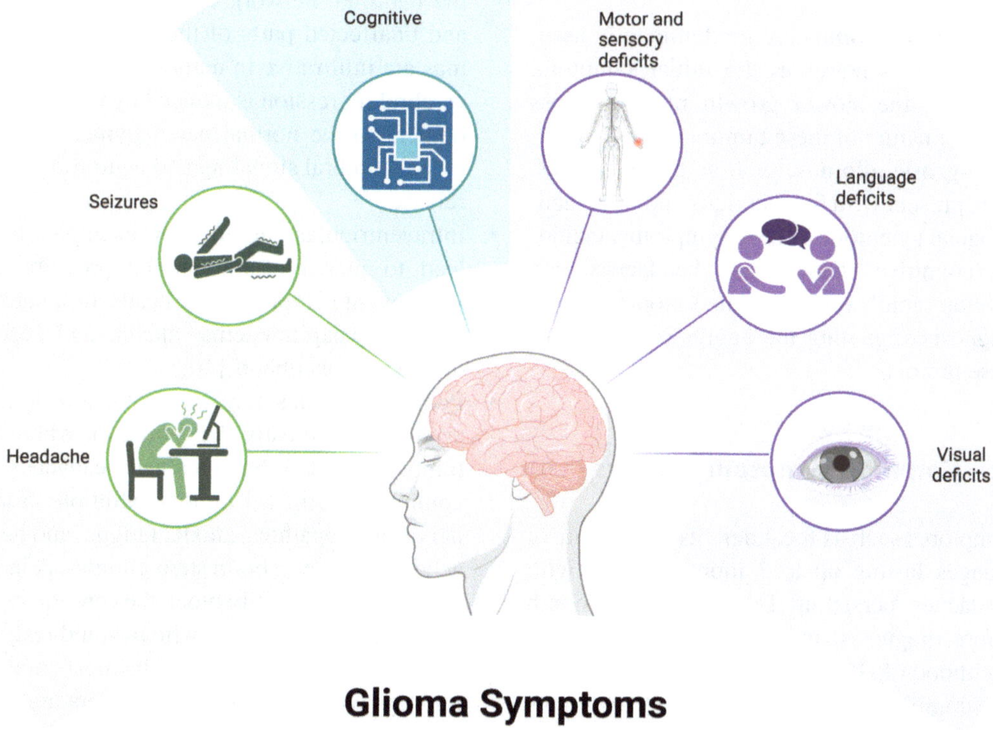

Fig. 4.1 Key symptoms of gliomas—this diagram illustrates the common symptoms associated with gliomas, including headaches, seizures, cognitive changes, and focal neurological deficits. Made with Biorender

4.4 Symptom Correlation with Tumor Characteristics

The symptoms exhibited by glioma patients can provide significant insights into the underlying tumor characteristics such as grade, location, and growth rate. These correlations are crucial for guiding diagnostic and therapeutic strategies. In gliomas, the size of the tumor and the extent of peritumoral edema are indeed related to the clinical presentation and symptomatology. The mass effect from the tumor itself can cause direct compression of adjacent brain structures, leading to focal neurological deficits that correspond to the affected brain region. Peritumoral edema, which is typically vasogenic due to the disruption of the blood–brain barrier, can exacerbate these symptoms by increasing intracranial pressure and causing additional mass effect. Edema in the white matter tracts can lead to more diffuse neurological deficits due to the disruption of fiber tracts that connect different brain regions. Studies have shown that preoperative peritumoral edema may not predict seizure outcome postoperatively, but long-term edema resolution is associated with improved seizure outcome. Advanced imaging techniques, such as diffusion tensor imaging (DTI) and functional MRI (fMRI), are being used to study the relationship between edema, tumor biology, and brain connectivity [18–21].

4.4.1 Symptom Patterns by Tumor Grade

- **Low-grade gliomas** are predominantly associated with seizures as the initial symptom, reflecting the slower growth rates and less invasive nature of these tumors [3].
- **High-grade gliomas**, such as glioblastomas, often present with focal deficits and other neurological symptoms. These symptoms, including cognitive changes and headaches, can develop rapidly, often within 3 months before diagnosis, signaling the aggressive nature of these tumors

4.4.2 Common Symptom Clusters

- Symptoms such as focal deficits and cognitive changes lasting up to 3 months, along with headaches persisting for up to one month before diagnosis, independently indicate the likelihood of HGGs [3].
- The combination of progressing focal deficits and worsening cognitive changes is a common symptom cluster among patients with glioblastoma [3, 11].
- Anaplastic gliomas exhibit symptoms and symptoms' evolution more quickly. Seizures are a common presentation of oligodendrogliomas. Because of the increased intracranial pressure and hydrocephalus caused by intraventricular lesions, headache, nausea, vomiting, papilloedema, ataxia, and vertigo are frequently experienced [10].

4.4.3 Symptoms Linked to Tumor Location

- Impairments in cognition are more common in glioma patients with dominant hemisphere tumors than in those with non-dominant hemisphere tumors, but cognitive deficits are not limited to the afflicted brain lobe [22–25]. This might be caused by the loss of integrity in the neuronal network connecting the injured and unaffected parts of the brain, since gliomas are infiltrative in nature and the systemic cerebral regression is induced by tumor development in the normal parenchyma, affecting global cerebral signaling and neurotransmitter release.
- Intraventricular tumors, for example, often lead to increased intracranial pressure and subsequent symptoms like headaches, nausea, vomiting, papilloedema, ataxia, and vertigo due to hydrocephalus [10].
- Pediatric gliomas may manifest in a wide variety of ways, mostly depending on where the tumor is located. Seizures and headaches are common in cortical tumors. Multiple cranial nerves neuropathies, ataxia, fatigue, and headaches common in brain stem gliomas. A larger tumor may eventually block the cerebral aqueduct or fourth ventricle, which would result in obstructive hydrocephalus. The most common findings with posterior fossa tumors are cerebellar symptoms and elevated intracranial pressure from obstructive hydrocephalus [26–30] (Fig. 4.2).

Damage to white and gray matter structures has been associated with declines in motor, cognitive, and visual functions in survivors of pediatric LGGs. Researchers used advanced structural and functional imaging techniques, such as diffusion tensor imaging and voxel-based morphometry, to explore these correlations [31, 32]. These observations highlight the complexity of symptomatology in glioma patients and underscore the importance of a thorough and nuanced assessment of symptoms in relation to tumor pathology. Understanding these correlations helps in anticipating the disease course and tailoring individualized treatment plans, enhancing the potential for positive outcomes.

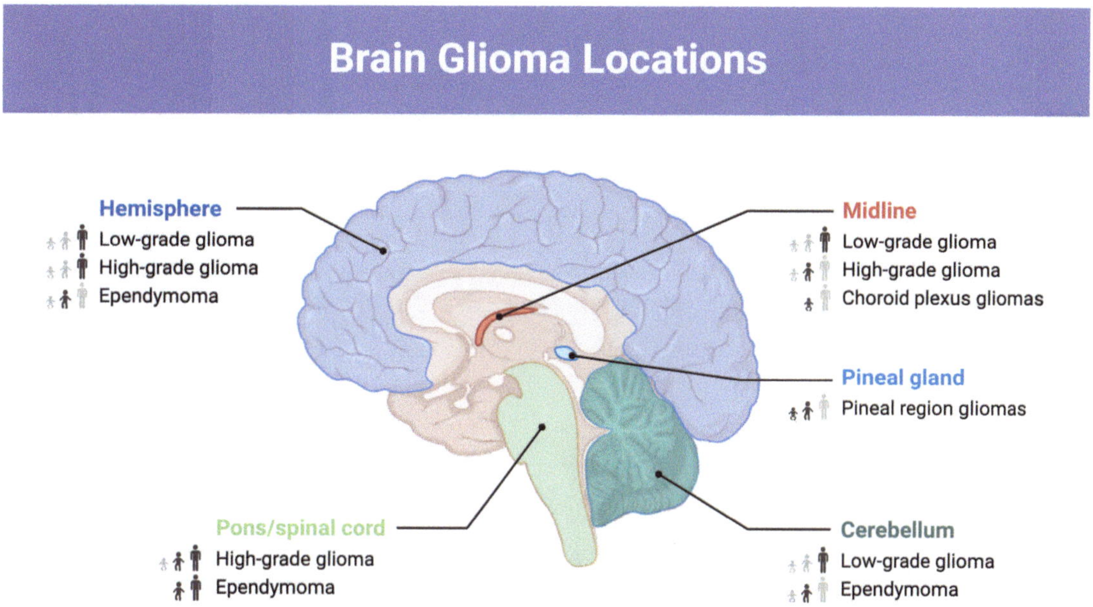

Fig. 4.2 Common glioma locations and associated age groups—this diagram illustrates typical glioma locations alongside the age groups most frequently affected, highlighting age-specific trends in tumor distribution. Made with Biorender

4.5 Pediatric Gliomas

According to the WHO classification, the majority of pediatric gliomas are benign, slowly developing lesions which are categorized as grade I or II (25–30% of all childhood CNS tumors). They have good overall survival with the current treatments and are essentially distinct from adult LGGs in that they seldom become malignant. Nonetheless, a substantial amount of gliomas evolve and expand quickly; as a result, they are still mostly fatal even after multiple treatment attempts, with the most severe cases being fatal in a matter of months [29, 33]. The brainstem (9%), cerebral hemispheres (17%), cerebellum (25%), and hypothalamic-chiasmatic area (40%) are among the most common sites for pediatric LGGs [29, 30, 34]. Children with LGGs may experience a long-term decline in their quality of life, as the condition can be considered chronic [29, 35]. In addition to nonspecific symptoms due to elevated intracranial pressure (like nausea, emesis, and increased head circumference), tumors often involve the optic pathway, presenting with visual dysfunction [28, 34, 36]. Optic gliomas are also associated with monocular or asymmetric nystagmus and optic atrophy [28]. Other common presentations of pediatric gliomas are motor deficits, altered coordination, epilepsy, and endocrine dysfunction [28, 30, 34]. An uncommon neurological condition called diencephalic syndrome, which is often characterized by euphoria and failure to thrive, may occur in children under three years old with hypothalamic LGGs. Since diencephalic syndrome is an extremely unusual cause of failure to thrive, pediatric LGG diagnosis is sometimes delayed when this is the main sign at presentation [37] (Fig. 4.3).

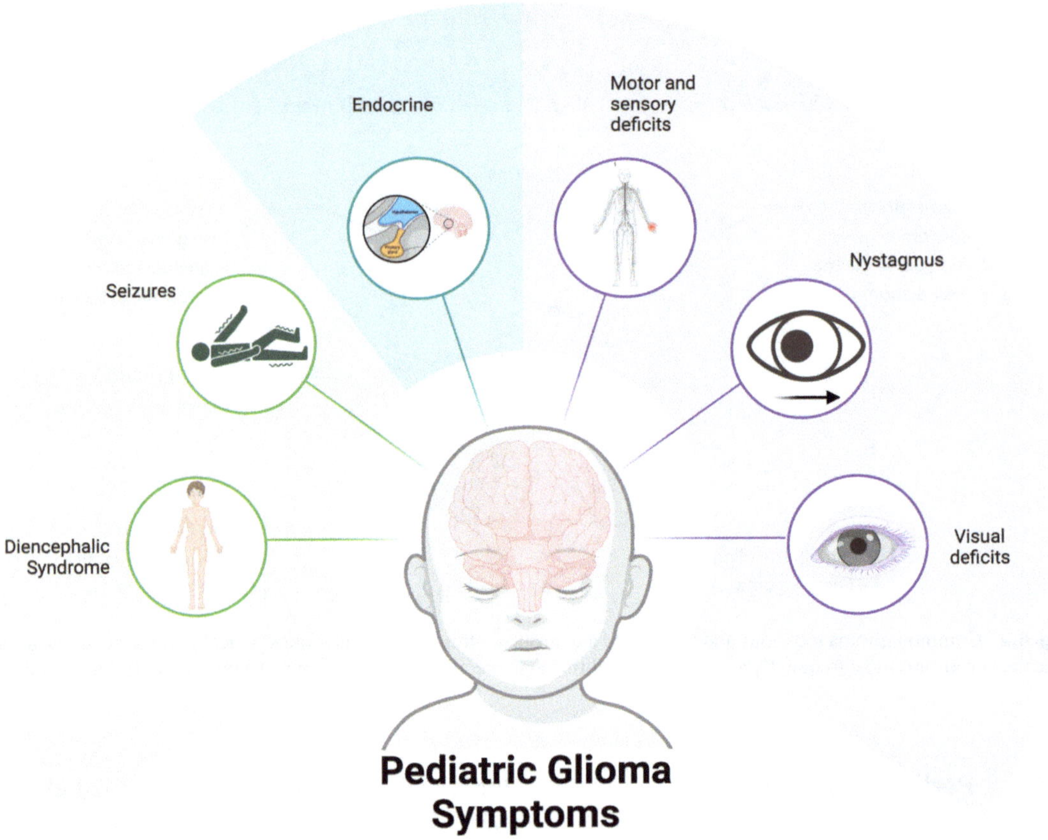

Fig. 4.3 Key symptoms of gliomas in pediatric patients—this diagram illustrates the common symptoms associated with gliomas in children, including seizures, endocrine dysfunctions, and focal neurological deficits. It also underlines the relevance of diencephalic syndrome, a rarer but relevant presentation

4.6 Prognostic Implications of Initial Symptoms

The relationship between symptoms and outcomes is multifaceted. For instance, preoperative motor or language deficits may predict a higher risk of postoperative neurological impairment, but they can also guide the use of intraoperative mapping to minimize functional loss [17, 38, 39]. Seizures at presentation may necessitate long-term antiepileptic management, and their control can significantly improve quality of life, but pharmacoresistence is common [9, 10]. Resective surgery, such as lobectomy or lesionectomy, can be highly effective, particularly in cases where a clear epileptogenic focus is identified and can be safely removed without compromising eloquent brain areas. Studies have shown that surgery can result in significantly higher rates of seizure freedom compared to continued medical management alone. In cases where resective surgery is not feasible or fails to control seizures, other treatment modalities may be considered. These include neuromodulation techniques such as vagus nerve stimulation (VNS), deep brain stimulation (DBS), and responsive neurostimulation (RNS). These therapies can reduce seizure frequency and severity in some patients with drug-resistant epilepsy. Additionally, dietary therapies such as the ketogenic diet or modified Atkins diet may be beneficial for some individuals, particularly children with specific epilepsy syndromes [40–44].

The presence of symptoms such as cognitive decline or neurological deficits may indicate a higher tumor grade or more aggressive behavior, potentially correlating with a poorer prognosis. Conversely, the absence of symptoms or the presence of isolated seizures may be more characteristic of LGGs. The return of epileptic seizures after a long seizure-free period can sometimes indicate disease progression before it is detectable through radiological methods[6, 45, 46]. Specifically seizures in LGG are strongly associated in prognosis and this topic will be discussed in more details in Chap. 7. Symptoms also influence the Karnofsky Performance Status (KPS), which is a measure of a patient's functional status and is used as a prognostic factor. A lower KPS score at diagnosis or before surgery can be associated with a worse outcome and shorter overall survival. The KPS is particularly valuable in oncology and neurosurgery because it helps in stratifying patients for clinical trials, making decisions about the aggressiveness of therapy, and in some cases, predicting outcomes.

However, the KPS does have limitations in the evaluation of symptoms:

- Lack of specificity: The KPS is a broad measure and does not capture specific neurological deficits or symptoms such as seizures, which can significantly impact a patient's quality of life.
- Subjectivity: The KPS is subject to the clinician's interpretation and may vary between observers. This can lead to inconsistencies in the assessment of a patient's performance status.
- Insensitivity to change: The KPS may not be sensitive enough to detect subtle changes in a patient's condition, especially in the context of neurological function.
- Non-comprehensive: The KPS does not account for all aspects of a patient's well-being, such as psychological, cognitive, and social factors.

Regarding the scenario of a patient with an optimal performance status without deficits but experiencing difficult-to-control seizures, a high KPS could be justified if the seizures do not significantly interfere with the patient's ability to carry out daily activities and self-care. However, this illustrates a limitation of the KPS, as it may not fully reflect the impact of the seizures on the patient's overall quality of life. In such cases, additional tools to measure seizure frequency and severity, as well as their impact on daily functioning, would provide a more comprehensive assessment of the patient's condition (Table 4.1).

According to a recent study, generalized symptoms, including confusion, memory loss, and hemiparesis were typically more persistent and often mistakenly believed to be a natural aspect of aging. These symptoms took longer to draw attention and lead to a conclusive diagnosis. Similar to seizure activity and communication

Table 4.1 Karnofski performance scale. The KPS ranges from 0 to 100, with higher scores indicating better functional status. A score of 100 signifies normal, no complaints, no evidence of disease. A score of 70 indicates that the patient is able to care for themselves but is unable to carry on normal activity or to do active work. A score of 50 suggests that the patient requires considerable assistance and frequent medical care

Score	Description
100	Normal, no complaints, no evidence of disease
90	Able to carry on normal activity; minor signs or symptoms of disease
80	Normal activity with effort; some signs or symptoms of disease
70	Cares for self; unable to carry on normal activity or do active work
60	Requires occasional assistance but is able to care for most personal needs
50	Requires considerable assistance and frequent medical care
40	Disabled; requires special care and assistance
30	Severely disabled; hospitalization indicated, death not imminent
20	Very sick; hospitalization necessary; active supportive treatment needed
10	Moribund, fatal processes progressing rapidly
0	Dead

impairments, visual loss or disruption prompted early intervention. Individuals who exhibit sudden or incapacitating symptoms are referred for treatment early and undergo more rapid scans and tests. Individuals with milder symptoms may go longer without being diagnosed, potentially jeopardizing surgical and radiotherapeutic interventions. Although individuals with incapacitating symptoms seemed to have a better prognosis during the first eighteen months, this difference did not last [47].

4.7 Treatment Implications

Initial symptoms of gliomas can significantly guide treatment planning by providing insights into the tumor's location, size, and potential impact on surrounding brain structures. Symptoms such as motor weakness, sensory changes, or aphasia can indicate the involvement of specific cortical areas or white matter tracts [5, 17, 22–24]. This information is critical for preoperative planning, including the use of neuronavigation and intraoperative mapping to maximize resection while preserving neurological function. The onset of seizures, particularly in LGGs, can suggest cortical involvement and may necessitate both antiepileptic medication management and consideration of the impact of surgery on seizure control. The semiology of the seizures can also help localize the tumor [9, 10]. Changes in cognition, personality, or behavior may indicate frontal lobe or other higher cortical involvement. Neuropsychological evaluation can be important for planning both the surgical approach and postoperative rehabilitation [22–25]. Headaches, nausea, vomiting, or papilledema can be signs of increased ICP due to tumor growth or obstructive hydrocephalus. Headaches associated with raised ICP typically worsen in the morning due to the supine position during sleep, which reduces venous outflow and CSF absorption, further exacerbating intracranial hypertension. The headache may also intensify with Valsalva maneuvers, bending over, or coughing [3, 4]. Papilledema, the optic disc swelling due to increased ICP, is a critical sign and can be observed during fundoscopic examination. It indicates that intracranial hypertension has been present for some time, as it typically takes hours to days to develop. Papilledema is a crucial indicator of hydrocephalus, with failure to detect it potentially leading to irreversible optic atrophy. However, its absence does not rule out elevated intracranial pressure (ICP), especially in cases involving brainstem and cerebellar tumors. These tumors can obstruct the third ventricle, the aqueduct of Sylvius, or the fourth ventricle, causing obstructive hydrocephalus. The likelihood of papilledema development is influenced by the duration of ICP elevation. Papilledema primarily results from axonal swelling due to raised ICP, which impairs axoplasmic flow. In cases of acute ICP elevation, both anterograde and retrograde axoplasmic flow are blocked [48–50]. Management may include medical therapies to lower ICP, such as osmotic diuretics (e.g., mannitol) or acetazolamide, corticosteroids to reduce vasogenic edema, but may also necessitate urgent surgical intervention to relieve pressure, sometimes requiring external ventricular drainage, ventriculoperitoneal shunt, decompressive craniectomy or endoscopic third ventriculostomy prior to tumor resection [51].

Visual field deficits or other visual disturbances can indicate involvement of the optic pathways. This may affect the surgical approach, such as choosing a transsphenoidal approach for tumors impacting the optic chiasm, and the need for ophthalmological assessment pre- and postoperatively [52]. Symptoms suggestive of endocrine dysfunction, such as diabetes insipidus or amenorrhea-galactorrhea syndrome, can indicate a tumor's impact on the hypothalamic-pituitary axis, guiding the need for endocrinological evaluation and management [53–55].

Rapidly progressing symptoms may suggest a more aggressive tumor phenotype, potentially guiding the urgency of intervention and the consideration of adjuvant therapies such as chemotherapy and radiation. The presence and severity of symptoms can correlate with the size and invasiveness of the tumor, which can impact the extent of resection achievable. For instance, a large tumor causing significant mass effect may be more amenable to gross total resection [56].

4.7.1 Influence on Adjuvant Therapy

The presence of certain symptoms may influence the timing and type of adjuvant therapy. For example, postoperative radiation may be considered more urgently in patients with aggressive symptoms suggestive of a HGG. In children diagnosed with LGGs associated with neurofibromatosis type 1, visual deficits are the primary criteria for initiating adjuvant treatment, taking precedence over radiographic progression [29, 36, 57–60]. Additional prevalent clinical manifestations that prompt the start of adjuvant treatment include dysmetria and weakness, which are associated with brainstem and motor circuit dysfunction [34]. Long-term chemotherapy has been associated with reduced motor performance in children with LGGs [61]. By identifying and addressing motor deficits earlier in the treatment process, targeted interventions such as physiotherapy and occupational therapy can be developed [62]. These interventions should focus on functional goals and enhancing the children's ability to perform activities of daily living, potentially mitigating the impact of these deficits during follow-up care.

4.7.2 Prognostic Implications

Certain symptoms at presentation, such as cognitive dysfunction or neurological deficits, may have prognostic implications that influence the overall treatment plan, including the aggressiveness of therapy and goals of care discussions. The Vineland Adaptive Behavior Scales II (VABS-II) categorizes its items into four primary domains: Communication, Daily Living Skills, Socialization, and Motor Skills, which together encompass a total of 11 subdomains and an overall Adaptive Behavior Composite Score (ABC) [27]. Initial findings using the Vineland Adaptive Behavior Scale for quantitatively assessing motor impairment in pediatric LGGs are promising, although the scale has not yet been incorporated into official guidelines [27]. Early-life motor development disorders may impede the acquisition of age-appropriate gross (walking and running) and fine motor abilities, which are necessary at crucial developmental stages of life [63] (Table 4.2). Early modest declines in visual acuity during therapy in pediatric patients with optic gliomas should be interpreted with caution, as they may reflect pre-existing damage rather than

Table 4.2 This table outlines the structure of the Vineland Adaptive Behavior Scales II (VABS-II)

Domain	Subdomain	Description
Communication	Receptive	Assesses the child's understanding of communicated information
	Expressive	Evaluates the child's ability to verbally communicate thoughts and needs
	Written (for children ≥3)	Measures skills in reading and writing
Daily living skills	Personal	Covers personal care activities like eating, dressing, and personal hygiene
	Domestic	Involves household tasks the child can perform, such as cleaning and helping out at home
	Community	Relates to how the child uses community resources and manages time, money, and other daily needs
Socialization	Interpersonal relationships	Describes the child's ability to interact and form relationships with others
	Play and leisure time	Assesses how the child engages in play and uses leisure time
	Coping skills	Evaluates the child's responsibility and sensitivity towards others
Motor skills	Gross	Focuses on the use of arms and legs for movement and coordination
	Fine	Involves using hands and fingers to manipulate objects

Table 4.3 This table provides an overview of how visual acuity measurements on the logMAR scale translate to more commonly known Snellen chart readings

logMAR value	Snellen equivalent	Description
−0.3	20/10	Vision significantly better than standard
−0.2	20/12.5	Excellent vision, better than standard
−0.1	20/16	Very good vision, above standard
0.0	20/20	Standard vision, considered "normal" vision
0.1	20/25	Slightly below standard vision
0.2	20/32	Mild vision loss
0.3	20/40	Moderate vision loss
0.4	20/50	Moderate vision loss
0.5	20/63	Noticeable vision loss
0.6	20/80	Considered low vision
0.7	20/100	Low vision, significant impairment
0.8	20/125	Severe vision loss
0.9	20/160	Severe vision loss
1.0	20/200	Legal blindness threshold in many countries

ongoing deterioration. A decrease of 0.2 logMAR is used as a criterion for visual worsening. However, if this occurs at the first on-therapy assessment (around 12 weeks) and the MRI shows the tumor is stable or responding, it is advisable to re-evaluate visual acuity within 4 weeks before confirming progressive visual disease. If subsequent testing shows stable vision, vision should be considered stable. Conversely, if there is further decline, then visual worsening should be noted. Vision monitoring should align with the imaging schedule, typically every 12 weeks, as per REiNS recommendations [34, 59, 64, 65] (Table 4.3).

4.8 Challenges in Predicting Prognosis Based on Clinical Onset

Predicting the prognosis from the clinical onset of gliomas is complicated by the diversity of these tumors and the variability in how patients present. Gliomas consist of a broad spectrum of tumors, each with unique histological grades and molecular characteristics. This variety complicates making broad prognostic assessments based solely on initial symptoms. For example, two patients may show similar symptoms initially but could have drastically different outcomes depending on specific molecular features like IDH mutation status or MGMT promoter methylation. Furthermore, glioma symptoms can differ greatly among patients, even with the same type and location of the tumor. Symptoms such as headaches or cognitive changes are often vague, making precise correlation with prognosis difficult. The interval from the appearance of symptoms to diagnosis can also vary, with delays potentially altering the prognosis. Additionally, the speed at which symptoms progress might offer some prognostic insights, although this is not consistently reliable. Factors such as the patient's age and their condition at the time of presentation are significant, yet they can be complicated by other health issues and might not directly reflect the tumor's initial presentation. While molecular markers are increasingly vital for prognosis and treatment decisions, they often do not manifest in clinical symptoms and their implications are typically revealed only after a surgical biopsy and molecular testing. A patient's psychological and social support networks can also impact their prognosis, although these factors are not directly connected to the initial clinical presentation.

4.8.1 Statistical and Methodological Limitations

Many prognostic models are based on retrospective data, which may not capture all variables affecting outcomes, and their direct applicability to individual patients can be limited. There is a shortage of information from primary care services regarding the development of symptoms, necessitating reliance on data from patients referred to secondary or tertiary care centers. However, in these specialized settings, it's hard to assess the predictive validity of symptoms due to selection bias. In addition, the positive predictive value of symptoms alone is very low [3]. While it is well recognized that brain tumors and their treatments can affect neurocognitive functions, it's hard to determine the types, severity, and progression of neurological impairments in these patients. Factors contributing to these deficits include age, coexisting conditions like diabetes and hypertension, and the use of various medications such as steroids, antiepileptic drugs, immunosuppressants, painkillers, and antibiotics for treating complications. Additionally, the presence of seizures, direct brain damage from the tumor, and the overall treatment regimen are also associated with neurological deficits. Patient features, such as personality changes, avoidance or adaptation, and lack of identification by medical staff and/or family members, can all lead to a delayed diagnosis. Addressing these challenges requires a multidisciplinary approach that includes thorough clinical assessments, advanced neuroimaging, surgical expertise, and molecular diagnostics. Prognostic models are now integrating a broader array of variables, including molecular biomarkers, to enhance accuracy. Nevertheless, personalized care for each patient is essential, as models provide guidance but cannot definitively determine outcomes.

4.9 Future Directions in Research

Emerging research points to intriguing associations between glioma symptoms and patient outcomes, though findings are rarely as indicative as those associated with biomarkers and often require further investigation. According to a study, patients with a better prognosis reported double vision, stress, and burnout far more frequently than patients with a worse prognosis; however, these differences not statistically significant [2]. Further research is needed to verify these findings and determine if there is a significant link between these symptoms and patient prognosis.

In a recent study, when compared to patients with subtler or slower-evolving symptoms, individuals with GBM who present with abrupt onset or highly debilitating symptoms seem to have a better prognosis in the first 18 months, but this difference disappears after this period [47]. The survival curves' early differences, nevertheless, were rather noticeable and could be worth more research.

Current research often focuses on postoperative neurocognitive deficits in glioma patients, making it challenging to isolate the impacts of the tumor from those of the treatment. There is a critical need for studies that examine neurocognitive disturbances prior to any surgical intervention. Such research could help clarify the extent to which the tumor itself contributes to cognitive impairment.

Standardizing neuropsychological testing could strengthen research on neurocognitive function (NCF), enabling formal meta-analyses and leading to more consistent outcome measures across studies. Findings suggest that many glioma patients experience cognitive decline before any anti-tumor treatment is administered, lending support to the hypothesis that the tumor itself plays a significant role in NCF dysfunction. The variation in the incidence and severity of cognitive impairments among untreated glioma patients remains poorly understood. Gaining a deeper insight into the causes and extent of tumor-related cognitive impairments could facilitate the development of more effective therapeutic and rehabilitative strategies. Moreover, it is essential to account for pre-existing cognitive impairments when assessing the cognitive impacts of various treatments. Understanding these baseline impairments can provide a clearer picture of how treatments affect neurocognitive outcomes and help tailor interventions that address both the tumor and its cognitive repercussions more effectively. Although important, patient-reported outcomes (such as quality of life), neuropsychological outcomes, and quantitative assessments of neurological functions (including language and motor functions) are not yet ready for inclusion in response evaluations for pediatric LGGs. However, these metrics should be incorporated as study objectives in clinical trials to further evaluate their impact on outcomes and treatment strategies. Overall, advancing our understanding of the relationship between glioma symptoms, treatment effects, and patient outcomes will require a comprehensive approach that includes improved research methodologies, enhanced standardization of assessments, and a focus on preoperative cognitive function. This holistic view will not only deepen our understanding of gliomas but also improve patient care through more personalized treatment strategies.

4.10 Conclusions

The symptoms of glioma provide critical insights into the tumor's characteristics, significantly impacting surgical planning, decisions regarding adjuvant therapy, and the overall prognostic outlook. However, the advent of molecular profiling has revolutionized the diagnostic process, offering a deeper and more refined understanding of the tumor's behavior and its implications for patient prognosis. This integration of clinical symptomatology with advanced molecular diagnostics and imaging enables a more targeted and effective approach to treatment, enhancing the precision of therapeutic strategies and potentially improving patient outcomes.

References

1. Pouratian N, Asthagiri A, Jagannathan J, Shaffrey ME, Schiff D. Surgery insight: the role of surgery in the management of low-grade gliomas. Nat Clin Pract Neurol. 2007;3:628–39. https://doi.org/10.1038/ncpneuro0634.
2. Peeters MCM, Dirven L, Koekkoek JAF, Gortmaker EG, Fritz L, Vos MJ, Taphoorn MJB. Prediagnostic symptoms and signs of adult glioma: the patients' view. J Neuro-Oncol. 2020;146:293–301. https://doi.org/10.1007/s11060-019-03373-y.
3. Rasmussen BK, Hansen S, Laursen RJ, Kosteljanetz M, Schultz H, Nørgård BM, Guldberg R, Gradel KO. Epidemiology of glioma: clinical characteristics, symptoms, and predictors of glioma patients grade I–IV in the the Danish Neuro-Oncology Registry. J Neuro-Oncol. 2017;135:571–9. https://doi.org/10.1007/s11060-017-2607-5.
4. Schankin C, Ferrari U, Reinisch V, Birnbaum T, Goldbrunner R, Straube A. Characteristics of brain tumour-associated headache. Cephalalgia. 2007;27:904–11. https://doi.org/10.1111/j.1468-2982.2007.01368.x.
5. Fang S, Li L, Weng S, Guo Y, Fan X, Jiang T, Wang Y. Altering patterns of sensorimotor network in patients with different pathological diagnoses and glioma-related epilepsy under the latest glioma classification of the central nervous system. CNS Neurosci Ther. 2023;29:1368–78. https://doi.org/10.1111/cns.14109.
6. Berntsson SG, Malmer B, Bondy ML, Qu M, Smits A. Tumor-associated epilepsy and glioma: are there common genetic pathways? Acta Oncol. 2009;48:955–63. https://doi.org/10.1080/02841860903104145.
7. Glantz MJ, Cole BF, Forsyth PA, Recht LD, Wen PY, Chamberlain MC, Grossman SA, Cairncross JG. Practice parameter: anticonvulsant prophylaxis in patients with newly diagnosed brain tumors. Neurology. 2000;54:1886–93. https://doi.org/10.1212/WNL.54.10.1886.
8. Beaumont A, Whittle IR. The pathogenesis of tumour associated epilepsy. Acta Neurochir. 2000;142:1–15. https://doi.org/10.1007/s007010050001.
9. Chang EF, Potts MB, Keles GE, Lamborn KR, Chang SM, Barbaro NM, Berger MS. Seizure characteristics and control following resection in 332 patients with low-grade gliomas. J Neurosurg. 2008;108:227–35. https://doi.org/10.3171/JNS/2008/108/2/0227.
10. Reni M, Mazza E, Zanon S, Gatta G, Vecht CJ. Central nervous system gliomas. Crit Rev Oncol

Hematol. 2017;113:213–34. https://doi.org/10.1016/j.critrevonc.2017.03.021.
11. Posti JP, Bori M, Kauko T, Sankinen M, Nordberg J, Rahi M, Frantzén J, Vuorinen V, Sipilä JOT. Presenting symptoms of glioma in adults. Acta Neurol Scand. 2015;131:88–93. https://doi.org/10.1111/ane.12285.
12. Barzilai O, Ben Moshe S, Sitt R, Sela G, Shofty B, Ram Z. Improvement in cognitive function after surgery for low-grade glioma. J Neurosurg. 2019;130:426–34. https://doi.org/10.3171/2017.9.JNS17658.
13. Guarracino I, Pauletto G, Ius T, Palese F, Skrap M, Tomasino B. Presurgical cognitive status in patients with low-grade glioma and epilepsy: testing the effects of seizures, antiseizure medications, and tumor localization. Brain Behav. 2022;12:2560. https://doi.org/10.1002/brb3.2560.
14. van Kessel E, Baumfalk AE, van Zandvoort MJE, Robe PA, Snijders TJ. Tumor-related neurocognitive dysfunction in patients with diffuse glioma: a systematic review of neurocognitive functioning prior to anti-tumor treatment. J Neuro-Oncol. 2017;134:9–18. https://doi.org/10.1007/s11060-017-2503-z.
15. Kölker S, Pawlak V, Ahlemeyer B, Okun JG, Hörster F, Mayatepek E, Krieglstein J, Hoffmann GF, Köhr G. NMDA receptor activation and respiratory chain complex V inhibition contribute to neurodegeneration in d-2-hydroxyglutaric aciduria. Eur J Neurosci. 2002;16:21–8. https://doi.org/10.1046/j.1460-9568.2002.02055.x.
16. Cairncross G, Wang M, Shaw E, Jenkins R, Brachman D, Buckner J, Fink K, Souhami L, Laperriere N, Curran W, Mehta M. Phase III trial of chemoradiotherapy for anaplastic oligodendroglioma: long-term results of RTOG 9402. J Clin Oncol. 2013;31:337–43. https://doi.org/10.1200/JCO.2012.43.2674.
17. Muir M, Gadot R, Prinsloo S, Michener H, Traylor J, Athukuri P, Tummala S, Kumar VA, Prabhu SS. Comparative study of preoperative functional imaging combined with tractography for prediction of iatrogenic motor deficits. J Neurosurg. 2022;139(1):65–72. https://doi.org/10.3171/2022.10.JNS221684.
18. Laajava J, Korja M. Peritumoral T2/FLAIR hyperintense MRI findings of meningiomas are not necessarily edema and may persist permanently: a systematic review. Neurosurg Rev. 2023;46:193. https://doi.org/10.1007/s10143-023-02094-1.
19. Zhang X, Zhang G, Wang Y, Huang H, Li H, Li M, Yang C, Li M, Chen H, Jing B, Lin S. Alteration of default mode network: association with executive dysfunction in frontal glioma patients. J Neurosurg. 2022;138:1512–21. https://doi.org/10.3171/2022.8.JNS22591.
20. Nestler U, Lutz K, Pichlmeier U, Stummer W, Franz K, Reulen H-J, Bink A. Anatomic features of glioblastoma and their potential impact on survival. Acta Neurochir. 2015;157:179–86. https://doi.org/10.1007/s00701-014-2271-x.
21. Gadot R, Khan AB, Patel R, Goethe E, Shetty A, Hadley CC, Harmanci AS, Klisch TJ, Yoshor D, Sheth SA, Patel AJ. Predictors of postoperative seizure outcome in supratentorial meningioma. J Neurosurg. 2022;137:515–24. https://doi.org/10.3171/2021.9.JNS211738.
22. Taphoorn MJ, Klein M. Cognitive deficits in adult patients with brain tumours. Lancet Neurol. 2004;3:159–68. https://doi.org/10.1016/S1474-4422(04)00680-5.
23. Reijneveld JC, Sitskoorn MM, Klein M, Nuyen J, Taphoorn MJB. Cognitive status and quality of life in patients with suspected versus proven low-grade gliomas. Neurology. 2001;56:618–23. https://doi.org/10.1212/WNL.56.5.618.
24. Klein M, Taphoorn MJB, Heimans JJ, van der Ploeg HM, Vandertop WP, Smit EF, Leenstra S, Tulleken CAF, Boogerd W, Belderbos JSA, Cleijne W, Aaronson NK. Neurobehavioral status and health-related quality of life in newly diagnosed high-grade glioma patients. J Clin Oncol. 2001;19:4037–47. https://doi.org/10.1200/JCO.2001.19.20.4037.
25. Klein M, Postma TJ, Taphoorn MJB, Aaronson NK, Vandertop WP, Muller M, van der Ploeg HM, Heimans JJ. The prognostic value of cognitive functioning in the survival of patients with high-grade glioma. Neurology. 2003;61:1796–8. https://doi.org/10.1212/01.WNL.0000098892.33018.4C.
26. Bilginer B, Narin F, Oguz KK, Uzun S, Soylemezoglu F, Akalan N. Benign cerebellar pilocytic astrocytomas in children. Turk Neurosurg. 2011;21:22–6.
27. van de Lande RS, Maurice-Stam H, Marchal JP, van Vuurden DG, Vandertop WP, Grootenhuis MA, Schouten-van Meeteren AYN. Adaptive behavior impaired in children with low-grade glioma. Pediatr Blood Cancer. 2019;66:27419. https://doi.org/10.1002/pbc.27419.
28. Chalil A, Ramaswamy V. Low grade gliomas in children. J Child Neurol. 2016;31:517–22. https://doi.org/10.1177/0883073815599259.
29. Sturm D, Pfister SM, Jones DTW. Pediatric gliomas: current concepts on diagnosis, biology, and clinical management. J Clin Oncol. 2017;35:2370–7. https://doi.org/10.1200/JCO.2017.73.0242.
30. de Blank P, Bandopadhayay P, Haas-Kogan D, Fouladi M, Fangusaro J. Management of pediatric low-grade glioma. Curr Opin Pediatr. 2019;31:21–7. https://doi.org/10.1097/MOP.0000000000000717.
31. de Blank P, Fisher MJ, Gittleman H, Barnholtz-Sloan JS, Badve C, Berman JI. Validation of an automated tractography method for the optic radiations as a biomarker of visual acuity in neurofibromatosis-associated optic pathway glioma. Exp Neurol. 2018;299:308–16. https://doi.org/10.1016/j.expneurol.2017.06.004.
32. Ailion AS, Hortman K, King TZ. Childhood brain tumors: a systematic review of the structural neuroimaging literature. Neuropsychol Rev. 2017;27:220–44. https://doi.org/10.1007/s11065-017-9352-6.
33. Gianno F, Giovannoni I, Cafferata B, Diomedi-Camassei F, Minasi S, Barresi S, Buttarelli FR, Alesi V, Cardoni A, Antonelli M, Puggioni C, Colafati GS,

Carai A, Vinci M, Mastronuzzi A, Miele E, Alaggio R, Giangaspero F, Rossi S. Paediatric-type diffuse high-grade gliomas in the 5th CNS WHO classification. Pathologica. 2022;114:422–35. https://doi.org/10.32074/1591-951X-830.
34. Fangusaro J, Witt O, Hernáiz Driever P, Bag AK, de Blank P, Kadom N, Kilburn L, Lober RM, Robison NJ, Fisher MJ, Packer RJ, Young Poussaint T, Papusha L, Avula S, Brandes AA, Bouffet E, Bowers D, Artemov A, Chintagumpala M, Zurakowski D, van den Bent M, Bison B, Yeom KW, Taal W, Warren KE. Response assessment in paediatric low-grade glioma: recommendations from the Response Assessment in Pediatric Neuro-Oncology (RAPNO) working group. Lancet Oncol. 2020;21:e305–16. https://doi.org/10.1016/S1470-2045(20)30064-4.
35. Armstrong GT, Conklin HM, Huang S, Srivastava D, Sanford R, Ellison DW, Merchant TE, Hudson MM, Hoehn ME, Robison LL, Gajjar A, Morris EB. Survival and long-term health and cognitive outcomes after low-grade glioma. Neuro-Oncology. 2011;13:223–34. https://doi.org/10.1093/neuonc/noq178.
36. Friedrich RE, Nuding MA. Optic pathway glioma and cerebral focal abnormal signal intensity in patients with neurofibromatosis type 1: characteristics, treatment choices and follow-up in 134 affected individuals and a brief review of the literature. Anticancer Res. 2016;36:4095. http://ar.iiarjournals.org/content/36/8/4095.abstract.
37. Tosur M, Tomsa A, Paul DL. Diencephalic syndrome: a rare cause of failure to thrive. BMJ Case Rep. 2017;6:220171. https://doi.org/10.1136/bcr-2017-220171.
38. Shetty P, Yeole U, Singh V, Moiyadi A. Navigated ultrasound-based image guidance during resection of gliomas: practical utility in intraoperative decision-making and outcomes. Neurosurg Focus. 2021;50:E14. https://doi.org/10.3171/2020.10.FOCUS20550.
39. Bander ED, Shelkov E, Modik O, Kandula P, Karceski SC, Ramakrishna R. Use of the train-of-five bipolar technique to provide reliable, spatially accurate motor cortex identification in asleep patients. Neurosurg Focus. 2020;48:E4. https://doi.org/10.3171/2019.11.FOCUS19776.
40. Lee KH, Lee Y-J, Seo JH, Baumgartner JE, Westerveld M. Epilepsy surgery in children versus adults. J Korean Neurosurg Soc. 2019;62:328–35. https://doi.org/10.3340/jkns.2019.0026.
41. Khan M, Paktiawal J, Piper RJ, Chari A, Tisdall MM. Intracranial neuromodulation with deep brain stimulation and responsive neurostimulation in children with drug-resistant epilepsy: a systematic review. J Neurosurg Pediatr. 2022;29:208–17. https://doi.org/10.3171/2021.8.PEDS21201.
42. Garcia JH, Morshed RA, Chung J, Millares Chavez MA, Sudhakar V, Saggi S, Avalos LN, Gallagher A, Young JS, Daras M, McDermott MW, Garcia PA, Chang EF, Aghi MK. Factors associated with preoperative and postoperative seizures in patients undergoing resection of brain metastases. J Neurosurg. 2023;138:19–26. https://doi.org/10.3171/2022.3.JNS212285.
43. Freund BE, Greco E, Okromelidze L, Mendez J, Tatum WO, Grewal SS, Middlebrooks EH. Clinical outcome of imaging-based programming for anterior thalamic nucleus deep brain stimulation. J Neurosurg. 2022;138:1008–15. https://doi.org/10.3171/2022.7.JNS221116.
44. Selner AN, Rosinski CL, Chiu RG, Rosenberg D, Chaker AN, Drammeh H, Esfahani DR, Mehta AI. Vagal nerve stimulation for epilepsy in adults: a database risk analysis and review of the literature. World Neurosurg. 2019;121:e947–53. https://doi.org/10.1016/j.wneu.2018.10.043.
45. Piepmeier J, Susan Christopher RN, Spencer D, Byrne T, Kim J, Knisel JP, Lacy J, Tsukerman L, Makuch R. Variations in the history and survival of patients with, supratentorial low-grade astrocytomas. Neurosurgery. 1996;38:872–9. https://doi.org/10.1097/00006123-199605000-00002.
46. Danfors T, Ribom D, Berntsson SG, Smits A. Epileptic seizures and survival in early disease of grade 2 gliomas. Eur J Neurol. 2009;16:823–31. https://doi.org/10.1111/j.1468-1331.2009.02599.x.
47. Yuile P, Dent O, Cook R, Biggs M, Little N. Survival of glioblastoma patients related to presenting symptoms, brain site and treatment variables. J Clin Neurosci. 2006;13:747–51. https://doi.org/10.1016/j.jocn.2005.10.011.
48. Lee HJ, Phi JH, Kim S-K, Wang K-C, Kim S-J. Papilledema in children with hydrocephalus: incidence and associated factors. J Neurosurg Pediatr. 2017;19:627–31. https://doi.org/10.3171/2017.2.PEDS16561.
49. Chou SY, Digre KB. Neuro-ophthalmic complications of raised intracranial pressure, hydrocephalus, and shunt malfunction. Neurosurg Clin N Am. 1999;10:587–608.
50. Hayreh SS. Pathogenesis of optic disc edema in raised intracranial pressure. Prog Retin Eye Res. 2016;50:108–44. https://doi.org/10.1016/j.preteyeres.2015.10.001.
51. Kienzler JC, Zakelis R, Marbacher S, Bäbler S, Schwyzer L, Remonda E, Fandino J. Changing the paradigm of intracranial hypertension in brain tumor patients: a study based on non-invasive ICP measurements. BMC Neurol. 2020;20:268. https://doi.org/10.1186/s12883-020-01837-7.
52. Bowman R, Walters B, Smith V, Prise KL, Handley SE, Green K, Mankad K, O'Hare P, Dahl C, Jorgensen M, Opocher E, Hargrave D, Thompson DA. Visual outcomes and predictors in optic pathway glioma: a single centre study. Eye. 2023;37:1178–83. https://doi.org/10.1038/s41433-022-02096-1.
53. Nagata Y, Inoshita N, Fukuhara N, Yamaguchi-Okada M, Nishioka H, Yamada S. Low-grade glioma of the neurohypophysis: clinical characteristics and surgical outcomes. World Neurosurg. 2018;114:e1225–31. https://doi.org/10.1016/j.wneu.2018.03.180.

54. Lea RW, Dawson T, Martinez-Moreno CG, El-Abry N, Harvey S. Growth hormone and cancer: GH production and action in glioma? Gen Comp Endocrinol. 2015;220:119–23. https://doi.org/10.1016/j.ygcen.2015.06.011.
55. Sani I, Albanese A. Endocrine long-term follow-up of children with neurofibromatosis type 1 and optic pathway glioma. Horm Res Paediatr. 2017;87:179–88. https://doi.org/10.1159/000458525.
56. Hu LS, D'Angelo F, Weiskittel TM, et al. Integrated molecular and multiparametric MRI mapping of high-grade glioma identifies regional biologic signatures. Nat Commun. 2023;14:6066. https://doi.org/10.1038/s41467-023-41559-1.
57. Widemann BC, Blakeley JO, Dombi E, Fisher MJ, Hanemann CO, Walsh KS, Wolters PL, Plotkin SR. Conclusions and future directions for the REiNS International Collaboration. Neurology. 2013;81:41–4. https://doi.org/10.1212/01.wnl.0000435748.79908.c5.
58. Fisher MJ, Belzberg AJ, de Blank P, De Raedt T, Elefteriou F, Ferner RE, Giovannini M, Harris GJ, Kalamarides M, Karajannis MA, Kim A, Lázaro C, Le LQ, Li W, Listernick R, Martin S, Morrison H, Pasmant E, Ratner N, Schorry E, Ullrich NJ, Viskochil D, Weiss B, Widemann BC, Zhu Y, Bakker A, Serra E. Children's Tumor Foundation conference on neurofibromatosis type 1, neurofibromatosis type 2, and schwannomatosis. Am J Med Genet A. 2016;176(2018):1258–69. https://doi.org/10.1002/ajmg.a.38675.
59. de Blank PMK, Fisher MJ, Liu GT, Gutmann DH, Listernick R, Ferner RE, Avery RA. Optic pathway gliomas in neurofibromatosis type 1: an update: surveillance, treatment indications, and biomarkers of vision. J Neuroophthalmol. 2017;37:S23–32. https://doi.org/10.1097/WNO.0000000000000550.
60. Avery RA, Ferner RE, Listernick R, Fisher MJ, Gutmann DH, Liu GT. Visual acuity in children with low grade gliomas of the visual pathway: implications for patient care and clinical research. J Neuro-Oncol. 2012;110:1–7. https://doi.org/10.1007/s11060-012-0944-y.
61. Hartman A, van den Bos C, Stijnen T, Pieters R. Decrease in peripheral muscle strength and ankle dorsiflexion as long-term side effects of treatment for childhood cancer. Pediatr Blood Cancer. 2008;50:833–7. https://doi.org/10.1002/pbc.21325.
62. Ryan DD, Kay RM. Orthopaedic issues in children and adolescents with central nervous system tumors. J Pediatr Rehabil Med. 2011;4:71–8. https://doi.org/10.3233/PRM-2011-0152.
63. Msall ME. Developing preschool surveillance tools for adaptive functioning: lessons for neuro-oncology. Eur J Paediatr Neurol. 2010;14:368–79. https://doi.org/10.1016/j.ejpn.2010.03.010.
64. Fisher MJ, Avery RA, Allen JC, Ardern-Holmes SL, Bilaniuk LT, Ferner RE, Gutmann DH, Listernick R, Martin S, Ullrich NJ, Liu GT. Functional outcome measures for NF1-associated optic pathway glioma clinical trials. Neurology. 2013;81:15–24. https://doi.org/10.1212/01.wnl.0000435745.95155.b8.
65. Pesce A, Armocida D, Paglia F, Palmieri M, Frati A, D'Andrea G, Salvati M, Santoro A. IDH wild-type glioblastoma presenting with seizure: clinical specificity, and oncologic and surgical outcomes. J Neurol Surg A Cent Eur Neurosurg. 2022;83(4):351–60. https://doi.org/10.1055/s-0041-1735515.

Update on Glioma's Neuroradiology

5

Andrea Romano, Allegra Romano, Giulia Moltoni, and Alessandro Bozzao

5.1 Introduction

The 2021 World Health Organization (WHO) classification of brain tumors incorporated the rapid advances in the molecular, genetic, and pathogenesis understanding of brain tumor pathogenesis, behavior, and treatment response [1–3]. It revolutionized brain tumor classification by placing great emphasis on molecular types and completely splitting adult-type and pediatric-type diffuse gliomas.

Neuroradiology, which specializes in diagnosing central nervous system (CNS) diseases, has simultaneously transformed its role by offering critical insights into the diagnosis, treatment, and management of glioma patients, which are important points to consider.

Magnetic resonance imaging (MRI) remains the leading imaging modality in patients with primary intra-axial brain tumors (BTs) [1]. Computed tomography (CT) has limited indications, predominantly in emergency settings such as for the detection of intratumoral acute hemorrhage or mass effects or less frequently for calcifications detection. The primary purposes of MRI at diagnosis include determining the lesion's size and location within the brain for treatment or biopsy planning, evaluating the mass effect and edema in surrounding healthy brain tissue, assessing the lesion's relationship with the ventricular system and brain vascular structures, and, with the help of other "functional" MRI sequences, suggesting a possible diagnosis [1].

Among the MRI sequences commonly used in clinical practice, FLAIR images are essential for identifying brain lesions of various origins. The T2-weighted (T2w) signal can reflect tissue density and potentially serve as an indicator of tumor cellularity: lesions with a low T2w signal are typically associated with higher cellularity. T2 hyperintensity, indicative of edema and infiltrative tumor tissue [4], often presents a diagnostic challenge.

Within a tumor, calcification or hemorrhagic components may be present; in this context, susceptibility-weighted imaging (SWI) can help in the differentiation between the two, as calcifications are diamagnetic and most hemorrhagic by-products are paramagnetic. Calcifications are commonly found in oligodendrogliomas (ODs) [5], although they can also be present in ependymomas and low-grade astrocytomas. Cystic components are more frequently observed in lower-grade gliomas, such as pilocytic astrocytoma. Conversely, intratumoral necrotic areas, which appear as regions lacking enhancement on post-gadolinium T1-weighted images, are more

A. Romano (✉) · A. Romano · G. Moltoni · A. Bozzao
NESMOS, Department of Neuroradiology, S. Andrea Hospital, University Sapienza, Rome, Italy
e-mail: andrea.romano@uniroma1.it

D. Armocida et al. (eds.), *Neurosurgery's Frontline Role in Gliomas Treatment*,
https://doi.org/10.1007/978-3-031-81850-9_5

common in high-grade tumors [6]. Ultimately, post-contrastographic enhancement is generally associated with higher tumor grade, although certain low-grade gliomas (LGG), such as pilocytic astrocytomas, commonly enhance while certain high-grade gliomas (HGG) may not [7].

In this chapter, the numerous applications of MRI sequences will be detailed and explicated, while simultaneously examining the primary pre- and intraoperative investigation methods utilized in neuroradiology.

5.2 Diffusion-Weighted Imaging (DWI)

Diffusion-weighted imaging (DWI) is based on the Brownian motion of water molecules in tissues.

Its apparent diffusion coefficient (ADC) reflects the corresponding microscopic tissue architecture, a crucial aspect of cancer imaging [8]. Indeed, ADC represents an indirect measurement of cellularity, as in solid tumors, an increase in cell density will result in lower ADC values [9]. Contrarily, cystic and necrotic areas present high ADC values due to higher free diffusion of water molecules in comparison to normal tissue as well as peritumoral edema. Additionally, DWI was shown to be useful in glioma grading, in assessing the growth potential of gliomas, and in suggesting clinical prognosis [10]. High-grade gliomas (HGGs) exhibit lower apparent diffusion coefficient (ADC) values compared to LGGs. This reduction in ADC values is indicative of increased cellular proliferation and malignancy [11]. Low tumor ADC is reported to be associated with shorter survival times [12].

5.3 Perfusion-Weighted Imaging (PWI)

Brain perfusion-weighted imaging (PWI), performed after intravenous administration of gadolinium, analyzes cerebral perfusion parameters by observing signal changes through a series of dynamic images post-bolus administration using two different techniques: dynamic susceptibility contrast (DSC) and dynamic contrast enhancement (DCE) techniques.

Arterial spin labeling (ASL) is a perfusion-weighted MR sequence that does not require exogenous contrast. It utilizes labeled blood water as the endogenous tracer, resulting in a non-invasive method of measuring brain perfusion. ASL applications in cerebrovascular diseases, neurodegenerative diseases, epilepsy, and recently neuro-oncology are becoming more promising [13].

In pseudo-continuous ASL (pcASL), continuous labeling is achieved through a sequence of rapidly repeating low-tip RF pulses and alternating sign (bipolar) magnetic field gradients also suitable for MR systems lacking continuous RF capabilities [14]. This train of short pulses is designed to invert the inflowing blood magnetization in an adiabatic or pseudo-steady-state manner. The blood is continuously inverted as it flows through a "labeling plane" in the inferior-superior direction [15].

Labeled water protons with negative magnetization mixes with the positive magnetization of static tissue water protons, resulting in a small signal intensity decrease of 1–2%. Images are obtained after a short time from the labeling process; this post-label delay (PLD), typically between 1 and 3 s, allows the visualization of blood in the parenchymal capillary phase. A control image of static tissue signal intensity is then obtained, and the label image is subtracted from the control image to produce a cerebral blood flow (CBF)-weighted difference image [16].

DSC-PWI is the most used and validated perfusion imaging technique, particularly for brain tumors [17]. The relative cerebral blood volume (rCBV) and the percentage of signal intensity recovery (PSR) derived from DSC-PWI provide information about neo-angiogenesis and tumor capillary permeability, respectively, information that can be used to characterize tumor type and grade and to distinguish primary tumor from metastasis and tumor recurrence from post-treatment changes.

In recent years, DCE-MRI has increasingly been used for a more accurate mapping of blood volumes in tumor lesions, as well as for tumor grading, differential diagnosis with other neoplasms, evaluation of post-treatment effects, or chemotherapic response monitoring.

This technique could potentially represent a better alternative to DSC, as there are pitfalls of DSC utility related to surgery and blood-dependent artifacts [18, 19].

The main parameters indicating increased tumor vascularity and BBB permeability are the area under contrast curve (AUC) and the Ktrans, respectively. Other DCE-derived parameters, Ve and Vp, represent the fractional volume of gadolinium-based contrast agents (GBCA) in the extravascular-extracellular space and the plasma space, respectively.

The main disadvantages of DCE are related to longer scanning time, reduced temporal resolution, complex post-processing and quantification of image; for these reasons, this technique is less often used in clinical practice and less frequently studied in the literature compared to DSC [20].

Contrarily, pseudo-continuous ASL (PCASL) has been demonstrated by several authors as a robust alternative to DSC-MRI in the evaluation of perfusion in gliomas, showing less susceptibility to artifacts [21–25]. Its utility in distinguishing glioma grading lies in capturing differences in tumor vascularity and perfusion characteristics by offering quantitative measures of tumor blood flow (TBF), including relative (normalized) and absolute tumor blood flow values (rTBF and TBF) [26]; it hence appears as a useful tool for clinicians to potentially differentiate between LGGs (less vascularized) and HGGs (more vascularized), aiding in treatment planning and clinical prognosis [26, 27] (Fig. 5.1).

So far, several studies have investigated the utility of ASL in glioma grading and differentiation.

Among these, Batalov et al. [28] demonstrated that ASL-derived CBF values were directly proportional to the grading with high sensitivity and specificity, particularly using small regions of interest. Similarly, meta-analyses by Kong et al. [29] and Alsaedi et al. [26] support ASL's potential in distinguishing HGGs from LGGs, with HGGs showing higher perfusion values. This likely reflects a direct correlation between ASL-derived perfusion parameters and histopathological vessel density, as found by Chatha et al. [16], supporting ASL's reliability in evaluating glioma vascularity (Fig. 5.2).

Among all the quantitative parameters that have been analyzed in the above-mentioned studies, rTBF may be a better index to grade gliomas [29].

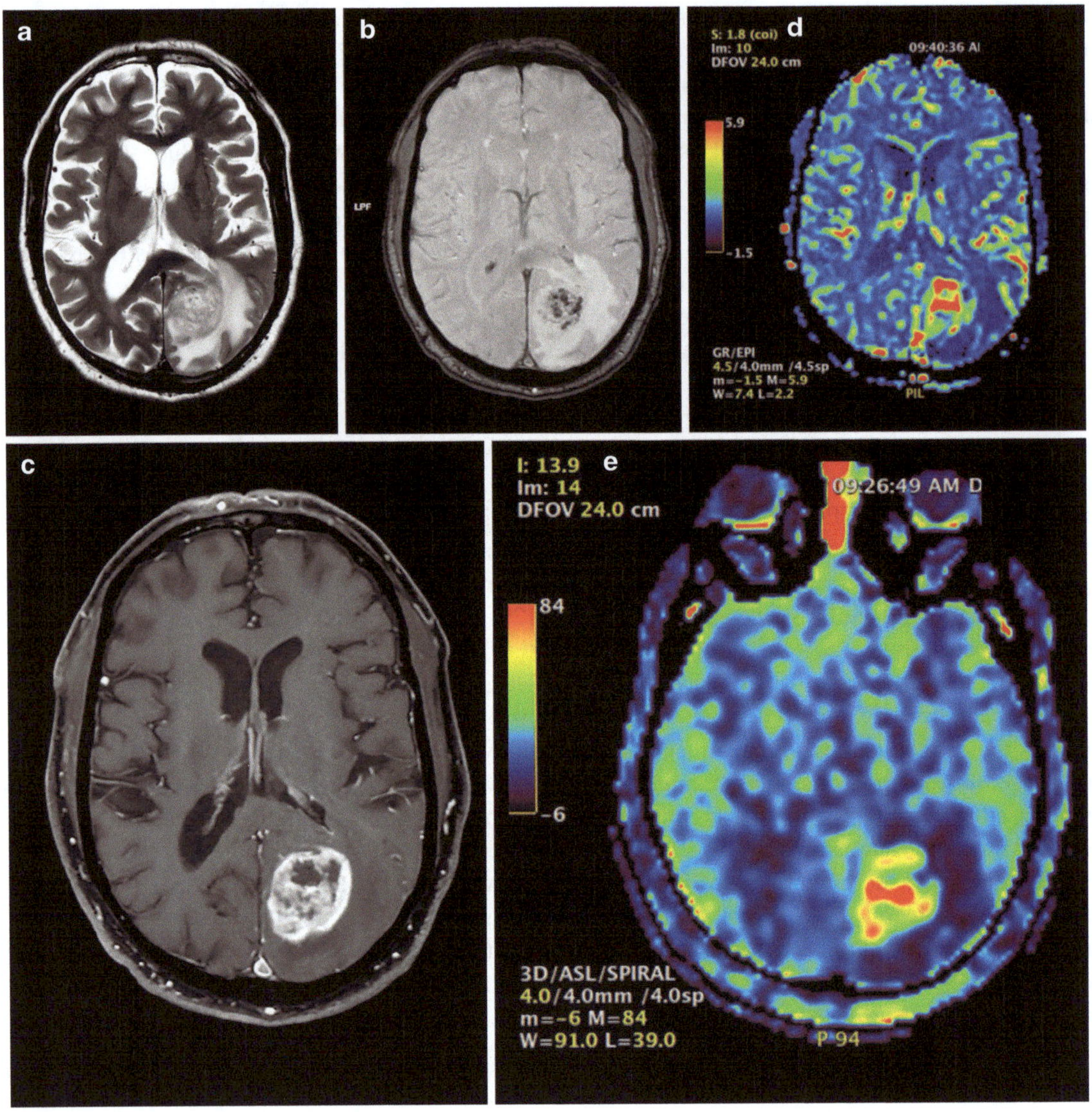

Fig. 5.1 High-grade glioma in left parieto-occipital region. Low signal in T2 (**a**), intratumoral bleeding in SWI (**b**), bright enhancement after gadolinium (**c**) and increased values of perfusional sequences (ASL, **d**; DSC, **e**) summarize the anaplastic condition of tumor

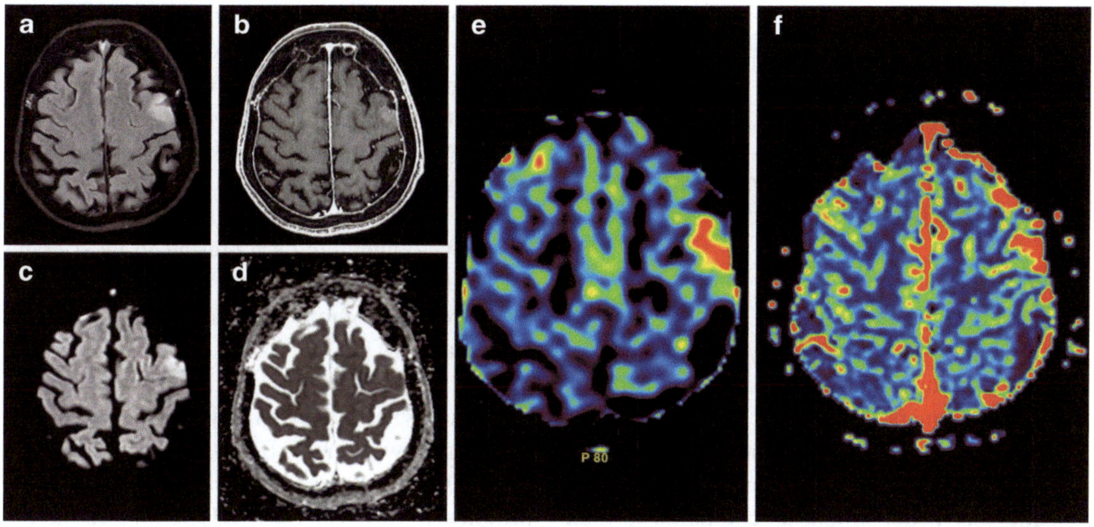

Fig. 5.2 Role of MR perfusion in tumor grading. Small cortical lesion in left frontal lobe (pre-rolandic area) with hyperintensity in FLAIR (**a**), low enhancement after gadolinium (**b**), restricted effects in DWI-ADC (**c**, **d**). Both ASL (**e**) and DSC (**f**) perfusion technique show increased values, better in ASL (**e**) (no confounded effects with cortical vessel as visible in DSC)

5.4 Spectroscopy

MR spectroscopy (MRS) is a non-invasive in vivo technique that measures biochemical parameters alteration in brain tissue. MR has been widely used in the field of neuro-oncology, as it is able to distinguish between primitive tumors from tumor mimics and other neoplasms, assess tumor malignancy, and monitor therapeutic outcomes. Nevertheless, due to the variability and heterogeneity of lesions, as well as the overlap between different tumor types and between neoplastic and non-neoplastic lesions, MRS should not be used alone for diagnosing brain lesions. It should always be combined with other conventional, morphological, and advanced MRI techniques.

Nearly all BTs show decreased NAA—because of the replacement of neuronal cells by tumoral, necrotic, and reactive tissues, and possibly reduced NAA synthesis, and increased levels of Cho, because of increased density of proliferating tumor cells [30–32].

Nevertheless, LGGs usually show either modest Cho elevation or NAA reduction, sometimes accompanied by increased mI and mI/Cr ratio. Moreover, LGGs typically lack Lac and Lip peaks, and consequently their presence in a tumor could potentially indicate a transformation to HGGs.

On the other hand, HGGs tend to have more dramatic MRS changes, including a marked increase in Cho and a decrease in Cr, NAA, and mI. Thus, higher Cho/Cr and lower NAA/Cho ratios suggest HGGs as opposed to LGGs. Conversely, pilocytic astrocytomas (despite their benign nature) present with a low NAA/Cho ratio, and occasionally low Cho levels in HGGs have been reported (probably related to necrotic areas) [30, 31].

Elevated Cho and reduced NAA levels can also help distinguish tumor regions from normal brain tissue beyond the enhancing lesion and guide tissue biopsy to the most aggressive part of the tumor.

High Cho/NAA and Cho/Cr ratios and the combined high Lac and Lip signal are associated with a higher risk of poor outcomes [31, 32]. Also, increased Cr was found to be a significant predictor for tumor progression, while gliomas with decreased Cr appeared to have longer progression-free times and delayed malignant transformation [33].

5.5 Radiogenomics and Genetic Profiles

5.5.1 IDH

The discovery of isocitrate dehydrogenase (IDH) mutations in the majority of grade II and III diffuse gliomas marked a significant advancement in the molecular characterization of these tumors [34, 35]. Gliomas with IDH mutations have a considerably better prognosis compared to their IDH wild-type (IDHwt) counterparts of the same lineage and grade. This finding also aids in identifying patient subgroups that are more responsive to chemotherapy [36].

Recent studies [37, 38] have refined this concept, suggesting that diffuse gliomas can be categorized into three subtypes based on a few key molecular markers: combined copy number alterations of chromosomal arms 1p and 19q, chromosomal arm 10q and chromosome 7, and the mutational status of the IDH, telomerase reverse transcriptase (TERT), tumor protein p53 (TP53), and alpha-thalassemia/mental retardation syndrome X-linked (ATRX) genes.

TERT and ATRX mutations are mutually exclusive and have diagnostic value: TERT mutations are diagnostic of oligodendroglioma (with 1p19q codeletion) or glioblastoma (without 1p19q codeletion), while TP53 mutations in the presence of IDH mutation are indicative of astrocytoma.

This molecular classification also contains more prognostic information than the classic histopathologic evaluation [37], according to which LGGs have a better prognosis than HGGs. However, irrespective of tumor grade, IDHwt tumors, even those histopathologically classified as low-grade, are biologically all the glioblastoma type (class 3) and have a poor prognosis [38].

The identification of isocitrate dehydrogenase (IDH) mutations is a pivotal event in the development of diffuse gliomas, found in nearly all 1p19q-codeleted tumors and other glioma types.

Tumors with IDH mutations can be classified into astrocytic (with TP53 mutations) and oligodendroglial (with 1p19q codeletion) categories, which are mutually exclusive [39, 40].

IDH mutations play a significant role in glioma development and are present in most grade II–III gliomas and secondary glioblastomas, but they are uncommon in primary glioblastomas (less than 5%) [41].

The presence of IDH mutations can help to distinguish secondary glioblastomas from primary ones, with grade II and III tumors harboring IDH mutations associated with better prognoses [40], whereas IDHwt tumors have a prognosis similar to primary glioblastomas. Tumors with IDH mutations are more often restricted to a single lobe [42]. Research by Wang et al. [43] indicated that low-grade IDH1-mutated gliomas are predominantly located in the frontal lobe, especially around the rostral extension of the lateral ventricles and near the left hippocampus.

On the other hand, Grade II–III IDHwt low-grade tumors more commonly have a multilobar, and frontotemporal-insular localization (86% vs 30%in IDH wt vs IDH-mutated tumors, respectively) [44]. This type of topographic distribution supports the well-known hypothesis that IDH-mutated gliomas could derive from specific distinct precursor cells localized in the subventricular region, the largest germinal region in the brain and lines the lateral ventricles and the hippocampus.

The presence of large portions of non-enhancing tumors in glioblastomas is reported to be strongly associated with IDH1 mutation [45]. The combination of this feature and frontal lobe localization, larger tumor size, and presence of cysts and satellite lesions is more common in IDH-mutated tumors.

With the advent of radiogenomics, efforts have combined to acquire non-invasive preoperative biomarkers that point to a specific diagnosis and thus allowing a tailored therapeutic approach.

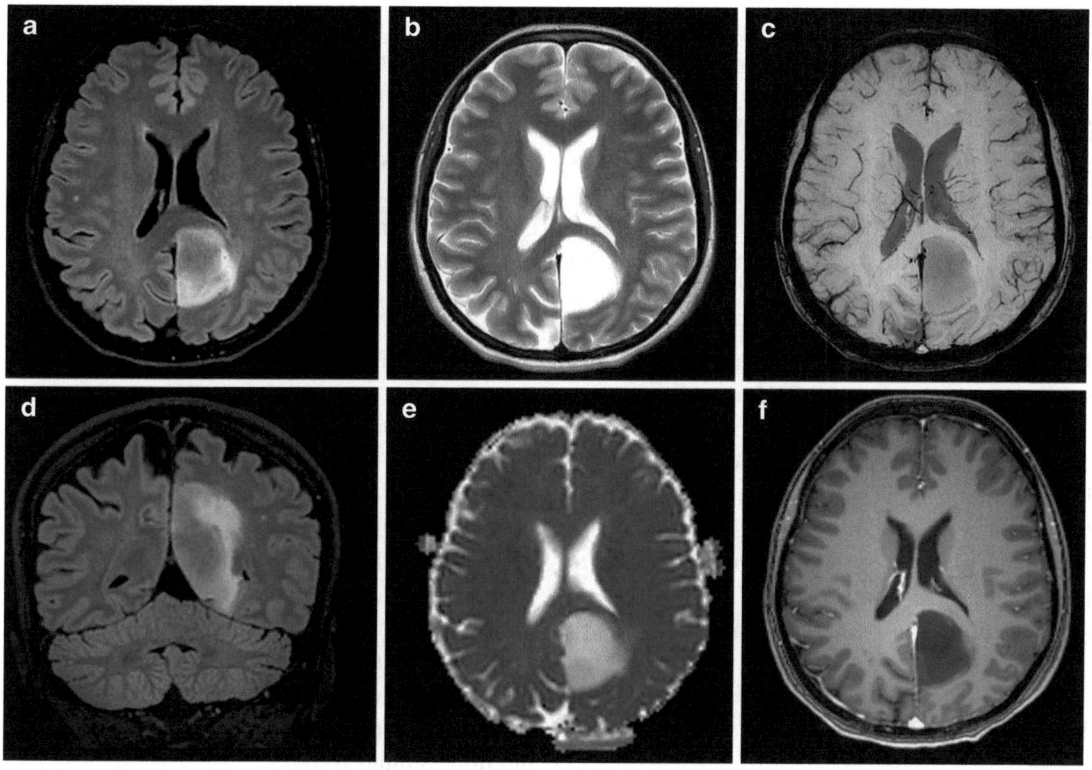

Fig. 5.3 Mismatch FLAIR-T2. Left deep parietal glioma with central hypointensity in T2 FLAIR (**a–d**) and homogeneous hyperintensity in T2 (**b**). No bleeding in SWI (**c**), no restriction in ADC (**e**), no enhancement after gadolinium (**f**). Low-grade glioma (diffuse astrocytoma IDH mutated)

The T2-fluid attenuated inversion recovery (T2-FLAIR) mismatch sign is one such example, being 100% specific for IDH-mutant 1p/19q non-codeleted gliomas [46–48] (Fig. 5.3).

Although this sign has low sensitivity, it serves as a surrogate marker for tumor molecular status.

The T2-FLAIR mismatch sign is characterized by: (1) a homogenous hyperintense signal on T2-weighted images; (2) attenuation of FLAIR signal intensity, with a bright peripheral rim [49].

This sign is a highly specific imaging marker for IDH-mutant non-codeleted LGGs and predicts not only the molecular type but also the tumor behavior and prognosis, as IDH mutation and 1p/19q codeletion status are associated with slower growth and better prognosis in LGGs [50].

The pathophysiology of the T2-FLAIR mismatch sign is not fully understood, but it is believed to correlate with abundant microcystic changes within the tumor [43].

Diffusion-weighted imaging (DWI) may offer some utility in distinguishing IDH-mutated from IDHwt tumors, although evidence is limited.

Elkhaled et al. [51] found a significant negative correlation between ADC and 2-HG levels detected with high-resolution "magic angle" spinning, which suggests that ADC maybe decreased in IDH-mutated tumors. IDH mutation can regulate hypoxia-inducible factor 1-alpha (HIF-1α), which is a driving force in tumorigenesis and angiogenesis, thus suppressing aggressive behavior (such as angiogenesis) [52]. Consistent with this, IDH-mutated status correlates with lower dynamic susceptibility contrast-cerebral blood volume (DSC-CBV) and cerebral blood flow (DSC-CBF) compared to IDHwt, with percentage of signal intensity recovery (PSR) being lower in IDHwt tumors. Dynamic contrast-enhanced (DCE) MRI studies report that IDH-mutated gliomas exhibit decreased Ktrans, Vp, Ve, and area under the curve (AUC) [52].

Among advanced MR imaging techniques, MR spectroscopy is particularly promising for identifying IDH-mutated tumors non-invasively. Normally, 2-HG is not detectable because its concentration is too low, but IDH mutations cause 2-HG to accumulate, increasing its concentration more than 100-fold (5–35 mM), making it detectable [53]. In vivo, MR spectroscopy has the great advantage of being entirely non-invasive and not requiring tissue from biopsy or resection. It may allow the follow-up of tumors treated with agents targeted against the IDH mutation.

Reliable detection in vivo, however, remains challenging because the 2-HG spectrum, consisting of multiplets at three locations, largely overlaps with abundant brain metabolites such as glutamate, glutamine, and g-aminobutyric acid at the largest 2.25-ppm multiplet, and N-acetyl aspartate at the 1.9-ppm multiplet.

5.5.2 TERT Promotion

Telomerase reverse transcriptase (TERT) serves as the catalytic subunit of telomerase, an enzyme critical for determining cell lifespan. Mutations in the TERT promoter led to unlimited proliferative capacity in tumor cells and have been observed in up to 80% of glioblastomas [54].

These mutations are associated with a worse prognosis thus requiring more aggressive treatment [55, 56]. Normal cells present with lower telomerase activity compared to tumor cells, consequently, targeted telomerase-inhibitor therapy has become over time more and more promising.

The combination of TERT promoter mutation and wild-type isocitrate dehydrogenase 1 (IDH1) is the most common genotype observed in glioblastoma. The percentage of necrosis was greater in TERT-mutated than in TERT-wild type. This is related to increased levels of epidermal growth factor receptor amplification, lower glycogen accumulation, and increased interleukin 6, which induces tumor angiogenesis and necrosis. Glioma patients with TERT promoter mutation are significantly older than those with wild-type TERT, and glioma prognosis is related to age at diagnosis [57].

It has been reported increased DSC-CBV, and DCE-Ktrans in EGFR-amplified GB [20] due to accelerated tumor angiogenesis. Higher expression of TERT was correlated to resistance to anti-growth signals and angiogenesis; this could be an explanation for the higher mean values of DSC-CBV, CBF, and DCE-Vp in TERTp mutant IDH-wt gliomas.

5.5.3 EGFR Mutation

The activation of the epidermal growth factor receptor (EGFR) pathway is a frequent molecular event in glioblastomas, with EGFR overexpression or amplification present in up to 50% of cases [58, 59]. Located on chromosome 7p12, EGFR amplification is more common in primary glioblastomas compared to secondary ones [60–62]. Restricted diffusion correlates with EGFR amplification, suggesting diffusion analysis may help predict EGFR amplification status in glioblastomas [63].

The EGFRvIII mutation is tumor-specific and absent in normal tissues. Radiomic signatures for EGFRvIII mutation in glioblastomas include higher relative cerebral blood volume (rCBV), lower apparent diffusion coefficient (ADC), higher fractional anisotropy (FA), lower T2-FLAIR, and a more variable spatial pattern [64]. Tumors with this mutation typically overlap the frontoparietal lobes, whereas EGFRvIII-negative tumors are more commonly found in the temporal lobe.

5.5.4 MGMT

O6-Methylguanine-DNA methyltransferase (MGMT) is a DNA repair enzyme coded by a gene on chromosome 10q26 [65]. High MGMT levels in cancer cells reduce the efficacy of alkylating chemotherapy. Epigenetic silencing of the MGMT gene through promoter methylation results in decreased MGMT expression, leading to reduced DNA repair, increased DNA damage, and cell death, thus enhancing sensitivity to alkylating agents. IDH mutations cause a CpG island hypermethylation phenotype, often including the MGMT promoter. Therefore, IDH-mutated tumors frequently show MGMT promoter methylation [66, 67]. Approximately, 50% of newly diagnosed glioblastomas exhibit MGMT methylation [65].

Ellingson et al. [68] observed a higher prevalence of methylated tumors in the left hemisphere, mainly in the temporal lobe, while unmethylated tumors were more common in the right hemisphere. This partially aligns with Eoli et al.'s findings, which noted methylated tumors in the parietal and occipital lobes and unmethylated tumors in the temporal lobes [69]. Mixed nodular enhancement is often seen in methylated glioblastomas, with rim enhancement more common in unmethylated tumors [69, 70]. Most studies report no differences in edema, although Ellingson et al. noted lower volumes of T2 abnormalities in methylated tumors [68].

Methylated tumors seem to exhibit imaging features indicative of lower cellularity (e.g., low maximum CT attenuation, high minimum ADC ratio) and greater white matter destruction (low minimum FA ratio) [71]. Authors of other studies also noted a positive relationship between mean ADC and methylation ratio, and Romano et al. [72] reported high sensitivity (84%) and specificity (91%) to distinguish methylated from unmethylated tumors at a cutoff minimum ADC of 0.8×1023 mm^2/s [73]. The ADC is highly sensitive to the effects of the inadvertent inclusion of (micro) cysts and necrosis, which increase the ADC and may obscure subtle reductions in the ADC in the solid tumor components.

A lower degree of perfusion in methylated (n = 16) compared with unmethylated (n = 9) tumors (mean rCBV ratio, 5.4 vs 9.5, respectively) was reported by Ryoo et al. [74]. By using dynamic contrast-enhanced MR imaging, Ahn et al. [75] found an increase in the volume transfer constant (Ktrans) in methylated compared with unmethylated glioblastomas, which not only has diagnostic implications but also may be of more fundamental interest.

Increased Ktrans may be a marker of the high permeability of the blood vessel wall under certain conditions (e.g., low cerebral blood flow), which, in turn, potentially enhances the delivery of drugs across the blood–brain barrier. These findings are consistent with those from mouse models.

5.6 The Role of Neuroradiology in the Pre-surgical Planning

The extent of resection is crucial for the prognosis of patients with both HGGs and LGGs.

Various techniques have been developed to enhance the neurosurgeon's capability to perform a maximal safe resection. These techniques include fluorescence guidance, direct electrical stimulation (DES), intraoperative imaging, and preoperative functional imaging methods such as functional MRI (fMRI) and diffusion tensor imaging (DTI) [76].

5.6.1 fMRI

Over the past 20 years, fMRI has become a valuable tool for non-invasive mapping of brain function, to guide surgical resections to reduce complications [77]. Indeed, unlike the standard DES brain mapping techniques, one advantage of fMRI is that it can be performed preoperatively for surgical decision-making; moreover, it is a non-invasive technique that allows a wide mapping of brain areas beyond those limited areas exposed by craniotomy [78].

fMRI uses a blood oxygen level-dependent (BOLD) signal, which relies on the deoxyhemoglobin-to-oxyhemoglobin ratio. After activation of a specific brain, there is consequent increased local perfusion because of capillary vasodilation, with an increase in the metabolic demand of the active brain region. Consequently, the increasing level of oxyhemoglobin relative to deoxyhemoglobin increases the T2* signal, and this phenomenon can be reported on imaging using a T2*change-sensitive MR sequences. Importantly, the BOLD signal change serves as a proxy for neuronal activity and is predicated on a predictable vascular response to neuronal activity (neurovascular coupling) [78].

Mapping of BOLD signal changes during the performance of a particular task is referred to as task-based fMRI (tb-fMRI). Conversely, resting-state fMRI (rs-fMRI) examines spontaneous brain activity at rest, capturing BOLD images without any tasks performed by the patient [79].

Despite these advantages, the adoption of single-subject rs-fMRI has been limited in clinical medicine because of several barriers: the effect of tumors on this signal source is not well understood; rs-fMRI lacks the specificity of tb-fMRI; the processing and analysis of rs-fMRI is much more complex, and there is currently no reference standard.

Another challenge in the interpretation of fMRI is related to pathologic changes. Tumor infiltration, angiogenesis, and perilesional edema can decrease the BOLD signal in functionally intact tissue, resulting in false-negative results, as well as in the presence of blood products that cause signal loss and image distortion [80].

In patients undergoing resection, false-negative results can be problematic because the assumption of an eloquent region no longer having function could lead to substantial harm [81]. Indeed, fMRI is best suited to help identify targets for intraoperative mapping rather than being relied on solely for preoperative decision-making, as the literature reports a high prevalence of false-negative activation and the possibility of false-positive activation.

Validation of clinical fMRI against the reference standard of DES is crucial. The literature reports varying degrees of concordance between fMRI and DES, influenced by patient characteristics and task selection. There is high concordance between the techniques for sensorimotor functions (with sensitivity at 84.6% and specificity at 77.8%), but less so for cognitive functions such as language (with sensitivity at 67% and specificity at 55%). One explanation for this variability is that tb-fMRI is an activation technique, while DES is an inhibition or disruption technique. Furthermore, tb-fMRI activates all brain regions involved in task performance, but not all these regions are necessarily critical for function or may be easily compensated for if damaged [76]. This condition represents a debated argument in literature. Overall, fMRI and rs-fMRI currently seem inadequate for standalone preoperative cortical functional mapping. A significant reason for the limited sensitivity and specificity of both fMRI and rs-fMRI compared to DES is that DES provides a more direct assessment of neuronal function, while the fMRI BOLD signal is inherently an indirect measure [75–77].

5.6.2 MR Tractography

DTI assesses the water diffusion characteristics of neural tissue and can be utilized to estimate functionally significant anatomical white matter tracts (WMT) in the brain.

In neuro-oncology, specifically for intracranial tumor diagnosis and treatment, DTI is well known for its aid in planning neurosurgical interventions [79, 82], defining areas to excise and areas to avoid [83, 84], potentially differentiating tumor pathology before surgery [85, 86], intraoperative estimation of brain shift [86], improving location/orientation targeting for DES sites [79, 87], improving postoperative functionality scores [88], assessing postoperative morbidity and mortality using preoperative information [89–91] (Fig. 5.4), and so on.

Incorporating tractography in presurgical planning is beneficial for both neurosurgeon and patient as it improves defining the boundaries between eloquent areas and tumor, helping to formulate a patient-specific approach, and thereby reducing the risk of postoperative neurological deficits. Studies have demonstrated that tractography is useful in selecting the optimal surgical approach for corticectomy by assessing the impact of potential access routes on WMT [92, 93]. During surgical planning, DTI provides critical information about tumor proximity to WMT [94], the impact of the tumor on these tracts, and the extent of tumor invasion into surrounding tissues [95–97].

An additional advantage of DTI in surgical planning is its role in defining the resection boundary, balancing between maximal lesion excision, and the preservation of functional tissue.

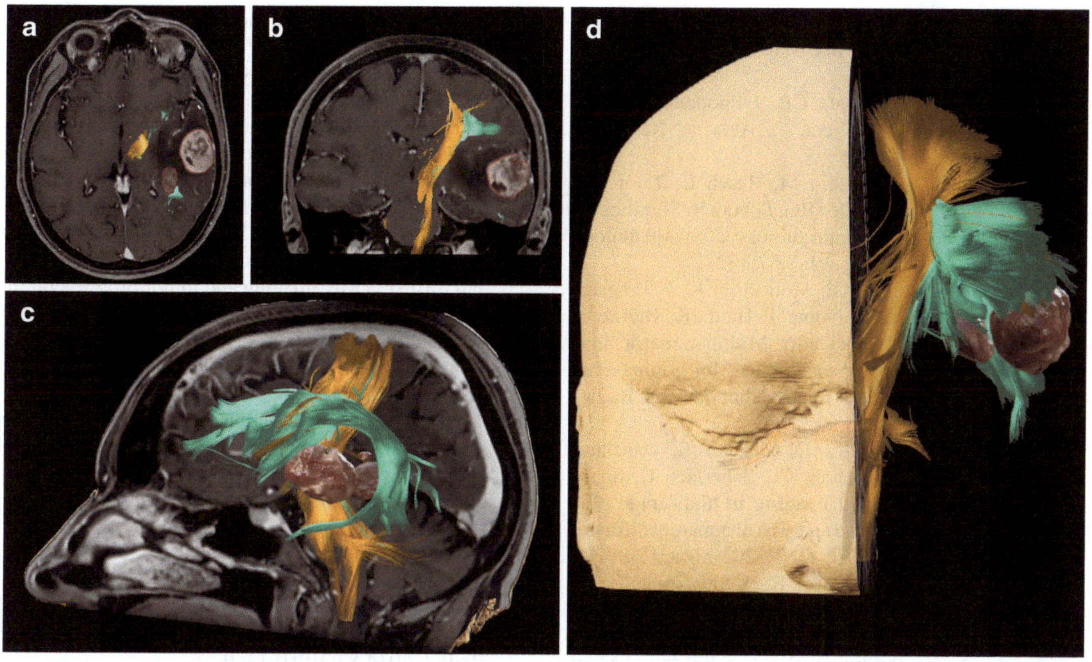

Fig. 5.4 Preoperative planning. Left temporo-opercular glioma. Tractographic reconstructions of arcuate fasciculum (green) and cortico-spinal tract (yellow) visible on axial (**a**), coronal (**b**) planes and on tridimensional images (**c**, **d**) show relationship between deep portion of the lesion and arcuate fasciculum. No contact is evident between cortico-spinal tract and glioma

A "functional" approach that combines preoperative fMRI and DTI scans with intraoperative neurophysiological monitoring shows promise as the current standard for managing brain lesions. Brain shift is known to affect the reliability of preoperatively generated DDT [98]. This hurdle can be reduced by updating tractography through intraoperative imaging. Although both DTI and DTT present many advantages and have shown their utility in approximating the geometry of WMT in neurosurgical interventions, it is well known that they present a limited ability to resolve multiple fibers and appear susceptible to partial volume effects [99].

Advanced diffusion imaging sequences include diffusion spectrum imaging (DSI), high angular resolution diffusion imaging (HARDI), DKI, and Crossing Fiber Angular Resolution Intra-voxel structure (CFARI). The combination of HARDI and Q-ball imaging is effective for improving the resolution of tractography, especially in regions with crossing fiber populations showing more complex structures than DDT. Emerging applications of DTI and DTT demonstrate that preoperative, non-invasive mapping of eloquent cortical regions and functionally relevant WMT, used alongside intraoperative tools like DES and navigated transcranial magnetic stimulation (nTMS), can reduce postoperative deficits and improve quality of life and overall survival in glioma patients [100].

References

1. Mabray MC, Barajas RF, Cha S. Modern brain tumor imaging. Brain Tumor Res Treat. 2015;3:8–23.
2. Osborn AG, Louis DN, Poussaint TY, Linscott LL, Salzman KL. The 2021 World Health Organization classification of tumors of the central nervous system: what neuroradiologists need to know. AJNR Am J Neuroradiol. 2022;43:928–37.
3. Iv M, Bisdas S. Neuroimaging in the era of the evolving WHO classification of brain tumors, from the AJR special series on cancer staging. AJR Am J Roentgenol. 2021;217:3–15.

4. Claes A, Idema AJ, Wesseling P. Diffuse glioma growth: a guerilla war. Acta Neuropathol. 2007;114:443–58.
5. Leonardi MA, Lumenta CB. Oligodendrogliomas in the CT/MR-era. Acta Neurochir. 2001;143:1195–203.
6. Kondziolka D, Bernstein M, Resch L, Tator CH, Fleming JF, Vanderlinden RG, Schutz H. Significance of hemorrhage into brain tumors: clinicopathological study. J Neurosurg. 1987;67:852–7.
7. Garzón B, Emblem KE, Mouridsen K, Nedregaard B, Due-Tønnessen P, Nome T, Hald JK, Bjørnerud A, Håberg AK, Kvinnsland Y. Multiparametric analysis of magnetic resonance images for glioma grading and patientsurvival time prediction. Acta Radiol. 2011;52:1052–60.
8. Gihr G, Horvath-Rizea D, Hekeler E, Ganslandt O, Henkes H, Hoffmann KT, Scherlach C, Schob S. Diffusion weighted imaging in high-grade gliomas: a histogram-based analysis of apparent diffusion coefficient profile. PLoS ONE. 2021;16:e0249878.
9. Ellingson BM, Malkin MG, Rand SD, Connelly JM, Quinsey C, LaViolette PS, Bedekar DP, Schmainda KM. Validation of functional diffusion maps (fDMs) as a biomarker for human glioma cellularity. J Magn Reson Imaging. 2010;31:538–48.
10. Gihr G, Horvath-Rizea D, Kohlhof-Meinecke P, Ganslandt O, Henkes H, Härtig W, Donitza A, Skalej M, Schob S. Diffusion weighted imaging in gliomas: a histogram-based approach for tumor characterization. Cancer. 2022;14:3393.
11. Kang XW, Xi YB, Liu TT, Wang N, Zhu YQ, Wang XR, Guo F. Grading of glioma: combined diagnostic value of amide proton transfer weighted, arterial spin labeling and diffusion weighted magnetic resonance imaging. BMC Med Imaging. 2020;20:50.
12. Poussaint TY, Vajapeyam S, Ricci KI, Panigrahy A, Kocak M, Kun LE, Boyett JM, Pollack IF, Fouladi M. Apparent diffusion coefficient histogram metrics correlate with survival in diffuse intrinsic pontine glioma: a report from the Pediatric Brain Tumor Consortium. Neuro-Oncology. 2016;18:725–34.
13. Chatha G, et al. The utility of arterial spin labelled perfusion-weighted magnetic resonance imaging in measuring the vascularity of high grade gliomas - a prospective study. Heliyon. 2023;9(7):e17615.
14. Nezamzadeh M, et al. Improved pseudo-continuous arterial spin labeling for mapping brain perfusion. J Magn Reson Imaging. 2010;31(6):1419–27.
15. Haller S, et al. Arterial spin labeling perfusion of the brain: emerging clinical applications. Radiology. 2016;281(2):337–56.
16. Amukotuwa SA, Yu C, Zaharchuk G. 3D pseudo-continuous arterial spin labeling in routine clinical practice: a review of clinically significant artifacts. J Magn Reson Imaging. 2016;43(1):11–27.
17. Chakravorty A, Steel T, Chaganti J. Accuracy of percentage of signal intensity recovery and relative cerebral blood volume derived from dynamic susceptibility-weighted, contrast-enhanced MRI in the preoperative diagnosis of cerebral tumours. Neuroradiol J. 2015;28:574–83.
18. Xi YB, Kang XW, Wang N, Liu TT, Zhu YQ, Cheng G, Wang K, Li C, Guo F, Yin H. Differentiation of primary central nervous system lymphoma from high-grade glioma and brain metastasis using arterial spin labeling and dynamic contrast-enhanced magnetic resonance imaging. Eur J Radiol. 2019;112:59–64.
19. White ML, Zhang Y, Yu F, Shonka N, Aizenberg MR, Adapa P, Jaffar Kazmi SA. Post-operative perfusion and diffusion MR imaging and tumor progression in high-grade gliomas. PLoS ONE. 2019;14:e0213905.
20. Van Santwijk L, Kouwenberg V, Meijer F, Smits M, Henssen D. A systematic review and meta-analysis on the differentiation of glioma grade and mutational status by use of perfusion-based magnetic resonance imaging. Insights Imaging. 2022;13:102.
21. Jaganmohan D, et al. A pictorial review of brain arterial spin labelling artefacts and their potential remedies in clinical studies. Neuroradiol J. 2021;34(3):154–68.
22. Cebeci H, et al. Assesment of perfusion in glial tumors with arterial spin labeling; comparison with dynamic susceptibility contrast method. Eur J Radiol. 2014;83(10):1914–9.
23. Warmuth C, Gunther M, Zimmer C. Quantification of blood flow in brain tumors: comparison of arterial spin labeling and dynamic susceptibility-weighted contrast-enhanced MR imaging. Radiology. 2003;228(2):523–32.
24. Ma H, et al. Three-dimensional arterial spin labeling imaging and dynamic susceptibility contrast perfusion-weighted imaging value in diagnosing glioma grade prior to surgery. Exp Ther Med. 2017;13(6):2691–8.
25. Järnum H, et al. Perfusion MRI of brain tumours: a comparative study of pseudo-continuous arterial spin labelling and dynamic susceptibility contrast imaging. Neuroradiology. 2010;52(4):307–17.
26. Alsaedi A, et al. The value of arterial spin labelling in adults glioma grading: systematic review and meta-analysis. Oncotarget. 2019;10(16):1589–601.
27. ElBeheiry AA, Abdel-Latif AA-B, Abbas M, Ismail AS. Arterial spin labeling in the grading of brain gliomas: could it help? Egypt J Radiol Nucl Med. 2020;51:235.
28. Batalov AI, et al. 3D pCASL-perfusion in preoperative assessment of brain gliomas in large cohort of patients. Sci Rep. 2022;12(1):2121.
29. Kong L, et al. A meta-analysis of arterial spin labelling perfusion values for the prediction of glioma grade. Clin Radiol. 2017;72(3):255–61.
30. Currie S, Hadjivassiliou M, Craven IJ, Wilkinson ID, Griffiths PD, Hoggard N. Magnetic resonance spectroscopy of the brain. Postgrad Med J. 2013;89:94–106.
31. Horská A, Barker PB. Imaging of brain tumors: MR spectroscopy and metabolic imaging. Neuroimaging Clin N Am. 2010;10:293–310.

32. Hourani R, Horská A, Albayram S, Brant LJ, Melhem E, Cohen KJ, Burger PC, Weingart JD, Carson B, Wharam MD, et al. Proton magnetic resonance spectroscopic imaging to differentiate between nonneoplastic lesions and brain tumors in children. J Magn Reson Imaging. 2006;23:99–107.
33. Hu J, Salzillo TC, Sailasuta N, Lang FF, Bhattacharya P. Interrogating IDH mutation in brain tumor: magnetic resonance and hyperpolarization. Top Magn Reson Imaging. 2017;26:27–32.
34. van den Bent MJ, Dubbink HJ, Marie Y, et al. IDH1 and IDH2 mutations are prognostic but not predictive for outcome in anaplastic oligodendroglial tumors: a report of the European Organization for Research and Treatment of Cancer Brain Tumor Group. Clin Cancer Res. 2010;16(5):1597–604.
35. Parsons DW, Jones S, Zhang X, et al. An integrated genomic analysis of human glioblastoma multiforme. Science. 2008;321(5897):1807–12.
36. Cairncross JG, Wang M, Jenkins RB, et al. Benefit from procarbazine, lomustine, and vincristine in oligodendroglial tumors is associated with mutation of IDH. J Clin Oncol. 2014;32(8):783–90.
37. Reuss DE, Sahm F, Schrimpf D, et al. ATRX and IDH1-R132H immunohisto-chemistry with subsequent copy number analysis and IDH sequencing as a basis for an "integrated" diagnostic approach for adult astrocytoma, oligodendroglioma and glioblastoma. Acta Neuropathol. 2015;129(1):133–46.
38. Labussière M, Di Stefano AL, Gleize V, et al. TERT promoter mutations in gliomas, genetic associations and clinico-pathological correlations. Br J Cancer. 2014;111(10):2024–32.
39. Cohen AL, Holmen SL, Colman H. IDH1 and IDH2 mutations in gliomas. Curr Neurol Neurosci Rep. 2013;13(5):345.
40. Wang Y, Zhang T, Li S, et al. Anatomical localization of isocitrate dehydrogenase 1 mutation: a voxel-based radiographic study of 146 low-grade gliomas. Eur J Neurol. 2015;22(2):348–54.
41. Yan H, Parsons DW, Jin G, et al. IDH1 and IDH2 mutations in gliomas. N Engl J Med. 2009;360(8):765–73.
42. Qi S, Yu L, Li H, et al. Isocitrate dehydrogenase mutation is associated with tumor location and magnetic resonance imaging characteristics in astrocytic neoplasms. Oncol Lett. 2014;7(6):1895–902.
43. Tay KL, Tsui A, Phal PM, Drummond KJ, Tress BM. MR imaging characteristics of protoplasmic astrocytomas. Neuroradiology. 2011;53(6):405–11.
44. Metellus P, Coulibaly B, Colin C, et al. Absence of IDH mutation identifies a novel radiologic and molecular subtype of WHO grade II gliomas with dismal prognosis. Acta Neuropathol. 2010;120(6):719–29.
45. Carrillo JA, Lai A, Nghiemphu PL, et al. Relationship between tumor enhancement, edema, IDH1 mutational status, MGMT promoter methylation, and survival in glioblastoma. AJNR Am J Neuroradiol. 2012;33(7):1349–55.
46. Batchala PP, Muttikkal TJE, Donahue JH, Patrie JT, Schiff D, Fadul CE, et al. Neuroimaging-based classification algorithm for predicting 1p/19q-codeletion status in IDH-mutant lower grade gliomas. AJNR Am J Neuroradiol. 2019;40:426–32.
47. Broen MP, Smits M, Wijnenga MM, Dubbink HJ, Anten MH, Schijns OE, et al. The T2-FLAIR mismatch sign as an imaging marker for non-enhancing IDH-mutant, 1p/19q-intact lower-grade glioma: a validation study. Neuro-Oncology. 2018;20:1393–9.
48. Patel SH, Poisson LM, Brat DJ, Zhou Y, Cooper L, Snuderl M, et al. T2-FLAIR mismatch, an imaging biomarker for IDH and 1p/19q status in lower-grade gliomas: a TCGA/TCIA project. Clin Cancer Res. 2017;3:6078–85.
49. Aliotta E, Dutta SW, Feng X, et al. Automated apparent diffusion coefficient analysis for genotype prediction in lower grade glioma: association with the T2-FLAIR mismatch sign. J Neuro-Oncol. 2020;149(2):325–35.
50. van den Bent MJ, Brandes AA, Taphoorn MJ, et al. Adjuvant procarbazine, lomustine, and vincristine chemotherapy in newly diagnosed anaplastic oligodendroglioma: long-term follow-up of EORTC brain tumor group study 26951. J Clin Oncol. 2013;31(3):344–50.
51. Lu J, Li X, Li H. Perfusion parameters derived from MRI for preoperative prediction of IDH mutation and MGMT promoter methylation status in glioblastomas. Magn Reson Imaging. 2021;83:189–95.
52. Stumpo V, Guida L, Bellomo J, Van Niftrik CHB, Sebök M, Berhouma M, Bink A, Weller M, Kulcsar Z, Regli L, et al. Hemodynamic imaging in cerebral diffuse glioma-part B: molecular correlates, treatment effect monitoring, prognosis, and future directions. Cancer. 2022;14:1342.
53. Andronesi OC, Kim GS, Gerstner E, et al. Detection of 2-hydroxyglutarate in IDH- mutated glioma patients by in vivo spectral-editing and 2D correlation magnetic resonance spectroscopy. Sci Transl Med. 2012;4(116):116ra4.
54. Killela PJ, Reitman ZJ, Jiao Y, et al. TERT promoter mutations occur frequently in gliomas and a subset of tumors derived from cells with low rates of self-renewal. Proc Natl Acad Sci USA. 2013;110:6021–6.
55. Spiegl-Kreinecker S, Lötsch D, Ghanim B, et al. Prognostic quality of activating TERT promoter mutations in glioblastoma: interaction with the rs2853669 polymorphism and patient age at diagnosis. Neuro-Oncology. 2015;17:1231–40.
56. Simon M, Hosen I, Gousias K, Rachakonda S, Heidenreich B, Gessi M, Schramm J, Hemminki K, Waha A, Kumar R. TERT promoter mutations: a novel independent prognostic factor in primary glioblastomas. Neuro-Oncology. 2015;17:45–52.
57. Yamashita K, Hatae R, Akio H, Togao O, Kikuchi K, Momosaka D, Yamashita Y, Kuga D, Hata N, Yoshimoto K, Suzuki S, Iwaki T, Iihara K, Honda H. Predicting TERT promoter mutation using MR

images in patients with wild-type IDH1 glioblastoma. Diagn Interv Imaging. 2019;100(7-8):411–9.
58. Lal A, Glazer CA, Martinson HM, et al. Mutant epidermal growth factor receptor up-regulates molecular effectors of tumor invasion. Cancer Res. 2002;62:3335–9.
59. Schlegel J, Merdes A, Stumm G, et al. Amplification of the epidermal-growth-factor-receptor gene correlates with different growth behaviour in human glioblastoma. Int J Cancer. 1994;56:72–7.
60. Ohgaki H, Kleihues P. Genetic pathways to primary and secondary glioblastoma. Am J Pathol. 2007;170:1445–53.
61. Halatsch ME, Schmidt U, Behnke-Mursch J, et al. Epidermal growth factor receptor inhibition for the treatment of glioblastoma multiforme and other malignant brain tumours. Cancer Treat Rev. 2006;32:74–89.
62. Ramis G, Thomas-Moya E, Fernandez de Mattos S, et al. EGFR inhibition in glioma cells modulates Rho signaling to inhibit cell motility and invasion and cooperates with temozolomide to reduce cell growth. PLoS One. 2012;7:e38770.
63. Young RJ, Gupta A, Shah AD, Graber JJ, Schweitzer AD, Prager A, Shi W, Zhang Z, Huse J, Omuro AMP. Potential role of preoperative conventional MRI including diffusion measurements in assessing epidermal growth factor receptor gene amplification status in patients with glioblastoma. AJNR Am J Neuroradiol. 2013;34(12):2271–7.
64. Akbari H, et al. In vivo evaluation of EGFRvIII mutation in primary glioblastoma patients via complex multiparametric MRI signature. Neuro-Oncology. 2018;20(8):1068–79.
65. Hegi ME, Diserens AC, Gorlia T, et al. MGMT gene silencing and benefit from temozolomide in glioblastoma. N Engl J Med. 2005;352(10):997–1003.
66. Noushmehr H, Weisenberger DJ, Diefes K, et al. Identification of a CpG island methylator phenotype that defines a distinct subgroup of glioma. Cancer Cell. 2010;17(5):510–22.
67. Turcan S, Rohle D, Goenka A, et al. IDH1 mutation is sufficient to establish the glioma hypermethylator phenotype. Nature. 2012;483(7390):479–83.
68. Ellingson BM, Cloughesy TF, Pope WB, et al. Anatomic localization of O6-methyl- guanine DNA methyltransferase (MGMT) promoter methylated and unmethylated tumors: a radiographic study in 358 de novo human glioblastomas. NeuroImage. 2012;59(2):908–16.
69. Eoli M, Menghi F, Bruzzone MG, et al. Methylation of O6-methylguanine DNA methyltransferase and loss of heterozygosity on 19q and/or 17p are overlapping features of secondary glioblastomas with prolonged survival. Clin Cancer Res. 2007;13(9):2606–13.
70. Drabycz S, Roldán G, de Robles P, et al. An analysis of image texture, tumor location, and MGMT promoter methylation in glioblastoma using magnetic resonance imaging. NeuroImage. 2010;49(2):1398–405.
71. Moon WJ, Choi JW, Roh HG, Lim SD, Koh YC. Imaging parameters of high grade gliomas in relation to the MGMT promoter methylation status: the CT, diffusion tensor imaging, and perfusion MR imaging. Neuroradiology. 2012;54(6):555–63.
72. Romano A, Calabria LF, Tavanti F, et al. Apparent diffusion coefficient obtained by magnetic resonance imaging as a prognostic marker in glioblastomas: correlation with MGMT promoter methylation status. Eur Radiol. 2012;23(2):513–20.
73. Sunwoo L, Choi SH, Park CK, et al. Correlation of apparent diffusion coefficient values measured by diffusion MRI and MGMT promoter methylation semiquantitatively analyzed with MS-MLPA in patients with glioblastoma multiforme. J Magn Reson Imaging. 2013;37(2):351–8.
74. Ryoo I, Choi SH, Kim JH, et al. Cerebral blood volume calculated by dynamic susceptibility contrast-enhanced perfusion MR imaging: preliminary correlation study with glioblastoma genetic profiles. PLoS One. 2013;8(8):e71704.
75. Ahn SS, Shin NY, Chang JH, et al. Prediction of methylguanine methyltransferase promoter methylation in glioblastoma using dynamic contrast-enhanced magnetic resonance and diffusion tensor imaging. J Neurosurg. 2014;121(2):367–73.
76. Azad TD, Duffau H. Limitations of functional neuroimaging for patient selection and surgical planning in glioma surgery. Neurosurg Focus. 2020;48:1–5.
77. Lakhani DA, Sabsevitz DS, Chaichana KL, et al. Current state of functional MRI in the presurgical planning of brain tumors. Radiology. 2023;5:1–10.
78. Castellano A, Cirillo S, Bello L, Riva M, Falini A. Functional MRI for surgery of gliomas. Curr Treat Options Neurol. 2017;19(10):34.
79. Silva MA, See AP, Essayed WI, Golby AJ, Tie Y. Challenges and techniques for presurgical brain mapping with functional MRI. Neuroimage Clin. 2017;17:794–803.
80. Barkhof F, Haller S, Rombouts SA. Resting-state functional MR imaging: a new window to the brain. Radiology. 2014;272(1):29–49.
81. Thickbroom GW, Byrnes ML, Morris IT, Fallon MJ, Knuckey NW, Mastaglia FL. Functional MRI near vascular anomalies: comparison of cavernoma and arteriovenous malformation. J Clin Neurosci. 2004;11(8):845–8.
82. Vassal F, Schneider F, Nuti C. Intraoperative use of diffusion tensor imaging-based tractography for resection of gliomas located near the pyramidal tract: comparison with subcortical stimulation mapping and contribution to surgical outcomes. Br J Neurosurg. 2013;27:668–75.
83. Sollmann N, Kelm A, Ille S, Schröder A, Zimmer C, Ringel F, et al. Setup presentation and clinical outcome analysis of treating highly language-eloquent

gliomas via preoperative navigated transcranial magnetic stimulation and tractography. Neurosurg Focus. 2018;44:E2. https://doi.org/10.3171/2018.3.focus1838.
84. Essayed WI, Zhang F, Unadkat P, Cosgrove GR, Golby AJ, O'Donnell LJ. White matter tractography for neurosurgical planning: a topography-based review of the current state of the art. NeuroImage Clin. 2017;15:659–72. https://doi.org/10.1016/j.nicl.2017.06.011.
85. Farshidfar Z, Faeghi F, Mohseni M, Seddighi A, Kharrazi HH, Abdolmohammadi J. Diffusion tensor tractography in the presurgical assessment of cerebral gliomas. Neuroradiol J. 2014;27:75–84. https://doi.org/10.15274/NRJ-2014-10008.
86. Caverzasi E, Papinutto N, Castellano A, Zhu AH, Scifo P, Riva M, et al. Neurite orientation dispersion and density imaging color maps to characterize brain diffusion in neurologic disorders. J Neuro-Oncol. 2016;26:494–8. https://doi.org/10.1111/jon.12359.
87. Romano A, D'Andrea G, Calabria LF, et al. Pre- and intraoperative tractographic evaluation of corticospinal tract shift. Neurosurgery. 2011;69:696–704.
88. Ostrý S, Belšan T, Otáhal J, Beneš V, Netuka D. Is intraoperative diffusion tensor imaging at 3.0T comparable to subcortical corticospinal tract mapping? Neurosurgery. 2013;73:797–807. https://doi.org/10.1227/NEU.0000000000000087.
89. Barbosa BJAP, Dimostheni A, Teixeira MJ, Tatagiba M, Lepski G. Insular gliomas and the role of intraoperative assistive technologies: results from a volumetry-based retrospective cohort. Clin Neurol Neurosurg. 2016;149:104–10. https://doi.org/10.1016/j.clineuro.2016.08.001.
90. Meyer EJ, Gaggl W, Gilloon B, Swan B, Greenstein M, Voss J, et al. The impact of intracranial tumor proximity to white matter tracts on morbidity and mortality: a retrospective diffusion tensor imaging study. Neurosurgery. 2017;80:193–200. https://doi.org/10.1093/neuros/nyw040.
91. Caverzasi E, Hervey-Jumper SL, Jordan KM, Lobach IV, Li J, et al. Identifying preoperative language tracts and predicting postoperative functional recovery using HARDI q-ball fiber tractography in patients with gliomas. J Neurosurg. 2015;125:33–45. https://doi.org/10.3171/2015.6.jns142203.
92. Zhu FP, Wu JS, Song YY, Yao CJ, Zhuang DX, Xu G, et al. Clinical application of motor pathway mapping using diffusion tensor imaging tractography and intraoperative direct subcortical stimulation in cerebral glioma surgery: a prospective cohort study. Neurosurgery. 2012;71:1170–83. https://doi.org/10.1227/NEU.0b013e318271bc61.
93. Romano NA, Minniti AG, Mastronardi L, Ferrante L, Fantozzi LM, Bozzao A. Pre-surgical planning and MR-tractography utility in brain tumour resection. Eur Radiol. 2009;19:2798–808. https://doi.org/10.1007/s00330-009-1483-6.
94. Zakaria H, Haider S, Lee I. Automated whole brain tractography affects preoperative surgical decision making. Cureus. 2017;9:e1656. https://doi.org/10.7759/cureus.1656.
95. Sunaert S. Presurgical planning for tumor resectioning. J Magn Reson Image. 2006;23:887–905. https://doi.org/10.1002/jmri.20582.
96. Celtikci E, Celtikci P, Fernandes-Cabral DT, Ucar M, Fernandez-Miranda JC, Borcek AO. High-definition fiber tractography in evaluation and surgical planning of thalamopeduncular pilocytic astrocytomas in pediatric population: case series and review of literature. World Neurosurg. 2017;98:463–9. https://doi.org/10.1016/j.wneu.2016.11.061.
97. Yu CS, Li KC, Xuan Y, Ji XM, Qin W. Diffusion tensor tractography in patients with cerebral tumors: a helpful technique for neurosurgical planning and postoperative assessment. Eur J Radiol. 2005;56:197–204. https://doi.org/10.1016/J.EJRAD.2005.04.010.
98. Dimou S, Battisti RA, Hermens DF, Lagopoulos J. A systematic review of functional magnetic resonance imaging and diffusion tensor imaging modalities used in presurgical planning of brain tumour resection. Neurosurg Rev. 2013;36:205–14. https://doi.org/10.1007/s10143-012-0436-8.
99. Maesawa S, Fujii M, Nakahara N, Watanabe T, Wakabayashi T, Yoshida J. Intraoperative tractography and motor evoked potential (MEP) monitoring in surgery for gliomas around the corticospinal tract. World Neurosurg. 2010;74:153–61. https://doi.org/10.1016/j.wneu.2010.03.022.
100. Zhang H, Wang Y, Lu T, Qiu B, Tang Y, Ou S, et al. Differences between generalized q-sampling imaging and diffusion tensor imaging in the preoperative visualization of the nerve fiber tracts within peritumoral edema in brain. Neurosurgery. 2013;73:1044–53.; discussion 1053. https://doi.org/10.1227/NEU.0000000000000146.

Modern Surgical Planning for Intracranial Surgery

6

Daniele Armocida, Fulvio Tartara, Riccardo Boccaletti, Antonio Santoro, and Michele Lanotte

6.1 Introduction

"Surgery starts from the time of the visit and ends when the patient goes home," most neurosurgeons have heard this warning at least once during their residency. This recommendation served as a warning to follow the patient throughout the process of care by paying attention to the preparation for surgery and especially to the postoperative management in the department. Nowadays, with the great implementation of diagnostics, clinical decision-making, operating room instrumentation, and new technologies this warning is as relevant as ever to reality.

Surgical approaches tailored to an individual patient's anatomy and pathology have become standard in neurosurgery. Precise preoperative planning of these procedures, however, is necessary to achieve an optimal therapeutic effect. Therefore, multiple radiological imaging modalities are used prior and during surgery to delineate the patient's anatomy and neurological function [1]. This makes the three main operative variables that undoubtedly impact patient prognosis improvable: reduced surgical timing, the extent of tumor resection, and preservation of neurological functions. It is therefore not surprising that the first important step in successful surgical planning is precisely the organization of the operating room and its operating staff.

D. Armocida (✉)
Neurosurgery Unit, Dept. Neuroscience "Rita Levi Montalcini", Università degli studi di Torino, Torino, TO, Italy
e-mail: danielearmocida@yahoo.it

F. Tartara · R. Boccaletti
Neurosurgical Department, Ospedale Maggiore University of Parma, Parma, Italy

A. Santoro
Neurosurgery Division, Human Neurosciences Department, "La Sapienza" University, Rome, RM, Italy

M. Lanotte
Neuroscience Department "Rita Levi Montalcini", Neurosurgery Unit, Università degli Studi di Torino, Turin, Italy

6.2 The neurosurgical Operating Room

The operating room (OR) is the financial nexus of modern hospitals, accounting for up to 40% of a hospital's costs and 60–70% of revenue [2]; it also represents an important interface between surgeons, patients, consultants, and the community. With significant revenue at stake and operating costs conservatively estimated at $15–50/min [3, 4] every professional care provider has a strong vested interest in maximizing OR efficiency (Fig. 6.1) [5]. Beyond simple financial savings, improving OR efficiency can have myriad secondary benefits, including improved patient safety; increased OR throughput; and

D. Armocida et al. (eds.), *Neurosurgery's Frontline Role in Gliomas Treatment*,
https://doi.org/10.1007/978-3-031-81850-9_6

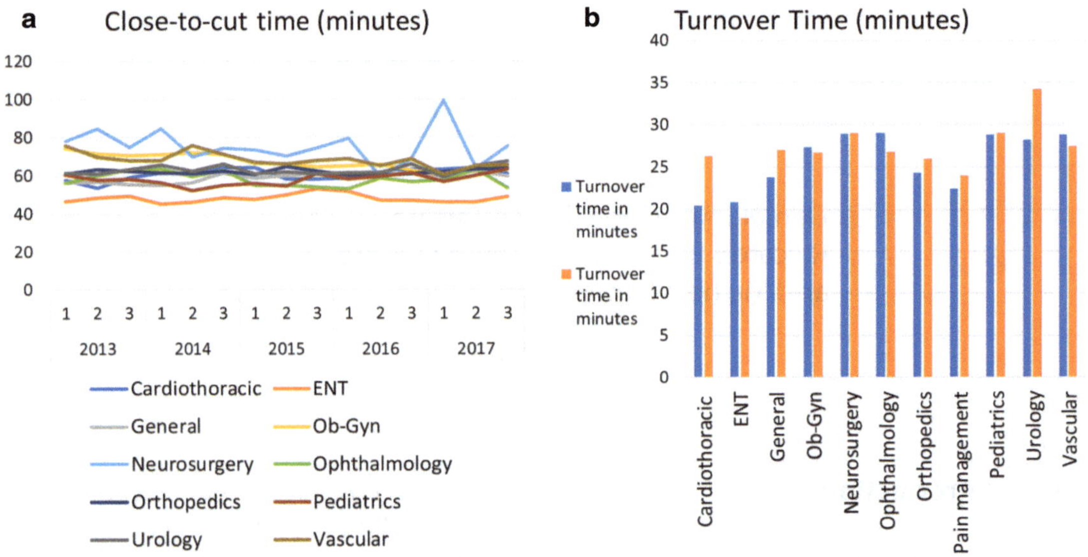

Fig. 6.1 The average operating room (OR) preparation time from the moment of patient admission to the actual beginning of the procedure, expressed as close-to-cut time, and its evolution over the years. This was compared with the average room turnover times at the end of the procedure. It is evident that compared to other medical disciplines, neurosurgery OR has larger procedure preparation times in relation to overlapping turnover times

improved patient, surgeon, and staff satisfaction [6].

OR environments are known for being complex and comprising multilayered social interactions, unpredictability, low tolerance for errors, and high expectations [2]. A significant portion of this complexity arises from the unpredictable nature of the environment. Factors such as patients not adhering to preoperative instructions regarding timeliness, fasting periods, or medical clearance may result in last-minute cancellations. To improve efficiency during the intraoperative phase, it is crucial to have adequately trained staff, proper instrumentation, and equipment, and necessary materials. Conducting a surgical time-out can help identify and prevent potential sources of delay, but timeouts are not always comprehensive [7]. Preference cards for instruments and equipment are a common source of problems for most surgeons. One solution is to streamline the instrumentation and equipment used for standard procedures by all surgeons at a particular center [8].

The considerable number of specialized instruments and personnel required for glioma surgery is noteworthy. The presence of the intra-operative microscope, neuronavigator, endoscope, ultrasonic aspirator device, intra-operative ultrasound, Tullium laser, system of monitors, nursing staff, surgeons, specialists, neurophysiologist, and psychologist in cases of awake surgery, can make the operating space extremely crowded (Fig. 6.2) [9]. The use of digital tools, including the recreation or introduction of new technologies, has altered the traditional methods of neurosurgery [10]. Therefore, it is essential to have a clear understanding of the operating room organization and instrumentation, including the impact on efficiency, time, cost, and patient outcomes, before scheduling surgery. Prolonged operative time has been linked to postoperative complications across various neurosurgical procedures [11], leading to the exploration of modified surgical approaches and techniques to enhance efficiency, starting from preoperative planning.

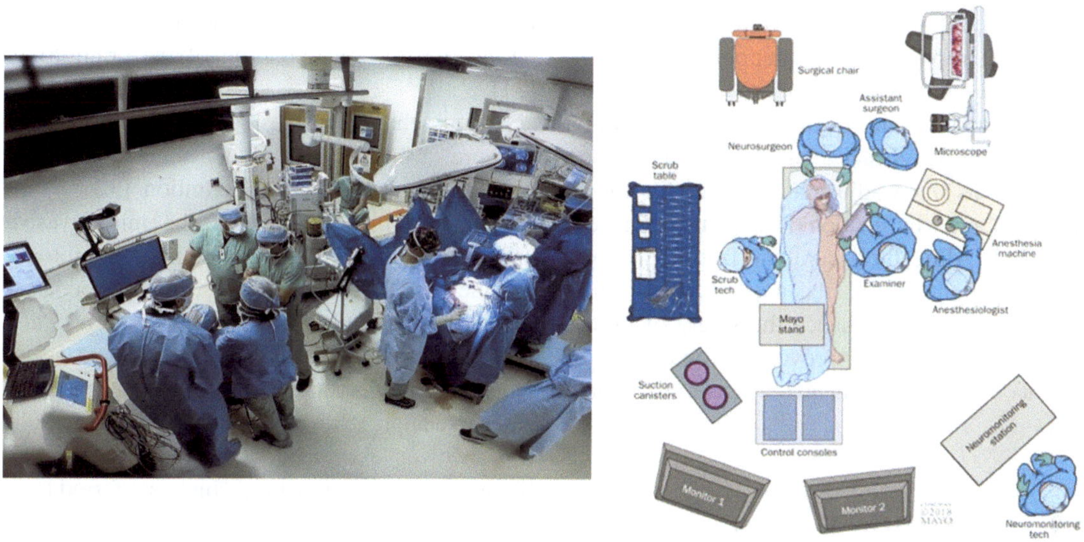

Fig. 6.2 The complexity and crowding of the neurosurgery OR, with its numerous stakeholders, including surgeons, nurses, technicians, equipment, and dedicated staff

6.3 Pre-operative and Intra-operative Imaging

Correct and detailed preoperative planning is one of the most important prerequisites for successful surgery and requires years to master and understand [7, 9, 12]. The difficulty comes from transforming the two-dimensional preoperative radiological black-and-white data into a three-dimensional (3D) image in the surgeon's mind, a view that represents the surgical position of the patient, small cranial exposure, and distortion of the normal anatomy caused by the lesion [13]. However, developing a three-dimensional perception of the surgical approach is traditionally performed by mentally fusing multiple modalities. Therefore, the concurrent 3D visualization of these datasets can significantly improve the planning process [1]. Images from every modality can be examined on a Picture Archiving and Communication System (PACS), and successfully, tumor resection can be assisted intraoperatively by new imaging resources integrated into the surgical microscope [2].

Gliomas pose a significant challenge to neurosurgeons due to their inability to differentiate the tumor from surrounding brain tissue, making it crucial to have an accurate imaging-guided approach [14]. The lack of visual distinction between brain structures complicates surgical planning, necessitating an evidence-based approach to achieve optimal outcomes. In patients with glioma, achieving both functional preservation and extensive lesion removal is difficult without visible structures [15]. To avoid leaving behind residual tumor cells, surgeons may inadvertently destroy surrounding healthy tissue. Alternatively, incomplete resection may be performed to preserve neurological function, leading to suboptimal outcomes. Several intraoperative adjuvant techniques have been developed to help surgeons push the boundaries of the extent of resection (EOR) while maintaining safety [16]. Fluorescence-guided surgery is the most commonly used modern adjuvant technique for brain tumors, allowing for intraoperative delineation of diseased and normal brains, thus improving maximal safe resection. The most widely used fluorophores are 5-aminolevulinic acid (5-ALA) and sodium fluorescein (SFL), which have different spectrophotometric properties, mechanisms of action, and considerations for their use [13, 14, 17]. When combined with other surgical adjuvant strategies such as neuronavigation, intraoperative ultrasound, intraoperative MRI, awake resection, and/or electrophysiological mapping/monitoring, fluorescence-guided resection can further improve resection quality with regard to EOR and safety. More recently, virtual reality (VR) has been developed as a new adjuvant technique for border definition and examination of the extent of resection [18]. Altogether, computerization at each level of patient care has been affected by digital technology to help enhance the safety of procedures and thereby improve the outcomes of patients undergoing neurosurgical procedures [10].

6.4 Approach Planning

Based on these adjuvant strategies, it is necessary to approach the tumor precisely and safely. The basic principle of modern neurosurgery is precise lesion localization, resulting in a minimally invasive approach [9–12]. To achieve this goal, various methods have been developed to define the correct position of the craniotomy and are considered standard in today's neurosurgical armamentarium. The correct position of the craniotomy and the study of the anatomical relations of the lesion with the neural structures around it are of great importance for oncological neurosurgery [19]. Many craniometric references have been correlated with different underlying gyri and sulci, and accurate knowledge of these references is helpful for assessing the extracranial projection of intracranial lesions [20, 21].

Therefore, the use of surgical navigation systems is becoming an increasingly important part of planning and performing intracranial surgery [16, 22–24]. This method is very useful and accurate, but the main problem is the brain shift during surgery [25–27]. In addition to the benefits of neuronavigation in tumor localization, tumor resection control, skull base surgery, or in procedures close to functionally important structures, several studies have pointed out that one of the most valuable applications of neuronavigation is craniotomy localization [28, 29]. Wagner et al. [30] showed that in 40% of cases that had been operated on using intraoperative neuronavigation, the system was only needed to correctly define the size and position of the craniotomy [31].

Often, what the neurosurgeon actually needs is a more accurate three-dimensional image for proper surgical trajectory definition [32–36]. In the modern natural trend of the mini-invasive approach, reducing the size of both the craniotomy and the skin flap has advantages, such as good cosmetic outcomes, lower patient discomfort, and reduced costs. In glioma surgery, in contrast to emergency surgery and tumors of the basicranium, extensive approaches with extensive bone demolition are given less consideration in favor of smaller, highly targeted approaches, which is referred to as the keyhole approach [30, 31].

Key-hole approaches have been widely reported for aneurysm surgery and functional neurosurgery and have recently been introduced for the treatment of intra-axial tumors [30, 37].

In the last decade, a minimally invasive approach, entailing linear skin incision and a few centimeters craniotomy (Fig. 6.3) [38] followed by microsurgical tumor removal, has been performed in selected cases [39]. To date, mini-craniotomy has not been routinely used, particularly for large and superficial lesions, where inadequate control of the brain-tumor interface may be a concern [11, 36, 37]. Until now, most studies were retrospective in nature and involved selected groups of tumors. Furthermore, in procedures requiring intraoperative neurophysiological monitoring, issues might arise from insufficient exposure of the eloquent cortex for mapping or monitoring purposes [37]. The specific anatomy and pathology of an individual patient can be precisely visualized using modern diagnostic tools. This allows us to establish a detailed surgical plan and determine the exact anatomic pathway for optimal surgical access. Based on well-defined access, surgical dissection can be performed while creating a minimally traumatizing cranial opening and avoiding exploratory dissection [40]. The basis for ensuring the best trajectory in the keyhole approach is patient positioning, which ensures the best viewing angle and comfort for the surgeon [41]. The prone, lateral, and anterior head

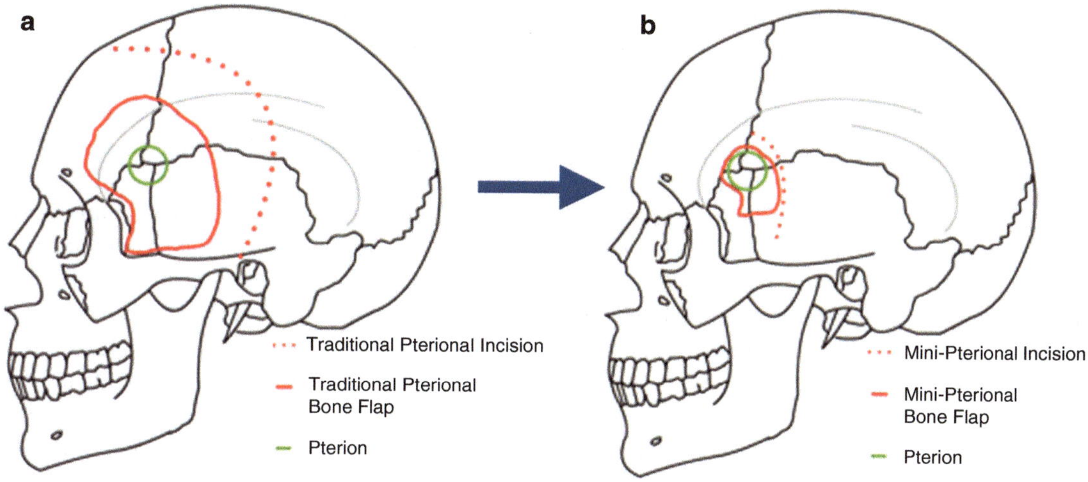

Fig. 6.3 The difference between a classical pterional approach and a minimally invasive keyhole approach in terms of skin incision and craniotomy size

positions, park-bench position, and semi-sitting positions are widely used to ensure the best and safest access. Furthermore, now with the recent studies, it has in fact been shown that most post-operative complications (surgical or otherwise) were comparable between head positioning, concluding that, both sitting and horizontal positions can be used safely in cranial surgeries [31].

The position and course of the surgical approach play the most important role in minimally invasive keyhole neurosurgery, and it is complemented by the use of carefully chosen instruments and the recognition of small technical details to avoid intraoperative confusion or space constraints during dissection [35, 42]. Performing keyhole craniotomy clearly defined the dimensions of the surgical corridor toward the target. Craniotomy must be placed accurately and exactly in the right position to avoid intraoperative difficulties or disorientation [43]. Two preconditions for a precisely placed craniotomy are important: (a) Distinguished preoperative approach planning. The smaller the craniotomy, the greater the need for precise planning and exact implementation of the plan because it is extremely difficult to change the surgical corridor during the procedure.

Trajectory planning in image-guided keyhole neurosurgery is usually performed by manual selection of 2D axial, sagittal, and/or coronal cross sections of preoperative CT/MRI head scans [44]. This requires the surgeon to mentally identify and reconstruct complex 3D structures, such as blood vessels, eloquent brain areas, and the ventricular system, and to derive spatial relationships between these structures and their trajectory [45]. Thus, evaluation of expected treatment risks is a complex, challenging, and time-consuming task, even for experienced neurosurgeons. Although spatial visualization and segmentation of critical brain structures are sometimes used to enhance the neurosurgeon's spatial perception, the tool insertion trajectory is still selected manually. Trajectory selection does not incorporate quantitative trajectory-specific measures and/or visualization of nearby critical structures and does not consider the expected surgical localization error [45–47]. This problem is being overcome by the acquisition and study of detailed multimodal imaging series, including high-resolution structural magnetic resonance imaging (MRI), f-MRI, diffusion tensor imaging (DTI), and detailed arterial and venous vascular imaging. These imaging studies may then be reconstructed and matched on a 3D surgical planning neuronavigator to plan the approach in a stereoscopic environment, which displays surgically relevant structures in a virtual 3D space. This enables the simulation of intraoperative viewpoints, and hence, the exploration of the surgical site even before the actual surgery has started.

One of the most important drawbacks of keyhole procedures is their difficulty in intraoperative orientation. Incorrect placement of the surgical tool may result in undesired outcomes such as nondiagnostic tissue samples, ineffective treatment, and temporary or permanent neurological damage. The concomitant intraoperative use of ultrasound, intraoperative computed tomography, and MRI with navigation systems may be helpful if the limited cranial opening leads to a structurally complex and hard-to-understand situation [45, 46].

The second drawback is the narrow viewing angle and almost coaxial control of the dissection as a result of the small and individually tailored approach. If the craniotomy is too small, conventional microinstruments are difficult to use because they may strike the craniotomy site. For this reason, the development and intraoperative use of novel microinstruments, such as scissors, grasping and coagulating forceps, clip appliers, etc., has been an important step in advancing keyhole surgery. In particular, slim tube-shaft designed tools allow unhindered manipulation even through limited keyhole craniotomies [48]. When planning the approach and estimating craniotomy, it is critical to know what instruments will be used, whether a microscope or exoscope is needed, and to request an appropriately sized ultrasonic aspirator handpiece (Fig. 6.4) [48].

The third and most likely central difficulty of keyhole approaches is the loss of intraoperative light and sight because limited craniotomy causes a significant reduction in intraoperative optical control. However, neurosurgeons must be able to recognize both normal anatomical structures to avoid damage and abnormal structures to remove them [38]. To bring light into the surgical field

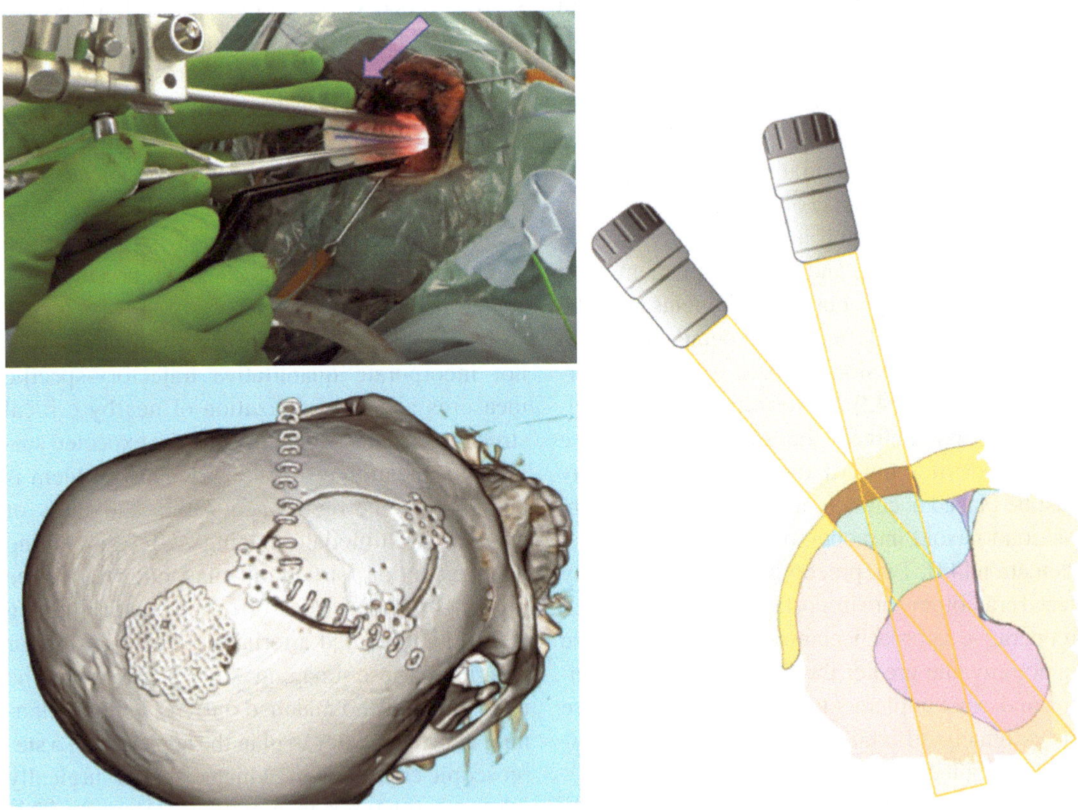

Fig. 6.4 The advantages and disadvantages of a minimally invasive keyhole approach, with the benefits of obtaining a small craniotomy and surgical corridor, but the risk of a poorly illuminated and inaccessible surgical field for large, multifocal tumors

and control manipulation at the depth of the operating field, surgical microscopes can be effectively supported by the optical properties of modern endoscopes. The advantages of endoscopes are (1) increased light intensity, (2) extended viewing angle, and (3) clear depiction of close-up details.

The endoscope is particularly suited for obtaining a detailed view of the structures in the shadow of the light beam of the microscope (Fig. 6.5) [5]. Thus, in situations during microsurgical dissection, where additional visual information of the target area is desired or when avoidance of retraction of superficial structures

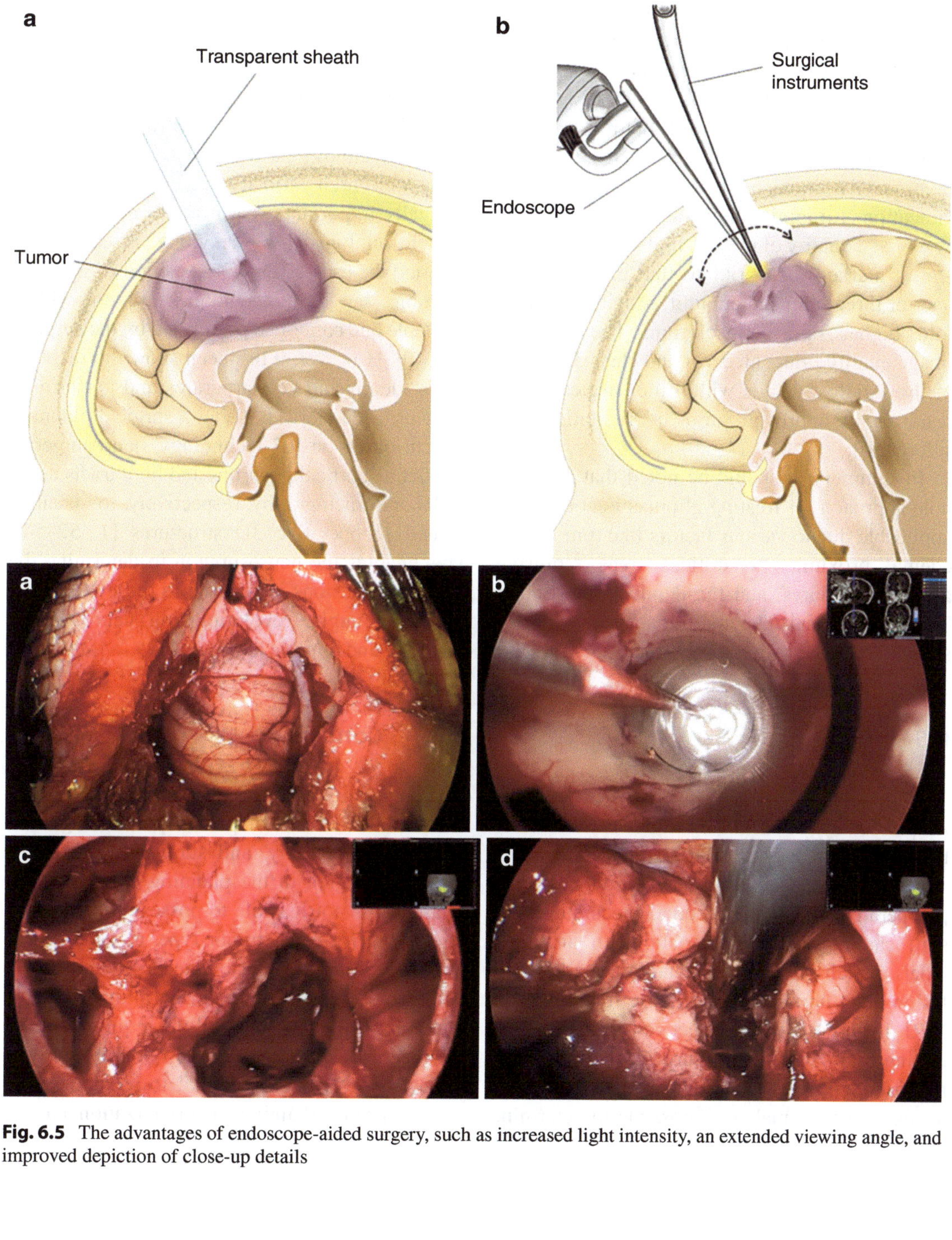

Fig. 6.5 The advantages of endoscope-aided surgery, such as increased light intensity, an extended viewing angle, and improved depiction of close-up details

is recommended, an endoscope may be introduced into the surgical site [49]. Rigid lens scopes in these cases are recommended because only instruments with rigid shafts can be controlled precisely, and because, at least at present, only lens scopes offer acceptable image quality. Endoscopes with angled shafts are preferred because the camera attached to the eyepiece does not interfere with the visual field of the microscope or hinder surgical manipulation. Different degrees of angulation of the front lens offer viewing angles of 0, 30, 45, and 70°. Recently, the intraoperative use of full-definition (HD) image quality has offered a new area in endoscopic neurosurgery with an increased range of indications for minimally invasive neurosurgery. The image quality of the full-high-definition system is markedly superior to that of a standard one- or three-chip camera unit, providing a fivefold higher optical resolution. The brilliant image quality offers an exact and clear depiction of the smallest details within the surgical field, resulting in improved surgical orientation and safety [50].

In summary, it should be noted that the keyhole approach for treating gliomas is not always applicable due to various factors like tumor size, edema, proximity to critical areas requiring awake procedures, and the depth of the tumor. These factors make the traditional approach more suitable in certain situations.

6.5 The Value of Intraoperative MRI

As previously stated, during tumor resection and the subsequent loss of cerebrospinal fluid, brain shift occurs, causing neuronavigation based on preoperative imaging to become inaccurate. Brain shift causes significant variations in anatomic labels, which often render anatomic markers for lesion sites unreliable. Currently, intraoperative MRI (iMRI) is the most effective method for correcting brain shift during surgery. iMRI enables neurosurgeons to objectively assess the extent of lesion resection, making it possible to determine whether the surgery should be continued or terminated [12]. The function and role of iMRI will be discussed in more detail in Chap. 13.

Recently, intraoperative virtual reality (VR) has been introduced, which allows neurosurgeons to visualize 3-dimensional (3D) images of lesions and their associated functional structures during surgery. This technique combines two manipulation techniques and can be interactively explored with a personal computer, where the content of the image can be moved in different directions or zoomed in or out using keys or a mouse-pad [51]. Over the past few decades, medical applications of VR technology have rapidly developed, from being a research curiosity to a commercially and clinically important area of medical informatics and technology [4]. Previous research has reported the use of 3D reconstruction for surgical planning, but these techniques are not widely available and cannot be performed by the surgeon [18, 40]. However, it has been shown to be helpful in identifying key structures and performing safer procedures [21]. Using a surgical planning system based on VR technology, neurosurgeons can define cortical positions and fiber tracts using fMRI and tractography, respectively, to visualize related preoperative 3D structures [1, 52–54]. This enables the neurosurgeon to determine the position of lesions in relation to these structures from any angle, revolutionizing neurosurgical planning and approach [55].

6.6 Conclusion

The contemporary era of glioma surgery necessitates the inclusion of patient positioning, skin incision, craniotomy, and surgical exposure of the target region in the planning and execution phases. It is not feasible to possess standardized equipment for every tumor type, as each procedure is unique and customized to the patient's specific needs. To summarize, a multitude of technological aids can fulfill the requirements of neurosurgeons to guarantee optimal surgical results. However, it is crucial to recognize that without proper planning and organization, having an abundance of instruments in the operating room may result in confusion, wasted time, and expensive procedures.

References

1. Beyer J, Hadwiger M, Wolfsberger S, Bühler K. High-quality multimodal volume rendering for preoperative planning of neurosurgical interventions. IEEE Trans Vis Comput Graph. 2007;13(6):1696–703. https://doi.org/10.1109/TVCG.2007.70560.
2. Healey T, El-Othmani MM, Healey J, Peterson TC, Saleh KJ. Improving operating room efficiency, part 1: general managerial and preoperative strategies. J Bone Jt Surg Rev. 2015;3(10):1–10.
3. Macario A. What does one minute of operating room time cost? J Clin Anesth. 2010;22:233–6.
4. Kaye AD, McDowell JL, Diaz JH, et al. Effective strategies in improving operating room case delays and cancellations at an academic medical center. Top Periop Med. 2015;6:24–9.
5. Sakata T, Tanikawa M, Yamada H, Fujinami R, Nishikawa Y, Yamada S, Mase M. Minimally invasive treatment for glioblastoma through endoscopic surgery including tumor embolization when necessary: a technical note. Front Neurol. 2023;14:1170045. https://doi.org/10.3389/fneur.2023.1170045.
6. Rothstein DH, Raval MV. Operating room efficiency. Semin Pediatr Surg. 2018;27(2):79–85. https://doi.org/10.1053/j.sempedsurg.2018.02.004.
7. Parikh N, Gargollo P, Granberg C. Improving operating room efficiency using the six sigma methodology. Urology. 2021;154:141–7. https://doi.org/10.1016/j.urology.2021.02.049. Epub 2021 May 11.
8. Skarda DE, Rollins M, Andrews S, McFadden M, Barnhart D, Meyers R, Scaife E. One hospital, one appendectomy: the cost effectiveness of a standardized doctor's preference card. J Pediatr Surg. 2015;50(6):919–22.
9. Quinones-Hinojosa A, et al. Brain mapping. In: Section II: intraoperative brain mapping: part 1: awake. 9 awake craniotomy operating room setup and surgical instruments. New York: Thieme; 2020. https://doi.org/10.1055/b-0040-174327.
10. Abdelwahab MG, Cavalcanti DD, Preul MC. Role of computer technology in neurosurgery. Minerva Chir. 2010;65(4):409–28.
11. Short HL, Fevrier HB, Meisel JA, Santore MT, Heiss KF, Wulkan ML, Raval MV. Defining the association between operative time and outcomes in children's surgery. J Pediatr Surg. 2017;52(10):1561–6.
12. Hou Y, Li Y, Li Q, Yu Y, Tang J. Full-course resection control strategy in glioma surgery using both intraoperative ultrasound and intraoperative MRI. Front Oncol. 2022;12:955807. https://doi.org/10.3389/fonc.2022.955807. PMID: 36091111; PMCID: PMC9453394.
13. Navarro-Bonnet J, Suarez-Meade P, Brown DA, Chaichana KL, Quinones-Hinojosa A. Following the light in glioma surgery: a comparison of sodium fluorescein and 5-aminolevulinic acid as surgical adjuncts in glioma resection. J Neurosurg Sci. 2019;63(6):633–47. https://doi.org/10.23736/S0390-5616.19.04745-3.
14. Zhang ZZ, Shields LB, Sun DA, Zhang YP, Hunt MA, Shields CB. The art of intraoperative glioma identification. Front Oncol. 2015;5:175. https://doi.org/10.3389/fonc.2015.00175. PMID: 26284196; PMCID: PMC4520021.
15. Armocida D, Pesce A, Palmieri M, D'Andrea G, Salvati M, Santoro A, Frati A. Periventricular zone involvement as a predictor of survival in glioblastoma patients: a single centre cohort-comparison investigation concerning a distinct clinical entity. Interdiscip Neurosurg. 2021;25:101185. https://doi.org/10.1016/j.inat.2021.101185.
16. Orringer DA, Golby A, Jolesz F. Neuronavigation in the surgical management of brain tumors: current and future trends. Expert Rev Med Devices. 2012;9:491–500.
17. Coburger J, Wirtz CR. Fluorescence guided surgery by 5-ALA and intraoperative MRI in high grade glioma: a systematic review. J Neuro-Oncol. 2019;141:533–46. https://doi.org/10.1007/s11060-018-03052-4.
18. Sun GC, Wang F, Chen XL, et al. Impact of virtual and augmented reality based on intraoperative magnetic resonance imaging and functional neuronavigation in glioma surgery involving eloquent areas. World Neurosurg. 2016;96:375–82. https://doi.org/10.1016/j.wneu.2016.07.107.
19. Mandel M, Amorim R, Paiva W, Prudente M, Teixeira MJ, Andrade AF. 3D preoperative planning in the ER with osiriX®: when there is no time for neuronavigation. Sensors. 2013;13:6477–91.
20. Ribas GC, Yasuda A, Ribas EC, Nishikuni K, Rodrigues AJ. Surgical anatomy of microneurosurgical sulcal key points. Neurosurgery. 2006;59:177–210.
21. Casey SO, Rubinstein D, Lillehei KO, Alberico RA, Ozsvath RR, Cajade-Law AG, et al. Integral and shell-MIP display algorithms in MR and CT three-dimensional models of the brain surface. AJNR Am J Neuroradiol. 1998;19:1513–21.
22. Mandel M, Amorim R, Paiva W, Prudente M, Teixeira MJ, Andrade AF. 3D preoperative planning in the ER with OsiriX®: when there is no time for neuronavigation. Sensors. 2013;13(5):6477–91. https://doi.org/10.3390/s130506477.
23. Watanabe E, Watanabe T, Manaka S, Mayanagi Y, Takakura K. Three-dimensional digitizer (neuronavigator): new equipment for computed tomography-guided stereotaxic surgery. Surg Neurol. 1987;27:543–7.
24. Cho JM, Kim EH, Kim J, Lee SK, Kim SH, Lee KS, et al. Clinical use of diffusion tensor image-merged functional neuronavigation for brain tumor surgeries: Review of preoperative, intraoperative,

and postoperative data for 123 cases. Yonsei Med J. 2014;55:1303–9.
25. Nabavi A, Black PM, Gering DT, Westin CF, Mehta V, Pergolizzi RS, et al. Serial intraoperative magnetic resonance imaging of brain shift. Neurosurgery. 2001;48:787–97.
26. Nimsky C, Ganslandt O, Cerny S, Hastreiter P, Greiner G, Fahlbusch R. Quantification of, visualization of, and compensation for brain shift using intraoperative magnetic resonance imaging. Neurosurgery. 2000;47:1070–9.
27. Roberts DW, Hartov A, Kennedy FE, Miga MI, Paulsen KD. Intraoperative brain shift and deformation: a quantitative analysis of cortical displacement in 28 cases. Neurosurgery. 1998;43:749–58.
28. Woerdeman PA, Willems PW, Noordmans HJ, Tulleken CA, van der Sprenkel JW. Application accuracy in frameless image-guided neurosurgery: a comparison study of three patient-to-image registration methods. J Neurosurg. 2007;106:1012–6.
29. Oishi M, Fukuda M, Ishida G, Saito A, Hiraishi T, Fujii Y. Presurgical simulation with advanced 3-dimensional multifusion volumetric imaging in patients with skull base tumors. Neurosurgery. 2011;68:188–99.
30. Spena G, Panciani PP, Nicolosi F, Fontanella M. Minimally invasive subfrontal route for the resection of medial temporal region intrinsic tumors. Acta Neurochir. 2015;157:1971–4.
31. Rath GP, Bithal PK, Chaturvedi A, Dash HH. Complications related to positioning in posterior fossa craniectomy. J Clin Neurosci. 2007;14(6):520–5. https://doi.org/10.1016/j.jocn.2006.02.010.
32. Fischer G, Stadie A, Schwandt E, Gawehn J, Boor S, Marx J, Oertel J. Minimally invasive superficial temporal artery to middle cerebral artery bypass through a minicraniotomy: benefit of three-dimensional virtual reality planning using magnetic resonance angiography. Neurosurg Focus. 2009;26:E20.
33. Ganslandt O, Behari S, Gralla J, Fahlbusch R, Nimsky C. Neuronavigation: concept, techniques and applications. Neurology. 2002;50:244–55.
34. Recinos PF, Raza SM, Jallo GI, Recinos VR. Use of a minimally invasive tubular retraction system for deep-seated tumors in pediatric patients. J Neurosurg Pediatr. 2011;7:516–21.
35. Stadie AT, Kockro RA, Reisch R, Tropine A, Boor S, Stoeter P, Perneczky A. Virtual reality system for planning minimally invasive neurosurgery. Technical note. J Neurosurg. 2008;108:382–94.
36. Enchev YP, Popov RV, Romansky KV, Marinov MB, Bussarsky VA. Cranial neuronavigation-a step forward or a step aside in modern neurosurgery. Folia Med. 2008;50:5–10.
37. Szelényi A, Bello L, Duffau H, Fava E, Feigl GC, Galanda M, Neuloh G, Signorelli F, Sala F. Intraoperative electrical stimulation in awake craniotomy: methodological aspects of current practice. Neurosurg Focus. 2010;28:E7.
38. Burks JD, Conner AK, Bonney PA, Archer JB, Christensen B, Smith J, Safavi-Abbasi S, Sughrue ME. Management of intracranial meningiomas using keyhole techniques. Cureus. 2016;8:e588.
39. Paolini S, Severino R, Mancarella C, et al. Mini-craniotomy for intra-axial brain tumors: a comparison with conventional craniotomy in 306 patients harboring non-dural based lesions. Neurosurg Rev. 2022;45(4):2983–91. https://doi.org/10.1007/s10143-022-01811-6.
40. Perneczky A, Reisch R. Multiple aneurysms treated via frontal interhemispheric approach. In: Kobayashi S, editor. Neurosurgery of complex vascular lesions and tumors. Stuttgart: Thieme; 2005. p. 7–11.
41. Perneczky A, Reisch R. Key hole approaches in neurosurgery. Volume I. Concept and surgical technique. Wien: Springer; 2008.
42. Reisch R, Stadie A, Kockro R, Gawish I, Schwandt E, Hopf N. The minimally invasive supraorbital subfrontal key-hole approach for surgical treatment of temporomesial lesions of the dominant hemisphere. Minim Invasive Neurosurg. 2009;52:163–9.
43. Corvino S, Armocida D, Offi M, Pennisi G, Burattini B, Mondragon AV, Esposito F, Cavallo LM, de Notaris M. The anterolateral triangle as window on the foramen lacerum from transorbital corridor: anatomical study and technical nuances. Acta Neurochir. 2023;165(9):2407–19. https://doi.org/10.1007/s00701-023-05704-5.
44. Spiriev T, Nakov V, Laleva L, Tzekov C. OsiriX software as a preoperative planning tool in cranial neurosurgery: a step-by-step guide for neurosurgical residents. Surg Neurol Int. 2017;8:241.
45. Navkar NV, Tsekos NV, Stafford JR, Weinberg JS, Deng Z. Visualization and planning of neurosurgical interventions with straight access. In: Navab N, Jannin P, editors. Proceedings of first international conference on information processing in computer-assisted interventions, lecture notes in computer science. New York: Springer; 2010. p. 1–11.
46. Tirelli E, Momi D, Borghese NA, Ferrigno G. An intelligent atlas-based planning system for keyhole neurosurgery. Int J Comput Assist Radiol Surg. 2009;4(Suppl. 1):S85–6.
47. Brunenberg J, Vilanova A, Visser-Vandewalle V, Temel Y, Ackermans L, Platel B, ter Haar Romeny BM. Automatic trajectory planning for deep brain stimulation: a feasibility study. In: Ayache N, Ourselin S, editors. Proceedings of 10th international conference on medical image computation and computer assisted intervention, lecture notes in computer science 4791. New York: Springer; 2007. p. 584–92.
48. Watanabe T, Iwami K, Kishida Y, Nagatani T, Yatsuya H, Miyachi S. Combined exoscopic and endoscopic two-step keyhole approach for intracranial meningiomas. Curr Oncol. 2022;29(8):5370–82. https://doi.org/10.3390/curroncol29080426.
49. D'Angelo L, Armocida D, Sampirisi L, Paglia F, Berra LV, Santoro A. Role of endoscopic surgical

biopsy in diagnoses of intraventricular/periventricular tumors: review of literature including a monocentric case series. Acta Neurol Belg. 2020;120(3):517–30. https://doi.org/10.1007/s13760-020-01299-1.
50. Reisch R, Stadie A, Kockro RA, Hopf N. The keyhole concept in neurosurgery. World Neurosurg. 2013;79(2):e9–e13. https://doi.org/10.1016/j.wneu.2012.02.024.
51. Alaraj A, Charbel FT, Birk D, Tobin M, Luciano C, Banerjee PP, et al. Role of cranial and spinal virtual and augmented reality simulation using immersive touch modules in neurosurgical training. Neurosurgery. 2013;72(1):115–23.
52. Lu JF, Zhang J, Wu JS, Yao CJ, Zhuang DX, Qiu TM, et al. Awake craniotomy and intra- operative language cortical mapping for eloquent cerebral glioma resection: preliminary clinical practice in 3.0 T intraoperative magnetic reso- nance imaging integrated surgical suite. Chin J Surg. 2011;49:693–8.
53. Hunt R, Scarpace L, Rock JP. Intraoperative augmented reality for complex glioma resection: a case report. Cureus. 2024;16(4):e57717. https://doi.org/10.7759/cureus.57717.
54. Ragnhildstveit A, Li C, Zimmerman MH, Mamalakis M, Curry VN, Holle W, Baig N, Uğuralp AK, Alkhani L, Oğuz-Uğuralp Z, Romero-Garcia R, Suckling J. Intra-operative applications of augmented reality in glioma surgery: a systematic review. Front Surg. 2023;10:1245851. https://doi.org/10.3389/fsurg.2023.1245851.
55. Kirkman MA, Ahmed M, Albert AF, Wilson MH, Nandi D, Sevdalis N. The use of simulation in neurosurgical education and training. J Neurosurg. 2014;121:228–46.

Part II

Part II

7 The Role of Surgery Along the Diffuse Low-Grade Glioma Timeline: Insights into Surgical Paradigms

Tamara Ius, Chiara Bertolotti, Edoardo Agosti, Daniele Bagatto, and Pier Paolo Panciani

7.1 Introduction

Supratentorial diffuse low-grade glioma (DLGG), classified as World Health Organization (WHO) Grade II tumors, are an heterogeneous group of slowly growing intrinsic brain tumors derived from glial cell lines [1].

DLGG are relative rare tumors accounting for 6.4% of all adult primary CNS tumors, with a predicted incidence in the USA of 0.51 and 0.25 per 100,000 per year for astrocytomas and oligodendrogliomas, respectively [2].

As high-grade gliomas (HGG), the risk factors for the growth of DLGG are mostly unknown, except a prior history of exposure to ionizing radiation. Nonetheless, a small percentage of cases are believed to be caused by well-known hereditary tumor predisposition syndromes, such as Lynch syndrome, Li-Fraumeni syndrome, and neurofibromatosis type 1 [3].

T. Ius (✉)
Academic Neurosurgery, Department of Neurosciences, University of Padova, Padova, Italy
e-mail: tamara.ius@gmail.com

C. Bertolotti · D. Bagatto
Unit of Neuroradiology, Department of Diagnostic Imaging, University Hospital of Udine, Udine, Italy

E. Agosti · P. P. Panciani
Division of Neurosurgery, Department of Medical and Surgical Specialties, Radiological Sciences and Public Health, University of Brescia, Brescia, Italy

Compared with HGG (WHO grade 3 and 4), patients typically present at a younger age, with the peak incidence between ages 35 and 44 years [2].

Most DLGG patients present with epileptic seizures, with over 50% experiencing pharmacoresistant seizures. Uncontrolled, tumorrelated epilepsy significantly reduces quality of life, contributes to cognitive decline, and increases morbidity [4, 5].

Focal neurologic deficits are less common than in high-grade gliomas, probably in relation with the slower but continuous growth rate (average rate of 4 mm/year) [6, 7].

Indeed, DLGG show a progressive infiltrative nature along white matter tracts, without altering their function but limiting the feasibility of radical or supramarginal surgical resection [8–11].

Another consequence of their infiltrative nature is the presence of tumor cell outside the radiologically visible tumor; this feature implies that, despite the often rather well-defined margins on MRI, these invasive cells will likely undergo malignant transformation (MT) [12, 13].

Overall, MT occurs over several years, with a the timeline that widely varies among patients: this evidence highlights the importance of individualized treatment and close monitoring to detect early radiological changes [14].

Median survival for patients with low-grade gliomas ranges from 5 to 13 years and depends on specific histology and molecular features.

D. Armocida et al. (eds.), *Neurosurgery's Frontline Role in Gliomas Treatment*,
https://doi.org/10.1007/978-3-031-81850-9_7

The epidemiological rarity of DLGG, combined with the long survival rates of patients and advances in molecular diagnostics, has made it challenging to design and complete large, high-quality, prospective studies. In spite of the lack of Class I evidence, surgery has become increasingly important only in recent years, assuming a central role in DLGG managment. Indeed, maximal safe resection currently represents the first step in DLGG workflow [15].

Significant advancements have been made in understanding glioma progression and clinical variability, supported by the WHO's updated pathological classification that incorporates molecular markers. For a comprehensive understanding of this subject matter, readers are encouraged to explore Chap. 3 where it is extensively covered.

In addition, new MRI techniques enhance diagnostic and prognostic capabilities, shifting treatment from a "wait and watch" approach to proactive intervention. Insights into the molecular and genetic aspects of gliomas have led to personalized treatment strategies, including targeted therapies and adjuvant treatments. This review aims to provide a comprehensive understanding of current surgical and multistage treatment strategies for DLGG, encompassing the latest advancements in diagnostic techniques, molecular profiling, and individualized therapeutic approaches.

7.2 Low-Grade Glioma Evolution Over Time

DLGG are progressive primary brain tumor where four evolution stages can be recognized (see Fig. 7.1). First, glioma-initiating cells undergo neoplastic transformation, acting as the biological inception of the tumor. This occult stage is characterized by a "nascent glioma" that does not cause any clinical symptoms and probably even remains below the routine magnetic resonance imaging (MRI) detection limit. Second, at a certain stage, the glioma becomes detectable on MRI while the patient remains asymptomatic; this phase is known as the clinically silent stage. During this period, gliomas can be incidentally discovered on brain MRI, as in healthy volunteers or in trauma patients requiring brain imaging. Third, the glioma begins to cause clinical symptoms, typically presenting as an epileptic seizure, marking the onset of the symptomatic period. The glioma finally changes during the fourth period from a relatively slow-growing condition to a more aggressive form that characterized by neo-angiogenesis and malignant progression. In the final stage of evolution, the tumor grows and spreads, resulting in the patient's death [16–18].

To date, oncologic therapy has failed to cure patients with DLGG, but a significant delay of malignant transformation (MT) and death from disease can be achieved by appropriate and timely treatment [16, 17].

With regards to tumor kinetics, the rate of spontaneous tumor expansion, shown by a growth curve of mean glioma diameter over time generated from successive MRIs, predicts long-term prognosis in DLLG patients, and the continuous tumor growth suggests increased WM infiltration, limiting the possible EOR [18, 19].

Growth kinetics diverge significantly among DLGG cases at diagnosis, ranging from less than 1 mm/year to 8 mm/year. Growth rates greater than 8 mm/year indicate a higher risk of malignant transformation [7]. Identifying DLGG with rapid growth during the pre-therapeutic phase provides insight into the best time to initiate therapy, including incidental DLGG patients [19, 20]. This assessment remains critical throughout post-treatment surveillance, guiding decisions on additional therapeutic measures; it is particularly true in cases of incomplete tumor resection, when rapid residual tumor growth may demand earlier re-operation, even in asymptomatic patients [21].

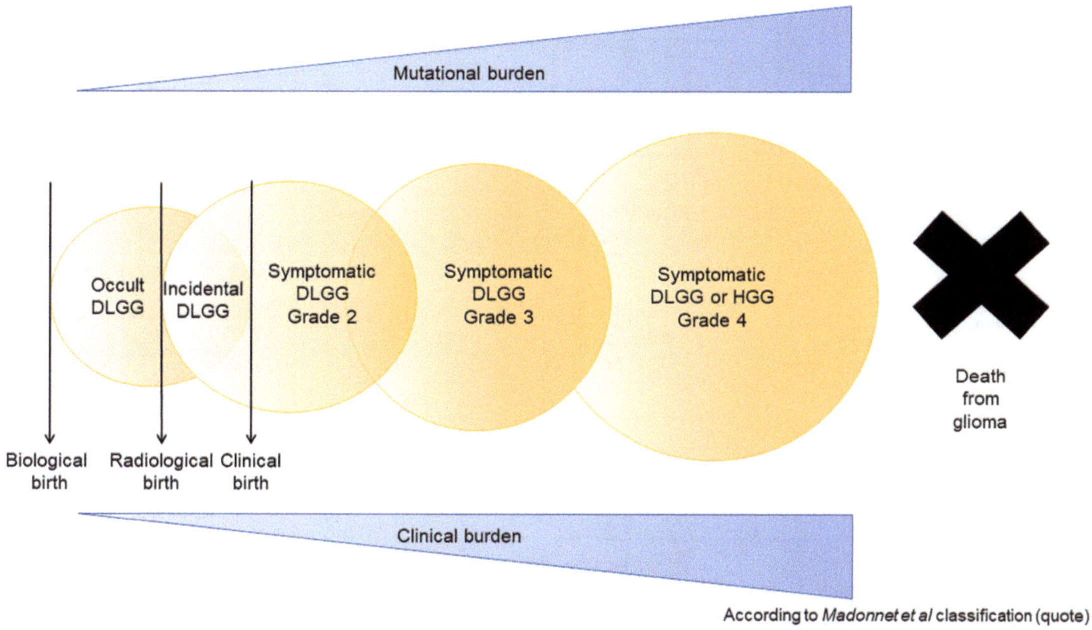

Fig. 7.1 Timeline of the evolution of DLGG from occult, to incidental, to its malignant counterpart. DLGG evolution over time according the gliomagenesis model [16]. *DLGG* diffuse low-grade glioma, *HGG* high-grade glioma

DLGG can exhibit a great deal of individual variety, from little tumors to extensive gliomatosis, as well as unique patterns of progression in the brain, including a diffuse "migratory" pattern or a proliferative "bulky" pattern [14]. The EOR is hindered by gliomas' propensity to travel down subcortical fibers and the density of tumor cells in peripheral white matter pathways [21]. Glioma evolution is predicted by biomathematical models; nevertheless, treatment effects may cause patterns to alter, such as a shift from bulky to diffuse after incomplete resection [22]. Tumor development pattern affects the achievable EOR, which in turn affects OS and tumor-related epilepsy [9, 23]. Given that white matter connection influences neuroplasticity, an understanding of these patterns is essential for treatment decisions [14].

Advancements in glioma prognosis have resulted in an increasing number of young female glioma patients experiencing pregnancy despite their diagnosis. Current evidence does not indicate an elevated risk of glioma development during pregnancy [24]. However, alterations in glioma behavior during pregnancy have been documented, including increased tumor volume and growth rates, earlier symptom onset, and a higher incidence of seizures. In patients with low-grade glioma (LGG), specifically, pregnancy has been associated with dedifferentiation and tumor progression [24, 25].

7.3 The Role of Surgery

Although surgery plays a central role in the management of DLGG patients today (Fig. 7.2), its value has been discussed for many years. Recent volumetric studies have shown that achieving the maximum safe extent of tumoral resection (EOR)

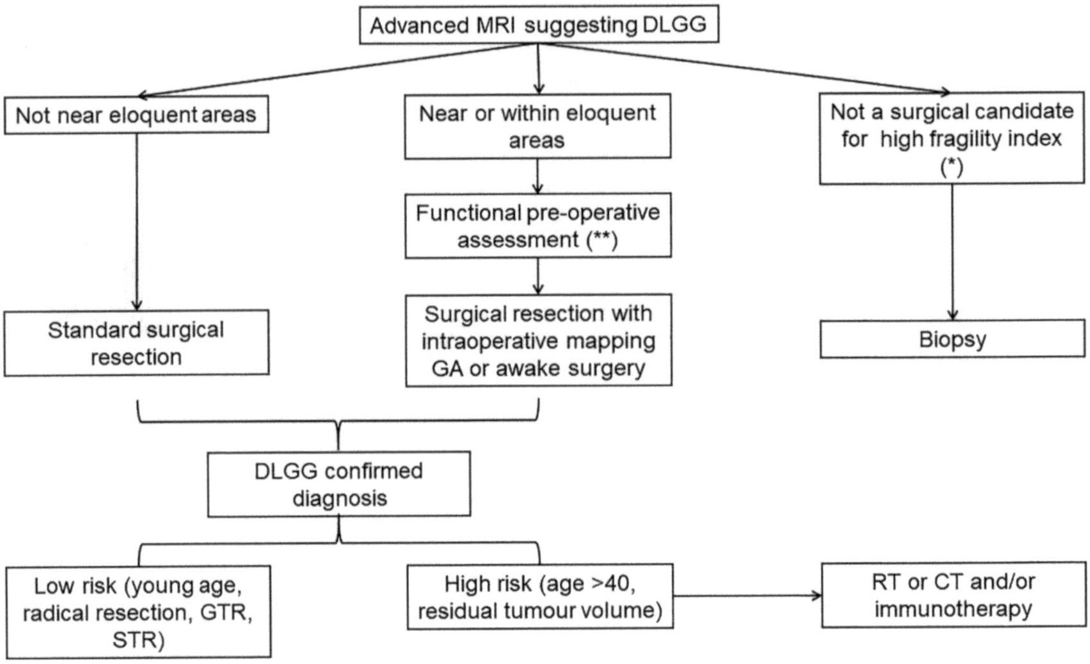

Fig. 7.2 Flowchart illustrating the multidisciplinary management approach for diffuse low-grade gliomas (DLGG), integrating surgical, oncological, and magnetic resonance findings. (*) elderly patient, poor clinical condition, comorbidity, deep-seated/eloquent tumor location such as basal ganglia or brainstem. (**) fMRI, DTI, TMS. *MRI* magnetic resonance imaging, *DLGG* diffuse low-grade glioma, *GA* general anesthesia, *GTR* gross total resection, *STR* supratotal resection, *R* radiotherapy, *CT* chemotherapy

is the primary treatment modality, which correlates with higher survival rates [9–11, 26, 27]. Over the last decade, qualitative descriptors of EOR, such as "gross total resection" (GTR) or "subtotal resection" (STR) have given way to a more exact and objective metric based on the following calculation: "EOR = (preoperative tumor volume − postoperative tumor volume)/preoperative tumor volume" [28, 29]. This systematic adjustment in tumor volume estimation improves comparability among surgical investigations and reduces reliance on surgeons' subjective opinions (Table 7.1).

The fundamental aim of DLGG surgery is to preserve functional integrity while obtaining maximum tumor resection. In the context of radical resection, intraoperative detection and preservation of eloquent cortical areas and subcortical functional connections are crucial for preserving quality of life limiting the risk of permanent deficits [30]. Personalized anatomic and functional planning along with intraoperative brain mapping technique are thus mandatory for optimal intraoperative management of these patients (Figs. 7.3 and 7.4).

Table 7.1 Predictive survival factors in DLGG patients undergoing surgery: a literature review according to the EOR

Study (year)	Number of cases (medium age, age interval)	Histology	EOR	OS	Predictive survival factors
Claus et al. (2005) [1]	156 (41.6)	Oligodendroglioma 95 Astrocytoma 35 Mixed 26	100% (56)	5 year 98.2%	Patients who underwent subtotal resection were at 1.4 times the risk of disease recurrence and at 4.9 times the risk of death relative to patients who underwent gross total resection
Smith et al. (2008) [2]	216 (38, 19–72)	Astrocytoma 93 Oligodendroglioma 91 Mixed 32	Group 1 100% (75) Group 2 90–99% (26) Group 3 70–89% (55) Group 4 41–69% (39) Group 5 0–40% (21)	5-years survival Group 1 98% Group 2 97% Group 3, 4, 5: nd	EOR ($p < 0.001$), log preoperative tumor volume ($p = 0.004$), postoperative tumor volume ($p = 0.03$) were predictive of OS Log preoperative tumor volume ($p <$ or $= 0.001$), postoperative tumor volume ($P = 0.035$) were predictive of PFS
Sanai et al. (2010) [3]	104	Grade III, IV 34 Grade II glioma 70	LGG, EOR = 91–100% (14) LGG EOR = <90% (56)	5 yrs OS for LGG • 100% EOR = 91–100% • 84% EOR = <90%	EOR was predictive of OS ($p = 0.017$) and PFS ($p = 0.0414$)
Skrap et al. (2012) [4]	66 non-enhancing insular glioma 53 LGG	Astrocytomas with gemistocytic foci: 2 Fibrillar astrocytomas: 34	EOR >90% (22) EOR 70–89% (30)	5 years OS 92% EOR >90% 82% EOR 70–89%	EOR ($p < 0.001$), [T2–T1] MRI volume ($p = 0.02$) predictive of OS
Ius et al. (2012) [5]	190 (37, 18–75)	Fibrillary astyrocytoma 98 Oligoastrocytoma 34 Oligodendroglioma 58	EOR >90% (91) EOR 70–89% (69)	5 years OS • 93% EOR >90% • 84% EOR 70–89%	EOR ($p = 0.001$), age ($p = 0.003$), histological subtype ($p = 0.005$), tumor growing pattern value ($p < 0.0001$) were predictive of OS. Histological subtype ($p = 0.003$), EOR ($p < 0.0001$), tumor growing pattern ($p < 0.0001$) were predictive of PFS
Nitta et al. (2013) [6]	153 (37, 15–76)	Astrocytoma 49 Oligoastrocytoma 45 Oligodendroglioma 59	EOR >90% (94) EOR <90% (59)	5 years OS • 98.4% EOR >90% • 89.7% EOR <90%	EOR predictive of OS ($p = 0.0096$) and PFS ($p = 0.0007$) in patients with diffuse astrocytoma

(continued)

Table 7.1 (continued)

Study (year)	Number of cases (medium age, age interval)	Histology	EOR	OS	Predictive survival factors
Capelle et al. (2013) [7]	1771 (37, 4–75)	"Grade II glioma" 1097 gliomas 674 LGG	EOR 100% (80) EOR 50–99% (418) EOR <50% (431)	5 years OS • 100% EOR 100% • 88% EOR 50-99% • 77% EOR <50%	Age >54 years (p = 0.008), tumour volume ($p < 0.0001$), KPS score ($p = 0.0057$)
Kaspera et al. (2013) [8]	68	Astrocytoma 46 Oligodendroglioma 5 Mixed 17	EOR >95% (21) EOR 80–95% (13) EOR <85% (34)	5 years OS • 100% >95% • 100% EOR 80-95% • 81% EOR <85%	Age ($p = 0.032$), rCBV ($p = 0.002$) were predictive of OS Preoperative tumor volume ($p = 0.005$), postoperative tumor volume ($p = 0.008$), the EOR ($p = 0.001$), rCBV ($p = 0.033$) were predictive of PFS
Snyder et al. (2014) [9]	93	All oligodendroglioma	EOR >90% (42) EOR <90% (51)	5 years OS • 90% EOR >90% • 87% EOR <90%	EOR predictive of OS ($p = 0.005$) and PFS ($p = 0.004$)
Coburger et al. (2016) [10]	288 (39, 18–75)	Astrocytoma 173 Oligodendroglioma 52 Mixed 63	EOR 100% (138) EOR <100% (149)	302 months EOR 100% 171 months EOR <100% with failed GTR 162 months for EOR <100% with intended STR	High-field iMRI ($P <$ 0.01) in eloquent location was negatively associated with GTR
Jungk et al. (2016) [11]	46 (35, 17–54)	Astrocytoma	100% (10) 90–99% (11) 41–89% (14) <40% (7)	NA	A greater EOR was prognostic for increased PFS (p = 0.031) and time to re-intervention (TTR) ($p = 0.03$) In IDH1 mutant patients, smaller residual tumor volumes were associated with increased TTR (p = 0.03)

(continued)

Table 7.1 (continued)

Study (year)	Number of cases (medium age, age interval)	Histology	EOR	OS	Predictive survival factors
Roelz et al. (2016) [12]	49 (41.5, 35–60)	Astrocytoma 18 Oligodendroglioma 12 Mixed 19	RTV <15 cm^3 (27) RTV >15 cm^3 (22)	5-years survival • 96% RTV <15 cm^3 • 64% RTV >15 cm^3	Initial resection yielded 5-years OS 82% A significant survival benefit was found for patients with an initial management by resection (5-year OS 82% vs. 54%). The survival benefit of patients with initial resection was reserved to patients with a residual tumor volume of less than 15 cm (3)
Eseonu et al. (2017) [13]	25 (54, 18–80)	"Grade II glioma"	EOR >90% (nd) EOR <90% (nd)	5 years survival • 100% EOR >90% • 90% EOR <90%	EOR predictive of OS ($P = 0.017$), PFS ($P = 0.039$), and malignant PFS ($P = 0.014$) 1p/19q codeletion predictive of PFS ($P = 0.014$)
Eseonu et al. (2017) [14]	109 (37, 19–74)	Astrocytoma 73 Oligodendroglioma 36	EOR 100% (34) EOR 90–99% (25) EOR 70–89% (24)	5 years survival • 95% EOR 100% • 92% EOR 90–99% • 82% EOR 70–89%	OR predictive of OS ($p = 0.029$) and PFS ($p = 0.018$). 1p/19q co-deletion predictive of MPFS ($p = 0.048$)
Patel et al. (2018) [15]	74	Astrocytoma 43 Oligodendroglioma 19 Mixed 12	Median EOR 57.6% Group 1 IDHmut 73.3% Group 2 IDHwt 27.8%	Group 1 95.2% Group 2 55%	Greater EOR independently prolonged MPFS and OS for wtIDH patients, but not for mtIDH patients
Wijnenga et al. (2018) [17]	228 (42, 34–51)	Oligodendroglioma 93 Astrocytoma IDHmut 112 Astrocytoma IDHwt 23	EOR 100% (35) EOR 90–99% (14) EOR 90–94% (22) EOR 41–89% (90) EOR 0–40% (67)	5 years survival • 94% EOR 100% • 91% EOR 90–99% • 84% EOR 90–94% • 88% EOR 41–89% • 56% EOR 0–40%	Postoperative volume predictive of OS ($p = 0.016$)/cm^3 increase in volume

(continued)

Table 7.1 (continued)

Study (year)	Number of cases (medium age, age interval)	Histology	EOR	OS	Predictive survival factors
Hameed et al. (2018) [16]	120 (48, 20–78)	Diffuse astrocytoma IDH1 mutant 56 Diffuse astrocytoma IDH1 wild-type 22 Diffuse astrocytoma NOS 5 Oligodendroglioma IDH1 mutant and 1p/19q-codeleted 25 Oligodendroglioma NOS 7 Oligoastrocytoma NOS 5	EOR >90% (93) EOR <90% (27)	Mean OS 68.51 months	Tumor location predictive of OS ($p = 0.003$) IDH1 associated with giant tumors ($p < 0.001$) EORs were achieved in anterior-zone LGGs ($p = 0.024$)
Ius et al. (2018) [18]	146	Diffuse astrocytoma IDH1 mutant 81 Diffuse astrocytoma IDH1 wild-type 8 oligodendroglioma IDHmut 1p19qcodel 57	Mean EOR 86% (49–100)	5 years survival 74%	KPS, EOR, IDH1 and IDH2 mutations ($p < 0.05$) Nuclear expression of p65 ($P = 0.028$), Ki67 ($P = 0.018$), age ($P = 0.030$), EOR ($P < 0.0001$), high infiltrative pattern index ($P = 0.021$), IDH1/2 mutation ($P < 0.0001$), IDH1/2 mutation and 1p/19q codeletion ($P < 0.0001$)
BØ et al. (2019) [19]	47 (43)	Diffuse astrocytoma IDH1 mutant 20 Diffuse astrocytoma IDH1 wild-type 7 Oligodendroglioma IDHmut 1p19qcodel 19 Oligodendroglioma NOS 1	EOR 100% (14) EOR 90–99% (14) EOR <90% (19)	Significantly better OS with postoperative tumor remnant of less than 10 ml (estimated 5-year survival 94% vs 53%, $p = 0.03$)	Tumour remnants <10 ml ($p = 0.03$)
Cesselli et al. (2019) [20]	241 (39, 19–75)	Diffuse astrocytoma IDH1 mutant 20 Diffuse astrocytoma IDH1 wild-type 7 Oligodendroglioma IDHmut 1p19qcodel 19	Median EOR 86% (range 28–100%)	Median OS: 66 months (range 13–23) Estimated 3-, 5-, and 10-year OS was 84.9%, 72.5%, and 36.8%, respectively	Age at surgery ($p = 0.0001$), tumour location ($p = 0.006$), post-operative volume ($p = 0.027$), EOR ($p = 0.008$)

(continued)

Table 7.1 (continued)

Study (year)	Number of cases (medium age, age interval)	Histology	EOR	OS	Predictive survival factors
Ius et al. (2021) [21]	288 (37.5, 18–74)	DLGG	Cases were stratified according to the surgical protocol that changed over time Group 1: DES; median EOR of 83% Group 2: DES plus functional MRI/DTI images fused on a NeuroNavigation system; median EOR of 88% Group 3: protocol 2 plus RTNT; median EOR 98%	3 years OS: 87.58% 5 years OS: 75.80% 10 years OS: 43.69%	Molecular class (p = 0.028), EOR (p = 0.018), preoperative tumor growing pattern (p = 0.004)
Rossi et al. (2021) [22]	460	LGG 347 IDH mutated 319 IDH wild type 28	Total resection obtained in 39% patients IDH1 mutated Supratotal resection in 35% patients IDH1-mutated	Median PFS in subtotal resection: 29 months (95% CI: 25–36), median PFS in total resection: 46 months (95% CI: 38–48) Median PFS in supratotal resection: 94.0%	EOR associated with PFS (hazard ratio, 0.03; 95% CI: 0.01–0.13)
Ius et al. (2022) [23]	267 (39, 18–71)	Diffuse astrocytoma IDH1/2 mutated 83 Diffuse astrocytoma IDH1/2 wild-type 34 Oligodendroglioma 115	Median EOR achieved: 95%	5 years OS 98.09% 10 years OS 93.2	Lower preoperative tumor volume (p = 0.001) and higher extent of resection (EOR) were predictive of OS (p = 0.037) Early surgery was predictive of TR (p = 0.028)
Hervey-Jumper et al. (2023) [24]	392	IDHmut grade 2 glioma	Three groups according to pre- and post-operative tumor volume	Median OS: 19.9 years	Tumor location (p = 0.02), radiation treatment (p = 0.02), IDH mutation (p < 0.0), ATRX mutation (p < 0.001), 1p19q codel (p < 0.001), p53 mut (p < 0.001)

(continued)

Table 7.1 (continued)

Study (year)	Number of cases (medium age, age interval)	Histology	EOR	OS	Predictive survival factors
Sauvageot et al. (2023) [25]	108 (36)	LGG (WHO grade 2 with possible foci of grade 3 transformation)	Mean extent of resection (EOR): 88.9% ± 7.0%	1 year FU: 100% 5 years FU 80% 10 years FU 58%	EOR > 90% (p = 0.047), residual tumoral volume >15 cm^3 ($p = 0.0058$), pathological features ($p = 0.02$)

OS overall survival, *PFS* progression-free survival, *EOR* extent of resection, *GTR* gross total resection, *STR* subtotal resection, *SUP* supratotal resection, *CR* complete resection, *NTR* near-total resection, *FU* follow up, *WHO* World Health Organization classification, *HGG* high-grade glioma, *HR* hazard ratio, *CI* confidence interval, *NA* not available data, *mut* mutant

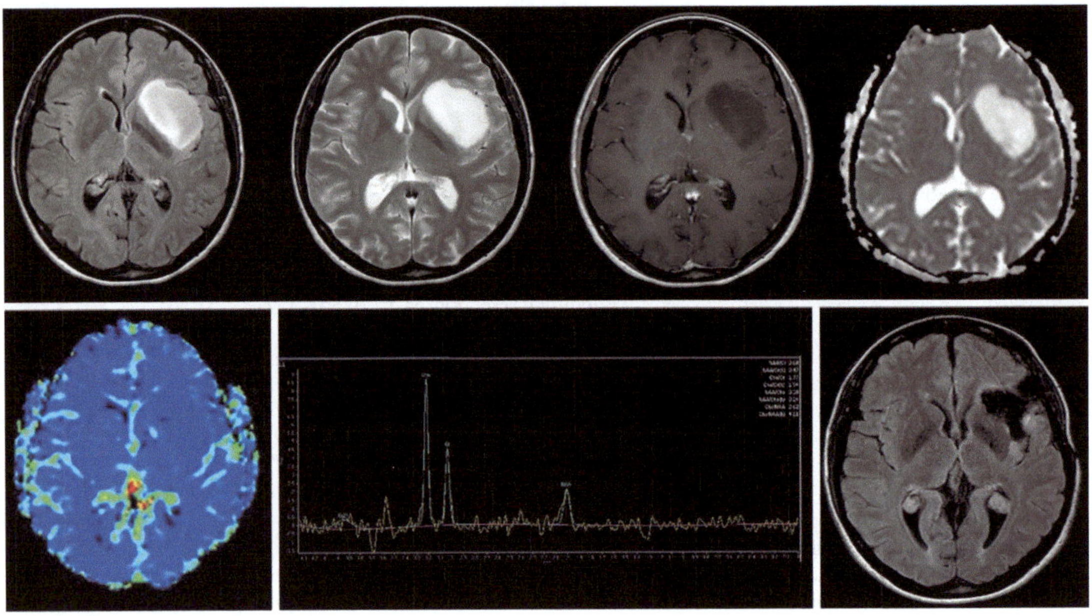

Fig. 7.3 Flowchart depicting the management pathway for incidentally discovered diffuse low-grade gliomas (DLGG) following MRI. *MRI* magnetic resonance imaging, *DLGG* diffuse low-grade glioma, *iDLGG* incidental diffuse low-grade glioma, *PET* positron emission tomography, *GTR* gross total resection, *STR* supratotal resection, *RT* radiotherapy, *CT* chemotherapy

Modern neurosurgical techniques rely on advanced methodologies and technologies such as frameless navigational systems, intraoperative imaging, navigated transcranial magnetic stimulation (nTMS), functional mapping, intraoperative neurophysiological monitoring, real-time neuropsychological testing (RTNT), and awake surgery [19]. The gold standard for brain mapping is represented by awake surgery, considering that it is the only method that permits a real-time direct identification of functional neural networks. Recent investigations have demonstrated that awake surgery (AS) combined with neuropsychological testing resulted in greater EOR and better quality of life for DLGGs involving language and extra-language functional networks [19, 20, 31–35].

Several studies have shown that surgery guided by awake mapping and real-time neuro-

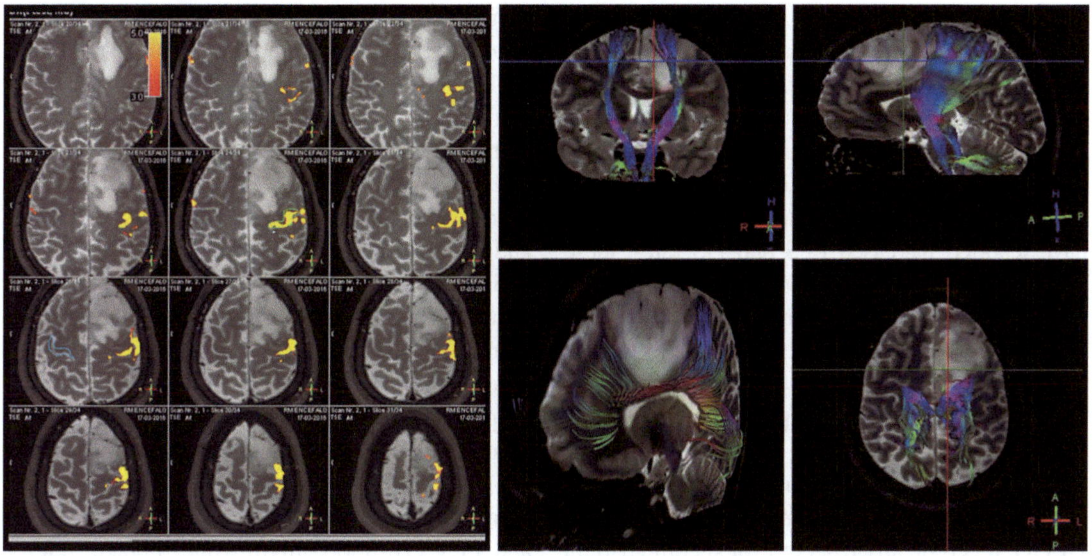

Fig. 7.4 Imaging of a left parietal cortical lesion consistent with an incidental low-grade glioma (LGG). The lesion is characterized by hyperintensity on FLAIR and T2-weighted sequences, lack of diffusion restriction on ADC, absence of significant post-contrast enhancement, and normal perfusion metrics. Spectroscopy findings further corroborate the glioma diagnosis with an altered Cho/NAA ratio. *FLAIR* fluid attenuated inversion recovery, *ADC* apparent diffusion coefficient

psychological testing (RTNT) associated with improved EOR and quality of life, particularly for DLGG affecting both language and extra-language functional networks [19]. While current research suggests that gross total resection is safe and possible, the validity of this statement requires prospective validation. Despite the ongoing emphasis on maximal safe resection in DLGG treatment, there is currently no agreement in the literature on a minimum EOR cut-off value linked with a survival benefit [15].

Furthermore, the impact of the molecular subtypes on EOR classes remains undetermined and the best postoperative treatment still debatable, especially in situations where radical resection is not functionally feasible [35].

Kavouridis et al. discovered that minor volumetric variations across distinct molecular classes influence prognosis [36]. Specifically, in IDH-mutant and IDH-wildtype astrocytoma subtypes, even a 1 cm^3 residual tumor can influence survival, but postoperative residuals greater than 8 cm^3 have an impact on survival in oligodendrogliomas. These findings suggest that postoperative clinical trials assessing adjuvant therapy for DLGG should be stratified by molecular subtype and EOR. Future multicenter studies are necessary to determine the EOR cut-off value, stratified by molecular class, that would benefit from adjuvant therapy, thus optimizing the surgical care of DLGG.

Recent clinical investigations have inquired into the role of supratotal resection (SupTR) in DLGG [37–39]. In this clinical context, SupTR comprises both GTR of the FLAIR signal and the removal of radiographically normal brain tissue surrounding the tumor. The rationale for SupTR is to eradicate invading cells near the radiographic margin of the tumor, as long as the neurologic risks are low [11, 37].

Yordanova et al. reported the first surgical series of SupTR in DLGG in 2011, arguing that it could improve progression-free survival (PFS) and overall survival (OS) outcomes for patients with these tumors [35]. In 2021, Rossi et al. published the largest study on the role of SupTR in DLGG [11]. The authors demonstrated that SupTR considerably improves PFS and OS while decreasing the risk of malignant transformation. Specifically, patients who underwent SupTR had longer PFS and OS than those who had less extensive resections, regardless of molecular class [11]. Despite these hopeful outcomes and developments in surgical procedures, there is still a major study gap on the relationship between the EOR and subsequent cognitive performance in DLGG patients. While preliminary studies from a limited number of canters have reported increased PFS and OS rates, these findings necessitate validation through prospective research involving larger patient cohorts [37–40].

7.4 The Role of Biopsy

Biopsy, as opposed to resection, represents a relatively infrequent approach in the management of DLGG. It is typically reserved for specific patient cohorts, such as elderly individuals, patients with compromised clinical status, significant comorbidities, or tumors located in eloquent areas or in deep-seated regions such as the basal ganglia or brainstem [41, 42].

The diagnostic accuracy and morbidity of stereotactic biopsy using frameless or framelink techniques are similar, with an overall cumulative morbidity and death rate of roughly 2% [43]. DLGG biopsy implies a considerable risk of underestimating the lesion grade, attributed to the extensive intra-tumoral heterogeneity of these lesions, which may harbor micro-foci of malignant transformation [42]. The primary objective of a neuropathological examination is to precisely assess the grade of the glioma. However, when stereotactic needle biopsy is utilized to collect tissue for diagnosis, there is a high risk of sample errors. Muragaki et al. found that 11% of cases resulted in over-grading of WHO grade I gliomas and 28% in under-grading of WHO grade III gliomas [42].

Notably, the integration of advanced imaging techniques (MRI spectroscopy, PET) in the neuronavigation system should be considered in order to increase the accuracy of the biopsy target [43]. Given that tumor biology is predominantly influenced by the most aggressive areas of the glioma, obtaining representative tissue samples is essential for histological diagnosis, prognostication, and treatment planning. However, the capability of MRI to visualize the most rapidly proliferating sections of DLGG is limited, particularly when the tumor lacks contrast enhancement. Ultimately, FDG (18 F-Fluorodeoxyglucose) and FLT ([18 F]deoxy-3fluorothymidine) PET scans typically yield negative results in DLGG and do not provide information on the regional variability of metabolic activity within these tumors. Radiolabeled amino acids demonstrate increased uptake in the majority of diffuse low-grade gliomas, facilitating the optimization of biopsy targeting and reducing the occurrence of non-diagnostic biopsies from nonspecifically altered tissue. Biopsy-controlled studies have revealed correlations between MET (methyonine) and FET (18-fluoroethyltirosine) uptake, micro-vessels proliferation, and cell density in non-contrast-enhancing gliomas; particularly, vascular density is frequently associated with early malignant transformation in gliomas [44–46].

The role of amino acid PET in identifying metabolic hotspots in DLGG for biopsy targeting has been poorly investigated in the current literature [47, 48]. It remains unclear whether the highest amino acid uptake in low-grade gliomas corresponds to the most aggressive tumor regions, necessitating further investigation in future research [49].

In closing, similarly to brain metastases, identifying actionable targets in newly diagnosed and recurrent gliomas is a growing area of research. This emphasizes the importance of minimally invasive yet highly successful approaches for gathering diagnostic material, especially in cases where open microsurgical resection is not functionally possible (e.g., brain stem gliomas) or in situations where diagnosis is the only goal [43, 50].

7.5 Incidental Diffuse Low-Grade Glioma

Incidental diffuse low-grade gliomas (iDLGG) are gliomas detected unintentionally during imaging studies performed for reasons unrelated to suspected brain pathology, such as routine MRI scans for conditions like headaches, trauma, or as part of research studies involving healthy volunteers. This subset of low-grade gliomas is exceptionally rare, with estimated occurrences ranging from 0.04% to 0.2% in the general population [51, 52].

The natural history of iDLGG prior to detection remains poorly understood, and the optimal clinical management of these cases has garnered increasing interest in recent literature. While some recent studies advocate for early surgical resection even in iDLGG cases, the therapeutic approach remains a subject of debate [11, 22, 23, 26, 27] (see Fig. 7.5).

Various studies propose using MRI to monitor tumor growth and guide surgical decisions based on changes in tumor volume; conversely, other research advocates for an immediate surgical approach after conducting second-level diagnostic imaging, including spectroscopic MR [20, 53] (see Fig. 7.6).

A recent multinational study, encompassing the largest cohort of surgically treated iDLGG, revealed a notable 10-year estimated overall survival (OS) rate of 93.2%, significantly surpassing that of symptomatic DLGG. Remarkably, larger preoperative tumor volume independently predicted overall survival, showing an inverse relationship with extent of resection. Tumor recurrence was observed in 38.73% of patients, with earlier surgical intervention significantly delaying recurrence. These findings emphasize the need to treat incidental low-grade gliomas as actively growing tumors rather than inert lesions, emphasizing the crucial role of timely surgical management [52].

7.6 Second Surgery at Tumor Recurrence

It is important to underline that surgery, even in instances of "supratotal" resection, cannot cure DLGG; in addition, considering the invasive nature of DLGG, tumor recurrence (TR), even after radical resection, is nearly certain despite enhancements in long-term outcomes resulting

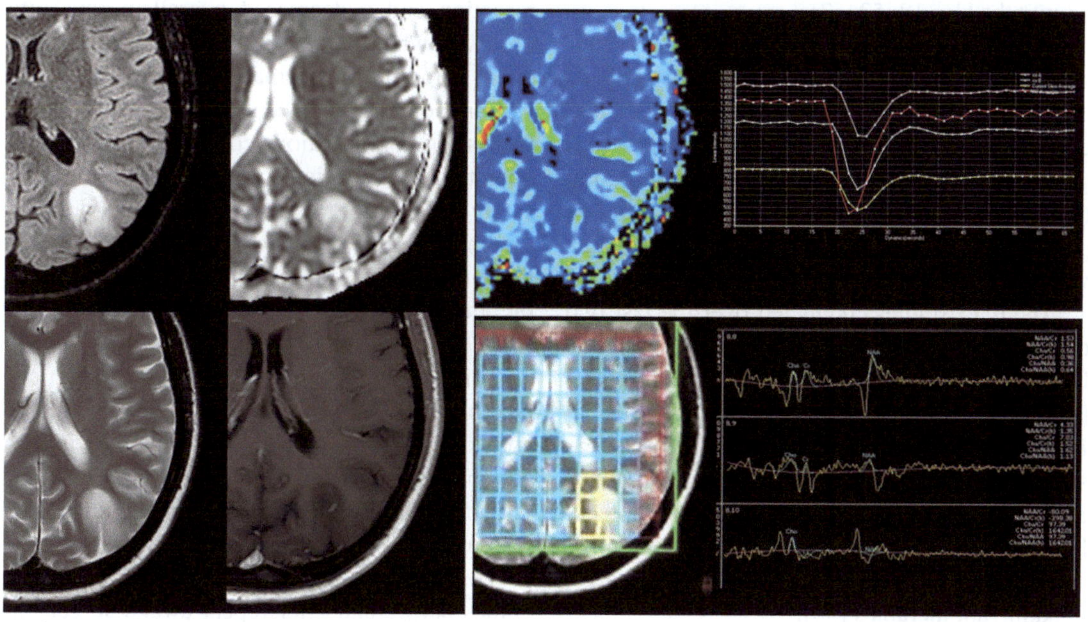

Fig. 7.5 The imaging studies collectively indicate a successful surgical resection of the left parietal low-grade glioma. Postoperative FLAIR and T2-weighted images show a significant reduction in the hyperintense signal associated with the lesion. The absence of contrast enhancement on post-gadolinium T1-weighted images and normal perfusion metrics further support the effective removal of the tumor. Spectroscopy findings corroborate the lack of significant residual tumor activity. *FLAIR* fluid attenuated inversion recovery

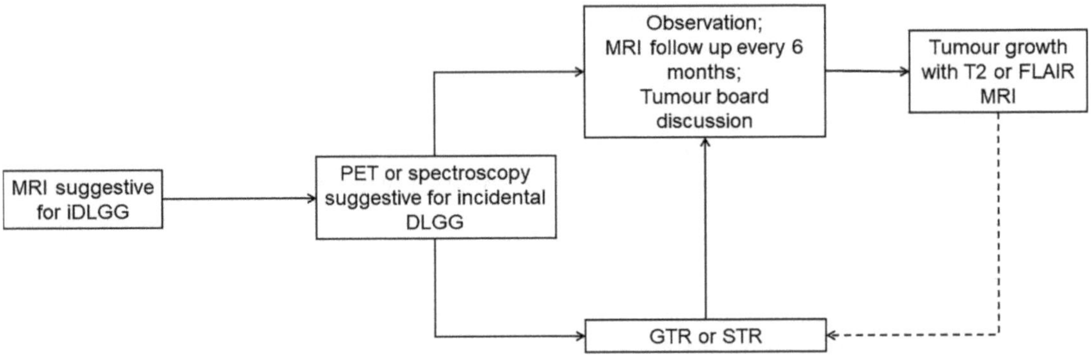

Fig. 7.6 Functional MRI (fMRI) of the patient's motor cortex showing activation in the right hand area during movement tasks, with clusters of activation in the pre-central gyrus. Diffusion tensor imaging (DTI) tracking illustrates the corticospinal tract and corpus callosum fibers

from proactive surgical interventions [32, 37]. According to Yordanova et al., tumor removal guided by FLAIR-weighted images prevented malignant transformation, without adjuvant treatment [35]; however, due to the persistence of isolated tumoral cells well beyond the discernible "glioma" on MRI, 26% of patients experienced recurrence, with a mean delay of approximately 38 months [16, 18, 52, 53].

Recently, reoperations are increasingly considered for patients with DLGG, especially as they are often young, actively employed, and engaged in long-term project [32]. Evidence suggests that achieving maximal extent of resection (EOR) for recurrent DLGG can improve progression-free survival (PFS) and overall survival (OS) [54–58].

About 15 studies conducted over the last two decades have shown that reoperations improve long-term oncological and functional results [14], implying repeated surgery for recurrent DLGG if extensive or near-total resection is feasible [59]. Furthermore, surgery at recurrence allows for histological reassessment and molecular updates, which aid in refining the diagnosis and in guiding future treatment decisions, including adjuvant therapies [30].

Ahmadi et al. observed a significantly OS among patients who underwent a second total resection in the event of relapse without malignant transformation, compared to those who had a single complete resection [60]. Similarly, Shofty et al. discovered that the median time to transformation was significantly prolonged following reoperation (14.4 years), compared to a control group that did not undergo a second surgery (3.5 years, $p = 0.0002$) [58]; the rate of histologically confirmed malignant transformation at reoperation is notably high, ranging between 19% and 74%. Furthermore, a lesser extent of resection and a decreased overall survival are observed when reoperation is performed subsequent to tumor transformation [54, 56–58, 60].

Functionally, repeated surgeries do not elevate the risk of complications compared to the initial operation. All surgical instances confirmed the safety of multiple resections, demonstrating a low incidence of permanent neurological impairment from 0% to 8.5%, which is comparable to the morbidity rate of the initial surgery [54, 56–59].

This trend has been confirmed even in particular brain regions such as eloquent sensorimotor cortex, language structures, and the insula. Notably, these results were obtained by employing intraoperative electrical mapping in awake patients in most of the study groups [54, 57, 61].

Two recent studies investigated cognitive outcomes before and after repeat awake surgery in DLGG patients. They concluded that re-operation in crucial brain regions, along with a comprehensive neuropsychological examination and real-time neurophysiological monitoring, is a safe and successful therapeutic method for recurrent gliomas. Despite the minor risk of neurocognitive impairment associated with re-operation, it is recommended to prioritize early re-intervention over postponing surgery [62, 63].

The modern approach to maximal safe resection in DLGG aims to reduce malignant transformation and extend survival by limiting tumor cell mutations. Early tumor progression, particularly within a year of resection, is linked to poorer outcomes and may predict aggressive tumor behavior, highlighting its importance as a prognostic marker [58].

Overall, these studies highlight that surgery remains a viable option for recurrent or relapsed DLGG, providing therapeutic and diagnostic benefits. The "Multistage Individualized Therapeutic Approach" proposed by Duffau and Taillandier emphasizes the role of surgery at various stages of disease evolution, stressing the importance of tailored management strategies to improve outcomes in patients with recurrent or relapsing DLGG [32].

7.7 Diffuse Low-Grade Glioma and Tumor-Related Epilepsy

Seizure is the most common initial symptom in supratentorial DLGG patients, with a frequency of 60–90% [64]. Tumor-related epilepsy (TRE) often manifests as focal or focal-to-bilateral tonic-clonic seizures, with over 50% of patients showing drug-resistance, severely affecting their quality of life [5, 64]. Effective management of seizure outcomes is crucial in the care of DLGG patients due to their younger age and long potential survival times [65, 66].

Recent studies have suggested that epileptogenesis and tumor growth in DLGG may share common pathogenic pathways, implying that the two conditions are related aspects of a single disease process. Interestingly, glioma-related epilepsy has been linked to a number of genetic abnormalities, including mutations in the isocitrate dehydrogenase genes (IDH1 and IDH2), which are present in between 70% and 80% of cases with DLGG. Due to the capacity for IDH-mutated glioma cells to infiltrate and envelop neurons within the gray matter, these mutations are linked to metabolic alterations that could promote the epileptogenesis [4, 67–69].

Emerging evidence indicates that epileptogenesis and tumor growth are interrelated, with seizures and glioma progression influencing each other [70–77]. Although seizures often recur during malignant progression, their impact on clinical outcomes and their temporal relationship with tumor progression in DLGG are not completed understood.

A growing body of surgical literature is provindig the role of the extent of resection on seizure outcome in this scenario (Table 7.2). In a pioneering volumetric investigation, Xu et al. showed that an EOR >80% corresponds to a threshold for long-term seizure independence [70].

A larger, methodologically sound multicenter study later by Still et al. showed that postoperative seizure control in individuals with supratentorial DLGG was more likely when EOR was 91% and/or the residual tumor volume was approximately 19 c [69].

In 2014, Ius et al. demonstrated that greater percent of tumor resection and decreasing post-operative tumor volume resulted in increased rates of Engel I classification in insular DLGG [67]. In a subsequent study in 2020, the same authors used area under the receiver operating curve (AUROC) analysis to determine that an EOR of 85% predicted Engel IA (completely seizure-free since surgery) classification with a 72.9% accuracy [23].

In addition, hippocampectomy and corticectomy, combined with lesionectomy, have been shown to improve seizure control in patients with temporal DLGG and intractable preoperative epilepsy [74]. Intraoperative electrocorticography (ECoG) aids in identifying irritative cortical areas with interictal spikes, improving postoperative seizure outcomes in pharmacoresistant cases [75]. However, the accuracy of neurophysiological approaches to detect distant epileptogenic foci and track epileptic activity spread remains low [78]. New prospective studies combining intraoperative direct electrical stimulation (DES) and ECoG are needed to optimize surgical outcomes.

Table 7.2 Tumor-related epilepsy outcome in DLGG: a literature review according to the EOR

Authors (year)	No. of cases (mean age, age interval)	Histology	EOR%	Clinical onset	Postoperative Seizures (Engel class I and (%)	Factors related to seizure outcome
Chang et al. (2008) [1]	332 (39.3, 16–95)	All grade II Astrocytoma 129 (38.9%) 95 (28.6%) 109 (32.8%)	Surgical data available for 253 pts: Subtotal 141 (56%) GTR 83 (33%) Biopsy 24 (9%)	Seizures 269 (81%)	6 months FU available for 137 pts Class I 110 (80.3%) FU at 12 months available for 114 pts Class I 90 (78.9%)	GTR vs STR/biopsy for seizure control: odds ratio 16, 95% confidence interval 2.2–124, p = 0.0064) Seizure recurrence after initial postoperative seizure control associated with tumor progression ($p = 0.001$)
You et al. (2012) [2]	508 (38.1, 16–72)	229 astrocytomas (45.1%), 48 oligodendroglioma (9.4%) 231 oligoastrocytoma (45.5%)	GTR 120 (36.5%) STR 209 (63.5%)	Seizures 350 (68.9%)	At 6months FU Class I 65.3% At 12 months FU Class 1 62.5%	Secondary generalized seizure (P 5.006), calcification on MRI ($p = 0.031$), gross total resection than after subtotal resection ($P <$ 0.0001) were associated with favourable prognosis
Pallud et al. (2014) [3]	1509 (<30 years = 390 cases 30–45 years = 726 cases)	327 astrocytoma 781 oligoastrocytoma 280 mixed glioma 121 missing	<100 cm^3 808 cases (53.54%) >100 cm^3 346 cases (22.92%), missing cases 355 (23, 54)	NA	NA	Gender, tumour location within functional areas, tumour volume, growth velocity, cortical location, histopathological subtype, molecular markers
Liubinas et al. (2014) [4]	30 LGG	22 astrocytoma 6 oligoastrocytoma 1 mixed oligoastrocytoma and Protoplasmic Astrocytoma 1 oligodendroglioma	NA	Seizures 23 cases (76.66%)	NA	IDH1-R132H mutation
Mulligan et al. (2014) [5]	62 LGG	62 oligodendroglioma	NA	Seizures 48 cases (77.41%)	NA	1p19q co-deletion status, mutant IDH1-R132H expression, tumor location, or enhancement status
Ius et al. (2014) [6]	52 LGG	32 astrocytoma 11 oligoastrocytoma 9 oligodendroglioma	87% >90% 21 cases 70–89% 23 cases <70% 8 cases	NA	35 cases (67.30%)	EOR, difference between the preoperative T2- and T1-weighted MR images (ΔVT2T1)

Yang et al. (2015) [7]	112 (34, 39.8–42.2)	64 WHO II 58 WHO III 48 WHO IV	NA	Seizures 74 cases (42.3%)	NA	IDH ½ mutation
Zhong et al. (2015) [8]	311 (38)	140 astrocytoma 140 oligoastrocytoma 31 oligodendroglioma	NA	Seizures 183 cases (58.84%)	211 cases (67.84%)	IDH1/2 mutation
Chen et al. (2017) [9]	712 gliomas	77 WHO II 128 WHO III 507 WHO IV	NA	Seizures 276 cases (38.76%)	NA	1p/19q codeletion, and temporal lobe location, showed that IDH1mut was an independent correlate with seizures
Neal et al. (2018) [10]	100 (age 50.2 ± 17.5)	70 HGG 20 astrocytoma 10 oligoastrocytoma/ oligodendroglioma	15 PR 42 ST 37 GTR 6 unknown	Seizures 52 cases (52%)	58 cases (58%)	IDH1-R132H mutations are associated with a more severe phenotype of postoperative epilepsy
Xu et al. (2018) [11]	128 (40.8)	18 astrocytoma 86 oligodendroglioma 24 oligoastrocytoma	90–99% 64 cases 80–89% 11 cases	All presenting with seizures	105 cases (82.03%)	EOR
Roberts et al. (2018)	63 (34)	36 oligodendroglioma (57%) 27 astrocytoma (42.8%) 53 IDH mut (84%)	9 complete resection (50%) 6 near-total resection (33%) 3 sub-total resection (17%)	Seizures 45 (71%)	Median FU 43 months: class I 33 (73%)	GTR and NTR were associated with improved Engel class compared to STR
Yao et al. (2018)	108 (average btw 27 ± 14.2 and 25.4 ± 14.8)	23 astrocytoma 13 mixed oligoastrocytoma 24 oligodendroglioma 18 ganglioganglioma	54 pts GTR + ECoG guided epileptolegine locus 54 pts GTR only	All presenting with refractory seizures	Group I Class I 40 (74%) Group II Class I 21 (39%)	Tumor location, intraoperative ECoG monitoring
Still et al. (2019) [12]	346 (35)	48 astrocytoma 298 oligodendroglioma	100% 50 cases 90–99% 92 cases; 50–89% 134 cases <50% 70 cases	All presenting with seizures	227 cases (65.60%)	EOR and residual tumour volume

(continued)

Table 7.2 (continued)

Authors (year)	No. of cases (mean age, age interval)	Histology	EOR%	Clinical onset	Postoperative Seizures (Engel class I and (%)	Factors related to seizure outcome
Ius et al. (2020) [13]	155 (37, 18–73)	44 oligodendroglioma IDH1/2 mutated 1p-19q codeleted (28.39%) Astrocytoma IDH 1/2 mutated 1p-19q non-codeleted 93 (60.00%) Astrocytoma IDH 1/2 wild type 18 (11.61%)	88 (38–100)	Seizures	Class I 110 (7.097%)	Age ($p = 0.014$), EOR ($p = 0.030$), ΔT2T1 MRI index ($p = 0.016$) resulted as independent predictors of postoperative seizure control
Tan et al. (2023) [14]	87 (42.24, 14–50)	42 WHO II (48.3%) 45 WHO III (51.7%)	70.78 (56.4–84)	Seizures 36 (41.4%)	At 1 year FU Class IA 59 (74%) Class IB 9 (11.4%) Class IC 0 Class ID 2 (2.5%)	Perirolandic involvement (HR 0.10; 95% CI: 0.02e0.46; $p = 0.005$) and preoperative seizures (HR 0.14; 95% CI: 0.02e0.62; $p = 0.017$) conferred a lower likelihood of durable seizure control, whereas increased extent of resection (HR 1.07; 95% CI: 1.03e1.12; $p = 0.003$) enhanced the likelihood of seizure freedom
Bono et al. (2024) [73]	52 (39, 32–48)	28 WHO grade 2 (54%) 24 WHO 3 (46%)	13 SUP/CR (32%) 12 NTR (29%) 16 STR (39%)	Seizures 40 pts	At 1 year FU class I 38 (32–47)	MET PET–derived semiquantitative data. With higher TBRmax ($p = 0.0192$) and TBRmean ($p = 0.0128$) values related to uncontrolled seizures 1 year after surgery

OS overall survival, *PFS* progression-free survival, *EOR* extent of resection, *GTR* gross total resection, *STR* subtotal resection, *SUP* supratotal resection, *CR* complete resection, *NTR* near-total resection, *FU* follow up, *WHO* World Health Organization classification, *HGG* high-grade glioma, *HR* hazard ratio, *CI* confidence interval, *NA* not available data

Recently, Bono et al. demonstrated the potential of preoperative [11C]methionine PET in identifying epileptogenic foci outside the lesion and predicting postoperative seizure outcomes in temporal lobe low-grade gliomas. These findings suggest the utility of qualitative and semi-quantitative analysis of MET PET in delineating seizure characteristics during surgery, guiding the process of tumor resection and patient management [79].

With regards to glioma evolution over time, Mazzucchi et al. investigated the relationship between postoperative seizure outcome and survival in DLGG patients [80]. Through their clinical retrospective study, the authors revealed a noteworthy association between the persistence of seizures after tumor removal and decreased survival rates in this patient population. This finding aligns with and extends upon previous research that has identified seizures as a prognostic factor in glioma patients. For example, a study by Pallud et al. demonstrated that the presence of preoperative seizures and early surgical resections were associated with favorable outcomes in patients with low-grade glioma, highlighting the relevance of seizure management in improving patient prognosis [4]. Furthermore, the study by Englot et al. provided evidence suggesting that seizures may influence glioma biology, potentially affecting tumor growth and progression [72]. Specifically, patients who continued to experience seizures postoperatively exhibited markedly poorer survival rates compared to those who became seizure-free following surgery. These results highlight the detrimental effect of persistent seizures on the prognosis of DLGG patients, emphasizing the importance of effectively managing postoperative seizure control to improve overall survival outcomes. In light of these findings, Mazzucchi et al.'s study underscores the importance of comprehensive seizure management strategies in the treatment of DLGG patients, not only for improving quality of life but also for potentially extending survival outcomes [80]. Furthermore, it enhances the need for further investigation into the underlying mechanisms linking seizures and glioma biology to inform more effective therapeutic approaches in the future.

7.8 Malignant Transformation

DLGG patients may preserve occupational and cognitive performance for long time. However, this stability can be deceiving, as DLGGs eventually advance unpredictably toward malignant forms, indicating a pivotal and irreversible stage in their development. The unpredictable timing of this malignant change hampers decisions about when to engage therapeutically, potentially leading to arbitrary choices [13].

Recognizing the non-linear and unpredictable progression of malignant transformation (MT) is crucial for developing effective treatments, given the potential neurological risks associated with interventions like surgery or radiotherapy. Studies report a wide range, from 25% to 72%, in the frequency of DLGG MT, highlighting its variable and likely multifaceted nature. Previous research has focused largely on general prognostic factors established before the 2016 WHO classification update, such as premotor or insular areas, Karnofsky performance score (KPS) above 80, age under 50, and tumor diameter less than 4 cm [8].

DLGG, with heterogeneous molecular, clinical, and histological characteristics, present a not fully understood natural history ranging from indolent to biologically aggressive behavior that inevitably culminates in neurological decline and death due to malignant transformation [19].

Currently, there are no integrated analyses in the literature that combine data on EOR and molecular classes for DLGG in light of the 2021 WHO classification on large case series.

Satar et al. conducted a robust well-designed systematic analysis to investigate various parameters associated with the DLGG MT, including tumor volume and expansion velocity, regional blood flow and topography, clinical features, and tissue-based post-surgery prognosticators [13]. The authors detected 33 qualifying articles, including 5672 patients and detecting 10 prognosticators for MT: (1) presentation with epileptic seizures, (2) velocity of tumor growth (VDE) >8 mm/year, (3) VDE >4 mm/year, (4) rCBV >1.75, (5) PTV ≥5 cm (65 ml), (6) PTV ≥100 ml, (7) cortical involvement, (8) IDH-wt, (9) TP53 mutation, and (10) TMZ monotherapy [13].

Tumor volume and expansion velocity were recurrently identified as crucial factors, despite showing different numerical thresholds in several studies [2, 9, 19, 81].

For example, a "nearly-randomized" trial by Roelz et al. reported that survival benefit was recorded in patients with residual tumor volume of <15 cm^3; conversely, those whose residual volumes did not meet this threshold had outcomes similar to those who underwent biopsy only instead of surgery [6, 82].

The role of velocity of tumor growth (VDE) was highlighted in different studies, with thresholds ranging from ≥4 mm/year to ≥12 cm/year. Studies showed that DLGG with VDE ≥12 cm/year are rare, with accepted thresholds typically set at ≥4 mm and ≥8 mm/year, the latter indicating worse prognostication [6].

As it comes to the extent of resection (EOR), several studies suggested that a minimum EOR of >90% of the original volume as needed for a definite survival benefit. Moreover, residual tumor volumes post-surgery were largely associated with varying degrees of survival benefit, with larger volumes correlating with poorer outcomes [81].

Furthermore, also regional blood flow, quantified by relative cerebral blood flow (rCBF), was linked to malignant transformation (MT). A threshold of rCBF = 1.742 showed a favorable combination of sensitivity and specificity for predicting MT; in addition, cortical and subventricular zone (SVZ) involvement were independently associated with MT [83].

In conclusion, several factors such as tumor volume, growth rate, regional blood flow, clinical characteristics, and tissue-based markers are critical in forecasting the transformation of DLGG into malignant forms. Comprehending these elements can facilitate the development of more effective and proactive treatment approaches to enhance the prognosis of DLGG patients.

7.9 Future Perspectives

Advancements in surgical techniques, intraoperative mapping modalities, and adjuvant therapies have significantly improved outcomes for patients with diffuse DLGG. However, the field continues to evolve, with ongoing research and innovative approaches paving the way for future advancements and personalized treatments.

One of the most exciting avenues for future research in DLGG lies in precision medicine and molecular profiling. Recent studies have highlighted the heterogeneity of DLGG, emphasizing the importance of molecular classification in predicting tumor behavior and treatment response. Integrating molecular information into clinical decision-making can enable personalized treatment strategies tailored to the specific molecular profile of each tumor. By identifying targetable molecular alterations and predictive biomarkers, precision medicine holds the potential to optimize therapeutic efficacy while minimizing treatment-related toxicity [84, 85].

Immunotherapy and targeted therapies represent promising avenues for the treatment of DLGGs. Immune checkpoint inhibitors, chimeric antigen receptor (CAR) T-cell therapy, and tumor-specific vaccines have shown encouraging results in preclinical and early clinical studies [86].

By harnessing the power of the immune system to recognize and eliminate tumor cells, immunotherapy offers a novel approach to combating DLGG. Similarly, targeted therapies directed against specific molecular pathways implicated in gliomagenesis hold promise for improving treatment outcomes. Continued research into novel immunotherapeutic agents and targeted inhibitors, as well as the development of combination strategies, will be critical for advancing the field [87].

Minimally invasive surgical techniques have gained traction in the management of DLGG, offering potential benefits such as reduced surgical morbidity and shorter recovery times. Emerging technologies, such as laser interstitial thermal therapy (LITT) and focused ultrasound, enable precise tumor ablation while minimizing damage to surrounding healthy tissue [88].

Furthermore, advances in intraoperative imaging modalities, such as intraoperative MRI and fluorescence-guided surgery, enhance the accuracy of tumor resection and facilitate maximal safe resection. Continued refinement of minimally invasive approaches and integration with adjunctive therapies will likely play a significant role in shaping the future of DLGG surgery.

The identification of reliable biomarkers for DLGG remains a key area of research. Liquid biopsies, which analyze circulating tumor DNA (ctDNA) and other biomarkers in peripheral blood, offer a non-invasive method for monitoring disease progression, predicting treatment response, and detecting early recurrence. By providing real-time information about tumor dynamics and evolution, liquid biopsies hold promise for guiding treatment decisions and improving patient outcomes [89].

7.10 Conclusions

DLGG remains a challenging entity in neuro-oncology. In the last decades, DLGG surgery has evolved into a dynamic field, characterized by a multidisciplinary approach aimed at optimizing oncological outcomes and preserving quality of life. Insights gleaned from navigating temporal challenges provide a roadmap for future advancements in DLGG management, emphasizing the importance of personalized treatment algorithms tailored to each patient's unique clinical trajectory. In the progression of DLGG glioma over time, surgery plays a crucial role at all stages, including incidental discoveries, symptomatic cases, and tumor recurrence.

The most recent WHO classification of gliomas includes genetic profiles as well as histological features, resulting in subclasses with distinct biological behaviors and prognostic outcomes. The emergence of molecular profiling has revolutionized DLGG classification, allowing for tailored treatment strategies and prognostication. Particularly, the incorporation of molecular markers into surgical decision-making has refined prognostic stratification and guided adjuvant therapy selection; new targeted therapies and immunotherapy involving the mutated IDH protein could improve the outcome in selected cases. In this evolving clinical setting, it is essential to emphasize that surgery plays a key and fundamental role for patients in all stages of glioma evolution—incidental, symptomatic, and tumor recurrence—by improving survival, controlling disease progression, preventing malignant transformation, and optimizing epileptological outcomes. This underscores the critical importance of achieving maximal safe resection in DLGG patients.

References

1. Louis DN, Perry A, Wesseling P, et al. The 2021 WHO classification of tumors of the central nervous system: a summary. Neuro-Oncology. 2021;23(8):1231–51. https://doi.org/10.1093/neuonc/noab106.
2. Ostrom QT, Cioffi G, Gittleman H, et al. CBTRUS statistical report: primary brain and other central nervous system tumors diagnosed in the United States in 2012–2016. Neuro-Oncology. 2019;21(5):1–100. https://doi.org/10.1093/neuonc/noz150.
3. Youssef G, Miller JJ. Lower grade gliomas. Curr Neurol Neurosci Rep. 2020;20(7):21. https://doi.org/10.1007/s11910-020-01040-8.
4. Pallud J, Audureau E, Blonski M, et al. Epileptic seizures in diffuse low-grade gliomas in adults. Brain. 2014;137(2):449–62. https://doi.org/10.1093/brain/awt345.
5. Ruda R, Bello L, Duffau H, Soffietti R. Seizures in low-grade gliomas: natural history, pathogenesis, and outcome after treatments. Neuro-Oncology. 2012;14(4):55–64. https://doi.org/10.1093/neuonc/nos199.
6. Pallud J, Mandonnet E, Duffau H, et al. Prognostic value of initial magnetic resonance imaging growth rates for World Health Organization grade II gliomas. Ann Neurol. 2006;60(3):380–3. https://doi.org/10.1002/ana.20946.
7. Pallud J, Blonski M, Mandonnet E, et al. Velocity of tumor spontaneous expansion predicts long-term outcomes for diffuse low-grade gliomas. Neuro-Oncology. 2013;15(5):595–606. https://doi.org/10.1093/neuonc/nos331.
8. Sanai N, Berger MS. Surgical oncology for gliomas: the state of the art. Nat Rev Clin Oncol. 2018;15(2):112–25. https://doi.org/10.1038/nrclinonc.2017.171.
9. Ius T, Isola M, Budai R, et al. Low-grade glioma surgery in eloquent areas: volumetric analysis of extent of resection and its impact on overall survival. A single-institution experience in 190 patients: clinical article. J Neurosurg. 2012;117(6):1039–52. https://doi.org/10.3171/2012.8.JNS12393.
10. Capelle L, Fontaine D, Mandonnet E, et al. Spontaneous and therapeutic prognostic factors in adult hemispheric World Health Organization Grade II gliomas: a series of 1097 cases: clinical article. JNS. 2013;118(6):1157–68. https://doi.org/10.3171/2013.1.JNS121.
11. Rossi M, Gay L, Ambrogi F, et al. Association of supratotal resection with progression-free survival, malignant transformation, and overall survival in lower-

grade gliomas. Neuro-Oncology. 2021;23(5):812–26. https://doi.org/10.1093/neuonc/noaa225.
12. Jakola AS, Bouget D, Reinertsen I, et al. Spatial distribution of malignant transformation in patients with low-grade glioma. J Neuro-Oncol. 2020;146(2):373–80. https://doi.org/10.1007/s11060-020-03391-1.
13. Satar Z, Hotton G, Samandouras G. Systematic review—time to malignant transformation in low-grade gliomas: predicting a catastrophic event with clinical, neuroimaging, and molecular markers. Neuro-Oncol Adv. 2021;3(1):vdab101. https://doi.org/10.1093/noajnl/vdab101.
14. Ng S, Duffau H. Brain plasticity profiling as a key support to therapeutic decision-making in low-grade glioma oncological strategies. Cancer. 2023;15(14):3698. https://doi.org/10.3390/cancers15143698.
15. Lombardi G, Barresi V, Castellano A, et al. Clinical management of diffuse low-grade gliomas. Cancer. 2020;12(10):3008. https://doi.org/10.3390/cancers12103008.
16. Mandonnet E, De Witt Hamer P, Pallud J, Bauchet L, Whittle I, Duffau H. Silent diffuse low-grade glioma: toward screening and preventive treatment? Cancer. 2014;120(12):1758–62. https://doi.org/10.1002/cncr.28610.
17. Youland RS, Schomas DA, Brown PD, et al. Changes in presentation, treatment, and outcomes of adult low-grade gliomas over the past fifty years. Neuro-Oncology. 2013;15(8):1102–10. https://doi.org/10.1093/neuonc/not080.
18. Mandonnet E, Delattre JY, Tanguy ML, et al. Continuous growth of mean tumor diameter in a subset of grade II gliomas. Ann Neurol. 2003;53(4):524–8. https://doi.org/10.1002/ana.10528.
19. Ius T, Mazzucchi E, Tomasino B, et al. Multimodal integrated approaches in low grade glioma surgery. Sci Rep. 2021;11(1):9964. https://doi.org/10.1038/s41598-021-87924-2.
20. Cesselli D, Ius T, Isola M, et al. Application of an artificial intelligence algorithm to prognostically stratify grade II gliomas. Cancer. 2019;12(1):50. https://doi.org/10.3390/cancers12010050.
21. Mandonnet E, Pallud J, Fontaine D, et al. Inter- and intrapatients comparison of WHO grade II glioma kinetics before and after surgical resection. Neurosurg Rev. 2010;33(1):91–6. https://doi.org/10.1007/s10143-009-0229-x.
22. Mandonnet E, Pallud J, Clatz O, et al. Computational modeling of the WHO grade II glioma dynamics: principles and applications to management paradigm. Neurosurg Rev. 2008;31(3):263–9. https://doi.org/10.1007/s10143-008-0128-6.
23. Ius T, Pauletto G, Tomasino B, et al. Predictors of postoperative seizure outcome in low grade glioma: from volumetric analysis to molecular stratification. Cancer. 2020;12(2):397. https://doi.org/10.3390/cancers12020397.
24. van Westrhenen A, Senders JT, Martin E, DiRisio AC, Broekman MLD. Clinical challenges of glioma and pregnancy: a systematic review. J Neuro-Oncol. 2018;139(1):1–11. https://doi.org/10.1007/s11060-018-2851-3.
25. Somma T, Bove I, Vitulli F, Cappabianca P, Pessina F, Alviggi C, Santi L, Della Pepa GM, Sabatino G, Olivi A, Ius T. Management and treatment of brain tumors during pregnancy: an Italian survey. J Neuro-Oncol. 2023;161(1):13–22. https://doi.org/10.1007/s11060-022-04215-0.
26. Sanai N, Polley MY, Berger MS. Insular glioma resection: assessment of patient morbidity, survival, and tumor progression. J Neurosurg. 2010;112(1):1–9. https://doi.org/10.3171/2009.6.JNS0952.
27. Coburger J, Merkel A, Scherer M, et al. Low-grade glioma surgery in intraoperative magnetic resonance imaging: results of a multicenter retrospective assessment of the German Study Group for Intraoperative Magnetic Resonance Imaging. Neurosurgery. 2016;78(6):775–86. https://doi.org/10.1227/NEU.0000000000001081.
28. Wijnenga MMJ, French PJ, Dubbink HJ, et al. The impact of surgery in molecularly defined low-grade glioma: an integrated clinical, radiological, and molecular analysis. Neuro-Oncology. 2018;20(1):103–12. https://doi.org/10.1093/neuonc/nox176.
29. Hervey-Jumper SL, Berger MS. Maximizing safe resection of low- and high-grade glioma. J Neuro-Oncol. 2016;130(2):269–82. https://doi.org/10.1007/s11060-016-2110-4.
30. Weller M, Van Den Bent M, Preusser M, et al. EANO guidelines on the diagnosis and treatment of diffuse gliomas of adulthood. Nat Rev Clin Oncol. 2021;18(3):170–86. https://doi.org/10.1038/s41571-020-00447-z.
31. Clark VE, Cahill DP. Extent of resection versus molecular classification: what matters when? Neurosurg Clin N Am. 2019;30(1):95–101. https://doi.org/10.1016/j.nec.2018.08.006.
32. Duffau H, Taillandier L. New concepts in the management of diffuse low-grade glioma: proposal of a multistage and individualized therapeutic approach. Neuro-Oncology. 2015;17(3):332–42. https://doi.org/10.1093/neuonc/nou153.
33. Duffau H. Is non-awake surgery for supratentorial adult low-grade glioma treatment still feasible? Neurosurg Rev. 2018;41(1):133–9. https://doi.org/10.1007/s10143-017-0918-9.
34. Szelényi A, Bello L, Duffau H, et al. Intraoperative electrical stimulation in awake craniotomy: methodological aspects of current practice. Neurosurg Focus. 2010;28(2):E7. https://doi.org/10.3171/2009.12.FOCUS09237.
35. Yordanova YN, Moritz-Gasser S, Duffau H. Awake surgery for WHO Grade II gliomas within "non-eloquent" areas in the left dominant hemisphere: toward a "supratotal" resection: clinical article. JNS.

2011;115(2):232–9. https://doi.org/10.3171/2011.3.JNS101333.
36. Kavouridis VK, Boaro A, Dorr J, et al. Contemporary assessment of extent of resection in molecularly defined categories of diffuse low-grade glioma: a volumetric analysis. J Neurosurg. 2019;133(5):1291–301. https://doi.org/10.3171/2019.6.JNS19972.
37. Duffau H. Long-term outcomes after supratotal resection of diffuse low-grade gliomas: a consecutive series with 11-year follow-up. Acta Neurochir. 2016;158(1):51–8. https://doi.org/10.1007/s00701-015-2621-3.
38. Rudà R, Angileri FF, et al. Italian consensus and recommendations on diagnosis and treatment of low-grade gliomas. An intersociety (SINch/AINO/SIN) document. J Neurosurg Sci. 2020;64(4):313–34. https://doi.org/10.23736/S0390-5616.20.04982-6.
39. Kreatsoulas D, Damante M, Gruber M, Duru O, Elder JB. Supratotal surgical resection for low-grade glioma: a systematic review. Cancer. 2023;15:2493. https://doi.org/10.3390/cancers15092493.
40. de Leeuw CN, Vogelbaum MA. Supratotal resection in glioma: a systematic review. Neuro-Oncology. 2019;21(2):179–88. https://doi.org/10.1093/neuonc/noy166.
41. Pedeutour-Braccini Z, Burel-Vandenbos F, Gozé C, et al. Microfoci of malignant progression in diffuse low-grade gliomas: towards the creation of an intermediate grade in glioma classification? Virchows Arch. 2015;466(4):433–44. https://doi.org/10.1007/s00428-014-1712-5.
42. Muragaki Y, Chernov M, Maruyama T, et al. Low-grade glioma on stereotactic biopsy: how often is the diagnosis accurate? Minim Invasive Neurosurg. 2008;51(5):275–9. https://doi.org/10.1055/s-0028-1082322.
43. Katzendobler S, Do A, Weller J, et al. Diagnostic yield and complication rate of stereotactic biopsies in precision medicine of gliomas. Front Neurol. 2022;13:822362. https://doi.org/10.3389/fneur.2022.822362.
44. Kracht LW, Friese M, Herholz K, et al. Methyl-[11C]-l-methionine uptake as measured by positron emission tomography correlates to microvessel density in patients with glioma. Eur J Nucl Med Mol Imaging. 2003;30(6):868–73. https://doi.org/10.1007/s00259-003-1148-7.
45. Stockhammer F, Plotkin M, Amthauer H, Van Landeghem FKH, Woiciechowsky C. Correlation of F-18-fluoro-ethyl-tyrosin uptake with vascular and cell density in non-contrast-enhancing gliomas. J Neuro-Oncol. 2008;88(2):205–10. https://doi.org/10.1007/s11060-008-9551-3.
46. Okita Y, Kinoshita M, Goto T, et al. 11C-methionine uptake correlates with tumor cell density rather than with microvessel density in glioma: a stereotactic image-histology comparison. NeuroImage. 2010;49(4):2977–82. https://doi.org/10.1016/j.neuroimage.2009.11.024.
47. Santo G, Laudicella R, Linguanti F, et al. The utility of conventional amino acid PET radiotracers in the evaluation of glioma recurrence also in comparison with MRI. Diagnostics. 2022;12(4):844. https://doi.org/10.3390/diagnostics12040844.
48. Bapuraj JR, Perni K, Gomez-Hassan D, Srinivasan A. Imaging surveillance of gliomas. Radiol Clin North Am. 2021;59(3):395–407. https://doi.org/10.1016/j.rcl.2021.01.006.
49. Rapp M, Heinzel A, Galldiks N, et al. Diagnostic performance of ^{18}F-FET PET in newly diagnosed cerebral lesions suggestive of glioma. J Nucl Med. 2013;54(2):229–35. https://doi.org/10.2967/jnumed.112.109603.
50. Ius T, Montemurro N, Lombardi G, et al. Decoding the puzzle: a multidisciplinary systematic review of adult brainstem glioma. Crit Rev Oncol Hematol. 2024;196:104261. https://doi.org/10.1016/j.critrevonc.2024.104261.
51. Eskandary H, Sabba M, Khajehpour F, Eskandari M. Incidental findings in brain computed tomography scans of 3000 head trauma patients. Surg Neurol. 2005;63(6):550–3. https://doi.org/10.1016/j.surneu.2004.07.049.
52. Ius T, Ng S, Young JS, et al. The benefit of early surgery on overall survival in incidental low-grade glioma patients: a multicenter study. Neuro-Oncology. 2022;24(4):624–38. https://doi.org/10.1093/neuonc/noab210.
53. Boetto J, Ng S, Duffau H. Predictive evolution factors of incidentally discovered suspected low-grade gliomas: results from a consecutive series of 101 patients. Neurosurgery. 2021;88(4):797–803. https://doi.org/10.1093/neuros/nyaa532.
54. Ius T, Pauletto G, Cesselli D, et al. Second surgery in insular low-grade gliomas. Biomed Res Int. 2015;2015:1–11. https://doi.org/10.1155/2015/497610.
55. Kaspera W, Majchrzak K, Bobek-Billewicz B, et al. Reoperations of patients with low-grade gliomas in eloquent or near eloquent brain areas. Neurol Neurochir Pol. 2013;47(2):116–25. https://doi.org/10.5114/ninp.2013.34399.
56. Ramakrishna R, Hebb A, Barber J, Rostomily R, Silbergeld D. Outcomes in reoperated low-grade gliomas. Neurosurgery. 2015;77(2):175–84. https://doi.org/10.1227/NEU.0000000000000753.
57. Morshed RA, Young JS, Han SJ, Hervey-Jumper SL, Berger MS. Perioperative outcomes following reoperation for recurrent insular gliomas. J Neurosurg. 2019;131(2):467–73. https://doi.org/10.3171/2018.4.JNS18375.
58. Shofty B, Haim O, Costa M, et al. Impact of repeated operations for progressive low-grade gliomas. Eur J Surg Oncol. 2020;46(12):2331–7. https://doi.org/10.1016/j.ejso.2020.07.013.

59. Uppstrom TJ, Singh R, Hadjigeorgiou GF, Magge R, Ramakrishna R. Repeat surgery for recurrent low-grade gliomas should be standard of care. Clin Neurol Neurosurg. 2016;151:18–23. https://doi.org/10.1016/j.clineuro.2016.09.013.
60. Rezvan A, Christine D, Christian H, et al. Long-term outcome and survival of surgically treated supratentorial low-grade glioma in adult patients. Acta Neurochir. 2009;151(11):1359–65. https://doi.org/10.1007/s00701-009-0435-x.
61. Southwell DG, Hervey-Jumper SL, Perry DW, Berger MS. Intraoperative mapping during repeat awake craniotomy reveals the functional plasticity of adult cortex. J Neurosurg. 2016;124(5):1460–9. https://doi.org/10.3171/2015.5.JNS142833.
62. Ng S, Lemaitre AL, Moritz-Gasser S, Herbet G, Duffau H. Recurrent low-grade gliomas: does reoperation affect neurocognitive functioning? Neurosurgery. 2022;90(2):221–32. https://doi.org/10.1227/NEU.0000000000001784.
63. Capo G, Skrap M, Guarracino I, et al. Cognitive functions in repeated glioma surgery. Cancer. 2020;12(5):1077. https://doi.org/10.3390/cancers12051077.
64. Rudà R, Bruno F, Pellerino A. Epilepsy in gliomas: recent insights into risk factors and molecular pathways. Curr Opin Neurol. 2023;36(6):557–63. https://doi.org/10.1097/WCO.0000000000001214.
65. Avila EK, Tobochnik S, Inati SK, et al. Brain tumor-related epilepsy management: a Society for Neuro-oncology (SNO) consensus review on current management. Neuro-Oncology. 2024;26(1):7–24. https://doi.org/10.1093/neuonc/noad154.
66. Pallud J, McKhann GM. Diffuse low-grade glioma-related epilepsy. Neurosurg Clin N Am. 2019;30(1):43–54. https://doi.org/10.1016/j.nec.2018.09.001.
67. Ius T, Pauletto G, Isola M, et al. Surgery for insular low-grade glioma: predictors of postoperative seizure outcome: clinical article. JNS. 2014;120(1):12–23. https://doi.org/10.3171/2013.9.JNS13728.
68. Neal A, Kwan P, O'Brien TJ, Buckland ME, Gonzales M, Morokoff A. IDH1 and IDH2 mutations in postoperative diffuse glioma-associated epilepsy. Epilepsy Behav. 2018;78:30–6. https://doi.org/10.1016/j.yebeh.2017.10.027.
69. Still MEH, Roux A, Huberfeld G, et al. Extent of resection and residual tumor thresholds for postoperative total seizure freedom in epileptic adult patients harboring a supratentorial diffuse low-grade glioma. Neurosurgery. 2019;85(2):E332–40. https://doi.org/10.1093/neuros/nyy481.
70. Xu DS, Awad AW, Mehalechko C, et al. An extent of resection threshold for seizure freedom in patients with low-grade gliomas. J Neurosurg. 2018;128(4):1084–90. https://doi.org/10.3171/2016.12.JNS161682.
71. Mehrotra A, Singh S, Kanjilal S, et al. Long-term epilepsy-associated tumors (LEATs): a single-center, retrospective series and review of literature on factors affecting the seizure outcome. World Neurosurg. 2020;144:e149–55. https://doi.org/10.1016/j.wneu.2020.08.036.
72. Englot DJ, Wang DD, Rolston JD, Shih TT, Chang EF. Rates and predictors of long-term seizure freedom after frontal lobe epilepsy surgery: a systematic review and meta-analysis: clinical article. JNS. 2012;116(5):1042–8. https://doi.org/10.3171/2012.1.JNS111620.
73. Nandoliya KR, Thirunavu V, Ellis E, et al. Preoperative predictors of post-operative seizure control in low-grade glioma: a systematic review and meta-analysis. Neurosurg Rev. 2024;47(1):94. https://doi.org/10.1007/s10143-024-02329-9.
74. Ghareeb F, Duffau H. Intractable epilepsy in paralimbic World Health Organization Grade II gliomas: should the hippocampus be resected when not invaded by the tumor? Clinical article. JNS. 2012;116(6):1226–34. https://doi.org/10.3171/2012.1.JNS112120.
75. Lombardi D, Marsh R, Tribolet N. Low grade glioma in intractable epilepsy: lesionectomy versus epilepsy surgery. In: Ostertag CB, Thomas DG, Bosch A, Linderoth B, Broggi G, editors. Advances in stereotactic and functional neurosurgery, vol. 12. Vienna: Springer; 1997. p. 70–4. https://doi.org/10.1007/978-3-7091-6513-3_13.
76. Huberfeld G, Vecht CJ. Seizures and gliomas—towards a single therapeutic approach. Nat Rev Neurol. 2016;12(4):204–16. https://doi.org/10.1038/nrneurol.2016.26.
77. Berntsson SG, Malmer B, Bondy ML, Qu M, Smits A. Tumor-associated epilepsy and glioma: are there common genetic pathways? Acta Oncol. 2009;48(7):955–63. https://doi.org/10.1080/02841860903104145.
78. Roessler K, Heynold E, Buchfelder M, Stefan H, Hamer HM. Current value of intraoperative electrocorticography (iopECoG). Epilepsy Behav. 2019;91:20–4. https://doi.org/10.1016/j.yebeh.2018.06.053.
79. Bono BC, Ninatti G, Riva M, et al. The role of preoperative [11C]methionine PET in defining tumor-related epilepsy and predicting short-term postoperative seizure control in temporal lobe low-grade gliomas. Neurosurg Focus. 2024;56(2):E6. https://doi.org/10.3171/2023.11.FOCUS23678.
80. Mazzucchi E, Vollono C, Pauletto G, et al. The persistence of seizures after tumor resection negatively affects survival in low-grade glioma patients: a clinical retrospective study. J Neurol. 2022;269(5):2627–33. https://doi.org/10.1007/s00415-021-10845-7.
81. Chaichana KL, McGirt MJ, Laterra J, Olivi A, Quiñones-Hinojosa A. Recurrence and malignant degeneration after resection of adult hemispheric low-grade gliomas: clinical article. JNS. 2010;112(1):10–7. https://doi.org/10.3171/2008.10.JNS08608.

82. Roelz R, Strohmaier D, Jabbarli R, et al. Residual tumor volume as best outcome predictor in low grade glioma – a nine-years near-randomized survey of surgery vs. biopsy. Sci Rep. 2016;6(1):32286. https://doi.org/10.1038/srep32286.
83. Kickingereder P, Sahm F, Radbruch A, et al. IDH mutation status is associated with a distinct hypoxia/angiogenesis transcriptome signature which is non-invasively predictable with rCBV imaging in human glioma. Sci Rep. 2015;5:16238. https://doi.org/10.1038/srep16238.
84. Agosti E, Zeppieri M, De Maria L, et al. Glioblastoma immunotherapy: a systematic review of the present strategies and prospects for advancements. Int J Mol Sci. 2023;24(20):15037. https://doi.org/10.3390/ijms242015037.
85. Ius T, Ciani Y, Ruaro ME, et al. An NF-κB signature predicts low-grade glioma prognosis: a precision medicine approach based on patient-derived stem cells. Neuro-Oncology. 2018;20(6):776–87. https://doi.org/10.1093/neuonc/nox234.
86. Goff SL, Morgan RA, Yang JC, et al. Pilot trial of adoptive transfer of chimeric antigen receptor-transduced T cells targeting EGFRvIII in patients with glioblastoma. J Immunother. 2019;42(4):126–35. https://doi.org/10.1097/CJI.0000000000000260.
87. Yuan B, Wang G, Tang X, Tong A, Zhou L. Immunotherapy of glioblastoma: recent advances and future prospects. Hum Vaccin Immunother. 2022;18(5):2055417. https://doi.org/10.1080/21645515.2022.2055417.
88. Scherschinski L, Jubran JH, Shaftel KA, et al. Magnetic resonance-guided laser interstitial thermal therapy for management of low-grade gliomas and radiation necrosis: a single-institution case series. Brain Sci. 2022;12(12):1627. https://doi.org/10.3390/brainsci12121627.
89. Pasqualetti F, Rizzo M, Franceschi S, Lessi F, Paiar F, Buffa FM. New perspectives in liquid biopsy for glioma patients. Curr Opin Oncol. 2022;34(6):705–12. https://doi.org/10.1097/CCO.0000000000000902.

Pediatric Gliomas in the Modern Era

8

Davide Luglietto, Sergio Capelli, Alessandro De Benedictis, Alessia Carboni, Andrea Carai, and Carlo Efisio Marras

8.1 Introduction

Pediatric gliomas are a common type of neoplastic lesion in the central nervous system (CNS), with unique characteristics in terms of distribution, incidence, diagnostic criteria, molecular-genetic profiling, and potential targeted therapies [1]. These lesions differ from adult gliomas, as the latest WHO classification allows them to be categorized into low-grade (LGG) and high-grade (HGG) gliomas. Each of these categories can be further subdivided based on molecular characteristics [2].

Beyond the clinical specifics of these glial pathologies in children, another classification can be made based on the anatomical configuration of the lesions. Therefore, we can identify three main categories, detailing for each the distinct surgical features and common technical-procedural aspects.

8.2 Pediatric Supratentorial Gliomas

Supratentorial gliomas are considered hemispheric lesions. The goal of treatment is radical resection, when safely possible, to obtain tissue for diagnosis and achieve maximum cytoreduction. For the majority of these lesions, achieving a gross total resection provides a significant survival advantage (Fig. 8.1).

Most pilocytic astrocytomas and other superficial gliomas can be resected grossly or near-grossly with acceptable risk. In some low-grade infiltrating gliomas that have not progressed, a biopsy followed by long-term imaging may be appropriate, as most of these lesions are unlikely to progress to high-grade tumors in childhood. In cases where a gross total resection is unlikely, subtotal resection can significantly decrease mass effect and potentially resolve hydrocephalus due to ventricular decompression [1].

D. Luglietto (✉)
Neurosurgery Unit, Bambino Gesù Children's Hospital, IRCCS, Rome, Italy

Department of Electrical Engineering and Information Technology (DIETI), University "Federico II", Naples, Italy
e-mail: davide.luglietto@opbg.net

S. Capelli
Division of Neurosurgery, Department of Medical and Surgical Specialties, Radiological Sciences and Public Health, University of Brescia, Brescia, Italy

Division of Neurosurgery, Department of Biotechnology and Life Sciences, University of Insubria, Varese, Italy

A. De Benedictis · A. Carai · C. E. Marras
Neurosurgery Unit, Bambino Gesù Children's Hospital, IRCCS, Rome, Italy

A. Carboni
Diagnostic and Interventional Neuroradiology and Vascular Anomalies Unit, Bambino Gesù Children's Hospital, IRCCS, Rome, Italy

D. Armocida et al. (eds.), *Neurosurgery's Frontline Role in Gliomas Treatment*,
https://doi.org/10.1007/978-3-031-81850-9_8

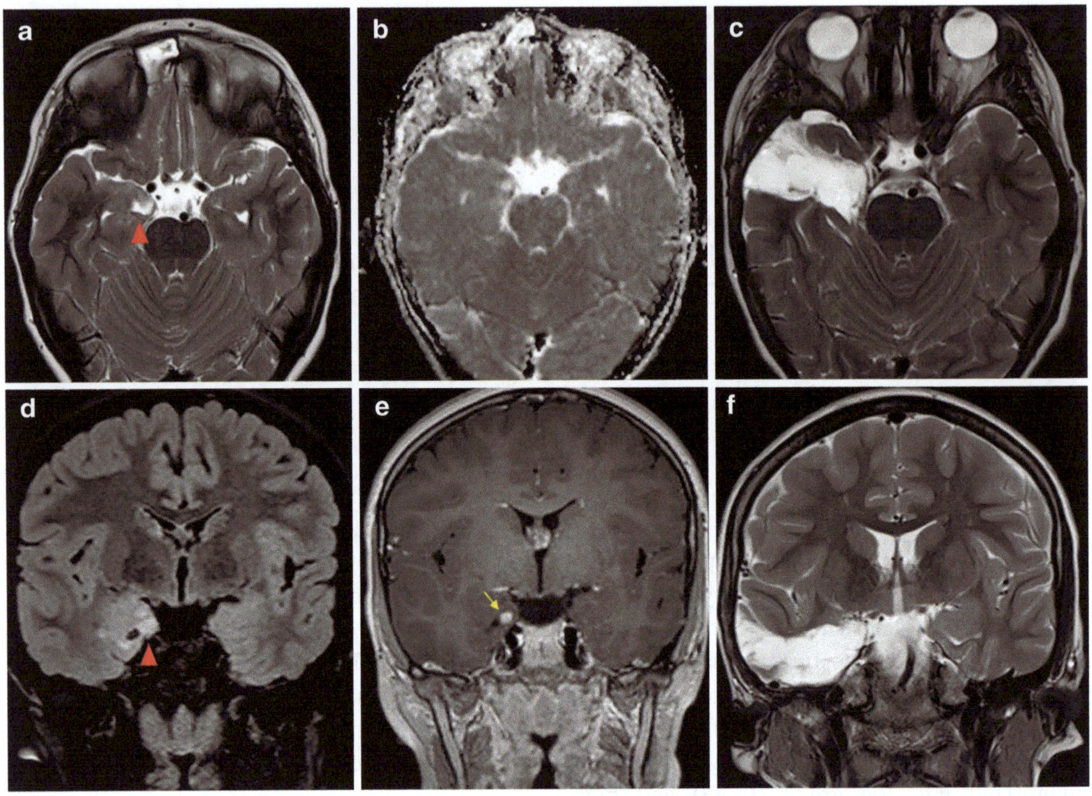

Fig. 8.1 Cortico-subcortical low-grade glioma (LGG) in the right temporo-mesial region. On axial T2-weighted (T2w) and coronal FLAIR MR images (**a**, **d**, arrow-head), the affected structures display a swollen appearance with a pseudo-cystic component. The lesion has a disomogeneous apparent diffusion coefficient (ADC) values on diffusion-weighted imaging (**b**). Coronal post-contrast T1-weighted image showing a region of pseudo-nodular contrast enhancement in the most mesial portion (**e**, arrow); areas of contrast enhancement (CE) are observed within the lesion, particularly posterior to the pseudo-cystic component and in the uncal region. Consequently, an anteromesial temporal lobe resection was performed. Axial and coronal T2w images showing the postoperative results (**c**, **f**)

For some deep tumors, such as those infiltrating deep nuclei or critical structures like optic pathway gliomas [3], and high-grade gliomas crossing the midline, a gross total resection or substantial cytoreduction may not be feasible. In these cases, a percutaneous image-guided stereotactic or robot-assisted biopsy can safely establish a diagnosis prior to adjuvant therapy [4].

For superficial or subcortical tumors that are not immediately under eloquent cortex, the most direct route is usually the most appropriate. For subcortical or deep lesions beneath critical areas of the brain, fMRI and diffusion tensor imaging can be very useful in selecting the safest path to a tumor. For tumors directly within or adjacent to eloquent cortex, a trans-sulcal approach may be the safest way of preserving function.

Tumors extending medially and toward the ventricular system can sometimes be resected using a trans-callosal or transventricular approach.

Tumors in the nondominant hemisphere which are extending laterally can be reached through trans-sylvian, trans-insular approach when the tumor spreads close to the cortical surface. Deep lesions in the dominant hemisphere may be approached through a posterior parietal or occipital way, avoiding the sensorimotor and speech pathways.

For LGG, a fairly sharp plane can be identified and followed while resecting the tumor, prior to centrally debulking the tumor mass [5].

Neuroendoscopic approaches are useful for removing low-grade lesions, such as optic pathway gliomas and subependymal giant astrocytomas (SEGA), through total, subtotal, or partial resections, as well as biopsies that restore cerebrospinal fluid circulation. In both endoscopic and open surgeries, ultrasonic aspirators (UA) are valuable for both low- and high-grade gliomas. UA allows for less invasive surgeries by reducing tumor mass from the inside, minimizing damage to surrounding brain tissue, blood vessels, and nerve fibers. This improves patient prognosis, shortens surgery time, reduces blood loss, and enhances overall surgical quality.

For HGG, where the margins may not be as sharply delineated, a central debulking of the tumor followed by intermittent dissection of the margins is frequently the best strategy for a maximal safe resection [4].

8.2.1 Intraoperative Tools

Various perioperative and intraoperative imaging techniques can help minimize surgical risks and aid in the removal of lesions previously considered unresectable. Firstly, the use of neuronavigation is mandatory in any surgical setting to ensure the safest possible execution of each surgical step. Diffusion tensor imaging (DTI) is helpful in preoperative visualization of white matter tracts, which can then be avoided during surgical resection. Functional MRI aids in the specific localization of critical eloquent brain areas near tumors or in the path of the planned approach for tumor resection. These imaging modalities are especially beneficial in young children where an awake craniotomy is not feasible for performing speech mapping.

From a neurophysiological perspective, intraoperative tools can help in understanding brain networks surrounding critical areas [6, 7]. This includes mapping the motor cortex, somatosensory evoked potential phase reversal, and subcortical pyramidal tract mapping and monitoring using transcranial motor evoked potentials (tcMEP), direct cortical motor evoked potentials (dcMEP), and electrocorticography (ECoG) [7].

Moreover, some instruments provide real-time feedback about anatomical features around the lesion, such as intraoperative MRI (iMRI) and intraoperative ultrasound (iUltrasound). The latter, an economically friendly tool, can overcome issues related to brain shift, offering the opportunity to identify and remove any residual tumor components.

Intraoperative ultrasound (ioUS) is commonly used in neurosurgery to assist with the resection of intracerebral diseases. While there are technical challenges, initial experiences indicate that ioUS has a satisfactory predictive ability compared to MRI studies. However, most existing evidence on ioUS applications in brain tumors comes from adult studies, which may not reflect the pediatric population. In the largest consecutive pediatric brain tumor resection series [8], histology was the only variable significantly associated with unexpected tumor residue on postoperative MRI; tumor location, patient positioning, age, and initial tumor volume did not significantly affect ioUS predictive ability. Therefore, in pediatric neurosurgical oncology, controlling the extent of resection is paramount. The integration of real-time intraoperative imaging with direct inspection of the microsurgical field, neuronavigation data, intraoperative monitoring information, and intraoperative ultrasound has the potential to significantly improve surgical orientation and outcomes (Fig. 8.2).

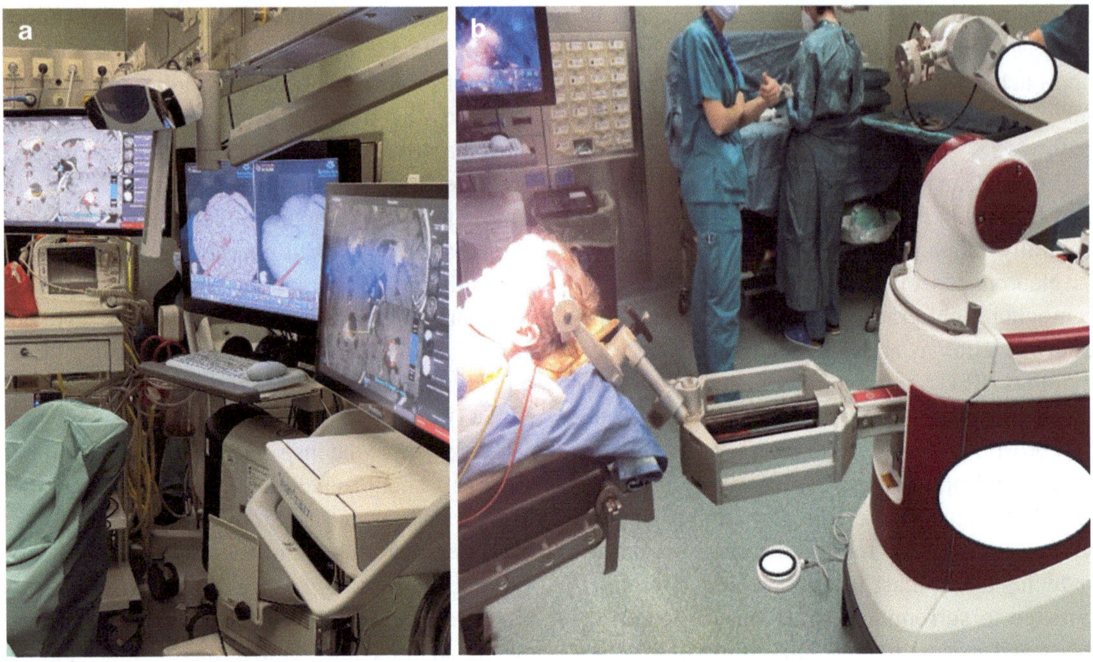

Fig. 8.2 (**a**) Intraoperative setting with VR (virtual reality) and neuronavigation; (**b**) Robot-assisted biopsy, intraoperative setting

8.2.2 Age Related Surgical Approaches

When discussing brain tumors in pediatric patients, it is essential to consider the unique issues related to different age groups, particularly during the infantile period, including newborns and the first year of life. These cases represent a rare subgroup of central nervous system neoplasms that pose significant challenges to neurosurgeons. Diagnosis is often delayed because intracranial hypertension progresses slowly due to the flexibility of cranial bones. Despite this, these lesions tend to exhibit more aggressive behavior (Fig. 8.3). Glial tumors are the most frequent subtype, and surgical resection remains the best therapeutic option. Surgical mortality and morbidity are estimated at 1–25% and 5–50%, respectively. However, surgery is still the first choice for large tumors to control hydrocephalus and obtain a histological sample [9].

Aiming for gross total resection is crucial, as its completeness is directly related to prognosis and outcome [10]. Although surgery is the main prognostic element, it may not always be possible to achieve a total resection due to the lesion's location. In such cases, a biopsy may be performed, and if necessary, a multiple-stage surgery must be taken into account [11, 12].

Nevertheless, young children diagnosed with CNS tumors face a high risk of long-term health complications, especially if under 4 years of age. There is a strong need for long-term support strategies tailored specifically to young children. These strategies include early screening for visual and hearing impairments as well as assessments for endocrine disorders and neuropsychological challenges, to provide appropriate support. Advances in treatment methods, such as targeted anti-tumor therapies and improvements in high-precision radiation techniques, hold promise for reducing treatment burdens and improving long-term outcomes for these children.

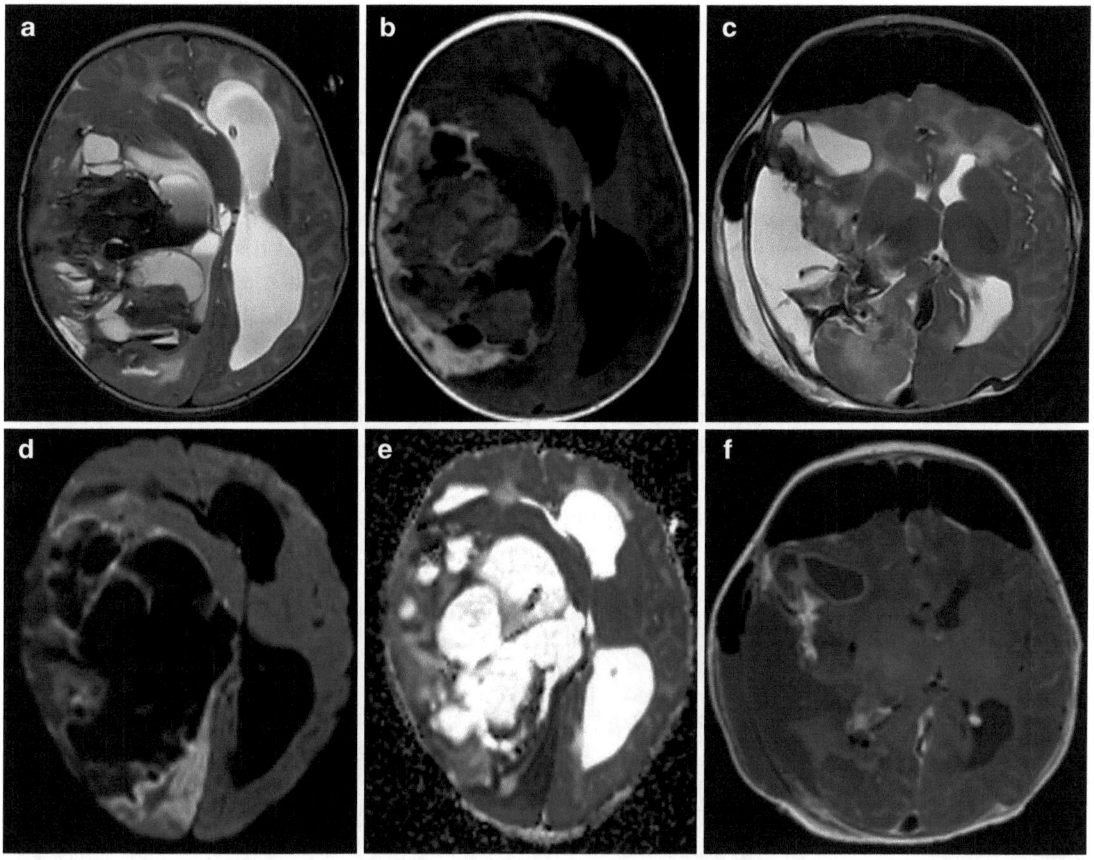

Fig. 8.3 Four-month-old patient diagnosed with a voluminous cerebral mass. Axial T2w image (**a**) exhibit a solid-multicystic mass with hemorrhagic changes and fluid-fluid levels within the cysts involving the fronto-temporo-parietal region of the right cerebral hemisphere. T1w post-contrast image (**b**) shows a peripherical contrast enhancement of the cyst and an intense contrast enhancement of the solid components, predominantly located in the superficial cortical and septal areas (infant HGG). The DWI (**d**) and ADC map (**e**) exhibit disomogeneous restriction of the tumor and high values on ADC of the right posterior parieto-mesial cerebral parenchyma due to the mass effect of the lesion. Axial T2w (**c**) and post-contrast T1w (**f**) images demonstrate postoperative results

8.3 Pediatric Cerebellar Gliomas

The posterior cranial fossa is the region where most CNS tumors in childhood are located. In particular, the cerebellum is often the site of intra-axial lesions of glial origin, especially low-grade ones such as pilocytic astrocytomas (PA). The primary treatment for these lesions is surgery aimed at gross total resection (GTR), often without the need for adjuvant therapies. Most low-grade gliomas (LGGs) identified in the cerebellum have a very good prognosis if a GTR is achieved. Unlike their adult counterparts, low-grade cerebellar gliomas in children have an excellent prognosis, and patients can maintain excellent quality of life [13].

Therefore, regardless of the specific histopathology, almost all cerebellar LGGs are managed with GTR if it can be performed safely. Adjunctive therapies are only employed in cases of partial or subtotal resection, recurrence, or when the tumors are unresectable [14]. On the other hand, high-grade gliomas (HGGs), which are more significant in the supratentorial and brainstem regions, have less impact at the cerebellar level [15].

8.3.1 Pilocytic Astrocytoma

The most frequent histological subtype of LGG in childhood is pilocytic astrocytoma (Fig. 8.4).

Its therapeutic management is modulated by the extent of resection achievable through different surgical approaches. Classically, with a suboccipital craniotomy and subsequent wide exposure of the cerebellar surface, any lesional area in this context can be reached transcortically. This surgical choice allows a clear demarcation from the surrounding parenchyma. Bipolar surgical aspiration or ultrasound may be used to resect the tumor. The cyst wall does not have to be resected if it is smooth and does not increase in volume on preoperative imaging examination. However, gross inspection should help the surgeon determine the need for resection of the cyst wall. In tumors, close to the fourth ventricle, a cottonoid can be placed along the floor to provide critical localization and protection of brainstem structures. After resection, it is necessary to carefully inspect the tumor bed and pay close attention to the "lip" of the cerebellum under the retractor blades, thus avoiding the persistence of small islands of residual tumor.

This route, although able to guarantee a more direct route to the lesion with ample exposure at the same time, does not guarantee the absence of risk in damaging surrounding cortical tissue and may compromise the postoperative course.

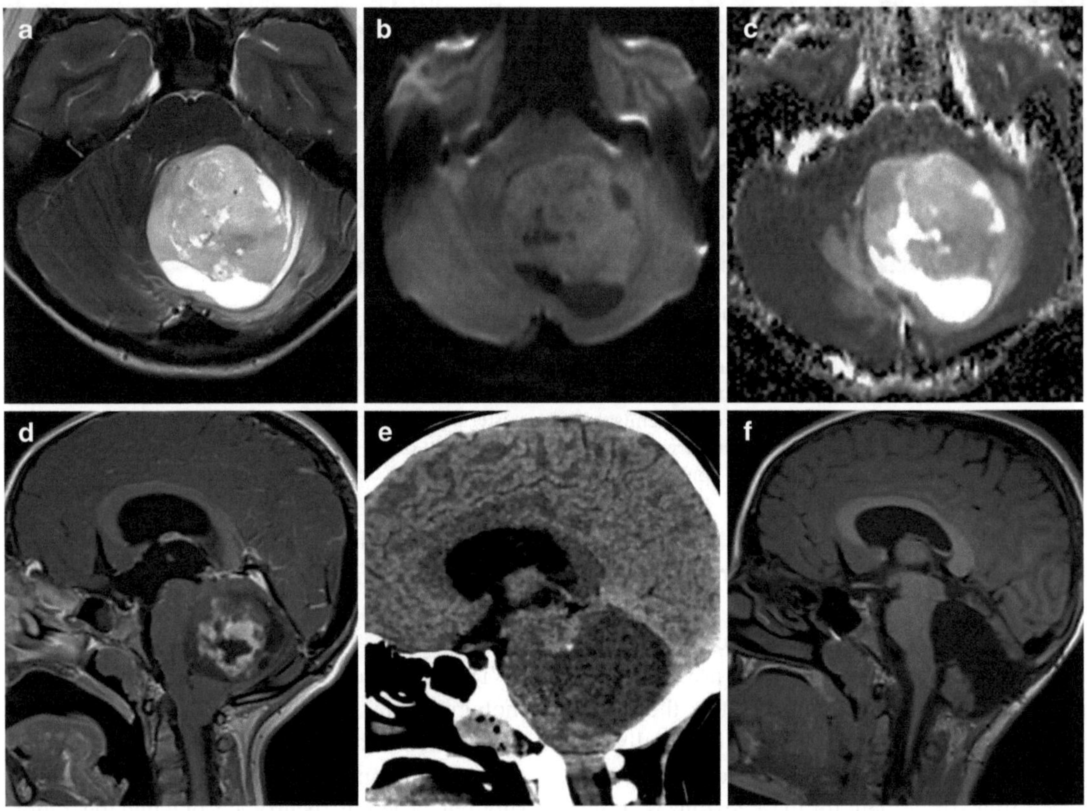

Fig. 8.4 Cerebellar solid-cystic mass, mildly edematous and centered in the left cerebellar hemisphere. The lesion has a heterogeneous appearance due to the presence of some predominantly peripheral cystic components and a more distinctly solid central component (T2w axial, **a**), characterized by heterogeneous contrast enhancement on T1w post-contrast image (**d**) without high values on ADC map (**b**, **c**) suggestive for LGG (pilocytic astrocytoma). Sagittal reconstruction on CT scan (**e**) after ETV and positioning of ventricular catheter with Rickham reservoir. Sagittal T1w image after tumor resection (**f**)

Alternative surgical approaches have therefore been proposed over time, especially in the case of lesions located in more complex areas such as the anterosuperior/superomedial cerebellar portion and the deep area adjacent to the fourth ventricle, precisely at the level of the superior, middle and inferior cerebellar peduncles.

In the former case, a possible surgical route is the trans-tentorial occipital interhemispheric approach [16, 17]. Originally conceived as a route for the pineal region, it soon became established as a surgical option for some cerebellar lesions.

In case of lesions involving the superior cerebellar surface, the best surgical route is the supracerebellar infratentorial one: the adoption of a natural anatomical route avoids sacrificing noble neurovascular structures. Moreover, with a good patient positioning (prone or sitting position) and the necessary bending of the head, it is possible to reach the deep structures until the identification of the internal cerebral veins toward the pineal region.

Reaching the cerebellar peduncles is related to possible postoperative complications such as cerebellar mutism syndrome, a common complication following surgical resection of childhood tumors arising in the posterior fossa. The risk of developing cerebellar mutism syndrome, as extensively discussed, is higher in case of: brainstem invasion, midline localization, tumor size >5 cm, left-handedness, incision of the vermis, diagnosis of medulloblastoma if compared with other lesions (LGGs) [18, 19]. It is possible to aim a surgical resection of a peduncle lesion through telovelar/transcerebellomedullary fissure approach [20–22]. As in the case of the supracerebellar infratentorial approach, the peculiarity of the telovelar approach is the adoption of anatomo-surgical corridors that do not damage or compromise the integrity of the cortical and eloquent structures.

8.4 Pediatric Brainstem Gliomas

The localization of a neoplastic lesion in the brainstem during pediatric age is not uncommon. Although the histology of such lesions may fall within benign criteria (e.g., low-grade gliomas such as exophytic pilocytic astrocytomas), any lesion in this region is considered aggressive due to its anatomical location. For obvious functional reasons, achieving a gross total resection in this area is challenging. As a result, the need for adjuvant therapies in a patient undergoing surgery for a lesion in an eloquent site significantly impacts quality of life and, consequently, overall survival.

Brainstem surgery by definition requires the use of a wide range of intraoperative neurophysiological monitoring. Dedicated neurophysiologic monitoring is possible for cranial nerves III, IV, V, VI, VII, IX, X, XI, and XII, along with brainstem auditory evoked potentials (BAEPs), cortical motor evoked potentials (MEPs), and somatosensory evoked potentials (SSEPs). Direct electromyographic simulation of the fourth ventricular floor can assist in the anatomic identification of nuclei and cranial nerves. Careful monitoring by the anesthesiology team of cardiac rate, rhythm, and blood pressure can reveal bradycardia, systolic pauses, or hypotension induced by manipulation near the nuclei of Vth cranial nerve and Xth cranial nerve. Short internuncial brainstem fibers (or association neurons) connecting the sensory nucleus of CN V to the dorsal motor nucleus of the vagus give rise to these effects, through the trigemino-cardiac reflex.

8.4.1 Exophytic-Focal Brainstem Tumors

In 25% of cases, exophytic lesions are the most amenable to surgery from a surgical point of view: in fact, if a maximal safe resection were to be achieved, the prognosis would improve drastically. For 3/4 of cases identifiable as LGG, (in the remaining HGG), exophytic tumors of the brainstem can be subjected to both surgical resection and debulking.

Surgery is most commonly performed via posterior fossa craniotomy and midline telovelar or transvermian approach, although a number of other approaches have been utilized when warranted, including the infratentorial supracerebellar route for lesions in the dorsal midbrain, endoscopic transventricular or open transventricular/trans-choroidal approaches for the rostral midbrain, lateral supracerebellar approaches for the lateral midbrain, retrosigmoid/presigmoid approaches for ventrolateral pontine lesions, and far-lateral/transcondylar approaches for lesions in the anterior/lateral surface (Fig. 8.5) [23, 24].

An entry point into the tumor is typically chosen where the mass arises in optimal proximity to the brainstem surface, with potential modification based on known points of safe brainstem entry such as the supra-collicular/infracollicular zones, suprafacial triangle, infrafacial triangle, posterior median sulcus, and many others [25, 26].

8.4.2 Diffuse Brainstem Tumors

Most pediatric brainstem lesions are malignant and lack precise boundaries. Consequently, minimal surgical intervention is necessary to obtain a tissue sample for histological analysis, enabling targeted therapy in light of recent therapeutic advancements.

Biopsies can be performed using various methods [27–30]. Currently, the most common approach is neuronavigation-guided stereotactic biopsy (frameless) [27]. Different surgical trajectories have been described, including precoronal (Fig. 8.6) and trans-cerebellar routes. It is beneficial to select a target with contrast enhancement whenever possible. In cases where the lesion lacks contrast enhancement, careful target selection is

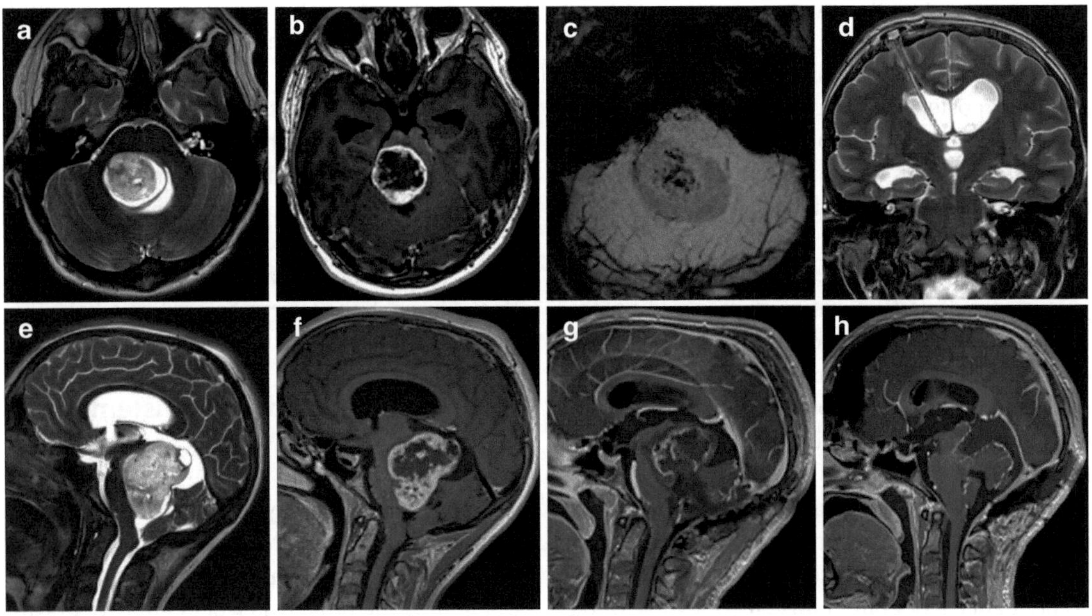

Fig. 8.5 Male 13 years with exophytic tumor of the posterior cranial fossa with triventricular hydrocephalus. Axial and sagittal T2w image (**a**, **e**) show a big solid-cystic mass with an exophytic dorsal brainstem component and multilobulated contours. The lesion appears markedly heterogeneous (**a**) due to the presence of solid and cystic areas, necrosis-like areas outlined by peripherical contrast enhancement on T1w images (**b**, **f**) and calcific/hemosiderin deposits visible on susceptibility weighted image (SWI; **c**), suggestive for LGG. The coronal T2w sequence shows the presence of ventricular catheter with Rickham reservoir after ETV. (**d**). Sagittal T1w post-contrast images exhibit the results after first surgery via suboccipital telovelar approach (**g**) and after 2nd surgery via supracerebellar infratentorial approach (**h**)

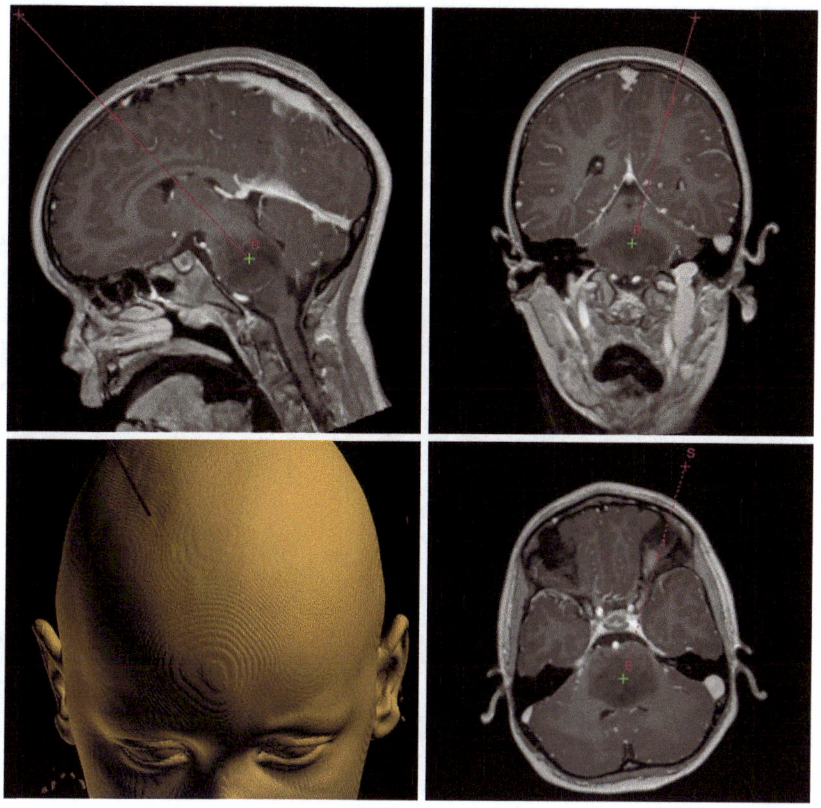

Fig. 8.6 Diffuse brainstem lesion. Robot-assisted biopsy, planning of a precoronal surgical approach

crucial to obtain multiple samples along the same trajectory. With the advent of increasingly precise and safe technologies, robot-assisted biopsies have been explored, demonstrating their feasibility, safety, and efficacy [28, 29].

If ventriculomegaly and/or hydrocephalus are present, and there is a targetable exophytic portion of the tumor within the interpeduncular and prepontine cistern, an endoscopic transventricular approach can be considered [30].

8.4.3 Cervicomedullary Tumors

In contrast to the always-malignant diffuse intrinsic tumors where surgery does not improve prognosis, cervicomedullary gliomas (CMGs) located in the low brainstem and upper cervical spinal cord are often histologically low-grade, indolent tumors (Fig. 8.7). These are suitable for surgical resection with potential clinical benefits. Surgery is generally considered of primary importance in treating CMGs, aiming to achieve maximal safe resection rather than gross total or subtotal resection due to the eloquence of the region [31]. The potential for surgical resection is influenced by the presence of a discrete margin between the tumor and surrounding tissue. These tumors may be approached via a posterior fossa craniotomy and variable-level cervical laminectomy, followed by a median myelotomy [32].

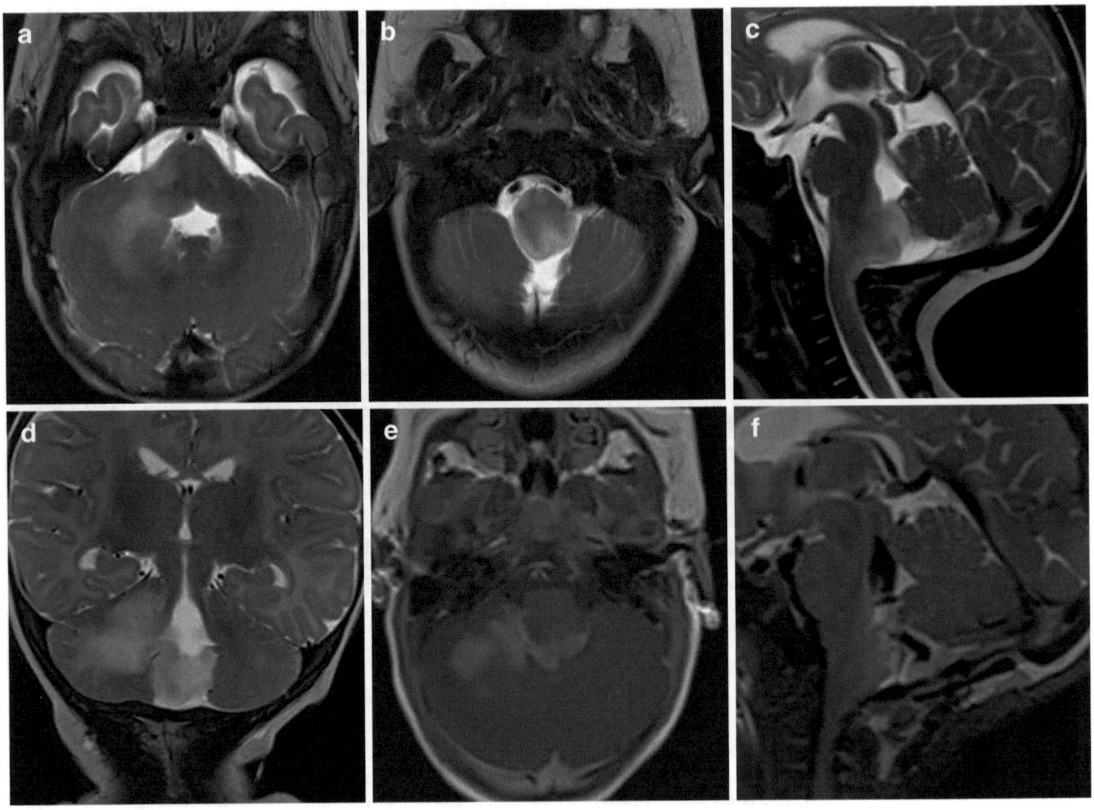

Fig. 8.7 3 month-old male diagnosed with LGG of the posterior cranial fossa. Axial, sagittal, and coronal T2w images (**a–d**) show ill-defined hyperintense pathological tissue involving middle and inferior right cerebellar peduncles, the cervical medulla up to C3 and the brainstem with a partially exophytic component on the dorsal side of the pons toward the fourth ventricle. The lesion is characterized by heterogeneous T2/FLAIR hyperintensity and limited areas of pathological contrast enhancement on T1w (**e**). T2 sagittal MRI post-biopsy via telovelar approach (**f**)

8.5 Pediatric Brain Tumor Biopsy

Despite the advantages of neurosurgery, the growing importance of molecular biology underscores the ongoing need to analyze surgical tissue to predict prognosis and guide therapy in pediatric brain tumors, particularly when open surgery is not indicated. Therefore, biopsy plays a crucial role in the therapeutic course of lesions that are not candidates for resection surgery due to their location in highly eloquent areas, such as optic pathway gliomas (OPGs), thalamic gliomas, and brainstem gliomas.

8.5.1 Stereotactic Biopsy in Pediatric Brainstem Lesions

Given the need to obtain histological samples to initiate targeted drug therapies, the neurosurgeon must offer a safe, minimally invasive and cost-effective sampling modality. Previously known as DIPGs, these lesions comprise 10% of pediatric brain tumors and are the leading cause of brain tumor–related mortality in children [33].

Until recent years, diagnosis was made using radiological findings alone, and neurosurgical intervention was indicated only to treat obstructive hydrocephalus. Later, a series of studies revealed that nearly 80% of DIPG cases harbor the H3-K27M mutation. The mutation is now considered pathognomonic for the new entity of H3 K27M-mutant diffuse midline glioma, which carries a WHO grade IV designation due to universally poor prognosis irrespective of histological features [34]. Lesional tissue is required for detection of the H3K27M mutation, which may be performed by immunohistochemistry or direct genetic sequencing.

For this kind of lesions involving the eloquent regions of the brainstem, whose open approach opens up the possibility of numerous risks and complications, highly precise stereotactic instruments are required to perform the biopsy safely.

Frame-based stereotaxy has historically been the gold standard for successfully performing these procedures. Recent studies have explored frameless procedures and new technologies such as robotic assistance to improve surgical workflow, reduce operative time, and perform other procedures such as ETV during the same surgery. Since the first use in 1985 [35], robotic assistance in brain lesion biopsies has advanced significantly, particularly with the introduction of MRI-guided stereotactic imaging. Enhanced accuracy, safety, and user-friendly features, like frameless surface registration, have made robotic assistance common in biopsy procedures. The two main approaches are trans-frontal and trans-cerebellar [36]. The trans-frontal route offers advantages, such as avoiding venous hypertension and preserving cranial nerve nuclei, especially in cases of H3K27 HGG, where brainstem anatomy is distorted [37, 38]. Robot-assisted precoronal needle biopsy allows for a single-stage procedure without moving the patient or using fiducial markers, offering high stability and eliminating the need for ionizing radiation [37]. The trans-cerebellar route provides a shorter trajectory and avoids key motor and sensory pathways [28]. Studies show good outcomes and low complication rates with robot-assisted neurosurgery, highlighting its role in safer, more accurate, and cost-effective biopsies [39–41].

8.5.2 New Technologies in Pediatric Gliomas Management

As technology evolves, neurosurgery increasingly utilizes advanced instrumentation to simplify procedures, making them less invasive and potentially safer. Virtual reality (VR) and augmented reality (AR) now allow both novice and experienced surgeons to interact with anatomical structures, customize surgical plans, and anticipate challenges based on individual anatomy. Among these innovations, laser interstitial thermal therapy (LITT) has also become prominent.

MR-guided LITT is a minimally invasive surgical technique that uses laser-induced heat to ablate pathological tissue (Fig. 8.8) [42]. Over the years, LITT has gained acceptance as an alternative to open resection for various conditions in both adults and children. Its key advantage is the ability to precisely target deep-seated lesions while minimizing damage to surrounding brain tissue. Initially developed for epilepsy surgery, LITT has become a promising option for treating pediatric brain tumors, especially low-grade gliomas (LGGs) [43, 44].

Studies show that LITT can be safely performed in children with LGGs, with low complication rates and preservation of neurological function [45]. Due to its minimally invasive nature, LITT is now the second most common indication for pediatric brain tumors after epilepsy surgery [46]. It not only minimizes harm to critical brain areas but also effectively reduces tumor volume during follow-up, making it a valuable tool in managing low-grade pediatric tumors [47].

LITT is particularly suitable for small, deep, non-cystic lesions. While a biopsy can be performed simultaneously, it may affect LITT's efficacy, so tissue sampling must be carefully considered. The long-term effects of LITT on pediatric LGGs, including the risk of malignant transformation, remain unclear. Further research is needed to evaluate its overall safety and effectiveness [45].

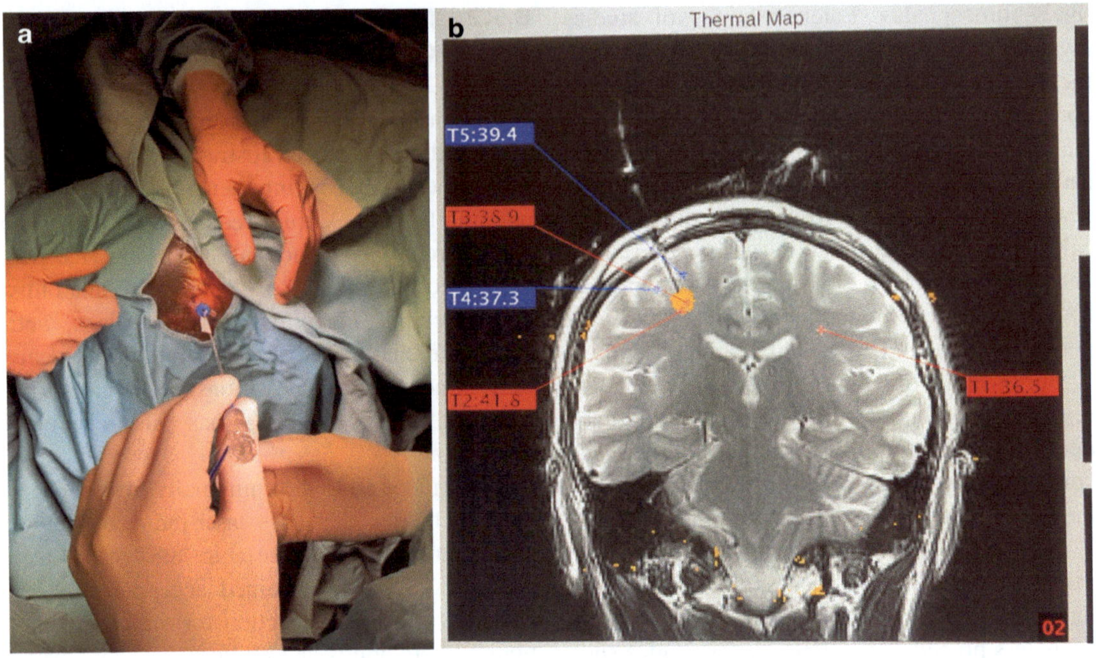

Fig. 8.8 (**a**) Intraoperative image, robot-assisted positioning of a laser fiber; (**b**) Intraoperative Thermal Map MRI during LITT for a supratentorial lesion located at the base of the precentral gyrus

8.6 Hydrocephalus Management in Pediatric Gliomas

The connection between hydrocephalus and pediatric brain tumors is well-established due to its impact on outcomes [48]. Pediatric tumor-related hydrocephalus (pTRH) occurs in over 70% of new cases, and more than 90% of children with infratentorial tumors [49]. Since the posterior fossa is the most common tumor site in children, resulting hydrocephalus is typically obstructive, especially with midline lesions [50]. Obstruction can arise from direct cerebrospinal fluid (CSF) blockage, protein shedding, or a combination of these factors [49].

Neurosurgical management prioritizes relieving intracranial hypertension before addressing the tumor to optimize outcomes and prepare for neuro-oncological trials. Pre-resection hydrocephalus management debates center on endoscopic third ventriculostomy (ETV) versus ventriculoperitoneal shunt (VPS). While shunts were previously routine, earlier diagnoses and improved imaging have shifted this approach [51]. Though a pre-craniotomy shunt can improve physiological conditions and postoperative outcomes [52], tumor resection often restores CSF flow, potentially eliminating the need for a permanent shunt [48]. Shunt complications, such as infections and malfunctions, can significantly impact quality of life [48].

Temporary CSF diversion, such as external ventricular drainage (EVD), poses risks of infection and hemorrhage [53, 54]. Approximately, 80% of children with advanced hydrocephalus and those under 3 years old will require a postoperative shunt [48]. Factors associated with shunt placement include younger age, midline tumors, severe ventricular enlargement, incomplete tumor resection, and prolonged EVD use [55, 56].

The obstructive nature of hydrocephalus in posterior fossa tumors supports the curative role of ETV. Pre-surgical ETV can alleviate intracranial hypertension and prevent post-surgical hydrocephalus [51–58]. However, hydrocephalus persists in about 30% of patients after tumor resection, often requiring permanent CSF diversion [59].

While lesion removal may restore CSF circulation, acute intracranial hypertension from subarachnoid hemorrhage and cerebellar swelling can occur [51]. Historically, VPS has been the standard treatment for hydrocephalus, but ETV offers the advantage of avoiding shunt-related complications, particularly in patients with limited survival prognosis [60, 61]. Research suggests both ETV and VPS are effective, but VPS may be favored in patients with high-grade lesions requiring rapid intervention due to ETV's higher early failure rate [62, 63].

Severe ventricular dilation at diagnosis is a predictor of persistent post-surgical hydrocephalus [64]. Given the obstructive nature of hydrocephalus, ETV is often preferred, though lesions extending into the prepontine cistern may lead to rapid ETV failure. In such cases, placing a ventricular catheter with a Rickham reservoir after ETV can allow for quick ventricular access and intracranial pressure monitoring, with VPS as a potential subsequent step.

Acknowledgments Work supported by #NEXTGENERATIONEU (NGEU) and funded by the Ministry of University and Research (MUR), National Recovery and Resilience Plan (NRRP), project MNESYS (PE0000006)—A Multiscale integrated approach to the study of the nervous system in health and disease (DN. 1553 11.10.2022).

References

1. Schaumann A, Hammar C, Alsleben S, et al. Neurosurgical treatment of pediatric brain tumors - results from a single center multidisciplinary setup. Childs Nerv Syst. 2024;40(2):381–93.
2. Gianno F, Giovannoni I, Cafferata B, et al. Paediatric-type diffuse high-grade gliomas in the 5th CNS WHO Classification. Pathologica. 2022;114(6):422–35.
3. Del Baldo G, Cacchione A, Dell'Anna VA, et al. Rethinking the management of optic pathway gliomas: a single center experience. Front Surg. 2022;9:890875. Published 2022 Jun 16.
4. Gonçalves FG, Alves CAPF, Vossough A. Updates in pediatric malignant gliomas. Top Magn Reson Imaging. 2020;29(2):83–94.
5. Sait SF, Giantini-Larsen AM, Tringale KR, Souweidane MM, Karajannis MA. Treatment of pediatric low-grade gliomas. Curr Neurol Neurosci Rep. 2023;23(4):185–99.
6. Sala F. Intraoperative neurophysiology in pediatric neurosurgery: a historical perspective. Childs Nerv Syst. 2023;39(10):2929–41.
7. Roth J, Korn A, Sala F, et al. Intraoperative neurophysiology in pediatric supratentorial surgery: experience with 57 cases. Childs Nerv Syst. 2020;36(2):315–24.
8. Carai A, De Benedictis A, Calloni T, et al. Intraoperative ultrasound-assisted extent of resection assessment in pediatric neurosurgical oncology. Front Oncol. 2021;11:660805.
9. Simone V, Rizzo D, Cocciolo A, et al. Infantile brain tumors: a review of literature and future perspectives. Diagnostics. 2021;11(4):670.
10. McGirt MJ, Chaichana KL, Gathinji M, et al. Independent association of extent of resection with survival in patients with malignant brain astrocytoma. J Neurosurg. 2009;110(1):156–62.
11. Toniutti M, Sasso AL, Carai A, et al. Central nervous system tumours in neonates: what should the neonatologist know? Eur J Pediatr. 2024;183(4):1485–97.
12. Ceglie G, Vinci M, Carai A, et al. Infantile/congenital high-grade gliomas: molecular features and therapeutic perspectives. Diagnostics. 2020;10(9):648.
13. Cicutti SE, Del Río RJ, Cáceres A, Gonzalez Ramos JD. Pediatric hemispheric cerebellar low-grade gliomas: clinical approach, diagnosis, and management challenges-experience at a tertiary care children's hospital. Childs Nerv Syst. 2024;40(8):2321–32.
14. Ge PF, Wang HF, Qu LM, Chen B, Fu S, Luo Y. Pilomyxoid astrocytoma in cerebellum. Chin J Cancer Res. 2011;23(3):242–4.
15. Das KK, Mehrotra A, Nair AP, et al. Pediatric glioblastoma: clinico-radiological profile and factors affecting the outcome. Childs Nerv Syst. 2012;28(12):2055–62.
16. Peters DR, VanHorn T, Karimian B, Wait SD. Occipital interhemispheric transtentorial approach in pediatric patients for lesions of the superomedial cerebellum: operative findings and results. Childs Nerv Syst. 2023;39(2):491–6.
17. Shirane R, Kumabe T, Yoshida Y, et al. Surgical treatment of posterior fossa tumors via the occipital transtentorial approach: evaluation of operative safety and results in 14 patients with anterosuperior cerebellar tumors. J Neurosurg. 2001;94(6):927–35.
18. Grønbæk JK, Wibroe M, Toescu S, et al. Postoperative speech impairment and surgical approach to posterior fossa tumours in children: a prospective European Multicentre Cohort Study. Lancet Child Adolesc Health. 2021;5(11):814–24.
19. Fabozzi F, Margoni S, Andreozzi B, et al. Cerebellar mutism syndrome: from pathophysiology to rehabilitation. Front Cell Dev Biol. 2022;10:1082947.
20. Matsushima K, Matsushima T. Telovelar/transcerebellomedullary fissure approach: giant distal posterior inferior cerebellar artery aneurysm, epidermoid cyst, and brainstem cavernoma: 2-dimensional operative video. Oper Neurosurg. 2023;25(6):e359–60.
21. Majchrzak H, Tymowski M, Majchrzak K, Stepień T. Surgical approaches to pathological lesions of the middle cerebellar peduncle and the lateral part of the pons - clinical observation. Neurol Neurochir Pol. 2007;41(5):436–44.

22. Kawashima M, Matsushima T, Nakahara Y, Takase Y, Masuoka J, Ohata K. Trans-cerebellomedullary fissure approach with special reference to lateral route. Neurosurg Rev. 2009;32(4):457–64.
23. Cavalheiro S, Yagmurlu K, da Costa MD, et al. Surgical approaches for brainstem tumors in pediatric patients. Childs Nerv Syst. 2015;31(10):1815–40.
24. Mahmoud AT, Enayet A, Alselisly AMA. Surgical considerations for maximal safe resection of exophytic brainstem glioma in the pediatric age group. Surg Neurol Int. 2021;12:310.
25. Cavalcanti DD, Preul MC, Kalani MY, Spetzler RF. Microsurgical anatomy of safe entry zones to the brainstem. J Neurosurg. 2016;124(5):1359–76.
26. Yang Y, van Niftrik B, Ma X, et al. Analysis of safe entry zones into the brainstem. Neurosurg Rev. 2019;42(3):721–9.
27. Joud A, Stella I, Klein O. Diffuse infiltrative pontine glioma biopsy in children with neuronavigation, frameless procedure: a single center experience of 10 cases. Neurochirurgie. 2020;66(5):345–8.
28. Di Rita A, Lenge M, Mantovani G, et al. Robot-assisted transcerebellar stereotactic approach to the posterior fossa in pediatric patients: a technical note. Childs Nerv Syst. 2023;39(9):2493–7.
29. Lu VM, Koester SW, Di L, et al. Frameless robotic-assisted biopsy of pediatric brainstem lesions: a systematic review and meta-analysis of efficacy and safety. World Neurosurg. 2023;169:87–93.
30. La Corte E, Babini M, Bortoluzzi G, Zucchelli M. Endoscopic transventricular biopsy in brainstem diffuse midline glioma: how I do it. Acta Neurochir. 2023;165(4):1099–103.
31. Trezza A, de Laurentis C, Biassoni V, et al. Cervicomedullary gliomas in pediatric age: a systematic review of the literature and tertiary care center experience. Pediatr Neurosurg. 2022;57(3):149–60.
32. Sandri A, Sardi N, Genitori L, et al. Diffuse and focal brain stem tumors in childhood: prognostic factors and surgical outcome. Experience in a single institution. Childs Nerv Syst. 2006;22(9):1127–35.
33. Cooney T, Lane A, Bartels U, et al. Contemporary survival endpoints: an International Diffuse Intrinsic Pontine Glioma Registry study. Neuro-Oncology. 2017;19(9):1279–80.
34. Khuong-Quang DA, Buczkowicz P, Rakopoulos P, et al. K27M mutation in histone H3.3 defines clinically and biologically distinct subgroups of pediatric diffuse intrinsic pontine gliomas. Acta Neuropathol. 2012;124(3):439–47.
35. Kwoh YS, Hou J, Jonckheere EA, Hayati S. A robot with improved absolute positioning accuracy for CT guided stereotactic brain surgery. IEEE Trans Biomed Eng. 1988;35(2):153–60.
36. Gupta M, Chan TM, Santiago-Dieppa DR, et al. Robot-assisted stereotactic biopsy of pediatric brainstem and thalamic lesions. J Neurosurg Pediatr. 2020;27(3):317–24. Published 2020 Dec 25.
37. Carai A, Mastronuzzi A, De Benedictis A, et al. Robot-assisted stereotactic biopsy of diffuse intrinsic pontine glioma: a single-center experience. World Neurosurg. 2017;101:584–8.
38. Puget S, Beccaria K, Blauwblomme T, et al. Biopsy in a series of 130 pediatric diffuse intrinsic Pontine gliomas. Childs Nerv Syst. 2015;31(10):1773–80.
39. Coca HA, Cebula H, Benmekhbi M, Chenard MP, Entz-Werle N, Proust F. Diffuse intrinsic pontine gliomas in children: interest of robotic frameless assisted biopsy. A technical note. Neurochirurgie. 2016;62(6):327–31.
40. Terrier L, Gilard V, Marguet F, Fontanilles M, Derrey S. Stereotactic brain biopsy: evaluation of robot-assisted procedure in 60 patients. Acta Neurochir. 2019;161(3):545–52.
41. De Benedictis A, Trezza A, Carai A, et al. Robot-assisted procedures in pediatric neurosurgery. Neurosurg Focus. 2017;42(5):E7.
42. Holste KG, Orringer DA. Laser interstitial thermal therapy. Neurooncol Adv. 2019;2(1):vdz035.
43. Tovar-Spinoza Z, Choi H. MRI-guided laser interstitial thermal therapy for the treatment of low-grade gliomas in children: a case-series review, description of the current technologies and perspectives. Childs Nerv Syst. 2016;32(10):1947–56.
44. Spacca B, Di Maurizio M, Grandoni M, Tempesti S, Genitori L. Laser interstitial thermal therapy (LITT) for pediatric patients affected by intracranial tumors. Front Neurol. 2023;14:1120286.
45. Strauss I, Gabay S, Roth J. Laser interstitial thermal therapy (LITT) for pediatric low-grade glioma-case presentations and lessons learned. Childs Nerv Syst. 2024;40(10):3119–27.
46. Zeller S, Kaye J, Jumah F, et al. Current applications and safety profile of laser interstitial thermal therapy in the pediatric population: a systematic review of the literature. J Neurosurg Pediatr. 2021;28(3):360–7.
47. Arocho-Quinones EV, Lew SM, Handler MH, et al. Magnetic resonance-guided stereotactic laser ablation therapy for the treatment of pediatric brain tumors: a multiinstitutional retrospective study. J Neurosurg Pediatr. 2020;26(1):13–21.
48. El-Ghandour NM. Endoscopic third ventriculostomy versus ventriculoperitoneal shunt in the treatment of obstructive hydrocephalus due to posterior fossa tumors in children. Childs Nerv Syst. 2011;27(1):117–26.
49. Yengo-Kahn AM, Dewan MC. Tumor-related hydrocephalus in infants: a narrative review. Childs Nerv Syst. 2021;37(11):3365–73.
50. Frisoli F, Kakareka M, Cole KA, Waanders AJ, Storm PB, Lang SS. Endoscopic third ventriculostomy prior to resection of posterior fossa tumors in children. Childs Nerv Syst. 2019;35(5):789–94.
51. Cinalli G, Ozek M, Saint-Rose C. Pediatric hydrocephalus. 2nd ed. Cham: Springer; 2019.
52. Albright L, Reigel DH. Management of hydrocephalus secondary to posterior fossa tumors. J Neurosurg. 1977;46(1):52–5.
53. Sainte-Rose C, Cinalli G, Roux FE, Maixner W, Chumas PD, Mansour M, Carpentier A, Bourgeois

M, Zerah M, Pierre-Kahn A, Renier D. Management of hydrocephalus in pediatric patients with posterior fossa tumors: the role of endoscopic third ventriculostomy. J Neurosurg. 2001;95:791–7.
54. Schmid UD, Seiler RW. Management of obstructive hydrocephalus secondary to posterior fossa tumors by steroids and subcutaneous ventricular catheter reservoir. J Neurosurg. 1986;65:649–53.
55. Lee M, Wisoff JH, Abbott R, Freed D, Epstein FJ. Management of hydrocephalus in children with medulloblastoma: prognostic factors for shunting. Pediatr Neurosurg. 1994;20:240–7.
56. Santos de Oliveira R, Barros Jucá CE, Valera ET, Machado HR. Hydrocephalus in posterior fossa tumors in children. Are there factors that determine a need for permanent cerebrospinal fluid diversion? Childs Nerv Syst. 2008;24:1397–403.
57. Bhatia R, Tahir M, Chandler CL. The management of hydrocephalus in children with posterior fossa tumors: the role of pre-resectional endoscopic third ventriculostomy. Pediatr Neurosurg. 2009;45:186–91.
58. Ruggiero C, Cinalli G, Spennato P, Aliberti F, Cianciulli E, Trischitta V, Maggi G. Endoscopic third ventriculostomy in the treatment of hydrocephalus in posterior fossa tumors in 362 children. Childs Nerv Syst. 2004;20:828–33.
59. Foreman P, McClugage S, Naftel R, et al. Validation and modification of a predictive model of postresection hydrocephalus in pediatric patients with posterior fossa tumors. J Neurosurg Pediatr. 2013;12(3):220–6.
60. Cochrane DD, Kestle JR. The influence of surgical operative experience on the duration of first ventriculoperitoneal shunt function and infection. Pediatr Neurosurg. 2003;38(6):295–301.
61. Morelli D, Pirotte B, Lubansu A, et al. Persistent hydrocephalus after early surgical management of posterior fossa tumors in children: is routine preoperative endoscopic third ventriculostomy justified? J Neurosurg. 2005;103(3 Suppl):247–52.
62. Dewan MC, Isaacs AM, Cools MJ, et al. Treatment of hydrocephalus following posterior fossa tumor resection: a multicenter collaboration from the Hydrocephalus Clinical Research Network. J Neuro-Oncol. 2023;163(1):123–32.
63. Dewan MC, Lim J, Shannon CN, Wellons JC 3rd. The durability of endoscopic third ventriculostomy and ventriculoperitoneal shunts in children with hydrocephalus following posterior fossa tumor resection: a systematic review and time-to-failure analysis. J Neurosurg Pediatr. 2017;19(5):578–84.
64. Tamburrini G, Pettorini BL, Massimi L, Caldarelli M, Di Rocco C. Endoscopic third ventriculostomy: the best option in the treatment of persistent hydrocephalus after posterior cranial fossa tumour removal? Childs Nerv Syst. 2008;24(12):1405–12.

New Advances in Glioblastoma Treatment

9

Raffaele De Marco, Andrea Bianconi, Roberta Rudá, Diego Garbossa, and Fabio Cofano

9.1 Introduction

Glioblastoma, formerly known as glioblastoma multiforme (GBM), is recognized as the most common and malignant primary brain tumor in adults. With the new World Health Organization (WHO) 2021 classification a greater emphasis has been placed on the molecular aspect of the neoplasm: indeed, some of those previously categorized as II and III grades (according to the WHO 2016 classification) that did not have the histological features of glioblastoma, namely central pseudopalisading necrosis and microvascular proliferation, are now considered isocitrate dehydrogenase (IDH)-wild type glioblastoma, if one among telomerase reverse transcriptase (TERT) promoter mutation, Epidermal Growth Factor Receptor (EGFR) amplification or gained of chromosomal and the entire loss of chromosome 10 (+7/−10 copy change) is confirmed during molecular testing [1]. This molecular aspect may define a glioma with "GBM signature" [*molecular Glioblastoma* (molGBM) in addition to *histological GBM* (histGBM)] that shares a similar malignant behavior and poor prognosis, questioning many of the results obtained from clinical trials in previous years. In this evolving world, which sees on the one hand important discoveries on the biology of these tumors, but on the other hand, few or no improvements on therapeutic strategies, this chapter will attempt to make a synopsis of the current strategies and future directions for the management of GBM.

R. De Marco (✉) · A. Bianconi · F. Cofano
Neuroscience Department "Rita Levi Montalcini", Neurosurgery Unit, Università degli Studi di Torino, Turin, Italy
e-mail: raffaele.demarco@unito.it

R. Rudá
Neuroscience Department "Rita Levi Montalcini", Neuro-oncology Unit, Università degli Studi di Torino, Turin, Italy

D. Garbossa
Neurosurgery Unit, Dept. Neuroscience "Rita Levi Montalcini", Università degli studi di Torino, Torino, TO, Italy

9.2 Epidemiology and Disease Burden

The incidence rates of GBM vary across different regions and countries, influenced by factors such as genetic predisposition, environmental exposures, healthcare infrastructure, and diagnostic practices. The global incidence of GBM ranges from approximately 0.59–5 cases per 100,000 person-years. This variation reflects both biological differences and disparities in healthcare systems and reporting practices, obtaining generally higher incidence rates in high-income countries due to better diagnostic capabilities and comprehensive cancer registries compared to lower and middle-income countries. Considering specific regions and adjusting by age, an age-standardized incidence rate (ASIR) of 3.19 per 100,000 indi-

D. Armocida et al. (eds.), *Neurosurgery's Frontline Role in Gliomas Treatment*,
https://doi.org/10.1007/978-3-031-81850-9_9

viduals has been calculated for GBM in United States (US) [2] with a great preponderance of males over females in the range 40–49 years [3]. In Europe, higher ASIR was reported for France, with 5.3 cases per 100,000 individuals [4] and United Kingdom 7.1 per 100,000 individuals [5], while in Italy, the incidence rate was of approximately 3.2–3.8 per 100,000, although regional differences in healthcare quality and access can influence these numbers [6, 7]. A positive trend in incidence was registered with advancing age along with a plateauing in people aged over 65 years, reaching an incidence of 13.2 cases per 100,000 in elderly people in US [8, 9].

The costs associated with the discovery of GBM pathogenesis and subsequent treatments can be both direct and indirect and may vary from country to country due to differences in healthcare systems. These costs can impact both the healthcare system and the country's production system, as they are linked to the need for treatment and the potential impact on an individual's functional autonomy, which may affect their ability to return to work [10–14]. In addition to economic costs, it is crucial to consider the effects of GBM diagnosis on the quality of life of patients and their caregivers. Although the median overall survival without age stratification can range from 12 to 20 months with multimodal treatment, at 5 years, only 6.8% of IDH-wt GBM patients are alive. Results from US data showed better overall survival (OS) at 1 year for patients under 50 years old, those with smaller tumors, and those who underwent a larger extent of resection (EOR). Additionally, better OS was observed for tumors with methylation of the methylguanine-DNA methyltransferase (MGMT) promoter, which influences the response to the first-line chemotherapeutic agent temozolomide (TMZ) [15–17]. Furthermore, irrespective of the country, receiving oncological treatment, specifically maximal safe resection ± chemoradiation therapy, has predictably shown a significant improvement in overall survival compared to biopsy and/or supportive care. Although a few studies have investigated differences between histGBM and molGBM, no significant difference in median OS has been found (molGBM had only a slightly longer OS) [18, 19]. In contrast, molGBM showed a significantly longer progression-free survival (PFS). Multifocal and multicentric GBMs are typically burdened with worse OS, generally reported to be less than 10 months.

9.3 GBM Biology: A Glimpse in the "Omics"

Heralded by the increased importance of the molecular aspect in the latest WHO classification, studies aimed at investigating the biology of the neoplastic glial cell and its surrounding environment are steadily increasing. Although thousands of studies focusing on the specific molecule or the impaired signaling pathway or the aberrant interaction with non-tumor cells have been published, results in the treatment of this pathology are still lagging behind.

A more comprehensive view has been delineated on the molecular mechanisms of this incurable malignancy integrating results from genomics, epigenomics, trascriptomics, proteomics, and other "omics" fields, in addition to discoveries on how the tumor cells interact with the surrounding microenviroment (Tables 9.1 and 9.2) [20, 21]. However, despite the characterization of specific mutations leading to cell proliferation, evasion from apoptosis and ultimately to cell immortality, the attempt to subclassifiy GBM according to molecular features has been evanescent due to the spatial and temporal heterogeneity highlighted in and between tumors [22–24].

Explanations of this intra- and inter-tumoral heterogeneity could be found in the hypothesis behind the tumorigenesis of GBM: facing two theories, "the clonal evolution model" and "the cancer stem cell model," an intriguing hypothesis has been sustained after the observation of similar mutations between Glioma Stem Cells (GSCs) of the GBM and the neural stem cells both located in the astrocytic ribbon of the subventricular zone distant from tumor [25]. The former are characterized by severe aberrations in the stem cells regulatory patterns, with upregulation of cell proliferation, stemness maintance, and cell survival while a downregulation is observed in differentiation, apoptosis, and cell cycle regulation [26]. Like the spreading of the firework when elevates

Table 9.1 Most important mutations of glioblastoma sorted by frequency. The process in which the product of that mutation/alteration is involved, is specified along to its contribution to tumorigenesis. A multilevel analysis referred as multiomics approach is specified

Mutation/ alteration	Involved process	Contribution to tumorigenesis	Multiomics information
TERT promoter mutation	Telomere maintenance	Increases telomerase expression, enabling unlimited cell division, and tumor immortality	Genomics: mutation detected by sequencing. Transcriptomics: increased TERT mRNA expression
CDKN2A/B deletion	Cell cycle regulation	Loss of CDKN2A/B disrupts cell cycle checkpoints, allowing uncontrolled cell division	Genomics: deletion detected by copy number variation analysis Transcriptomics: decreased mRNA expression of CDKN2A/B
EGFR amplification	Cell proliferation and survival	Enhances cell proliferation and survival signals, promoting tumor growth	Genomics: amplification detected by copy number variation analysis Transcriptomics: increased mRNA expression. Proteomics: overexpression of EGFR protein
MGMT promoter methylation	DNA repair	Reduces DNA repair capacity, making tumor cells more susceptible to alkylating agents	Epigenomics: promoter methylation detected by methylation assays Transcriptomics: reduced MGMT mRNA expression
EGFRvIII mutation	Cell proliferation and survival	Constitutively active receptor signaling, leading to uncontrolled cell proliferation	Genomics: mutation identified by sequencing Proteomics: presence of the EGFRvIII protein isoform
TP53 mutation	DNA repair, apoptosis	Loss of function leads to impaired DNA repair and evasion of apoptosis	Genomics: mutation detected by sequencing. Transcriptomics: altered expression of p53 target genes
PTEN deletion/ mutation	PI3K/AKT pathway regulation	Loss of PTEN results in unregulated PI3K/AKT signaling, promoting cell survival and proliferation	Genomics: deletion/mutation detected by sequencing and copy number analysis Proteomics: reduced PTEN protein levels
PDGFRA amplification	Cell proliferation and survival	Promotes autocrine or paracrine growth signaling, enhancing tumor cell proliferation and survival	Genomics: amplification detected by copy number variation analysis Transcriptomics: increased mRNA expression. Proteomics: overexpression of PDGFRA protein
NF1 mutation	RAS signaling	Loss of NF1 leads to increased RAS pathway activity, driving cell proliferation	Genomics: mutation detected by sequencing Proteomics: reduced NF1 protein levels Transcriptomics: altered RAS pathway gene expression
PIK3CA/ PIK3R1 mutations	PI3K/AKT pathway regulation	Activates the PI3K/AKT pathway, enhancing cell survival, growth, and proliferation	Genomics: mutation detected by sequencing Proteomics: altered levels of PI3K pathway proteins. Transcriptomics: Altered expression of PI3K pathway genes
CDK4/6 amplification	Cell cycle regulation	Promotes cell cycle progression by bypassing the G1 checkpoint	Genomics: amplification detected by copy number variation analysis Transcriptomics: increased mRNA expression. Proteomics: overexpression of CDK4/6 proteins

Table 9.2 Principal actors of tumor microenvironment (TME) involved in glioblastoma growth and diffusion

TME actor	Role in tumorigenesis	Mechanism of action
Tumor-associated macrophages (TAMs)	Promote tumor growth, invasion, and immunosuppression	Secrete cytokines and growth factors (e.g., IL-10, TGF-β) that suppress anti-tumor immune responses and promote angiogenesis
Myeloid-derived suppressor cells (MDSCs)	Suppress immune responses and promote tumor progression	Inhibit T cell activation and proliferation, secrete immunosuppressive molecules (e.g., arginase, ROS)
Regulatory T cells (Tregs)	Suppress anti-tumor immune responses	Produce immunosuppressive cytokines (e.g., IL-10, TGF-β), inhibit effector T cell function
Neutrophils	Promote tumor progression, angiogenesis, and immunosuppression	Promote tumor growth, invasion, angiogenesis, and immune evasion
Cancer-associated fibroblasts (CAFs)	Support tumor growth, invasion, and metastasis	Secrete extracellular matrix components, growth factors (e.g., VEGF, FGF), and cytokines that promote tumor cell proliferation and invasion
Endothelial cells	Promote tumor angiogenesis	Form new blood vessels (angiogenesis) in response to tumor-secreted VEGF, providing oxygen and nutrients to the tumor
Pericytes	Stabilize new blood vessels and support angiogenesis	Interact with endothelial cells to support vessel maturation and stability, secrete pro-angiogenic factors
Extracellular vesicles	Facilitate cell-cell communication, promote tumor growth and resistance	Small membrane-bound particles released by cells that can transfer proteins, lipids, and nucleic acids to recipient cell suppressing the immune response, promote angiogenesis, cell invasion or migration or transfer drug resistance
Extracellular matrix	Provides structural support and regulates cell behavior	Contains signaling molecules that promote cell adhesion, migration, and invasion, and modulates growth factor availability
Microglia	Support tumor growth, immune evasion, and neuroinflammation	Secrete cytokines and chemokines that modulate inflammation and support tumor cell survival and invasion
Mesenchymal stem cells (MSCs)	Support tumor growth and metastasis	Migrate to the tumor site and differentiate into CAFs, secrete immunomodulatory and pro-tumorigenic factors
Glioma stem cells (GSCs)	Drive tumor growth, resistance to therapy, and recurrence	Self-renewal, differentiation into various tumor cell types, and resistance to conventional therapies
Immune checkpoint molecules	Inhibit anti-tumor immune responses	Expression of PD-L1, CTLA-4, and other checkpoint molecules on tumor and immune cells suppresses T cell activity

in the sky, the migration of few cells can propagate and proliferate in the site where they reach the optimal environment to growth while contemporarly have accumulated more mutations compared to the cells from which they have originated in the first instance [27]. The same hypothesis has been advanced for recurrence as well. The latter occurrence, which is considered inevitable in the evolution of the disease, is profoundly intertwingled with interactions between tumors and other actors that constitutes the tumor microenvironment (TME) and the different niches inside and immediately outside from what is surgically and radiologically defined as GBM [28–31]. In fact, most GBMs recurs at the border of the surgical cavity even when a complete resection of the contrast-enhanced nodule is achieved [32, 33]. In this direction, many studies focused their attention on the area of brain that surrounds the contrast-enhanced nodule and extends several centimeters around it, which can appear normal at MRI and intraoperatively. The peritumor brain zone (PBZ) presents a different subset of niches, where the GSCs show a more invasive than proliferative behavior and all the actors sustain the same infiltrative process contributing to therapeutic resistance, recurrence, and progression [31].

9.4 Current Management of Glioblastoma

Surgery represents the pillar of treatment of GBM followed by radiotherapy and concomitant and adjuvant chemotherapy with temozolomide (TMZ) as per the Stupp Protocol (Fig. 9.1) [34, 35]. Although the diversity in tumor biology can influence the response to radiation and chemotherapy among patients and in the same patient, the only modifiable factor which is capable to afford an improvement in survival is related to surgery. Indeed, the extent of resection (EOR) independently correlates with PFS and OS [36–38]. Recently, new EOR classes have been introduced to better define this aspect among studies [39, 40]: supramaximal resection of contrast-enhanced (CE) tumor, complete resection (100%), near-total resection (95–99.9% + $\leq$1 cm^3 residual CE tumor), subtotal resection (80–94.9% + $\leq$5 cm^3 residual CE tumor), partial resection (<80% + $\geq$5 cm^3 residual CE tumor), and biopsy (no tumor reduction). Starting from these classes, no significant differences were found between complete and near-total resection nor between subtotal and partial resection. Therefore, analyzing data from 910 IDH-wt GBMs, 4 Response Assessment in Neuro-Oncology (RANO) classes of EOR have been found and validated prognostically: (1) supramaximal CE resection (0 cm^3 CE + $\leq$5 cm^3 residual non CE tumor), (2) maximal CE resection (comprehending both complete (0 cm^3 CE + $\geq$5 cm^3 residual non CE tumor) and near-total ($\leq$ 1 cm^3 residual CE tumor) CE resection), (3) submaximal CE resection (comprehending both subtotal ($\leq$5 cm^3 residual CE tumor), and (4) partial ($\geq$5 cm^3 residual CE tumor) CE resection) and finally biopsy [40]. A statistically significant difference both in PFS and OS were found between these classes. However, age, preoperative CE volume, tumor localization, MGMT promoter methylation status could interefere with the EOR in a real-world clinical setting as well as the pursuing of the onco-functional balance where preserving the functions should be preferred over pushing resection outside the traditional boundary of the tumor.

A radiation treatment is recommended in patient up to 70 years old in good clinical and neurological condition with a common scheme of 54–60 Gy given in 1.8–2 Gy fractions which is administered within 3–6 weeks from surgery [41]. Three-dimensional conformal radiation therapy (3D-CRT), or more recently, intensity-modulated radiation therapy (IMRT) or volumetric modulated arc therapy (VMAT), are used to deliver these doses to a gross tumor volume (GTR) delineated as the surgical cavity plus any residuals observed at contrast-enhanced T1-weighted MRI sequences or fluid-attenuated inversion recovery (FLAIR) intensities clearly visualized as tumor (excluding edema but including those area with infiltrating GBM cells of the PBZ, which are important for those tumors defined as molGBM) or aminoacids PET-based with meaningful biological tumor volume (BTV) [42]. The details of radiation treatment and advances are treated in Chap. 17. Unfortunately, the data from the real world on the newly diagnosed glioblastomas are discouraging with 18% of patients in Germany not being operated on and 5% not receiving any kind of treatment [43]. This percentage reaches 22% when it comes to the United States [44]. Furthermore, few data from China records showed an incredibly low rate of complete resection (36% of GTR) [45], and, for staying in Europe, around 20% of GBMs patients (1856) in France did not receive any other treatment after surgery in a study of 2008 [14].

9.4.1 Beyond the Contrast-Enhanced Nodule: What Should Be the Limit of Resection?

With an increasing number of evidence regarding the importance of the TME and the peritumoral zone, the surgical trend has been directed to involve in the resection also areas outside the contrast-enhanced nodule (which is used to calculate the percentage of Gross Total Resection) [46–49]. In order to reach ("at least") this goal, different tools can aid the surgeon to detect residual or to increase EOR: fluorescent dyes such as

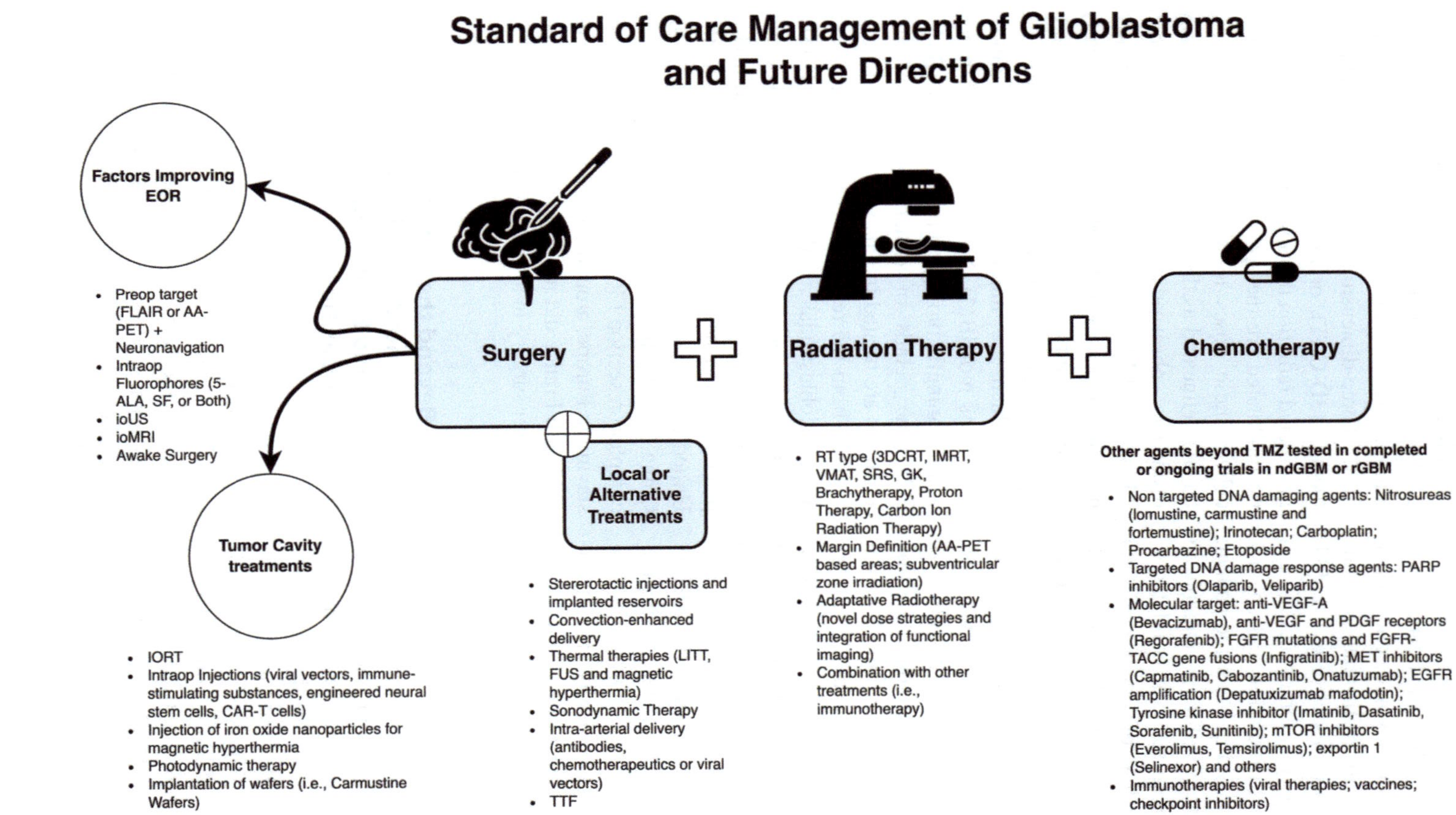

Fig. 9.1 Standard of care management of glioblastoma is graphically showed. Pillars of treatment (surgery, radiation therapy, and chemotherapy) are reported along with acquired advancements and new opportunities that have been or are being under investigation. *EOR* extent of resection, *FLAIR* fluid-attenuated inversion recovery, *AA-PET* amino acid positron emission tomography, *5-ALA* 5-aminolevulinic acid, *SF* sodium fluorescein, *ioMRI* intraoperative magnetic resonance imaging, *ioUS* intraoperative ultrasonography, *IORT* intraoperative radiation therapy, *CAR* chimaeric antigen receptor, *LITT* laser interstitial thermal therapy, *FUS* focused-ultrasonography, *3DCRT* 3-dimensional conformal radiation therapy, *IMRT* intensity-modulated radiation therapy, *VMAT* volumetric modulated arc therapy, *SRS* stereotactic radiosurgery, *GK* gamma-knife, *TMZ* temozolomide, *ndGBM* newly diagnosed glioblastoma, *rGBM* recurrentGBM, *PARP* poly (ADP-ribose) polymerase, *VEGF* vascular endothelial growth factor, *FGFR* fibroblast growth factor receptor, *TACC* transforming acidic coiled-coil (TACC), *EGFR* epidermal growth factor receptor, *PDGFR* platelet-derived growth factor receptor, *mTOR* mammalian target of rapamycin

5-aminolevulinic acid (5-ALA) and/or sodium fluorescein (SF) [50–54], intraoperative ultrasound (ioUS) for a real-time visualization of tumor bulk overcoming the problem of the brain-shift [55–57] and intraoperative MRI (ioMRI) [58–60]. Preferring a multimodal approach with contemporary use of more tools during surgery, ioMRI seems to help more than established fluorophores and ioUS in extending the resection to non-contrast enhancing (nCE) regions [61–63]. However, as per the others, few disadvantages follow this technique, such as poor spatial resolution, high cost and increased operation time, limiting its diffusion to few centers.

When targeting the nCE regions, most studies have investigated the role of T2 weighted sequences and FLAIR as methods to characterize those areas that can influence tumor recurrence, progression and resistance to therapies [64, 65]. Indeed, Yamahara et al. [64] found tumor cell infiltration or classical GBM features in 85% of samples from FLAIR hyperintensities and a similar amount of GSCs in both CE and nCE areas. Similarly, in the work from Barajas et al. [65], 81% of samples from nCE areas contained tumor cells which showed mild proliferative activity (around 4% of Ki-67) and absence of hypoxia. Another work, performing biopsy of nCE areas—specifically FLAIR hyperintensities areas—found regional differences in cell composition and a great representation of non-neoplastic cells that constitute the PBZ [66].

Since it is not easy to differentiate between reactive edema and tumor infiltration in T2/FLAIR hyperintensities, few studies have integrated information and variables from other MRI techniques or sequences [i.e., the choline to N-acetyl aspartate index (CNI) from MR spectroscopy or the relative cerebral blood volume (rCBV) from perfusion and apparent diffusion coefficient (ADC) from DWI] to better define the "meaningful" target in the nCE areas [65, 67–69].

A similar potential has been found in amino acid positron emission tomography (PET), with [methyl-11C]-L-methionine (Met), O-(2-[18F] fluoroethyl)-L-tyrosine (FET) or 18F-fluoro-L-dihydroxy-phenylalanine (FDOPA) which is now recommended in the surgical planning (especially in case of biopsy) or eventually in the definition of the GTV for radiation therapy [42, 70, 71]. Indeed, a more accurate identification of infiltrative areas outside the contrast-enhanced tumor borders could be delineated with this imaging technique [72–74], specifically targeting those GCSs of PBZ from which the tumor inevitably recurs [75].

In order to better characterize tumor tissue beyond what can be perceived under white-light or currently-used fluorophores, new tracers, such as EGFR antibody-conjugated IR dye (IRDye800) [76] and tozuleristide (BLZ-100) [77], have demonstrated their applicability in fluorescence-guided surgery and many others are being studied [78]. Furthermore, some optical devices (i.e., Raman Spectroscopy, Fourier-Transform Infrared Spectroscopy, Optical Coherence Tomography, and Diffuse Reflectance Spectroscopy) [116, 117] have been tested in human-based studies [79] providing real-time information about the molecular buildup of specific tissue and differentiating pathologic from normal tissue at tumor margins [80, 81].

However, indipendently from what the tumor border is, resection must avoid functional and eloquent areas, since a new neurological impairment could impact more on survival than EOR [37, 82]. Preoperative and intraoperative tools should be used in order to preserve this delicate, often conflicting, balance [83]: navigated transcranial magnetic stimulation (nTMS), magnetoencefaphalography (MEG), functional MRI (fMRI), diffusion tensor imaging (DTI) [84, 85], direct cortical stimulation with only motor evoked potentials or somatosensory potentials variations to map motor and somatosensory cortexes during asleep surgery or speech impairment to map language areas in awake surgery [86, 87].

Given the complexity of the brain, the variable locations of eloquent areas among patients and the potential of plasticity, the possibility to increase the EOR beyond the CE nodule could not be always achievable [88, 89]. In addition, the involvement in the resection of certain anatomical boundaries such as the ventricle wall is still debated, although the evidence of GCSs in the subventricular zone [90–93].

When the resection cannot extend over the CE border, other options have been explored in order to destroy pathological tissue or disrupt the brain–blood barriers, which is a known limit for reaching a therapeutic concentration of the post-operative chemotherapeutic or for an immune-response after surgery. In this regard, different strategies have been analyzed [94]: wafers of chemical agents (carmustine wafers were the most tested ones) left on the surface of the surgical cavity, or the placement of cannula for convection enhanced delivery to increase concentration of a drug, or lining the resection cavity with superparamagnetic iron oxide nanoparticles to perform magnetic hyperthermia. In case of deep-seated and/or eloquent lesions otherwise inoperable or for frail patients who would not tolerate craniotomy, alternative treatments have been explored: although much of the experience comes from studies on recurrent glioblastoma [84], stereotactic laser interstitial thermal therapy (LITT) or laser ablation have provided good results both on PFS and OS for newly diagnosed GBM as well [85, 95].

9.4.2 "Add Insult to Injury": Unresolved Issues in GBM Management

If the treatment for young adults (<65–70 years old) with good functional status and a lesion surgically prone for maximal safe resection is standardized (surgery + CRT), in case of elderly, multifocal/multicentric and recurrent GBMs no guideline seems to aid the multidisciplinary team of neurosurgeons, neurooncologists, and radiation therapists.

Indeed, the management of GBM in elderly patients poses unique challenges, as this population often has comorbid conditions and a generally poorer prognosis compared to younger patients, which could be justified by reduced treatment intensity since the higher risk of toxicity and lower tolerance, poor response to therapies—probably influenced by drugs interactions—and altered tumor biology [96–99]. Many researches have focused their attention on this aspect considering that half of newly diagnosed GBMs are >65 and almost a quarter are >70 years old. Furthermore, a positive trend is expected in the next years since the increase in life expectancy [96]. Although the age itself and the presence of comorbidities makes the surgical decision more difficult to take, meta-analysis (mostly retrospective studies) [100, 101] and randomized phase III trials [102, 103] have shown significantly better results in OS with GTR/maximal safe resection than biopsy. Where the surgical option is not feasible, both radiotherapy and chemotherapy alone have shown better results compared to the best supportive care [104, 105]. The possibility to offer both (hypofractionated or short course regimens for radiation therapy), even in the absence of cytoreduction surgery, resulted in better OS and PFS without increasing the risk of toxicity and worsening the quality of life [106].

Multicentric and multifocal GBMs, characterized by the presence of multiple tumor foci, represent a complex subset of GBM with distinct biological, clinical, and radiographic features [19]. These forms of GBM are associated with a worse prognosis compared to unifocal tumors. Treatment strategies lack of consensus, but, surgical resection, where feasible (even with multiple craniotomies [107]) followed by radiotherapy and chemotherapy, remains the cornerstone of treatment [108]. Due to obvious limitations in EOR related to the diffuse nature of these tumors, the adjunct of radiation therapy + TMZ despite the impossibilty of cytoreduction surgery have demonstrated an OS benefit [109]. Emerging therapies, including targeted molecular treatments and immunotherapy, are being explored to improve outcomes in these subtypes of GBM, but robust clinical guidelines are yet to be established.

Given the intrinsic nature of GBM, it inevitably recurs with a median interval of 7 months [34]. The prognosis is generally poor and no standardized treatment protocols have been defined. The management of recurrent GBM (rGBM) often involves a combination of re-resection, re-irradiation, and systemic therapies, enrolling patient in a clinical trial when eligible [11].

Results on re-resection could be influenced by selection biases: in fact, most of the reoperations were reported in patients who were younger, with better Karnofsky Performance Status (KPS) and with smaller tumor size. In addition to age, KPS and tumor size, also tumor location, pattern of recurrence (shorter time to progression or time-to-recurrence or recurrence during active therapy) and the possibility to reach gross total resection appeared to influence the decisional process [110, 111].

Considering that most of recurrences occur within 2–3 cm of the surgical cavity, which is also the high-dose radiation field, the role of re-irradiation seems controversial since the higher risk of toxicity. However, it can play a role with an appropriate patient selection [112, 113]. Furthermore, the combination with other therapies, namely Bevacizumab, a monoclonal antibody targeting the vascular endothelial growth factor (VEGF), seemed to impact positively on OS and the appearance of radionecrosis [114].

Advancements in molecular profiling have enabled more personalized approaches to treatment, identifying potential targets for novel therapies (Fig. 9.1) [115]: tyrosine kinase inhibitors (TKI), VEGF inhibitors, EGFR inhibitors, Platelet-Derived Growth Factors Receptor (PDGFR) inhibitors, MET receptor inhibitors, Fibroblast Growth Factor Receptor (FGFR), immunotherapy with immune checkpoint inhibitors, oncolytic viruses, therapeutic vaccines, and adoptive cell therapy (CAR-T cells therapy) have been tested in the last two decades.

9.5 Conclusions

GBM remains one of the most challenging malignancies to manage, characterized by its aggressive nature and poor prognosis despite advancements in multimodal treatments. The integration of novel imaging techniques and intraoperative tools has enhanced the precision of surgical resections, aiming to increase the extent of resection while preserving neurological function. Similarly, radiation therapy benefited by this integration in the planning. Despite these advancements, the inevitability of tumor recurrence highlights the importance of continued exploration into the tumor microenvironment and the development of new therapeutic strategies. Indeed almost 100 therapies are under evaluation, offering new hope through targeted therapies and immunotherapies.

References

1. Louis DN, Perry A, Wesseling P, et al. The 2021 WHO classification of tumors of the central nervous system: a summary. Neuro-Oncology. 2021;23:1231–51.
2. Ostrom QT, Price M, Neff C, Cioffi G, Waite KA, Kruchko C, Barnholtz-Sloan JS. CBTRUS statistical report: primary brain and other central nervous system tumors diagnosed in the United States in 2016-2020. Neuro-Oncology. 2023;25:IV1–IV99.
3. Schwartzbaum J, Harris R. Age at diagnosis and sex interact to modify primary malignant glioma incidence and survival. Neuro-Oncology. 2022;24:311.
4. Pouchieu C, Gruber A, Berteaud E, Ménégon P, Monteil P, Huchet A, Vignes JR, Vital A, Loiseau H, Baldi I. Increasing incidence of central nervous system (CNS) tumors (2000-2012): findings from a population based registry in Gironde (France). BMC Cancer. 2018. https://doi.org/10.1186/S12885-018-4545-9.
5. Wanis HA, Møller H, Ashkan K, Davies EA. The incidence of major subtypes of primary brain tumors in adults in England 1995-2017. Neuro-Oncology. 2021;23:1371–82.
6. Crocetti E, Trama A, Stiller C, et al. Epidemiology of glial and non-glial brain tumours in Europe. Eur J Cancer. 2012;48:1532–42.
7. Grochans S, Cybulska AM, Simińska D, Korbecki J, Kojder K, Chlubek D, Baranowska-Bosiacka I. Epidemiology of glioblastoma multiforme–literature review. Cancer. 2022;14:2412.
8. Chen B, Chen C, Zhang Y, Xu J. Recent incidence trend of elderly patients with glioblastoma in the United States, 2000-2017. BMC Cancer. 2021. https://doi.org/10.1186/S12885-020-07778-1.
9. Wang GM, Cioffi G, Patil N, et al. Importance of the intersection of age and sex to understand variation in incidence and survival for primary malignant gliomas. Neuro-Oncology. 2022;24:302–10.
10. Pöhlmann J, Weller M, Marcellusi A, Grabe-Heyne K, Krott-Coi L, Rabar S, Pollock RF. High costs, low quality of life, reduced survival, and room for improving treatment: an analysis of burden and unmet needs in glioma. Front Oncol. 2024;14:1368606.
11. Wen PY, Weller M, Lee EQ, et al. Glioblastoma in adults: a Society for Neuro-Oncology (SNO) and European Society of Neuro-Oncology (EANO)

consensus review on current management and future directions. Neuro-Oncology. 2020;22:1073–113.
12. Weller M, van den Bent M, Preusser M, et al. EANO guidelines on the diagnosis and treatment of diffuse gliomas of adulthood. Nat Rev Clin Oncol. 2020;183(18):170–86.
13. Hansen S, Rasmussen BK, Laursen RJ, Kosteljanetz M, Schultz H, Nørgård BM, Guldberg R, Gradel KO. Treatment and survival of glioblastoma patients in Denmark: The Danish Neuro-Oncology Registry 2009-2014. J Neuro-Oncol. 2018;139:479–89.
14. Fabbro-Peray P, Zouaoui S, Darlix A, et al. Association of patterns of care, prognostic factors, and use of radiotherapy-temozolomide therapy with survival in patients with newly diagnosed glioblastoma: a French national population-based study. J Neuro-Oncol. 2019;142:91–101.
15. Brown NF, Ottaviani D, Tazare J, Gregson J, Kitchen N, Brandner S, Fersht N, Mulholland P. Survival outcomes and prognostic factors in glioblastoma. Cancer. 2022. https://doi.org/10.3390/CANCERS14133161.
16. Blakstad H, Brekke J, Rahman MA, Arnesen VS, Miletic H, Brandal P, Lie SA, Chekenya M, Goplen D. Survival in a consecutive series of 467 glioblastoma patients: Association with prognostic factors and treatment at recurrence at two independent institutions. PLoS One. 2023. https://doi.org/10.1371/JOURNAL.PONE.0281166.
17. Ramos-Fresnedo A, Pullen MW, Perez-Vega C, et al. The survival outcomes of molecular glioblastoma IDH-wildtype: a multicenter study. J Neuro-Oncol. 2022;157:177–85.
18. Guo X, Gu L, Li Y, et al. Histological and molecular glioblastoma, IDH-wildtype: a real-world landscape using the 2021 WHO classification of central nervous system tumors. Front Oncol. 2023;13:1200815.
19. Baro V, Cerretti G, Todoverto M, et al. Newly diagnosed multifocal GBM: a monocentric experience and literature review. Curr Oncol. 2022;29:3472–88.
20. Takahashi S, Takahashi M, Tanaka S, et al. A new era of neuro-oncology research pioneered by multiomics analysis and machine learning. Biomolecules. 2021. https://doi.org/10.3390/BIOM11040565/S1.
21. Koh L, Novera W, Lim SW, Chong YK, Pang QY, Low D, Ang BT, Tang C. Integrative multi-omics approach to targeted therapy for glioblastoma. Pharmacol Res. 2022;182:106308.
22. Lee JK, Wang J, Sa JK, et al. Spatiotemporal genomic architecture informs precision oncology in glioblastoma. Nat Genet. 2017;494(49):594–9.
23. Dirkse A, Golebiewska A, Buder T, et al. Stem cell-associated heterogeneity in Glioblastoma results from intrinsic tumor plasticity shaped by the microenvironment. Nat Commun. 2019. https://doi.org/10.1038/s41467-019-09853-z.
24. Khalafallah AM, Huq S, Jimenez AE, Serra R, Bettegowda C, Mukherjee D. "Zooming in" on glioblastoma: understanding tumor heterogeneity and its clinical implications in the era of single-cell ribonucleic acid sequencing. Neurosurgery. 2021;88:477–86.
25. Lee JH, Lee JE, Kahng JY, et al. Human glioblastoma arises from subventricular zone cells with low-level driver mutations. Nature. 2018;5607717(560):243–7.
26. Nasrolahi A, Azizidoost S, Radoszkiewicz K, Najafi S, Ghaedrahmati F, Anbiyaee O, Khoshnam SE, Farzaneh M, Uddin S. Signaling pathways governing glioma cancer stem cells behavior. Cell Signal. 2023. https://doi.org/10.1016/J.CELLSIG.2022.110493.
27. Yoon SJ, Park J, Jang DS, et al. Glioblastoma cellular origin and the firework pattern of cancer genesis from the subventricular zone. J Korean Neurosurg Soc. 2020;63:26.
28. Hambardzumyan D, Bergers G. Glioblastoma: defining tumor niches. Trends Cancer. 2015;1:252.
29. Schiffer D, Annovazzi L, Casalone C, Corona C, Mellai M. Glioblastoma: microenvironment and niche concept. Cancer. 2019;11:5.
30. Bianconi A, Aruta G, Rizzo F, Salvati LF, Zeppa P, Garbossa D, Cofano F. Systematic review on tumor microenvironment in glial neoplasm: from understanding pathogenesis to future therapeutic perspectives. Int J Mol Sci. 2022. https://doi.org/10.3390/IJMS23084166.
31. Ballestín A, Armocida D, Ribecco V, Seano G. Peritumoral brain zone in glioblastoma: biological, clinical and mechanical features. Front Immunol. 2024;15:1347877.
32. Rapp M, Baernreuther J, Turowski B, Steiger HJ, Sabel M, Kamp MA. Recurrence pattern analysis of primary glioblastoma. World Neurosurg. 2017;103:733–40.
33. Yoo J, Yoon SJ, Kim KH, et al. Patterns of recurrence according to the extent of resection in patients with IDH-wild-type glioblastoma: a retrospective study. J Neurosurg. 2021;137:533–43.
34. Stupp R, Mason WP, van den Bent MJ, et al. Radiotherapy plus concomitant and adjuvant temozolomide for glioblastoma. N Engl J Med. 2005;352:987–96.
35. Stupp R, Hegi ME, Mason WP, et al. Effects of radiotherapy with concomitant and adjuvant temozolomide versus radiotherapy alone on survival in glioblastoma in a randomised phase III study: 5-year analysis of the EORTC-NCIC trial. Lancet Oncol. 2009;10:459–66.
36. Lacroix M, Abi-Said D, Fourney DR, et al. A multivariate analysis of 416 patients with glioblastoma multiforme: prognosis, extent of resection, and survival. J Neurosurg. 2001;95:190–8.
37. McGirt MJ, Mukherjee D, Chaichana KL, Than KD, Weingart JD, Quinones-Hinojosa A. Association of surgically acquired motor and language deficits on overall survival after resection of glioblastoma multiforme. Neurosurgery. 2009;65:463–9.
38. Brown TJ, Brennan MC, Li M, et al. Association of the extent of resection with survival in glioblastoma: a systematic review and meta-analysis. JAMA Oncol. 2016;2:1460–9.

39. Karschnia P, Vogelbaum MA, van den Bent M, Cahill DP, Bello L, Narita Y, Berger MS, Weller M, Tonn JC. Evidence-based recommendations on categories for extent of resection in diffuse glioma. Eur J Cancer. 2021;149:23–33.
40. Karschnia P, Young JS, Dono A, et al. Prognostic validation of a new classification system for extent of resection in glioblastoma: a report of the RANO resect group. Neuro-Oncology. 2023;25:940.
41. Weller M, van den Bent M, Hopkins K, et al. EANO guideline for the diagnosis and treatment of anaplastic gliomas and glioblastoma. Lancet Oncol. 2014. https://doi.org/10.1016/S1470-2045(14)70011-7.
42. Niyazi M, Andratschke N, Bendszus M, et al. ESTRO-EANO guideline on target delineation and radiotherapy details for glioblastoma. Radiother Oncol. 2023;184:109663.
43. Efremov L, Abera SF, Bedir A, Vordermark D, Medenwald D. Patterns of glioblastoma treatment and survival over a 16-years period: pooled data from the German Cancer Registries. J Cancer Res Clin Oncol. 2021;147:3381–90.
44. Aly A, Singh P, Korytowsky B, Ling YL, Kale HP, Dastani HB, Botteman MF, Norden AD. Survival, costs, and health care resource use by line of therapy in US Medicare patients with newly diagnosed glioblastoma: a retrospective observational study. Neurol Pract. 2020;7:164–75.
45. Woo PYM, Yau S, Lam T-C, et al. Patterns of care and survival of Chinese glioblastoma patients in the temozolomide era: a Hong Kong population-level analysis over a 14-year period. Neuro-Oncol Pract. 2023;10:50.
46. Incekara F, Koene S, Vincent AJPE, van den Bent MJ, Smits M. Association between supratotal glioblastoma resection and patient survival: a systematic review and meta-analysis. World Neurosurg. 2019;127:617–24.
47. Molinaro AM, Hervey-Jumper S, Morshed RA, et al. Association of maximal extent of resection of contrast-enhanced and non-contrast-enhanced tumor with survival within molecular subgroups of patients with newly diagnosed glioblastoma. JAMA Oncol. 2020;6:495.
48. Jackson C, Choi J, Khalafallah AM, Price C, Bettegowda C, Lim M, Gallia G, Weingart J, Brem H, Mukherjee D. A systematic review and meta-analysis of supratotal versus gross total resection for glioblastoma. J Neuro-Oncol. 2020;148:419–31.
49. Wach J, Vychopen M, Kühnapfel A, Seidel C, Güresir E. A systematic review and meta-analysis of supramarginal resection versus gross total resection in glioblastoma: can we enhance progression-free survival time and preserve postoperative safety? Cancer. 2023;15:1772.
50. Stummer W, Pichlmeier U, Meinel T, Wiestler OD, Zanella F, Reulen HJ. Fluorescence-guided surgery with 5-aminolevulinic acid for resection of malignant glioma: a randomised controlled multicentre phase III trial. Lancet Oncol. 2006;7:392–401.
51. Schwake M, Stummer W, Suero Molina EJ, Wölfer J. Simultaneous fluorescein sodium and 5-ALA in fluorescence-guided glioma surgery. Acta Neurochir. 2015;157:877.
52. Molina ES, Wölfer J, Ewelt C, Ehrhardt A, Brokinkel B, Stummer W. Dual-labeling with 5-aminolevulinic acid and fluorescein for fluorescence-guided resection of high-grade gliomas: technical note. J Neurosurg. 2017;128:399–405.
53. Acerbi F, Broggi M, Schebesch KM, et al. Fluorescein-guided surgery for resection of high-grade gliomas: a multicentric prospective phase II study (FLUOGLIO). Clin Cancer Res. 2018;24:52–61.
54. Zeppa P, De Marco R, Monticelli M, et al. Fluorescence-guided surgery in glioblastoma: 5-ALA, SF or both? Differences between fluorescent dyes in 99 consecutive cases. Brain Sci. 2022;12:555.
55. Trevisi G, Barbone P, Treglia G, Mattoli MV, Mangiola A. Reliability of intraoperative ultrasound in detecting tumor residual after brain diffuse glioma surgery: a systematic review and meta-analysis. Neurosurg Rev. 2020;43:1221–33.
56. Moiraghi A, Prada F, Delaidelli A, et al. Navigated intraoperative 2-dimensional ultrasound in high-grade glioma surgery: impact on extent of resection and patient outcome. Oper Neurosurg. 2020;18:363–73.
57. Incekara F, Smits M, Dirven L, Bos EM, Balvers RK, Haitsma IK, Schouten JW, Vincent AJPE. Intraoperative B-mode ultrasound guided surgery and the extent of glioblastoma resection: a randomized controlled trial. Front Oncol. 2021;11:1.
58. Hatiboglu MA, Weinberg JS, Suki D, Rao G, Prabhu SS, Shah K, Jackson E, Sawaya R. Impact of intraoperative high-field magnetic resonance imaging guidance on glioma surgery: a prospective volumetric analysis. Neurosurgery. 2009;64:1073–81.
59. Senft C, Bink A, Franz K, Vatter H, Gasser T, Seifert V. Intraoperative MRI guidance and extent of resection in glioma surgery: a randomised, controlled trial. Lancet Oncol. 2011;12:997–1003.
60. Napolitano M, Vaz G, Lawson TM, Docquier MA, van Maanen A, Duprez T, Raftopoulos C. Glioblastoma surgery with and without intraoperative MRI at 3.0T. Neurochirurgie. 2014;60:143–50.
61. Li YM, Suki D, Hess K, Sawaya R. The influence of maximum safe resection of glioblastoma on survival in 1229 patients: can we do better than gross-total resection? J Neurosurg. 2016;124:977–88.
62. Eyüpoglu IY, Hore N, Merkel A, et al. Supracomplete surgery via dual intraoperative visualization approach (DiVA) prolongs patient survival in glioblastoma. Oncotarget. 2016;7:25755–68.
63. Pessina F, Navarria P, Cozzi L, Ascolese AM, Simonelli M, Santoro A, Clerici E, Rossi M, Scorsetti M, Bello L. Maximize surgical resection beyond contrast-enhancing boundaries in newly diagnosed glioblastoma multiforme: is it useful and

safe? A single institution retrospective experience. J Neuro-Oncol. 2017;135:129–39.
64. Yamahara T, Numa Y, Oishi T, Kawaguchi T, Seno T, Asai A, Kawamoto K. Morphological and flow cytometric analysis of cell infiltration in glioblastoma: a comparison of autopsy brain and neuroimaging. Brain Tumor Pathol. 2010;27:81–7.
65. Barajas RF, Phillips JJ, Parvataneni R, et al. Regional variation in histopathologic features of tumor specimens from treatment-naive glioblastoma correlates with anatomic and physiologic MR imaging. Neuro-Oncology. 2012;14:942–54.
66. Gill BJ, Pisapia DJ, Malone HR, et al. MRI-localized biopsies reveal subtype-specific differences in molecular and cellular composition at the margins of glioblastoma. Proc Natl Acad Sci USA. 2014;111:12550–5.
67. Hu LS, Ning S, Eschbacher JM, et al. Multiparametric MRI and texture analysis to visualize spatial histologic heterogeneity and tumor extent in glioblastoma. PLoS One. 2015. https://doi.org/10.1371/JOURNAL.PONE.0141506.
68. Artzi M, Liberman G, Blumenthal DT, Aizenstein O, Bokstein F, Ben Bashat D. Differentiation between vasogenic edema and infiltrative tumor in patients with high-grade gliomas using texture patch-based analysis. J Magn Reson Imaging. 2018;48:729–36.
69. Lasocki A, Gaillard F. Non-contrast-enhancing tumor: a new frontier in glioblastoma research. Am J Neuroradiol. 2019;40:758–65.
70. Albert NL, Weller M, Suchorska B, et al. Response Assessment in Neuro-Oncology Working Group and European Association for Neuro-Oncology recommendations for the clinical use of PET imaging in gliomas. Neuro-Oncology. 2016;18:1199–208.
71. Law I, Albert NL, Arbizu J, et al. Joint EANM/EANO/RANO practice guidelines/SNMMI procedure standards for imaging of gliomas using PET with radiolabelled amino acids and [18 F] FDG: version 1.0. Eur J Nucl Med Mol Imaging. 2019;46:540–57.
72. Yang Y, He MZ, Li T, Yang X. MRI combined with PET-CT of different tracers to improve the accuracy of glioma diagnosis: a systematic review and meta-analysis. Neurosurg Rev. 2019;42:185–95.
73. Zhang-Yin JT, Girard A, Bertaux M. What does PET imaging bring to neuro-oncology in 2022? A review. Cancer. 2022. https://doi.org/10.3390/CANCERS14040879.
74. De Marco R, Pesaresi A, Bianconi A, Zotta M, Deandreis D, Morana G, Zeppa P, Melcarne A, Garbossa D, Cofano F. A systematic review of amino acid PET imaging in adult-type high-grade glioma surgery: a neurosurgeon's perspective. Cancer. 2023. https://doi.org/10.3390/CANCERS15010090.
75. Inoue A, Ohnishi T, Kohno S, et al. Met-PET uptake index for total tumor resection: identification of 11 C-methionine uptake index as a goal for total tumor resection including infiltrating tumor cells in glioblastoma. Neurosurg Rev. 2021;44:587–97.
76. Miller SE, Tummers WS, Teraphongphom N, et al. First-in-human intraoperative near-infrared fluorescence imaging of glioblastoma using cetuximab-IRDye800. J Neuro-Oncol. 2018;139:135–43.
77. Patil CG, Walker DG, Miller DM, et al. Phase 1 safety, pharmacokinetics, and fluorescence imaging study of tozuleristide (BLZ-100) in adults with newly diagnosed or recurrent gliomas. Neurosurgery. 2019;85:E641–9.
78. Chirizzi C, Pellegatta S, Gori A, Falco J, Rubiu E, Acerbi F, Bombelli FB. Next-generation agents for fluorescence-guided glioblastoma surgery. Bioeng Transl Med. 2023. https://doi.org/10.1002/BTM2.10608.
79. Burström G, Amini M, El-Hajj VG, Arfan A, Gharios M, Buwaider A, Losch MS, Manni F, Edström E, Elmi-Terander A. Optical methods for brain tumor detection: a systematic review. J Clin Med. 2024;13:2676.
80. Livermore LJ, Isabelle M, Bell IM, Edgar O, Voets NL, Stacey R, Ansorge O, Vallance C, Plaha P. Raman spectroscopy to differentiate between fresh tissue samples of glioma and normal brain: a comparison with 5-ALA–induced fluorescence-guided surgery. J Neurosurg. 2020;135:469–79.
81. Pekmezci M, Morshed RA, Chunduru P, et al. Detection of glioma infiltration at the tumor margin using quantitative stimulated Raman scattering histology. Sci Rep. 2021;111(11):1–11.
82. Aabedi AA, Young JS, Zhang Y, et al. Association of neurological impairment on the relative benefit of maximal extent of resection in chemoradiation-treated newly diagnosed isocitrate dehydrogenase wild-type glioblastoma. Neurosurgery. 2022;90:124.
83. Gerritsen JKW, Broekman MLD, De Vleeschouwer S, Schucht P, Nahed BV, Berger MS, Vincent AJ. Safe surgery for glioblastoma: recent advances and modern challenges. Neuro-Oncol Pract. 2022;9:364.
84. Montemurro N, Anania Y, Cagnazzo F, Perrini P. Survival outcomes in patients with recurrent glioblastoma treated with laser interstitial thermal therapy (LITT): a systematic review. Clin Neurol Neurosurg. 2020;195:105942.
85. Mohammadi AM, Sharma M, Beaumont TL, et al. Upfront magnetic resonance imaging-guided stereotactic laser-ablation in newly diagnosed glioblastoma: a multicenter review of survival outcomes compared to a matched cohort of biopsy-only patients. Neurosurgery. 2019;85:762.
86. Gerritsen JKW, Klimek M, Dirven CMF, de Hoop EO, Wagemakers M, Rutten GJM, Kloet A, Hallaert GG, Vincent AJ. The SAFE-trial: safe surgery for glioblastoma multiforme: awake craniotomy versus surgery under general anesthesia. Study protocol for a multicenter prospective randomized controlled trial. Contemp Clin Trials. 2020. https://doi.org/10.1016/J.CCT.2019.105876.
87. Gerritsen JKW, Dirven CMF, De Vleeschouwer S, Schucht P, Jungk C, Krieg SM, Nahed BV, Berger MS, Broekman MLD, Vincent AJPE. The

PROGRAM study: awake mapping versus asleep mapping versus no mapping for high-grade glioma resections: study protocol for an international multicenter prospective three-arm cohort study. BMJ Open. 2021. https://doi.org/10.1136/BMJOPEN-2020-047306.
88. Duffau H. Is supratotal resection of glioblastoma in noneloquent areas possible? World Neurosurg. 2014;82:e101–3.
89. Zigiotto L, Annicchiarico L, Corsini F, et al. Effects of supra-total resection in neurocognitive and oncological outcome of high-grade gliomas comparing asleep and awake surgery. J Neuro-Oncol. 2020;148:97–108.
90. Chaichana KL, McGirt MJ, Frazier J, Attenello F, Guerrero-Cazares H, Quinones-Hinojosa A. Relationship of glioblastoma multiforme to the lateral ventricles predicts survival following tumor resection. J Neuro-Oncol. 2008;89:219–24.
91. Mistry AM, Hale AT, Chambless LB, Weaver KD, Thompson RC, Ihrie RA. Influence of glioblastoma contact with the lateral ventricle on survival: a meta-analysis. J Neuro-Oncol. 2017;131:125–33.
92. Mistry AM, Kelly PD, Gallant J-N, Mummareddy N, Mobley BC, Thompson RC, Chambless LB. Comparative analysis of subventricular zone glioblastoma contact and ventricular entry during resection in predicting dissemination, hydrocephalus, and survival. Neurosurgery. 2019;85:E924–32.
93. Cofano F, Bianconi A, De Marco R, et al. The impact of lateral ventricular opening in the resection of newly diagnosed high-grade gliomas: a single center experience. Cancer. 2024;16:1574.
94. van Solinge TS, Nieland L, Chiocca EA, Broekman MLD. Advances in local therapy for glioblastoma - taking the fight to the tumour. Nat Rev Neurol. 2022;18:221–36.
95. De Groot JF, Kim AH, Prabhu S, et al. Efficacy of laser interstitial thermal therapy (LITT) for newly diagnosed and recurrent IDH wild-type glioblastoma. Neuro-oncology Adv. 2022. https://doi.org/10.1093/NOAJNL/VDAC040.
96. Holdhoff M, Chamberlain MC. Controversies in the treatment of elderly patients with newly diagnosed glioblastoma. J Natl Compr Cancer Netw. 2013;11:1165–73.
97. Bauchet L, Zouaoui S, Darlix A, De Champfleur NM, Ferreira E, Fabbro M, Kerr C, Taillandier L. Assessment and treatment relevance in elderly glioblastoma patients. Neuro-Oncology. 2014;16:1459–68.
98. Fiorentino A, Balducci M, De Bonis P, et al. Can elderly patients with newly diagnosed glioblastoma be enrolled in radiochemotherapy trials? Am J Clin Oncol Cancer Clin Trials. 2015;38:23–7.
99. Bruno F, Pellerino A, Palmiero R, Bertero L, Mantovani C, Garbossa D, Soffietti R, Rudà R. Glioblastoma in the elderly: review of molecular and therapeutic aspects. Biomedicines. 2022. https://doi.org/10.3390/BIOMEDICINES10030644.
100. Noorbakhsh A, Tang JA, Marcus LP, McCutcheon B, Gonda DD, Schallhorn CS, Talamini MA, Chang DC, Carter BS, Chen CC. Gross-total resection outcomes in an elderly population with glioblastoma: a SEER-based analysis: clinical article. J Neurosurg. 2014;120:31–9.
101. Almenawer SA, Badhiwala JH, Alhazzani W, et al. Biopsy versus partial versus gross total resection in older patients with high-grade glioma: a systematic review and meta-analysis. Neuro-Oncology. 2015;17:868–81.
102. Malmström A, Grønberg BH, Marosi C, et al. Temozolomide versus standard 6-week radiotherapy versus hypofractionated radiotherapy in patients older than 60 years with glioblastoma: the Nordic randomised, phase 3 trial. Lancet Oncol. 2012;13:916–26.
103. Wick W, Platten M, Meisner C, et al. Temozolomide chemotherapy alone versus radiotherapy alone for malignant astrocytoma in the elderly: the NOA-08 randomised, phase 3 trial. Lancet Oncol. 2012;13:707–15.
104. Keime-Guibert F, Chinot O, Taillandier L, et al. Radiotherapy for glioblastoma in the elderly. N Engl J Med. 2007;356:1527–35.
105. Pérez-Larraya JG, Ducray F, Chinot O, et al. Temozolomide in elderly patients with newly diagnosed glioblastoma and poor performance status: an ANOCEF phase II trial. J Clin Oncol. 2011;29:3050–5.
106. Perry JR, Laperriere N, O'Callaghan CJ, et al. Short-course radiation plus temozolomide in elderly patients with glioblastoma. N Engl J Med. 2017;376:1027–37.
107. Hassaneen W, Levine NB, Suki D, et al. Multiple craniotomies in the management of multifocal and multicentric glioblastoma: clinical article. J Neurosurg. 2011;114:576–84.
108. Armocida D, Pesce A, Di Giammarco F, Frati A, Salvati M, Santoro A. Histological, molecular, clinical and outcomes characteristics of multiple lesion glioblastoma. A retrospective monocentric study and review of literature. Neurocirugia. 2021;32(3):114–23. https://doi.org/10.1016/j.neucir.2020.04.003.
109. Haque W, Thong Y, Verma V, Rostomily R, Brian Butler E, Teh BS. Patterns of management and outcomes of unifocal versus multifocal glioblastoma. J Clin Neurosci. 2020;74:155–9.
110. Ringel F, Pape H, et al. Clinical benefit from resection of recurrent glioblastomas: results of a multicenter study including 503 patients with recurrent glioblastomas undergoing surgical resection. Neuro-Oncology. 2016;18:96–104.
111. Zhao YH, Wang ZF, Pan ZY, Péus D, Delgado-Fernandez J, Pallud J, Li ZQ. A meta-analysis of survival outcomes following reoperation in recurrent glioblastoma: time to consider the timing of reoperation. Front Neurol. 2019. https://doi.org/10.3389/FNEUR.2019.00286/XML/NLM.

112. Straube C, Kessel KA, Zimmer C, Schmidt-Graf F, Schlegel J, Gempt J, Meyer B, Combs SE. A second course of radiotherapy in patients with recurrent malignant gliomas: clinical data on re-irradiation, prognostic factors, and usefulness of digital biomarkers. Curr Treat Options in Oncol. 2019;20:1–14.
113. Knisely JPS, Fine HA. Reirradiation for recurrent glioblastoma: what we know and what we do not. J Clin Oncol. 2023;41:1183–8.
114. Kulinich DP, Sheppard JP, Nguyen T, Kondajji AM, Unterberger A, Duong C, Enomoto A, Patel K, Yang I. Radiotherapy versus combination radiotherapy-bevacizumab for the treatment of recurrent high-grade glioma: a systematic review. Acta Neurochir. 2021;163:1921–34.
115. Vaz-Salgado MA, Villamayor M, Albarrán V, et al. Recurrent glioblastoma: a review of the treatment options. Cancer. 2023;15:4279.
116. Tuncer MS, Salvati LF, Grittner U, et al. Towards a tractography-based risk stratification model for language area associated gliomas. NeuroImage Clin. 2021. https://doi.org/10.1016/J.NICL.2020.102541.
117. Salvati LF, De Marco R, Palmieri G, Minardi M, Massara A, Pesaresi A, Cagetti B, Melcarne A, Garbossa D. The relevant role of navigated tractography in speech eloquent area glioma surgery: single center experience. Brain Sci. 2021. https://doi.org/10.3390/BRAINSCI11111436.

Part III

Part III

The Neuro-Oncological Balance in the Modern Era

10

Daniele Armocida, Sergio Corvino, Antonio Santoro, Alessandro Pesce, and Alessandro Frati

10.1 Introduction

Over the last two decades, we assisted to a change in the paradigm of treatment of low-grade gliomas (LGG), shifting from a conservative "wait and see" strategy in asymptomatic patients to an early and aggressive active therapeutic approach in which the surgery plays a leading role [1, 2]. Current guidelines of treatment for gliomas at initial diagnosis recommend maximal safe tumor resection while preserving the neurological functions, followed by radio and chemotherapy based on tumor IDH status and grade [3].

The rationale behind this change in management comes from the better understanding of the natural history of the disease as well as from the better understanding of the brain plasticity mechanisms and the identification of several prognostic factors of overall survival, especially the extent of resection.

Historically, incidental LGG were considered benign lesions, with a slow and linear growth of 2.7–4 mm per year [4–6], thus were conservatively treated through seriate MRI until symptoms occurred [7]. Nowadays, it is known that LGG show peculiar molecular, clinical and histological features, exhibiting an exponential growth [8] and diffuse and infiltrating pattern [8, 9], with invasion of the central nervous system, especially the subcortical connectivity which accounts for the brain functions and whose injury results in "disconnection syndrome" and worsening of quality of life, accordingly. Their natural history ranges from an indolent to a biologically aggressive behavior, resulting finally in a progressive neurological decline and death secondary to malignant transformation which unpredictably but inexorably occurs [10–13]. Even when seriate imaging studies show unchanged findings, not-detectable background molecular mutations occur. Therefore, in the light of this date and con-

D. Armocida (✉)
Neurosurgery Unit, Dept. Neuroscience "Rita Levi Montalcini", Università degli studi di Torino, Torino, TO, Italy
e-mail: danielearmocida@yahoo.it

S. Corvino
Division of Neurosurgery, Department of Neuroscience, Reproductive and Odontostomatological sciences, Università degli Studi di Napoli Federico II, Naples, NA, Italy

A. Santoro
Neurosurgery Division, Human Neurosciences Department, "La Sapienza" University, Rome, RM, Italy

A. Pesce
Policlinico Tor Vergata (PTV), Neurosurgery Unit, Università degli Studi di Roma (Tor Vergata), Rome, RM, Italy

A. Frati
IRCCS "Neuromed", Pozzilli, IS, Italy

Neurosurgery Division, Human Neurosciences Department, "La Sapienza" University, Rome, RM, Italy

D. Armocida et al. (eds.), *Neurosurgery's Frontline Role in Gliomas Treatment*, https://doi.org/10.1007/978-3-031-81850-9_10

sidering that the overall survival is worst in secondary high-grade gliomas (median 2 years after progression) [14, 15] compared to that one of unchanged low-grade histology at recurrence [16], most authors suggested an early diagnosis and preventive tumor resection to improve the outcome of LGG patients [17, 18].

In addition to the early intervention, the extension of resection represents the main prognostic factors, with the maximal extent of resection which improves the overall survival [14, 19–24].

Finally, as brain gliomas arise from glial cells forming the subcortical white matter of the brain hemispheres, they can potentially involve every functional pathway of the cerebral hemispheres, with frequent location near o within the so-called eloquent areas [25]; therefore, it is worth to consider that surgical resection might account for postoperative severe and transient or permanent neurological deficits. In this setting, preservation of quality of life represents a priority.

In conclusion, gliomas' surgery should be *early*, *maximal*, and *safe*, aiming for an onco-functional balance.

10.1.1 Benefit–Risk Ratio of Therapeutic Strategy: The Onco-Functional Balance

The "Hamletic doubt" in glioma surgery is whether to favor the widest extent of resection to delay the malignant transformation and prolong the overall survival but risking postoperative neurological deficits or to favor the preservation of the neurological functions and the quality of life by limiting the extent of resection but at expense of a shorter overall survival. A longer life or a better quality of life?

Duffau attempted to solve this dilemma introducing the concept of "onco-functional balance," also named "functional neuro-oncology" to weight the value of the extent of resection versus the transitory or permanent neurological deterioration voluntarily generated by radical resection [9, 26, 27]. The goal of surgery is the maximal safe tumor resection while preserving the neurological functions, so to prioritize the extent of resection and the quality of life. For this purpose, the neurosurgeon should perform the surgical resection based on the cortico-subcortical functional and not oncological boundaries [9]. This surgical strategy requires three steps of knowledge [27].

First, the preoperative detailed knowledge of the individual cerebral anatomo-functional organization of each patient to remove the pathological cerebral tissue that can be functionally compensated by the cerebral plasticity along with neuropsychological training, without impairment of the quality of life. In this way, according to the importance of neurofunctional area involved by the tumor and the capability of that function to be compensated after removal, the neurosurgeon decides for a complete or incomplete surgical resection, tailoring the resection to each patient at each moment.

Second, the understanding of the individual subcortical brain connectivity during resection. It is important to map both horizontal cortico-cortical connectivity as well as cortico-subcortical connectivity to preserve the networks underlying the minimal common core of the brain.

Finally, the understanding of the individual functional brain remapping after resection (neuroplasticity) to assist the neurosurgeon in the preoperative decision-making in terms of surgical radicality.

In addition, in cases of incomplete tumor resection for functional reasons, Duffau proposes a multistage surgical approach, which accounts for a decreased risk of malignant transformation thanks to the initial tumor debulking, and a more extensive resection in the subsequent surgeries thanks to the functional remapping of the surgical field [9].

Recently, Duffau have proposed a further advance of this theory to optimize the onco-functional balance of glioma surgery, suggesting to switch from a "tumor mass excision" toward a connectome-based resection taking into account both relationships between the tumor and critical distributed circuits as well as the perpetual instability of the meta-network [28]. This functional mapping-guided surgery provided a maximization of the extent of resection, by introducing the concept of "supramaximal resection" in both low-

and high-grade gliomas, and allowed an improvement of the overall survival in LGG patients while preserving their quality of life [28].

We are thus faced with two important areas of insight in which surgical research must address: how to maximize the extent of resection and how to minimize brain functions damage.

10.1.2 Minimize Brain Functions Damage

The current gold standard to minimize the eloquent damage is direct cortical and subcortical stimulation during awake craniotomy or asleep motor mapping, which allow for the intraoperative identification of functional cortex and white matter tracts before and during tumor resection [29]. The detection of tumor location and the identification of eloquent areas are two crucial factors in the decision to use mapping techniques, and they can be preoperatively assessed through anatomical and functional methods.

Anatomical methods included MRI, DTI, resection probability maps, voxel-based analysis, functional atlases, graph theory, Brodmann anatomical locations [30], and the classification systems by Sawaya et al. [31], McGirt et al. [23], and Lima et al. [17]. Brodmann anatomical areas are suboptimal for preoperative decision-making in glioma treatment because, conversely from Sawaya and the Friedlein (FGA/B) grading systems, they do not distinguish essential (i.e., critically eloquent) functions from other functional areas, and they do not consider anatomical distortion caused by the lesion. The Friedlein grading system, however, predicts the resectability of the tumor, without considering surgical approaches with intraoperative mapping. Though, tumor eloquence does not necessarily correlate with resectability of the tumor, it serves to inform neurosurgeons about the level of caution that should be applied when operating in each area. Sawaya's grading system consists of three classes, of which class I and III have proven to be objective and easy to use, whereas the ambiguity of class II eloquence (near-eloquent brain) limits the clinical applicability of the system [22].

Functional methods included functional MRI (fMRI), diffusion tensor imaging (DTI), navigated transcranial magnetic stimulation (nTMS) and magnetoencephalography (MEG), fMRI-based-DTI, nTMS-based-DTI, multitask graph neural networks and presurgical grids, each with associated pros and cons. Since large interindividual variability exists in the distribution of eloquent areas, it may be expedient to assess eloquence with a patient-specific method, as is seen with fMRI, nTMS and MEG [20]. However, these techniques (1) are not yet part of the clinically standard preoperative procedure, (2) are not universally available and, (3) most importantly, do not always yield reproducible results. Therefore, a technique based on standard preoperative MRI would currently appear most practical. One elegant approach to use this imaging to predict post-operative outcomes is in the form of resection probability maps. Though these "maps" are especially useful to predict the extent of resection [9], they do not inform the surgeon about eloquence and risk of potential deficits. Second, whereas resection probability maps enable group analysis of results and comparison of outcomes between teams, they are not suitable for guiding resection in individual patients. A similar approach is presented by functional atlases based on results from intraoperative DES, thereby providing a map of critical eloquence. However, preferential locations of tumors, the extent of exposed cortex, and intraoperative time constraints currently hinder its feasibility, but this method might yield promising results.

Assessment of eloquence based on MRI or classification systems focuses on cortical structures and therefore provides no information on subcortical white matter tracts, except for the internal capsule. In contrast, diffusion tensor imaging fiber tracking (DTI-FT) provides subcortical information but lacks information about cortical structures. DTI-FT is non-invasive, but its accuracy can be diminished by peritumoral edema and large tumor size and when fibers cross, since only one direction can be detected per voxel. This last issue may be overcome by the novel tractography techniques Q-ball imaging (QBI) and constrained spherical deconvolution

(CSD), which estimate the distribution of diffusion and fiber orientation when one voxel contains multiple fiber orientations [14].

This wide array of available methods, together with interpersonal anatomical variability, tumor mass effects and neuroplasticity, has led to subjectivity and a lack of consensus on the definition and assessment method of tumor eloquence.

Some studies focused on specific eloquent functions such as language or motor function, yet others exclusively described cortical structures or white matter tracts, most focused solely on cortical structures.

In this way, some brain structures showed discrepancy regarding their classification between studies: the supplementary motor area (SMA), corpus callosum, insula and paralimbic structures, and hippocampus were classified as eloquent by some authors and as near or semi-eloquent by others.

Therefore, there is an urgent need to develop an assessment method that can transform the various broad and subjective definitions of eloquence into an objective and easily applicable and interpretable factor. Ideally, this factor should meet three criteria. First, the methods used should be easy to use and widely accessible in all settings. Second, it should be able to differentiate adequately between patient subgroups based on their baseline characteristics and surgical outcomes. Third, the classification system should be able to do so in a validation cohort, thereby improving its external generalizability.

10.1.3 Maximize Extent of Resection

As mentioned earlier, weighting the value of tumor cytoreduction versus neurological and neurocognitive worsening should be the main purpose when opting for a therapeutic option.

Early and maximal safe resection with the aim of improving both oncological and epileptological outcomes has been mainly proposed for diffuse low-grade glioma (DLGG) [23]. Lima et al. [17] recently proposed a further shift in the philosophy of treating asymptomatic gliomas toward a "preventive" maximal functional-based resection achieving similar functional and oncological results compared to incidental DLGG. Based on the surgical resection technique with margins at the intraoperative cortical and subcortical functional boundaries, 52.6% of the patients had a transient deficit. These excellent functional outcomes demonstrate the reproducibility and the safety of early maximal functional-based resection with cortical and subcortical direct electric stimulations within functional boundaries.

10.1.4 Neuroplasticity

Neuroplasticity is the ability of neural networks to compensate the functional consequences of an injury to the brain architecture [32], including traumatic brain injury, ischemic stroke, and brain tumors. The mechanisms that govern cerebral remodeling in the event of gliomas invasion remain poorly understood but are thought to involve biochemical, paracrine, and synaptic transmission in parallel to macroscale network remodeling, including local and brain-wide modulations of functional brain activities and volume inflations within associated cortical areas. Anatomical structures infiltrated by the tumor show a variable propensity for functional reallocation. A group of WM pathways and unimodal cortices composes the "minimal connectome," a common structure that displays a very low inter-individual variability and a minimal potential for plastic compensation. Consequently, delineating the pattern of tumor diffusion within critical WM tracts is a necessary step to predict the expected extent of resection in a surgical perspective and the expected neurocognitive declines following surgery or radiotherapy [30].

In addition, individualized approaches should also integrate each patient's wishes, professions, and cultural environment, which are the epicenters of modern, personalized "à la carte" oncological therapies. For instance, patients with specific professional activities at risk for legal or cultural reasons might benefit from different approaches, considering a certain rate of "cognitive compensation."

Neuropsychological assessments provide objective measures of plasticity efficiency. Such examinations should be repeated before/after each therapeutical step. Cognitive declines suggest severe functional damages within critical circuits that cannot be compensated anymore, due to saturation of neuroplasticity mechanisms and risk of immediate functional deficits in case of local surgery.

The time-dependent and non-linear characteristics of LGG-induced plasticity are the results of evolving patterns of neural activity and reallocations. Such modulations, integrated in a dynamic onco-functional framework, are named metaplasticity [30].

Nonetheless, total or supratotal resections cannot be achieved in all patients, due to obvious limitations of plasticity potential. Thus, assessing neuroplasticity potential via appropriate and routine clinic-radiological measures (i.e., degree of WM infiltration, velocity of expansion, cognitive compensation) is decisive to select eligible patients for extensive resections and to estimate the functional consequences regarding reasonable oncological goals. A notable impact of neuroplasticity potential on surgical resectability is that earlier management generally results in smaller tumor volumes, less infiltration within the critical cortical and WM tracts, and better cognitive compensation. This is the reason why incidental LGGs usually benefit from higher rates of supratotal resections, better oncological prognosis, higher rates of cognitive preservation, and resumption of professional activities after preventive surgery.

Importantly, LGG-induced plasticity potential is constantly evolving. At the early stage of the disease, broadcasted schemes of functional hyperconnectivity were observed and may represent predictive markers of cognitive resilience to surgical excision. Subsequently, cortical reorganizations may continue and open the door to resections of brain areas that were non-compensable during the first surgery and that were finally reallocated years or decades later. Therefore, neuroplasticity markers should be assessed longitudinally, with repetitive appreciations of WM infiltration, velocity of expansion, and serial neuropsychological examinations. Patients with high plastic potential and whose tumor volume can still be reduced under the 10-mL threshold should benefit from reoperation, given the excellent neurological and neuropsychological tolerance of iterative awake-guided resections and the long-term benefits in terms of overall survival, even when the tumor invades crossroads and challenging anatomical regions such as the insula [30].

10.1.5 The Velocity of Tumor Expansion

The velocity of the tumor is correlated with long-term clinical outcomes [33]. In addition, the kinetics of tumor growth has a significant impact on adaptative plastic mechanisms. This is the reason why acute neurological lesions (e.g., stroke or brain trauma) or rapidly evolving brain tumors (e.g., glioblastomas or metastases) have typically a lower rate of functional compensation. Likewise, accelerations of the tumor expansion may encourage clinicians to select a preventive strategy by urging a local treatment in case of focal proliferative pattern versus by favoring systemic treatments such as chemotherapy in case of rapid anisotropic diffusion toward WM tracts [25]. On the other hand, patients with the so-called high risk profiles (i.e., age >40 years and/or subtotal resection) with tumor residual <10 mL and low pre-therapeutic velocities of expansion should be considered for simple follow-up and vigilant MRI surveillance, since the low velocity of tumor expansion may favor evolving plasticity potentials and effective early reoperation strategies [30].

Furthermore, one of the most important goals of the management of diffuse LGGs is to maintain permanent control over lesion size to reduce the risk of malignant transformation (MT). Although most assessments of therapeutic response in glioma trials are based on the neuro-oncology (RANO) criteria (which consider the bidirectional 2D measurements performed on a single slice), the 3D fluid attenuated inversion recovery (FLAIR) volume is by far the most effective radiological measure to assess objective treatment response, with the highest inter-reader agreement and the highest levels of correlation with the risk of MT [31]. Importantly, both the pre- and post-therapeutic volumes have been recently revalidated as independent prognostic parameters across all histomolecular subclasses of gliomas, with an impact in terms of progression-free survival (post-surgical volume threshold <9.75 mL) and overall survival (post-surgical volume threshold <4.6 mL). Furthermore, although every mL of tumor removed has a long-term impact on the course of the disease, the 10 ± 5 mL volume threshold was consistently established as a strong prognosis factor associated with MT and clinical outcomes. Of note, current guidelines and ongoing trials do not account for this volume threshold and keep on employing the historical dichotomy between "low-risk" and "high-risk" LGG patients, with the age and a less-than-total gross resection as criteria to recommend early adjuvant therapies. Beyond the necessary need to integrate molecular mutations (e.g., IDH mutation, 1p19q codeletion, CDKN2A/B homozygous deletion), the arbitrary cutoff of 40 years and the lack of consideration of recent studies regarding the prognosis impact of the volumetric threshold reduce the scope of this dichotomy, and current oncological teams tend to defer adjuvant treatment in subcategories of "high-risk" profiles, including in selected patients with grade 3/4 foci [32, 33]. The aim of this attitude is to reduce the late adverse effects of oncological treatments (especially radiotherapy).

10.2 Conclusions

The constant interplay between gliomas and the central nervous system is a perpetually evolving neurobiological process that considerably modulates the impact of current therapeutic resources against gliomas, the prognosis, and the cognitive resilience of patients. Strikingly, it has been neglected by practical oncological guidelines. Thus, the first step to improve the efficiency of the current armamentarium would be to reintegrate objective radio-clinical markers of brain compensation into the decision-making strategies, to improve the long-term oncological and functional prognosis of patients who will benefit from numerous sequential, combined, and repeated therapeutic regimens throughout their oncological course. Future game-changing therapies should be developed with the main goal of reducing the migration of tumor cells toward axonal connectivity, which considerably restrains the plasticity potential. A second perspective would be to improve the identification of plasticity mechanisms, by means of multimodal objective neuroimaging tool and/or noninvasive brain mapping of cognitive compensation. A third perspective would be to potentiate neuroplastic reorganizations by surpassing the functional limits represented by the minimal connectome.

References

1. Aghi MK, Nahed BV, Sloan AE, Ryken TC, Kalkanis SN, Olson JJ. The role of surgery in the management of patients with diffuse low grade glioma: a systematic review and evidence-based clinical practice guideline. J Neuro-Oncol. 2015;125(3):503–30.
2. Ius T, Ng S, Young JS, et al. The benefit of early surgery on overall survival in incidental low-grade glioma patients: a multicenter study. Neuro-Oncology. 2022;24(4):624–38.
3. Miller JJ, Gonzalez Castro LN, McBrayer S, et al. Isocitrate dehydrogenase (IDH) mutant gliomas: a Society for Neuro-Oncology (SNO) consensus review on diagnosis, management, and future directions. Neuro-Oncology. 2023;25(1):4–25.
4. Gui C, Kosteniuk SE, Lau JC, Megyesi JF. Tumor growth dynamics in serially-imaged low-grade glioma patients. J Neuro-Oncol. 2018;139(1):167–75.
5. Mandonnet E, Delattre JY, Tanguy ML, et al. Continuous growth of mean tumor diameter in a subset of grade II gliomas. Ann Neurol. 2003;53(4):524–8.
6. Pallud J, Taillandier L, Capelle L, et al. Quantitative morphological magnetic resonance imaging follow-up of low-grade glioma: a plea for systematic measurement of growth rates. Neurosurgery. 2012;71(3):729–39; discussion 739-740.
7. Shah AH, Madhavan K, Heros D, et al. The management of incidental low-grade gliomas using magnetic resonance imaging: systematic review and optimal treatment paradigm. Neurosurg Focus. 2011;31(6):E12.
8. Opoku-Darko M, Eagles ME, Cadieux M, Isaacs AM, Kelly JJP. Natural history and growth patterns of inci-

dentally discovered diffusely infiltrating low-grade gliomas: a volumetric study. World Neurosurg. 2019;132:e133–9.
9. Duffau H, Mandonnet E. The "onco-functional balance" in surgery for diffuse low-grade glioma: integrating the extent of resection with quality of life. Acta Neurochir. 2013;155(6):951–7.
10. Satar Z, Hotton G, Samandouras G. Systematic review-time to malignant transformation in low-grade gliomas: predicting a catastrophic event with clinical, neuroimaging, and molecular markers. Neurooncol Adv. 2021;3(1):vdab101.
11. Claus EB, Walsh KM, Wiencke JK, et al. Survival and low-grade glioma: the emergence of genetic information. Neurosurg Focus. 2015;38(1):E6.
12. Jansen E, Hamisch C, Ruess D, et al. Observation after surgery for low grade glioma: long-term outcome in the light of the 2016 WHO classification. J Neuro-Oncol. 2019;145(3):501–7.
13. Thon N, Eigenbrod S, Kreth S, et al. IDH1 mutations in grade II astrocytomas are associated with unfavorable progression-free survival and prolonged postrecurrence survival. Cancer. 2012;118(2):452–60.
14. Capelle L, Fontaine D, Mandonnet E, et al. Spontaneous and therapeutic prognostic factors in adult hemispheric World Health Organization grade II gliomas: a series of 1097 cases: clinical article. J Neurosurg. 2013;118(6):1157–68.
15. Tom MC, Park DYJ, Yang K, et al. Malignant transformation of molecularly classified adult low-grade glioma. Int J Radiat Oncol Biol Phys. 2019;105(5):1106–12.
16. Narang AK, Chaichana KL, Weingart JD, et al. Progressive low-grade glioma: assessment of prognostic importance of histologic reassessment and MRI findings. World Neurosurg. 2017;99:751–7.
17. Lima GL, Zanello M, Mandonnet E, Taillandier L, Pallud J, Duffau H. Incidental diffuse low-grade gliomas: from early detection to preventive neuro-oncological surgery. Neurosurg Rev. 2016;39(3):377–84.
18. Duffau H. Long-term outcomes after supratotal resection of diffuse low-grade gliomas: a consecutive series with 11-year follow-up. Acta Neurochir. 2016;158(1):51–8.
19. Duffau H, Taillandier L. New concepts in the management of diffuse low-grade glioma: proposal of a multistage and individualized therapeutic approach. Neuro-Oncology. 2015;17(3):332–42.
20. Smith JS, Chang EF, Lamborn KR, et al. Role of extent of resection in the long-term outcome of low-grade hemispheric gliomas. J Clin Oncol. 2008;26(8):1338–45.
21. Sanai N, Berger MS. Glioma extent of resection and its impact on patient outcome. Neurosurgery. 2008;62(4):753–64; discussion 264-756.
22. Li YM, Suki D, Hess K, Sawaya R. The influence of maximum safe resection of glioblastoma on survival in 1229 patients: can we do better than gross-total resection? J Neurosurg. 2016;124(4):977–88.
23. McGirt MJ, Chaichana KL, Attenello FJ, et al. Extent of surgical resection is independently associated with survival in patients with hemispheric infiltrating low-grade gliomas. Neurosurgery. 2008;63(4):700–7. author reply 707-708
24. Jakola AS, Myrmel KS, Kloster R, et al. Comparison of a strategy favoring early surgical resection vs a strategy favoring watchful waiting in low-grade gliomas. JAMA. 2012;308(18):1881–8.
25. Duffau H, Capelle L. Preferential brain locations of low-grade gliomas. Cancer. 2004;100(12):2622–6.
26. Duffau H. Surgery of low-grade gliomas: towards a 'functional neurooncology'. Curr Opin Oncol. 2009;21(6):543–9.
27. Duffau H. The challenge to remove diffuse low-grade gliomas while preserving brain functions. Acta Neurochir. 2012;154(4):569–74.
28. Duffau H. Brain connectomics applied to oncological neuroscience: from a traditional surgical strategy focusing on glioma topography to a meta-network approach. Acta Neurochir. 2021;163(4):905–17.
29. Sanai N, Mirzadeh Z, Berger MS. Functional outcome after language mapping for glioma resection. N Engl J Med. 2008;358(1):18–27.
30. Ng S, Duffau H. Brain plasticity profiling as a key support to therapeutic decision-making in low-grade glioma oncological strategies. Cancers (Basel). 2023;15(14):3698. https://doi.org/10.3390/cancers15143698.
31. Sawaya R, Hammoud M, Schoppa D, et al. Neurosurgical outcomes in a modern series of 400 craniotomies for treatment of parenchymal tumors. Neurosurgery. 1998;42(5):1044–55; discussion 1055-1046.
32. Duffau H. Dynamic interplay between lower-grade glioma instability and brain metaplasticity: proposal of an original model to guide the therapeutic strategy. Cancers (Basel). 2021;13(19):4759. https://doi.org/10.3390/cancers13194759.
33. Pallud J, Blonski M, Mandonnet E, et al. Velocity of tumor spontaneous expansion predicts long-term outcomes for diffuse low-grade gliomas. Neuro-Oncology. 2013;15(5):595–606.

11 Glioma's Clinical Onset and Its Impact on Resection Goals and Decision-Making

Giuseppe Maria Della Pepa, Salvatore Marino, Grazia Menna, and Alessandro Olivi

This chapter emphasizes the importance of understanding the functional reserve of the patient and the limitations of various mapping and monitoring techniques. Effective surgical planning requires evaluating whether a deficit can be alleviated or whether surgery might lead to temporary or permanent worsening of the patient's condition. This assessment involves three main considerations: the potential for improvement in neurological function, the likelihood of temporary functional deterioration with eventual recovery, and the risk of irreversible deficits. Advanced imaging techniques, such as diffusion tensor imaging (DTI) and BOLD fMRI, play a crucial role in distinguishing between deficits caused by mass effect and those due to direct tumor infiltration. These modalities help in planning resections and predicting postoperative outcomes by providing detailed insights into functional areas and the extent of tumor impact. In high-grade gliomas, the strategy may involve partial resection or even a biopsy-only approach if it offers oncological benefit. For low-grade gliomas, where brain plasticity and functional reorganization are more pronounced, a more aggressive resection may be feasible. Ultimately, a comprehensive approach integrating patient-specific factors, tumor characteristics, and advanced imaging is essential for optimizing surgical outcomes and enhancing recovery.

11.1 Resection Goals and Decision-Making in Glioma Surgery

Gliomas, both high-grade and low-grade, present unique challenges in neurosurgical practice. The management of these tumors involves a delicate balance between achieving maximum tumor resection and preserving neurological function. While the primary goal is to extend survival, this must be weighed against the potential for surgery-induced deficits that could significantly impair the patient's quality of life [1]. The decision to proceed with surgery, especially in cases involving reoperation, is contingent upon multiple factors, including the extent of resection achievable without exacerbating existing neurological deficits. However, this must be balanced against the risk of significant postoperative complications, which are linked to a lower Karnofsky Performance Status (KPS) and can ultimately lead to a poor prognosis. Therefore, achieving a balance between extensive tumor resection and the risk of surgical complications is critical in modern neurosurgery. This balance is particularly

G. M. Della Pepa (✉) · S. Marino · G. Menna · A. Olivi
Department of Neurosurgery, Fondazione Policlinico Universitario Agostino Gemelli IRCCS, Catholic University of Rome, Rome, Italy
e-mail: giuseppemaria.dellapepa@policlinicogemelli.it

D. Armocida et al. (eds.), *Neurosurgery's Frontline Role in Gliomas Treatment*,
https://doi.org/10.1007/978-3-031-81850-9_11

challenging when dealing with gliomas located in eloquent brain areas [1, 2].

When a patient presents with a pre-existing neurological deficit at the time of diagnosis, the surgical approach requires even more careful consideration. In such cases, the presence of a deficit could itself serve as a contraindication for surgery. This is primarily due to the risk that further deterioration could lead to:

(a) Loss of patient autonomy, thereby compromising their ability to engage in postoperative treatments such as chemotherapy and radiation.
(b) An irreversible decline in quality of life, with little chance of recovery to baseline function.

The central question becomes: can surgery improve, stabilize, or potentially worsen the patient's current neurological status? The surgical team must predict whether a deficit can be alleviated through intervention or if surgery will lead to either temporary or permanent deterioration [1–3]. The decision-making process is driven by three key considerations:

- *Improving Neurological Function*: Evaluating whether the surgical intervention can alleviate a pre-existing deficit.
- *Temporary Deterioration with Recovery Potential*: Determining if a worsening of function is likely to be transient, with the expectation of eventual improvement.
- *Risk of Permanent Deficit*: Assessing whether surgery might lead to an irreversible loss of function and therefore should be avoided or carefully tailored.

These considerations guide the planning of glioma surgery, emphasizing the importance of integrating both patient-centric and disease-specific factors into surgical decision-making. Therefore, the surgeon must assess the aforementioned considerations and, in cases where there is a substantial risk of worsening the clinical condition, must evaluate what are the potential limits of resection, what technological tools are available to assess and eventually extend these limits, and always conduct a thorough assessment including the possibility of abstaining from surgery, especially if the risk of functional deterioration in the patient is significant in the context of a partial or incomplete resection. In the case of high-grade tumors, partial resection should be considered if it provides oncological benefit, and in some instances, a biopsy-only approach may be appropriate [4]. The risk of hemorrhagic progression in any remaining tumor tissue, especially if significant, should also be carefully considered. The final assessment must consider the patient's overall status in relation to potential adjuvant treatments. On one hand, a worsening neurological condition may deprive the patient of the opportunity for such treatments, rendering surgery oncologically ineffective. On the other hand, even partial resections may reduce mass effect and edema, thereby enabling the completion of radiotherapy cycles [4, 5].

11.2 Infiltration Vs. Mass Effect: Differentiating the Causes of Neurological Deficits

The clinical presentation and management of high-grade and low-grade gliomas differ significantly due to their distinct biological behaviors. High-grade gliomas are characterized by aggressive infiltration into surrounding brain structures. This infiltrative nature often leads to the destruction of white matter tracts, causing irreversible neurological deficits. In contrast, low-grade gliomas tend to grow more slowly and with a more defined border, which may allow for greater surgical resection with lower risk of neurological dysfunction. Additionally, the growth dynamics of these types of tumors promote structural reorganization and plasticity, which must be carefully studied and considered, particularly in terms of the potential for postoperative recovery over time. Interestingly, even large tumors in eloquent regions can sometimes be associated with minimal symptoms due to brain reorganization and neuronal plasticity [6–11].

Despite these differences, it is paramount not to oversimplify the relationship between tumor grade and the associated neurological deficits. The presence of a deficit does not automatically imply that the function is irrecoverable, even in high-grade gliomas. Differentiating between deficits caused by mass effect versus direct infiltration is critical in determining the potential for postoperative recovery. High-grade tumors often exert a mass effect on adjacent brain structures, contributing to neurological dysfunction through mechanisms such as:

- *Perilesional edema*: Swelling around the tumor that compresses surrounding tissues and functional bundles/cortical eloquent areas.
- *Cystic degeneration*: Fluid-filled areas within the tumor that displace functional brain tissue.
- *Structural displacement*: Significant shifts in normal brain functional anatomy due to tumor mass effect.

In these cases, surgery can relieve the mass effect, potentially leading to improvement in the patient's neurological status. Even when critical white matter tracts are infiltrated by the tumor, they are rarely completely destroyed, allowing for some degree of functional recovery postoperatively. Ultimately, it is important to note that the concept of eloquent areas has evolved. Recent neuropsychological, neuroimaging, and neuropsychiatric studies have demonstrated that functions critical to higher cognition are also located in regions previously considered non-eloquent [8–14].

11.3 Distinguishing Infiltration from Mass Effect: The Role of Advanced Imaging Techniques

Accurate preoperative assessment of the tumor's impact on neurological function is critical in planning glioma surgery. Differentiating between deficits caused by direct infiltration versus those resulting from mass effect can significantly influence surgical strategy [7, 8]. Preoperative planning is crucial in the management of gliomas in eloquent areas. Modern imaging techniques provide reliable information about the precise location of functional areas, which can vary between individuals due to several factors:

- *Inter-individual Differences*: While general anatomical landmarks exist to identify eloquent areas, the exact location can vary slightly between individuals. For instance, Broca's area can be located in the pars triangularis, pars opercularis, or ventral region of the precentral gyrus.
- *Tumor-induced Modifications*: Gliomas can infiltrate, disrupt, or displace functional areas from their natural locations.
- *Plasticity*: The brain's ability to reorganize functions following tumor growth and disruption of a functional area. In many cases, nearby cortical regions or contralateral areas compensate for a damaged area. While plasticity is commonly observed in low-grade gliomas, recent literature suggests it may also play a role in high-grade gliomas.

The main imaging techniques used to assess these informations include functional magnetic resonance imaging (fMRI) [15–17], diffusion tensor imaging (DTI) [18, 19], and transcranial magnetic stimulation (TMS) [20, 21]. Advanced imaging modalities, particularly DTI, play a crucial role in this assessment [19]. By analyzing the degree of tract distortion and fractional anisotropy (FA), it is possible to infer whether a deficit is more likely due to compressive effects or direct infiltration. Comparing these imaging findings to the contralateral, unaffected side provides additional context, helping to clarify whether surgical decompression might restore function [14, 22].

In cases where tractography indicates that critical pathways are displaced but largely intact, the potential for functional recovery through resection is higher. The distinction between neurological deficits caused by direct tumor infiltration versus those due to mass effect (e.g., edema, displacement, or compression) is crucial. Accurately identifying the source of the deficit has a significant impact on surgical strategy [23]. If a deficit is caused primarily by a mass effect, decompression surgery can lead to functional improvement. On the other hand, if a deficit is primarily due to direct infiltration, the goal may shift toward minimizing further damage rather than attempting complete resection [15, 16].

Conversely, when tractography suggests significant infiltration or destruction of tracts, the likelihood of reversing a neurological deficit through surgery is lower, necessitating a more conservative approach. Indeed, DTI is not only useful for surgical planning but also for predicting postoperative outcomes. By identifying the extent of tract infiltration and assessing which tracts are displaced but still functional, DTI allows for better prediction of recovery or worsening of neurological deficits following surgery [24]. This multimodal approach not only improves resection strategies but also contributes to better functional outcomes for patients, especially when integrated with real-time intraoperative feedback. Differentiating between mass effect and direct infiltration through the analysis of tract distortion and FA values provides critical insights for surgical planning [17–19, 24].

Although not yet a standard in neuroradiological assessment, the analysis of FA parameters—often compared with the contralateral "healthy" side—has proven helpful in distinguishing truly infiltrated fascicles from those that are merely compressed or displaced. However, the current state of DTI analysis has limitations, particularly in accurately studying bundles located near the tumor or in the presence of edema. Consequently, making a definitive assessment remains challenging and is inherently constrained by these technical limitations [18, 19, 24].

In addition, BOLD fMRI not only maps active regions but also helps distinguish between areas affected by tumor infiltration versus those impacted by mass effect. Regions with preserved BOLD activation despite clinical deficits suggest that these functions might recover after tumor debulking. Conversely, areas with diminished or absent BOLD signals, especially if they correlate with direct tumor invasion, indicate a higher likelihood of permanent deficits. Especially in cases of low-grade tumors, where disease characteristics in terms of interference on eloquent structures and growth dynamics is different, BOLD fMRI can provide insights into functional reserve and reorganization suggesting that a functional reorganization has occurred, increasing the likelihood of deficit recovery after surgery. This information helps neurosurgeons decide whether more aggressive resections are feasible without causing permanent deficits. Despite its usefulness, BOLD fMRI has limitations, such as susceptibility to artifacts and variability in patient cooperation during imaging. Additionally, BOLD signals can be altered by the presence of the tumor itself, making it challenging to interpret functional areas accurately. However, in a multimodal imaging approach, BOLD fMRI can play a critical role in differentiating reversible from permanent deficits in glioma patients. By assessing functional regions and identifying compensatory reorganization, BOLD imaging helps predict post-surgical outcomes and guides surgical strategy [15–19].

Furthermore, brain plasticity can lead to the relocation of functions to the contralateral hemisphere, a phenomenon particularly relevant in low-grade gliomas. Understanding these factors is essential for selecting the appropriate surgical strategy and predicting postoperative outcomes [19–21, 23, 24].

11.4 Intraoperative Strategy: Balancing the Limits of Surgical Resection and Exploiting Intraoperative Mapping/Monitoring Techniques

When neurological deficits are believed to be primarily due to perilesional edema or mass effect—particularly when significant mass effect from cystic degeneration is present—surgery should be considered as the first option. This approach can facilitate some degree of functional recovery, thereby improving the patient's overall functional status and increasing the likelihood of benefiting from postoperative adjuvant treatments. The approach to resection must be cautious yet calculated. For instance, in motor area gliomas, the preservation of function should be prioritized over maximal tumor removal when the risk of irreversible damage is high. In cases of existing deficits, stimulation parameters should be tailored to the specific patient context. For example, lower stimulation intensities may be used to avoid overestimating resectable tissue and to reduce the risk of causing false-negative results during intraoperative monitoring [25, 26].

The resection goals must be guided by the patient's functional reserve. In cases of preoperative deficits, the surgeon must assess the remaining functional reserve. If there is potential for recovery, such as when the deficit is due to edema or tract displacement, a more aggressive resection may be considered [26, 27]. Conversely, if the functional reserve is low and further damage could lead to severe impairment, a more conservative approach is warranted. Planning to leave a residual tumor may be a viable option, especially when resection approaches critical functional areas. In the case of high-grade tumors, partial resection should be considered if it is oncologically beneficial. In certain instances, a biopsy-only approach may be advisable [28]. Additionally, the potential for hemorrhagic evolution in any residual tumor, particularly if substantial, must always be carefully considered. In low-grade tumors, in cases where functional reorganization has already begun (e.g., partial shifts in language or motor function), the surgeon can leverage this knowledge to perform a more extensive resection in the affected area, relying on the brain's compensatory mechanisms [29]. BOLD fMRI and resting-state connectivity studies provide valuable information on whether such shifts are occurring preoperatively [16–19]. In this context, a comprehensive rehabilitation program is essential, particularly when there is potential for improvement after surgery. Early and aggressive rehabilitation can take advantage of the brain's plasticity, further enhancing recovery and potentially reversing some preoperative deficits [25].

Surgery should be guided as effectively as possible by properly implemented techniques for cortical and subcortical monitoring and mapping. In particular, when performing surgery on a patient with pre-existing deficits, the surgeon must be well-versed in the limitations of potential mapping and monitoring techniques. This knowledge is crucial for maximizing the information obtained, selecting the most appropriate monitoring technique for the case, and avoiding misinterpretation of neurophysiological data. Such misinterpretations could lead to premature termination of the surgery or, conversely, result in excessively aggressive surgical approaches. A correct surgical approach should identify the functional boundaries of the tumor. Tasks relevant to the functions of the affected areas should be performed until these functional boundaries are reached, ensuring maximal tumor resection while preserving critical neurological functions [25–27].

In cases where awake surgery is deemed feasible, the approach offers unparalleled precision in balancing tumor resection with functional preservation. However, it requires careful patient selection and optimization of awake protocols. In cases of pre-existing deficits (e.g., reducing cognitive load or focusing on simpler tasks), optimization of awake protocols is key to ensuring that intraoperative feedback remains reliable [28]. However, when patients already present with significant motor or speech deficits, the utility of awake surgery may be limited. For example, patients with pre-existing motor weakness might be unable to provide reliable feedback during critical stages of the procedure. Additionally, the risk of mistaking a supplementary motor area (SMA) syndrome from a proper deficit must be considered in an awake setting [27–29]. In cases not amenable to an awake procedure, general anesthesia can offer valuable information. It should be underlined that for motor functions, a fine-tuned monitoring in general anesthesia can offer reliable information also in cases of severe pre-existing deficits [30]. In an asleep setting, it should be considered that effective surgery in motor areas requires the simultaneous optimization of both mapping and monitoring techniques

[31–33]. A common challenge is the occurrence of false-negative results in neurophysiological monitoring, where preserved MEPs may give a false sense of security regarding the integrity of motor pathways. In some cases, a drop in MEPs is noted, yet subsequent subcortical monopolar stimulation still elicits responses in the corresponding muscle groups [32]. This phenomenon suggests that axonal activation distal to the injury site may still be occurring, even if the pathway upstream is compromised. Such findings highlight the inherent limitations of relying solely on MEPs, especially when attempting to monitor both upper and lower limbs simultaneously.

11.5 Conclusions

The decision to proceed with glioma surgery, especially in cases with pre-existing neurological deficits, involves careful consideration of multiple factors including tumor type, location, and potential impact on function. Advanced imaging techniques such as DTI and fMRI play a crucial role in assessing the relationship between tumor infiltration and mass effect, guiding surgical planning, and predicting postoperative outcomes. Balancing the goals of maximal tumor resection with the preservation of neurological function is key to achieving optimal patient outcomes in glioma management.

References

1. Orringer D, Lau D, Khatri S, et al. Extent of resection in patients with glioblastoma: limiting factors, perception of resectability, and effect on survival. J Neurosurg. 2012;117(5):851–9. https://doi.org/10.3171/2012.8.JNS12234.
2. Sanai N, Berger MS. Operative techniques for gliomas and the value of extent of resection. Neurotherapeutics. 2009;6(3):478–86. https://doi.org/10.1016/j.nurt.2009.04.005.
3. Kahn E, Lane M, Sagher O. Eloquent: history of a word's adoption into the neurosurgical lexicon. J Neurosurg. 2017;127(6):1461–6. https://doi.org/10.3171/2017.3.JNS17659.
4. D'Angelo L, Armocida D, Sampirisi L, Paglia F, Berra LV, Santoro A. Role of endoscopic surgical biopsy in diagnoses of intraventricular/periventricular tumors: review of literature including a monocentric case series. Acta Neurol Belg. 2020 Jun;120(3):517–30. https://doi.org/10.1007/s13760-020-01299-1.
5. Chohan MO, Flores RA, Wertz C, Jung RE. "Non-eloquent" brain regions predict neuropsychological outcome in tumor patients undergoing awake craniotomy. PLoS One. 2024;19(2):e0284261. https://doi.org/10.1371/journal.pone.0284261.
6. Ius T, Pignotti F, Della Pepa GM, Bagatto D, Isola M, Battistella C, Gaudino S, Pegolo E, Chiesa S, Arcicasa M, La Rocca G, Olivi A, Skrap M, Sabatino G. Glioblastoma: from volumetric analysis to molecular predictors. J Neurosurg Sci. 2022;66(3):173–86. https://doi.org/10.23736/S0390-5616.20.04850-X. Epub 2020 Feb 4.
7. Ius T, Mazzucchi E, Tomasino B, Pauletto G, Sabatino G, Della Pepa GM, La Rocca G, Battistella C, Olivi A, Skrap M. Multimodal integrated approaches in low grade glioma surgery. Sci Rep. 2021;11(1):9964. https://doi.org/10.1038/s41598-021-87924-2.
8. Giordano C, Sabatino G, Romano S, Della Pepa GM, Tufano M, D'Alessandris QG, Cottonaro S, Gessi M, Balducci M, Romano MF, Olivi A, Gaudino S, Colosimo C. Combining magnetic resonance imaging with systemic monocyte evaluation for the implementation of GBM management. Int J Mol Sci. 2021;22(7):3797. https://doi.org/10.3390/ijms22073797.
9. Menna G, Caccavella VM, Olivi A, Della Pepa GM. Letter: presurgical identification of patients with glioblastoma at risk for cognitive impairment at 3-month follow-up. Neurosurgery. 2021;88(5):E488. https://doi.org/10.1093/neuros/nyab045.
10. Della Pepa GM, Caccavella VM, Menna G, Ius T, Auricchio AM, Chiesa S, Gaudino S, Marchese E, Olivi A. Machine learning-based prediction of 6-month postoperative Karnofsky performance status in patients with glioblastoma: capturing the real-life interaction of multiple clinical and oncologic factors. World Neurosurg. 2021;149:e866–76. https://doi.org/10.1016/j.wneu.2021.01.082.
11. Manini I, Caponnetto F, Dalla E, Ius T, Della Pepa GM, Pegolo E, Bartolini A, La Rocca G, Menna G, Di Loreto C, Olivi A, Skrap M, Sabatino G, Cesselli D. Heterogeneity matters: different regions of glioblastoma are characterized by distinctive tumor-supporting pathways. Cancers (Basel). 2020;12(10):2960. https://doi.org/10.3390/cancers12102960.
12. Ius T, Somma T, Altieri R, Angileri FF, Barbagallo GM, Cappabianca P, Certo F, Cofano F, D'Elia A, Della Pepa GM, Esposito V, Fontanella MM, Germane A, Garbossa D, Isola M, La Rocca G, Maiuri F, Olivi A, Panciani PP, Pignotti F, Skrap M, Spena G, Sabatino G. Is age an additional factor in the treatment of elderly patients with glioblastoma? A new stratification model: an Italian multicenter study. Neurosurg Focus. 2020;49(4):E13. https://doi.org/10.3171/2020.7.FOCUS20.
13. Ricciardi L, Sturiale CL, Scerrati A, Stifano V, Somma T, Ius T, Trungu S, Acqui M, Raco A, Miscusi M,

Della Pepa GM. Aminolevulinic acid false-positive rates in newly diagnosed and recurrent glioblastoma: do pseudoprogression and radionecrosis play a role? A meta-analysis. Front Oncol. 2022;12:848036. https://doi.org/10.3389/fonc.2022.848036.
14. Brennan NP, Peck KK, Holodny A. Language mapping using fMRI and direct cortical stimulation for brain tumor surgery: the good, the bad, and the questionable. Top Magn Reson Imaging. 2016;25(1):1–10. https://doi.org/10.1097/RMR.0000000000000074.
15. Glover GH. Overview of functional magnetic resonance imaging. Neurosurg Clin N Am. 2011;22(2):133–9, vii. https://doi.org/10.1016/j.nec.2010.11.001.
16. Otten ML, Xu L, Hu X, et al. Functional magnetic resonance imaging and diffusion tensor imaging in glioma surgery: prediction of postoperative deficits. J Neurosurg. 2012;116(3):538–46.
17. Harris RJ, Luppino R, Gorrell S, et al. Assessment of functional connectivity in brain tumor patients using resting-state fMRI: preoperative and postoperative considerations. Front Hum Neurosci. 2014;8:547.
18. Mazzucchi E, La Rocca G, Ius T, Sabatino G, Della Pepa GM. Multimodality imaging techniques to assist surgery in low-grade gliomas. World Neurosurg. 2020;133:423–5. https://doi.org/10.1016/j.wneu.2019.10.120.
19. Chang LC, Chao LL, Toga AW, et al. The application of diffusion tensor imaging to predict the motor recovery of glioma surgery patients. NeuroImage Clin. 2019;24:102074.
20. Groppa S, Oliviero A, Eisen A, et al. A practical guide to diagnostic transcranial magnetic stimulation: report of an IFCN committee. Clin Neurophysiol. 2012;123(5):858–82. https://doi.org/10.1016/j.clinph.2012.01.010.
21. Sollmann N, Fuss-Ruppenthal S, Zimmer C, Meyer B, Krieg SM. Investigating stimulation protocols for language mapping by repetitive navigated transcranial magnetic stimulation. Front Behav Neurosci. 2018;12:197. https://doi.org/10.3389/fnbeh.2018.00197.
22. Friederici AD. The brain basis of language processing: from structure to function. Physiol Rev. 2011;91(4):1357–92. https://doi.org/10.1152/physrev.00006.2011.
23. Armocida D, Pesce A, Palmieri M, D lmieri G, Salvati M, Santoro A, Frati A. Periventricular zone involvement as a predictor of survival in glioblastoma patients: a single centre cohort-comparison investigation concerning a distinct clinical entity. Interdiscip Neurosurg. 2021;25:101185. https://doi.org/10.1016/j.inat.2021.101185.
24. Mori S, Zhang J. Principles of diffusion tensor imaging and its applications to basic neuroscience research. Neuron. 2006;51(5):527–39. https://doi.org/10.1016/j.neuron.2006.08.012.
25. Menna G, Marino S, Valeri F, et al. Diffusion tensor imaging in detecting gliomas sub-regions of infiltration, local and remote recurrences: a systematic review. Neurosurg Rev. 2024;47(1):301. https://doi.org/10.1007/s10143-024-02529-3.
26. Duffau H. Contribution of brain mapping in surgery for low-grade gliomas: towards a 'functional neurooncology'. Curr Opin Oncol. 2005;17(6):543–50.
27. Bello L, Gambini A, Castellano A, et al. Intraoperative functional mapping and monitoring for surgery of gliomas in motor areas: the experience with awake surgery and the integration of preoperative data with intraoperative findings. Neuro-Oncology. 2010;12(2):95–104.
28. Marino S, Menna G, Bilgin L, et al. "False friends" in language subcortical mapping: a systematic literature review. World Neurosurg. 2024;190:350–361.e20. https://doi.org/10.1016/j.wneu.2024.06.156.
29. Salvati M, Armocida D, Pesce A, Palmieri M, Venditti E, D'Andrea G, Frati A, Santoro A. No prognostic differences between GBM-patients presenting with postoperative SMA-syndrome and GBM-patients involving cortico-spinal tract and primary motor cortex. J Neurol Sci. 2020;419:117188. https://doi.org/10.1016/j.jns.2020.117188.
30. Szelényi A, Bello L, Duffau H, et al. Intraoperative electrical stimulation in awake craniotomy: methodological aspects of current practice. Neurosurg Focus. 2010;28(2):E7. https://doi.org/10.3171/2009.12.FOCUS09237.
31. Ries SK, Piai V, Perry D, et al. Roles of ventral versus dorsal pathways in language production: an awake language mapping study. Brain Lang. 2019;191:17–27. https://doi.org/10.1016/j.bandl.2019.01.001.
32. Della Pepa GM, Di Domenico M, Ceccarelli GM, et al. Stereoscopic monitoring technique for motor area tumors. World Neurosurg. 2024;188:117–23. https://doi.org/10.1016/j.wneu.2024.05.056.
33. Armocida D, Berra LV, Frati A, Santoro A. Radiological and surgical aspects of polymorphous low-grade neuroepithelial tumor of the young (PLNTY). Acta Neurol Belg. 2023;123(2):327–40. https://doi.org/10.1007/s13760-023-02231-z.

Surgical Management of Deep-Seated Gliomas

12

Jacopo Bellomo, Simone Olei, Stefanos Voglis, Christiaan H B Van Niftrik, and Carlo Serra

12.1 Introduction

Unlike cancers affecting other solid organs, brain tumors grow within the context of complex neural circuitry. The adult brain is composed of nearly one billion neurons and over one trillion network connections. Consequently, regardless of location, all intrinsic brain tumors interface with nervous system structures [1].

Deep-seated gliomas pose a formidable challenge to neurosurgeons due to their proximity to critical neural structures (e.g., thalamus, hypothalamus, basal ganglia, internal capsule, midbrain) and vascular structures (e.g., basal arteries of the brain). Additionally, their distance from the lateral hemispheric surfaces makes them more difficult to access for surgical resection.

Lateral transcortical approaches to these regions under neurophysiological monitoring are reported in the literature with acceptable results in terms of motor function and language [2, 3]. However, the system of white matter fibers surrounding the central core of the brain conceals a great variety and complexity of functions that cannot be reduced to motion and language alone. The neuropsychological impact of glioma surgery or the consequences of extensive brain resections on complex networks, such as those involved in memory, personality, or other higher functions, cannot be predicted in a deterministic way. This is due to both the brain's organizational complexity and significant inter-individual variability [4, 5]. A similar perspective can be applied to the cerebellum. Though it was long perceived to be a region of limited importance, primarily involved in the regulation of motor control, evolving evidence supports its role in a range of cognitive processes, including executive decision-making, language, emotional processing, and working memory [6].

This poses a fundamental question to the surgeon: what is truly eloquent in the brain? Are

Jacopo Bellomo and Simone Olei contributed equally with all other contributors.

J. Bellomo (*) · S. Voglis · C. H B Van Niftrik
C. Serra
Department of Neurosurgery, University Hospital Zurich, Zurich, Switzerland

Clinical Neuroscience Center (KNZ), Neuroscience Center (ZNZ), University of Zurich, Zurich, Switzerland
e-mail: jacopo.bellomo@usz.ch

S. Olei
Department of Neurosurgery, University Hospital Zurich, Zurich, Switzerland

Clinical Neuroscience Center (KNZ), Neuroscience Center (ZNZ), University of Zurich, Zurich, Switzerland

Department of Neurosurgery, IRCCS Humanitas Research Hospital, Milan, Italy

D. Armocida et al. (eds.), *Neurosurgery's Frontline Role in Gliomas Treatment*,
https://doi.org/10.1007/978-3-031-81850-9_12

there brain areas that can be sacrificed without significant consequences?

12.2 What Is Truly Eloquent?

The word "eloquence" derives from the Latin eloquens, the present participle of eloqui, meaning "to speak out." Certain brain regions, where injury from intrinsic brain tumors and their associated perilesional edema or surgery disrupts network dynamics (referred to as "functional neural networks"), are considered eloquent cerebral structures due to their identifiable and measurable neurological consequences. The definition of eloquent areas implies a dichotomy with non-eloquent or silent areas, whose sacrifice or injury should cause no direct harm to the patient. However, historic reports demonstrate that damage to one brain area may result in secondary degeneration of distant areas connected to it [7]. Moreover, the brain's surface is extensively folded, with over two-thirds of its area located deep within sulci and fissures. Consequently, stimulation of the brain surface cannot reliably map brain function. The cerebellum displays similar anatomical convolutions, with even longer and deeper sulci and fissures [8, 9]. Many brain functions, such as memory storage and retrieval, emotional connections, and complex visuo-spatial abilities, are dispersed across different areas, highly interconnected, and subject to various modulation factors [10]. Consequently, the definition of an eloquent brain area in the literature varies significantly, from detailed anatomical descriptions to well-characterized neurological functional areas (such as motor, sensory, visual, and auditory regions) [11].

Regardless of whether the true function of the so-called silent areas is known or unknown or whether any physical or mental abnormality can be directly identified following damage, every healthy area of the brain should be preserved out of a principle of caution—the ancient principle of primum non nocere ("first, do no harm").

If every part of the brain must be considered eloquent, how can deep-seated lesions be approached? When confronting a brain tumor, it is essential to discern its natural planes of growth and identify its nutritional base while showing the utmost respect for surrounding healthy tissue. Creating a channel directly from the brain surface through normal brain tissue may sometimes be the shortest and fastest way to approach a brain tumor. However, this cannot be done without crossing the normal white matter between the surface and the target. Wide corticectomies may facilitate the approach and dissection of large deep lesions but sacrifice healthy cortical tissue, which may not be directly involved in the disease and should be spared. To preserve neurological function, reducing the size of a corticectomy and the length of an intraparenchymal surgical corridor as much as possible is essential. The preferable strategy is to get close to the target by traveling through the natural pathways provided by nature: the arachnoidal spaces, which surround the whole brain and extend to the deepest structures [12].

A surgical corridor that descends along a cistern, sulcus, or fissure, approximates the target, and allows precise and careful microsurgical dissection of the tumor through a small corticectomy, may be the best strategy to minimize parenchymal loss and intraoperative bleeding. Additionally, opening the liquoral spaces allows the release of cerebrospinal fluid (CSF), providing an opportunity for deep access with minimal brain retraction and compression of surrounding gyri [13].

In clinical neurosurgery, there must be a balance between the relative survival benefits associated with maximal resection and the functional impairments established by tumor network integration and oncological therapies. This process is often called "onco-functional balance."

12.3 Pathoclisis: Tumor Predilection Areas

In order to apply these concepts to glioma surgery, a full comprehension of normal white matter anatomy has to be supported by an excellent knowledge of some trends of behavior displayed by the disease [8].

The theory that glial tumors have a predilection to originate from specific anatomical areas has been the object of intense studies and can be traced down in literature since the 1890s [14]. Already at the end of the nineteenth century, mainly based on autopsy results, the neurologist M. Allen Starr (1854–1932) recognized and demonstrated that there was a propensity of tumors to rest within different cerebral tissues in different patients. He observed that certain parts of the brain have a special tendency in developing intrinsic tumors: the cerebral axis and the cerebellum in children and the cerebral cortex in adults [15]. Along the twentieth century, reports from neurologists and neurosurgeons confirmed these observations and pointed to the existence of preferential sites of origin of brain tumors in a vast majority of series, especially referring to glioblastoma [16, 17].

In the 1980s, Yaşargil observed that gliomas show preferential sites of origin beneath homotypical isocortex. Limbic and paralimbic systems, caudate nucleus, thalamus, hypothalamus, and brainstem are frequently hit by these tumors. He supposed that each brain region might have a specific differential vulnerability to specific pathologies, a term known as "pathoclisis," which would influence both its site of origin and its pattern of growth, observing that phylogenetically older cortex is also the most resistant to the development of intrinsic tumors. By describing an extensive patient series, he showed how gliomas in different sites have repeatable patterns of development and may be targeted through fissural approaches with good functional outcome. A detailed knowledge of anatomy and tumor behavior, a skillful microsurgical technique and surgical respect for healthy brain tissue play a pivotal role in leading to good patient outcomes [14].

Later studies showed that oncogene initiation and promotion in gliomas may be more likely to occur in regions with a more recent phylogenetical history (e.g., association cortex) or in older regions of the brain that are constantly active creating new information (e.g., the memory and limbic system) [18].

According to a number of evidence, some patterns emerge in the development and growth of intrinsic tumors. Gliomas of the neocortex arise most frequently in the white matter adjacent to heteromodal association areas (prefrontal, occipito-temporal, and occipito-parietal cortex) [19]. Gliomas arising in the transitional zones are common, but more often in paleocerebral than archicerebral zones. In the basal ganglia, thalamus, and hypothalamus, gliomas tend to arise within the intranuclear white matter. Tumors of the head of the caudate nucleus show a tendency to grow medially (toward the lateral ventricle) or laterally (toward the insula and the corona radiata) but never show diffusion along the caudate nucleus itself [19]. Tumors of the limbic and paralimbic system (allocortex and mesocortex) show the same tendency to remain confined into their own system, and do not invade neocortical zones [20].

Intrinsic cerebellar tumors also show predilection sites: gliomas show a strong tendency in involving the vermian area and the hemispheres. These areas belong to the neocerebellum, the phylogenetically most recent cerebellar area [14]. On the other hand, gliomas do not typically arise in the flocculo-nodular lobe, which belongs to the archicerebellum, the one with the oldest phylogenetic history. Moreover, cerebellar gliomas show a peculiar tendency to expand medially toward the vermis but rarely infiltrate to the contralateral side. The superior and inferior cerebellar peduncles are usually spared and do not allow extension of cerebellar tumors, while lesions of the middle part of the hemisphere may extend into and along the middle cerebellar peduncle to infiltrate the pons, and vice versa [21]. Overall, glial tumors tend to remain confined within their phylogenetic or architectonic zone of origin and do not invade adjacent territories with different phylogeny and different architecture and function. This concept can be exploited in planning and realizing safe surgery [14].

12.4 Surgical Principles: Cisterns and Fissures

The knowledge of biological patterns of glial tumors in relation to the white matter of the brain can greatly facilitate the planning of an appropriate surgical strategy. Advanced imaging techniques, such as DTI and MRI tractography, allow a study of anatomical relationships between tumor and highly eloquent white matter tracts (e.g., the cortico-spinal tract). The direct locations of some cerebral functions can even be predicted with functional imaging (e.g., functional MRI). However, imaging studies do not allow to acquire all possible information on eloquent brain structures, since the brain should be considered eloquent in its entirety: to some extent, knowledge of surgical anatomy and microsurgical skills cannot be replaced by any other tool [22]. Deep seated tumors may show a tendency to surface within a cistern, a sulcus, a fissure or a ventricle, introducing another important factor from which advantage can be taken to preserve neurological function [8]. The fundamental task of the surgeon is choosing, by every case, the appropriate surgical strategy to remove a lesion without sacrifice of healthy tissue (Fig. 12.1).

12.4.1 The Sylvian Fissure

The Sylvian fissure is a prominent and deep sulcus that spans the inferior and lateral surfaces of the brain, extending from the anterior perforated substance to the supramarginal gyrus [12, 13]. It acts as a boundary, separating the frontal and parietal lobes from the temporal lobe, with the insula forming the floor of the fissure. Structurally, the Sylvian fissure is divided into two sections: the anterior (stem) and the posterior (insulo-opercular) compartments. The stem begins inferiorly at the anterior perforated substance, near the ambient gyrus of the uncus, and runs laterally between the orbital gyri and the temporal pole. Two side branches of the stem include the temporal incisura and the fronto-orbital limb. As the

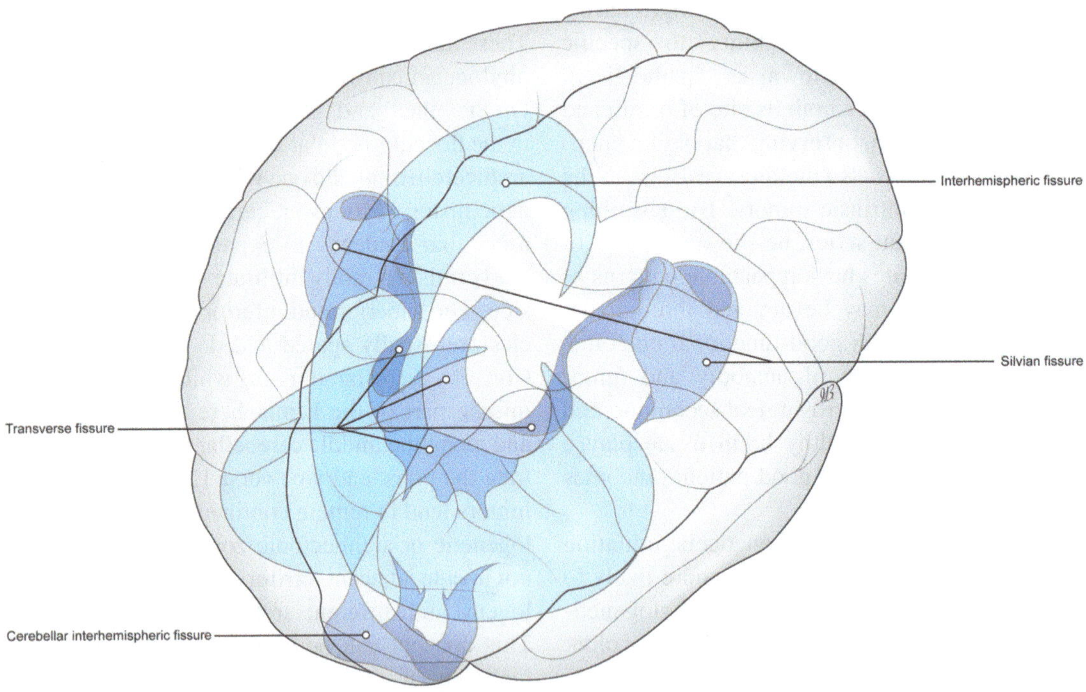

Fig. 12.1 Configuration of the main supratentorial and infratentorial fissures of the brain: transverse fissure, Sylvian fissure, cerebellar interhemispheric fissure, and interhemispheric fissure. [Adapted from Microneurosurgery Volume IIIA (Yaşargil [13]; Thieme; p. 303)]

stem reaches the brain's lateral surface, it branches into the horizontal, ascending, and posterior rami. The intersection of these three rami is termed the "Sylvian point." The horizontal and ascending rami subdivide the inferior frontal gyrus (F3) into the pars orbitalis, pars triangularis, and pars opercularis. The posterior ramus delineates the separation of the frontal and parietal lobes from the temporal lobe, creating the Sylvian line. The supramarginal gyrus curves over the superior boundary of the posterior ramus [23].

12.4.2 The Interhemispheric Fissure

The interhemispheric fissure divides the cerebral hemispheres, extends from the frontal to the occipital poles in the median plane, and it is divided longitudinally by the falx cerebri. The interhemispheric fissure continues anteriorly in the lamina terminalis cistern, posteriorly in the transverse fissure, and in the corpus callosum cistern over the corpus callosum [12, 13].

12.4.3 The Transverse Fissure

The term "transverse fissure" was passed on by Yaşargil and refers to the cisternal spaces occupying the tentorial incisura [13]. This fissure embraces the midbrain and extends around the thalamus and the diencephalon, medial to the uncus, and parahippocampal gyrus on both sides. It represents a natural plane of access to the posterior thalamus and subsplenial area, to the pineal region, to the almost entire lateral, postero-lateral, and posterior midbrain and to the medial-basal temporal region [23].

This space originates posteriorly to the midbrain on the midline, anterior to the superior cerebellar cistern. Here, the Galen cistern, the pineal cistern, and the quadrigeminal cistern form an interconnected space giving origin, on each side, to two orthogonal and specular limbs.

The superior (vertical) limb of the fissure runs close to the midline between the splenium and the pineal body: it constitutes the velum interpositum cistern, a space that runs forward between the fornix and tela choroidea superiorly, and the supero-lateral aspect of the thalamus inferiorly, reaching as far as the posterior border of the foramen of Monro [24].

The inferior (horizontal) limb is represented by the natural posterior to anterior progression of the cisterns of the tentorial incisura: the ambient and crural cisterns, running between the midbrain and the medial-basal aspect of the temporal lobe. The crural cistern communicates anteriorly with the interpeduncular cistern and laterally with the Sylvian fissure, below the anterior perforated substance, creating a continuous liquoral pathway [25].

Important anatomical structures can be found along these spaces. Besides the basal and internal cerebral veins, which follow the course of the horizontal and vertical limb, respectively, the transverse fissure contains the posterior cerebral artery, the medial posterior and lateral posterior choroidal arteries, the hippocampal and posterior temporal branches of the PCA, the thalamo-geniculate and collicular arteries, the SCA and its terminal branches, the IVth and Vth cranial nerves [25].

12.4.4 The Cerebellar Interhemispheric Fissure

This is an unusual term also passed on by Yaşargil to describe the vallecula cerebelli, a liquoral space located at the suboccipital cerebellar surface, dividing the inferior portion of the two cerebellar hemispheres, lodging the inferior part of the vermis (tuber, pyramid, uvula, nodule) which covers the foramen of Magendie. This space can be followed anteriorly underneath the tonsils or between the tonsils and the vermis and leads to the tela choroidea and inferior medullary velum. It continues inferiorly into the Cisterna Magna, where the foramen of Magendie opens [26].

The vallecula can be exploited to access the IVth ventricle. It provides a gateway to a surgical corridor that, through the tela choroidea and the inferior medullary velum, leads to the floor of the IV ventricle and the dorsal brainstem without transgressing the vermis. Opening this space underneath the tonsils leads to the calamus scriptorius and exposes with ease the inferior portion of the rhomboid fossa, while accessing between the uvula and the tonsil provides a steeper trajectory leading as far as the inferior aqueduct and superior medullary velum [27]. The lateral recesses can be exposed until the opening of the foramen of Luschka [28].

12.5 Deep-Seated Gliomas from the Surgeon's Point of View

Deep brain targets have a close relationship with vital neural and vascular structures. The thalamus, the hypothalamus, the basal ganglia, the internal capsule, the midbrain and deep branches of the cerebral arteries represent delicate anatomical relationships of deep gliomas, and to reach them may be a demanding task [29, 30] (Fig. 12.2).

Moreover, lateral transcortical approaches require crossing eloquent white matter fibers of the cerebral or cerebellar hemisphere, carrying further risk for neurological function. Nonetheless, transcortical approaches are widely adopted for the approach of deep-seated pathology. When planning a transcortical approach to a deep target, the side of the lesion usually plays a fundamental role, because white matter fibers in the non-dominant hemisphere are frequently considered more expendable than those in the dominant hemisphere [31–33].

However, crossing white matter fibers, even when they are not associated with directly measurable or elicitable neurological functions, always harbors a risk for neurological disfunction. Normal brain parenchyma should not be sacrificed whenever possible. By means of arachnoidal navigation, deep lesions can be targeted with limited necessity of parenchymal damage, with the highest possible preservation of neurological function. The deepest fissures and the convoluted sulci surrounding the whole brain parenchyma allow the surgeon, after exposition of the superficial cortex, to approximate the deep basal cisterns, the basal forebrain, the corpus callosum, the brainstem, and the medial-basal temporal region from different directions with a bloodless and safe technique, respectful of neurological function [34].

The interconnection of the liquoral spaces surrounding the lateral hemispheric surfaces with those of the basal cisterns and the ventricles allows the surgeon to reach deep targets from different directions, avoiding transparenchymal routes and preserving white matter fibers surrounding the lesion [8]. So, with a relatively small access through the corpus callosum, exposed via an interhemispheric route, the lateral ventricle and the correspondent thalamic surface can be easily accessed. If the callosotomy is placed anterior enough (at the transition between the body and genu of the corpus callosum, allowing an approach steep enough), the foramen of Monro can be reached to enter the third ventricle, reaching as far as the upper cerebral aqueduct without opening the choroidal fissure or sacrificing brain parenchyma [35]. To reach the inferior portion of the aqueduct, a completely different route can be selected, leading to the target through an uvulo-tonsillar telovelar approach or, when a more steep upward direction is required, a tonsillo-biventral fissural approach [36], without any change in surgical principles and without violation of cerebellar parenchyma.

In a similar way, navigation of the anterior basal cisterns can lead to the anterior portion of the third ventricle via the lamina terminalis without any transgression of neural structures [37], and the same surgical route may lead to the interpeduncular fossa and anterior midbrain [38] or to the basal forebrain, as a gateway to lesions involving the anterior thalamus or basal ganglia as well as lesions extending from the anterior insula, the orbital gyri or the medial-basal temporal lobe [39].

The medial-basal temporal region may be targeted from an anterior trans-sylvian approach, which allows direct access to the amygdalo-hippocampal region without damaging lateral temporal parenchyma. When the posterior parahippocampal region must be reached, this can be done through a paramedian infratentorial supra-

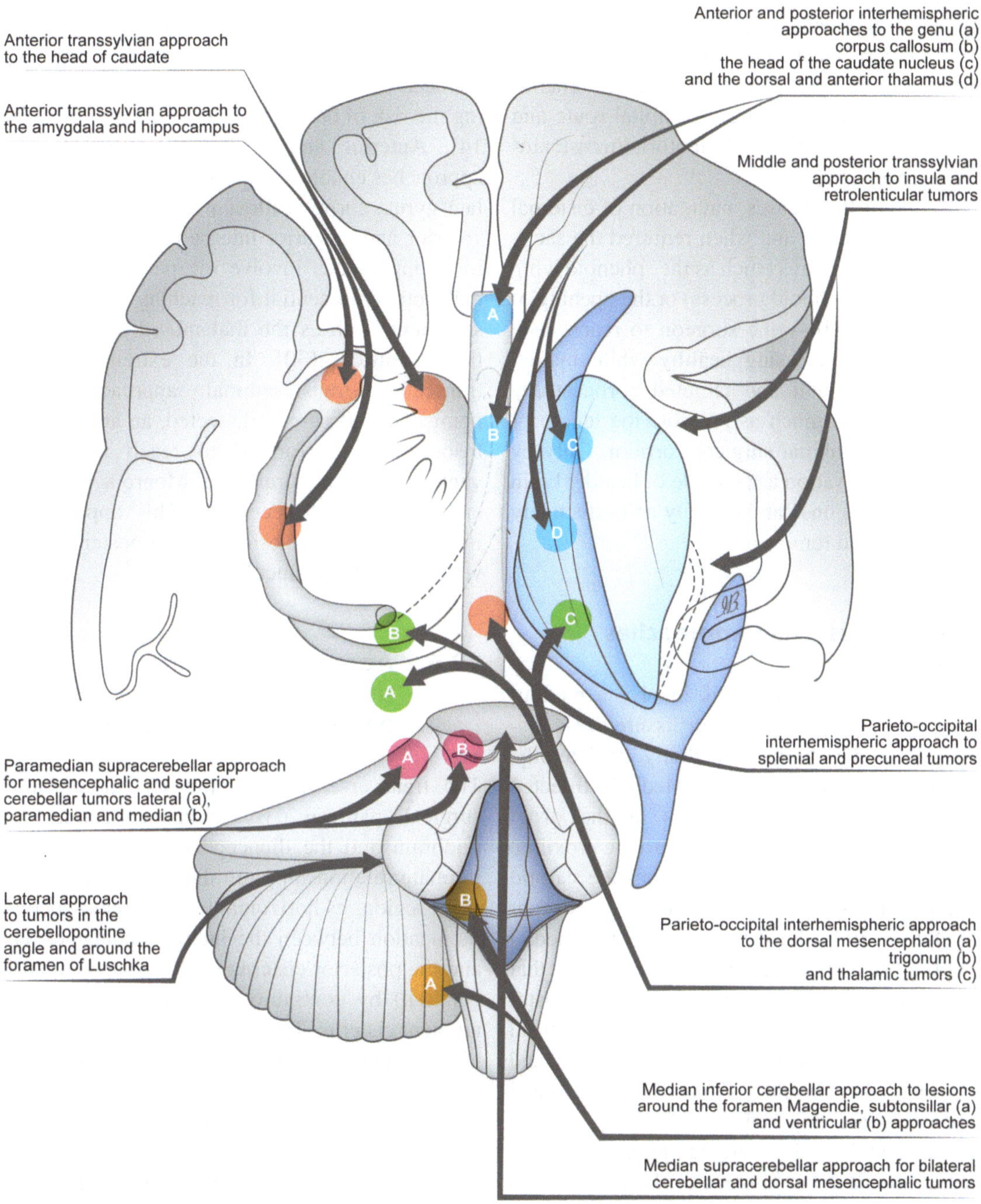

Fig. 12.2 Fissural approaches to deeply located brain tumor lesions. (1a) Anterior transsylvian approach to the head of caudate. (1b) Anterior transsylvian approach to the amygdala and hippocampus. (2) Anterior and posterior interhemispheric approaches to the genu (a), corpus callosum (b), the head of the caudate nucleus (c), and the dorsal and anterior thalamus (d). (3a, b) Middle and posterior transsylvian approach to insula and retrolenticular tumors. (4) Parieto-occipital interhemispheric approach to the dorsal mesencephalon (a), trigonum (b), and thalamic tumors (c). (5) Parieto-occipital interhemispheric approach to splenial and precuneal tumors. (6) Median supracerebellar approach for bilateral cerebellar and dorsal mesencephalic tumors. (7) Paramedian supracerebellar approach for mesencephalic and superior cerebellar tumors lateral (a), paramedian and median (b). (8) Lateral approach to tumors in the cerebellopontine angle and around the foramen of Luschka. (9) Median inferior cerebellar approach to lesions around the foramen Magendie, subtonsillar (a) and ventricular (b) approaches. [Adapted from Microneurosurgery Volume IVA (Yaşargil [14]; Thieme; p. 75)]

cerebellar approach [40]. Approaches to posterior midbrain (tectal plate), pulvinar and pineal region may be realized both from an interhemispheric transtentorial parieto-occipital route and from a supracerebellar infratentorial/transtentorial approach [41].

In each of these cases, navigation of cisternal and fissural spaces, and when required the sacrifice of bone structures (such as the sphenoid wing or the posterior clinoid process) or the opening of the tentorium, allow the surgeon to reach deep targets without crossing healthy white matter, performing a small and targeted corticectomy and reducing as much as possible the length of the intraparenchymal surgical corridor. Only by as much preservation as possible of healthy brain tissue, deep lesions can be safely and effectively approached and removed.

12.5.1 Transsylvian Approaches

The transsylvian approaches involve a meticulous dissection of the Sylvian fissure. This dissection can be directed medially or laterally, depending on the target area. Medially directed subarachnoid dissection begins at the distal Sylvian cistern and proceeds toward the proximal Sylvian cistern, ultimately reaching the carotid cistern. This approach allows access to deeper structures within the brain, such as the medial temporal region. Subarachnoid dissection that progresses in the other direction (laterally, posteriorly, and superiorly) involves splitting the distal Sylvian fissure, opening the operculum, and exposing the insula. Transsylvian surgical approaches are important for exposing insular, opercular and insulo-opercular gliomas, orbitofrontal gliomas, and gliomas of the medio-basal temporal region (hippocampus, amygdala, planum temporale gliomas) [8, 14].

12.5.2 Interhemispheric Approaches

Interhemispheric approaches involve the meticulous dissection of the interhemispheric fissure, providing access to midline brain structures. These approaches leverage the natural separation between the cerebral hemispheres, minimizing the need for excessive brain retraction and reducing the risk of damage to eloquent brain areas [8, 14]. Anterior and posterior interhemispheric approaches enable to expose lesions of the cingulate gyrus, corpus callosum and precuneus. The anterior and posterior interhemispheric transcallosal approaches involve the performance of a callosotomy, essential for reaching deep midline structures such as the thalamus, hypothalamus, third ventricle [30]. In the extreme anterior transcallosal-transforaminal approach, interhemispheric fissure is dissected, an anterior callosotomy is performed to reach the lateral ventricle, and the foramen of Monro is identified and enlarged, if necessary. This approach is important to reach lesions of the posterior third ventricle and aqueduct [42].

12.6 Approaches around the Transverse Fissure and the Tentorial Fissure

The transverse fissure represents an essential surgical pathway. By circumnavigating the midbrain and the diencephalon and having an intimate relationship with the medial-basal temporal region, its horizontal branch creates a communication between the interpeduncular cistern and the posterior cisterns (Galen, pineal, quadrigeminal) by continuity through the crural and ambient cisterns. The horizontal branch communicates antero-laterally with the Sylvian fissure and postero-laterally with the cerebello-mesencephalic fissure. Thus, this space surrounds the base of the brain and is accessible from an anterior, lateral, or posterior direction. Moreover, the vertical branch leads to the heart of the ventricular system, conducing as far as the foramen of Monro [24, 25].

This space can be approached posteriorly to reach lesions located along or near the midline: intrinsic tumors of the pineal region, tectal region, and posterior midbrain, along with tumors of the pulvinar and posterior thalamus can be safely reached through a median or perimedian supracerebellar infratentorial/transtentorial approach. This approach was introduced for pineal tumors by Stein in 1971 at the beginning of the microsurgical era, after the first pioneristic attempts by Krause, Brunner, and Rorschach in 1911. The supracerebellar corridor is specifically designed for tumors with main infratentorial extension and can offer a wide surgical space avoiding morbidity related to parietal and occipital retraction during supratentorial approaches [43–45].

More extensive lesions, exceeding the limits of the midline, may not be sufficiently controlled by this route. Superior transtentorial routes can overcome this limitation. The parieto-occipital transtentorial approach can be of choice for lesions located around the suboccipital portion of the tentorium, including also the quadrigeminal plate, posterior part of thalamus, tentorial surface of the cerebellum, posterior falx, lesions around the tentorial incisura, and the splenium itself [41].

Traditionally, the medial-basal temporal region has been approached via the Sylvian fissure. Trans-sylvian approaches to this region consent excellent surgical results in glioma surgery, with a low rate of approach-related neurological deficits. This technique was described by Wieser and Yaşargil in the treatment of temporal lobe epilepsy in a seminal study in 1982, and since then has been deeply studied. [46] The use of this route in tumor surgery allows for targeted approaches and preservation of neocortical structures and white matter of the temporal lobe [47].

However, for lesions reaching far posteriorly or widely involving the fusiform gyrus, this approach may not allow for adequate exposure and resection and damage to the optic radiations may be a major issue [48].

To address this problem, in 2012 Türe proposed the paramedian supracerebellar transtentorial approach, which allows the exposure of the entire length of the medial-basal temporal region, including the whole of the parahippocampal and fusiform gyri. Through this approach, gliomas of these areas can be safely resected under direct visual control, avoiding infraction and damage to the optic pathways [49]. Navigation of the supracerebellar space can be performed from the semi-setting position, to allow the cerebellum to fall with gravity and avoiding any unnecessary retraction. Preservation, whenever possible during the approach, of the tentorial bridging veins adds an additional caution, since there is no way to determine whether a bridging vein can be sacrificed without complications due to alterations of deep venous drainage [50].

When considering approaches to midbrain gliomas, it is important to consider that the whole outer surface of the midbrain is in contact with the subarachnoid space. This means that virtually any midbrain tumor can be reached through either a trans-cisternal or trans-callosal trans-ventricular approach. The choice of the approach may be greatly assisted by DTI imaging. Following the same surgical principle as above, different areas of the midbrain may be reached with minimal parenchymal damage via a trans-sylvian, interhemispheric transcallosal, interhemispheric transtentorial subsplenial, paramedian supracerebellar transtentorial or trans-uvulo-tonsillar telo-velar approach [51].

12.7 Approaches to the Fourth Ventricle and the Posterior Brainstem

The cerebellum is a highly eloquent organ. In addition to his fundamental role in motor control, it takes part to a variety of cognitive processes, to speech and language regulation, to working memory tasks, to the perception of music and rhythm and related operational tasks, and to processing of emotions [6]. The cerebellum has been implicated in neuropsychiatric disorders typically related to cerebral cortex and basal ganglia, and although non-motor cerebellar functions are mediated by the cerebellar hemispheres and their connections with the thalamus, an increasing importance is attributed to the role of the vermis [52]. Cerebellar mutism is a well-known complication after surgery for cerebellar tumors especially in children, and its pathogenetic mechanism is likely due to the damage occurring to the proximal efferent cerebellar pathways, including the dentate nucleus, the superior cerebellar peduncle, and its decussation in the mesencephalic tegmentum (Wernekink decussation) [53]. Damage to the superior cerebellar peduncles and Wernekink decussation in the caudal midbrain may cause rare complications such as Wernekink commissural syndrome and Holmes tremor [54, 55].

The surgeon should care for the utmost preservation of cerebellar parenchyma and cerebellar peduncles, and the afferent and efferent connections of the cerebellar gray nuclei should be preserved whenever possible. Approaches to the IVth ventricle and posterior brainstem should take careful consideration of that to reduce the risk of approach-related complications.

Arachnoidal approaches around the cerebellum offer a solution to these issues, allowing safe approaches to deep lesions involving the IV ventricle and posterior brainstem. Intracerebellar sulci course parallel to the folia and can be followed to the vermis without damage to cerebellar tissue. Moreover, the fissures dividing the cerebellum from the brainstem allow access, through a postero-lateral route, to the whole length of the brainstem itself, to the main vessels providing blood supply to the cerebellum, and to the entry and exit zones of the cranial nerves. Approaches through the cerebello-medullary fissure led to the certebello-pontin angle with a short and safe arachnoidal pathway [14].

The importance of the vallecula has already been mentioned: it represents the gateway to the fourth ventricle and permits to avoid transvermian routes. Intrinsic tumors originating at the posterior brainstem surface and approaching the foramen of Magendie can be easily accessed via a sub-tonsillar telo-velar approach, as well as lesions of the posterior surface of the medulla and inferior half of the rhomboid fossa, extending laterally to the lateral recesses and foramen of Luschka. Lesions involving the superior portion of the rhomboid fossa, extending up to the aqueduct and superior medullary velum can be approached through the vallecula via a tonsillo-uvular or tonsillo-biventral route, with removal of the posterior arch of C1 to facilitate the working angle [27]. Progressive CSF release during these approaches, starting from the cisterna magna or the cerebello-medullary fissure, allows progressive cerebellar relaxation and dynamic retraction without the need for excessive manipulations [8].

The horizontal fissure displays a particularly important role in the approach to deep seated lesions abutting the fourth ventricle or localizing in the deep cerebellar hemisphere. All major cerebellar fissures reach deeply inside the hemisphere, coursing parallel to the cerebellar folia and approaching the deep gray nuclei. Dissection of the horizontal fissure from the suboccipital cerebellar surface leads to the fourth ventricle with a minimal corticectomy and provides efficient visualization of the upper fourth ventricle without incision both inferior vermis and the tela choroidea and inferior medullary velum [56].

12.8 Surgical Outcomes

12.8.1 Surgery of Insular Gliomas

In a recently published consecutive series of 79 patients with insular gliomas treated using trans-sylvian surgical approaches, an extent of resection (EOR) of ≥90% was achieved in 30 cases (38%), while an EOR of <90% was achieved in 49 cases (62%). In the early postoperative period, new neurological deficits were observed in 31 patients (39.2%), and in 5 patients (6.3%), these deficits persisted up to 3 months. Tumor location in zone II, according to the Berger-Sanai classification, was significantly associated with a lower likelihood of achieving an EOR of ≥90% [57].

12.8.2 Surgery of Thalamic Gliomas

In a large, consecutive series of 92 patients with thalamic tumors (88% of which were gliomas) treated by a single surgeon using endoscopic-assisted approaches—including the anterior interhemispheric transcallosal, posterior interhemispheric transtentorial subsplenial, perimedian supracerebellar transtentorial, and perimedian contralateral supracerebellar suprapineal approaches—gross total resection (GTR) was achieved in 66% of cases with no surgical mortality observed. Most patients (59.8%) experienced an improvement in their functional performance status, while new permanent neurological deficits occurred in 8.7% of patients [30].

12.8.3 Surgery of Aqueduct Gliomas

The extreme anterior interhemispheric transcallosal approach has proven to be both effective and safe for the resection of pure aqueduct gliomas. In a recently published surgical series involving four patients, complete resection was achieved without any associated mortality or morbidity. All patients recovered and were neurologically intact at the 3-month postoperative follow-up. None experienced recurrence or required adjuvant therapy [29].

12.8.4 Surgery of Brainstem Gliomas

The brainstem is an extremely eloquent structure, and for a long time, most surgeons have advocated that it should not be violated. At earlier times, brainstem gliomas were all considered to be a single entity, and little was known of the true heterogeneous nature of these lesions. This was the main factor against surgical attempts. [58] Starting from the early twentieth century, reports began to appear of attempts of surgery for brainstem lesions. In 1910, Zenner performed a surgical exploration on a pediatric patient with a supposed brainstem glioma. While a pioneer in his approach, the patient died quickly after surgery [59]. Its work took its steps from the observation of earliest surgeons attempting surgery at the posterior fossa [15, 17, 60]. Cushing published in 1930 and 1931 his own experience in the treatment of tumors involving the cerebellum and the brainstem [61, 62], advocating that tumor debulking, tissue diagnosis, and management of hydrocephalus were the best treatment options for these lesions. Cushing's results showed a noteworthy reduction of surgical complications and mortality, which were capital achievements for the time. Nonetheless, the limitations of clinical and radiologic diagnosis in understanding the complexity of the anatomical nuances of these lesions, and the frequently fatal postoperative course, made tumor diagnosis and palliative decompression the main goal of surgery for the following decades. Matson stated, in 1969, that regardless of specific histology, brainstem gliomas must be classified as malignant tumors since "their location in itself renders them inoperable" [63].

It was only in the 1960s that the first pioneer Authors reported prolonged survivals, in the order of 10–25 years, on patients operated for brainstem gliomas [64, 65], followed by an increasing number of other series until the 1980s–1990s [66–68]. So, over the twentieth century, it became increasingly evident that brainstem gliomas were not all classifiable as diffuse tumors, but they included different entities with very different prognostic outcomes [69]. The fundamental distinction between focal and diffuse brainstem gliomas finally arose. More and more cases were being reported, tumor localization incrementally improved, and imaging techniques allowed for subtype classification and localization in an unprecedented way. The use of microsurgical techniques slowly moved the management of these lesions forward. Patients with reported focal lesions were depicted as having good outcomes, further tempting surgeons to attempt resections [58, 67, 70].

In the 1990s, Yaşargil presented the outcome of his surgical series on brainstem gliomas, showing how microsurgical techniques applied to brainstem gliomas may lead to an excellent neurological outcome with acceptable surgical risks, particularly when dealing with benign and focal tumors [8]. He claimed that an accurate study of the tumor topography and morphology, together with a careful study of the surrounding structures and the uttermost care in microsurgical preservation of healthy tissue and vessels are the milestones for the surgical approach to these tumors, which are operable. The surgeon should take care to "read" the tumor and its natural growth pattern, to individuate the natural routes leading to it and follow them to the target. Though many standard safe entry zones have been described for brainstem access [71], in many instances, the tumor itself tends to surface at a specific point in the brainstem, and this creates a natural safe entry zone to start the resection. Every single tumor may behave differently in this regard. Modern technological advances have allowed further evolution in the surgical management of these lesions [72] and they will be discussed in Chaps. 13 and 15.

12.9 Conclusions

Due to its complex functional organization, the whole brain should be considered eloquent, and the utmost care should be taken in avoiding removal of healthy brain tissue and vascular damage. However, surgical treatment of deep-seated intrinsic brain tumors is feasible, and requires a full comprehension of white matter anatomy, mastery of microsurgical arachnoidal dissection and skillful planning to tailor the best surgical strategy for the patient.

References

1. Hervey-Jumper SL, Berger MS. Introduction: surgical management of eloquent area tumors. Neurosurgery. 2020;87(6):1076–7. https://doi.org/10.1093/neuros/nyaa358.
2. Benet A, et al. Surgical assessment of the insula. Part 1: surgical anatomy and morphometric analysis of the transsylvian and transcortical approaches to the insula. J Neurosurg. 2016;124(2):469–81. https://doi.org/10.3171/2014.12.jns142182.
3. Hervey-Jumper SL, et al. Surgical assessment of the insula. Part 2: validation of the Berger-Sanai zone classification system for predicting extent of glioma resection. J Neurosurg. 2016;124(2):482–8. https://doi.org/10.3171/2015.4.jns1521.
4. Duffau H. The challenge to remove diffuse low-grade gliomas while preserving brain functions. Acta Neurochir. 2012;154(4):569–74. https://doi.org/10.1007/s00701-012-1275-7.
5. Yordanova YN, et al. Awake surgery for WHO grade II gliomas within 'noneloquent' areas in the left dominant hemisphere: toward a 'supratotal' resection. J Neurosurg. 2011;115(2):232–9. https://doi.org/10.3171/2011.3.jns101333.
6. Sankey EW, et al. Perioperative assessment of cerebellar masses and the potential for cerebellar cognitive affective syndrome. World Neurosurg. 2020;144:222–30. https://doi.org/10.1016/j.wneu.2020.09.048.
7. Block F, et al. Inflammation in areas of remote changes following focal brain lesion. Prog Neurobiol. 2005;75(5):342–65. https://doi.org/10.1016/j.pneurobio.2005.03.004.
8. Yaşargil MG. Microneurosurgery, vol. IVB. Thieme; 1996.
9. García-Cabezas MÁ, et al. The structural model: a theory linking connections, plasticity, pathology, development and evolution of the cerebral cortex. Brain Struct Funct. 2019;224(3):985–1008. https://doi.org/10.1007/s00429-019-01841-9.
10. Kandel E, et al. Principles of neural science. 5th ed. New York: McGraw-Hill; 2013.
11. Rammeloo E, et al. Preoperative assessment of eloquence in neurosurgery: a systematic review. J Neuro-Oncol. 2023;165(3):413–30. https://doi.org/10.1007/s11060-023-04509-x.
12. Yaşargil MG. Microneurosurgery, vol. I. New York: Thieme; 1985.
13. Yaşargil MG. Microneurosurgery, vol. IIIA. New York: Thieme; 1987.
14. Yaşargil MG. Microneurosurgery, vol. IVA. New York: Thieme; 1993.
15. Starr A. Brain surgery. New York: William Wood & Company; 1893.
16. Russell DS, Rubinstein LJ. Pathology of tumours of the nervous system. 5th ed. London: Arnold; 1989.
17. Jallo GI, et al. Brainstem gliomas. Childs Nerv Syst. 2004;20(3):143–53. https://doi.org/10.1007/s00381-003-0870-6.
18. Donaldson SS, et al. Advances toward an understanding of brainstem gliomas. J Clin Oncol. 2006;24(8):1266–72. https://doi.org/10.1200/jco.2005.04.6599.
19. Vogt C, Vogt O. Erkrankungen der Großhirnrinde im Lichte der Topistik, Pathoklise und Pathoarchitektonik. J Psychol Neurol. 1922;28:1–171.
20. Yaşargil MG, et al. Tumours of the limbic and paralimbic systems. Acta Neurochir. 1992;118(1–2):40–52. https://doi.org/10.1007/bf01400725.
21. Recinos PF, et al. Brainstem tumors: where are we today? Pediatr Neurosurg. 2007;43(3):192–201. https://doi.org/10.1159/000098831.
22. Quinones-Hinojosa A, Chaichana KL, Mahato D. Brain mapping. Indications and techniques. New York: Thieme; 2019.
23. Ammirati M, et al. Comparison of different infratentorial—supracerebellar approaches to the posterior and middle incisural space: a cadaveric study. J Neurosurg. 2002;97(4):922–8. https://doi.org/10.3171/jns.2002.97.4.0922.
24. Tubbs RS, et al. The velum interpositum revisited and redefined. Surg Radiol Anat. 2007;30(2):131–5. https://doi.org/10.1007/s00276-007-0293-2.
25. Rhoton AL. Rhoton's cranial anatomy and surgical approaches. 2019. ci.nii.ac.jp/ncid/BA65387500.

26. Spierer R. The debated neuroanatomy of the fourth ventricle. J Anat. 2023;243(4):555–63. https://doi.org/10.1111/joa.13885.
27. Brogna C, et al. Medial-tonsillar telovelar approach for resection of a superior medullary velum cerebral cavernous malformation: anatomical and tractography study of the surgical approach and functional implications. Acta Neurochir. 2020;163(3):625–33. https://doi.org/10.1007/s00701-020-04418-2.
28. Ghali MGZ. Telovelar surgical approach. Neurosurg Rev. 2019;44(1):61–76. https://doi.org/10.1007/s10143-019-01190-5.
29. Serra C, Türe U. The extreme anterior interhemispheric transcallosal approach for pure aqueduct tumors: surgical technique and case series. Neurosurg Rev. 2021;45(1):499–505. https://doi.org/10.1007/s10143-021-01555-9.
30. Serra C, et al. Microneurosurgical removal of thalamic lesions: surgical results and considerations from a large, single-surgeon consecutive series. J Neurosurg. 2020;135(2):458–68. https://doi.org/10.3171/2020.6.jns20524.
31. Arseni C. Tumors of the basal ganglia: their surgical treatment. AMA Arch NeurPsych. 1958;80(1):18. https://doi.org/10.1001/archneurpsyc.1958.02340070036003.
32. Rangel-Castilla L, Spetzler RF. The 6 thalamic regions: surgical approaches to thalamic cavernous malformations, operative results, and clinical outcomes. J Neurosurg. 2015;123(3):676–85. https://doi.org/10.3171/2014.11.jns14381.
33. Wong T-T, et al. Clinical considerations and surgical approaches for low-grade gliomas in deep hemispheric locations: thalamic lesions. Childs Nerv Syst. 2016;32(10):1895–906. https://doi.org/10.1007/s00381-016-3148-5.
34. Chandra PS. Diffuse intrinsic pontine gliomas: will there ever be a light at the end of the dark tunnel? Neurol India. 2023;71(1):2. https://doi.org/10.4103/0028-3886.314592.
35. Türe U, et al. The transcallosal—transforaminal approach to the third ventricle with regard to the venous variations in this region. J Neurosurg. 1997;87(5):706–15. https://doi.org/10.3171/jns.1997.87.5.0706.
36. Tanriover N, Ulm AJ, et al. Comparison of the transvermian and telovelar approaches to the fourth ventricle. J Neurosurg. 2004;101(3):484–98. https://doi.org/10.3171/jns.2004.101.3.0484.
37. Giussani C, Di Cristofori A. Lamina terminalis fenestration: an important neurosurgical corridor. Handb Clin Neurol. 2021;180:217–26. https://doi.org/10.1016/b978-0-12-820107-7.00014-8.
38. Giammattei L, et al. Basal cisternostomy for severe TBI: surgical technique and cadaveric dissection. Front Surg. 2022;9:915818. https://doi.org/10.3389/fsurg.2022.915818.
39. Serra C, Akeret K, et al. A white matter fiber microdissection study of the anterior perforated substance and the basal forebrain: a gateway to the basal ganglia? Oper Neurosurg (Hagerstown). 2018;17(3):311–20. https://doi.org/10.1093/ons/opy345.
40. Schramm J, Aliashkevich AF. Temporal mediobasal tumors: a proposal for classification according to surgical anatomy. Acta Neurochir. 2008;150(9):857–64. https://doi.org/10.1007/s00701-008-0013-7.
41. Katyal A, et al. Occipital transtentorial approach for pineal region lesions: addressing the controversies in conventional teaching. Surg Neurol Int. 2021;12:503. https://doi.org/10.25259/sni_168_2021.
42. Munoz-Gualan AP, et al. The extreme anterior interhemispheric transcallosal approach for pure aqueduct Tumors: an anatomical study. Turk Neurosurg. 2023;33(5):840–6. https://doi.org/10.5137/1019-5149.JTN.42429-22.3.
43. Mottolese C, et al. Supracerebellar infratentorial approach for pineal region tumors: our surgical and technical considerations. Neurochirurgie. 2015;61(2–3):176–83. https://doi.org/10.1016/j.neuchi.2014.02.004.
44. Krause F. Chirurgie des Gehirns und Ruckenmaks. London: Wellcome Library; 1908.
45. Krause F. Chirurgie des Gehirns und Rückenmarks nach eigenen Erfahrungen. Vol. 2. Urban & Schwarzenberg; 1911.
46. Wieser HG, Yaşargil MG. Selective amygdalohippocampectomy as a surgical treatment of mesiobasal limbic epilepsy. Surg Neurol. 1982;17(6):445–57. https://doi.org/10.1016/s0090-3019(82)80016-5.
47. Serra C, Akeret K, Staartjes VE, et al. Safety of the paramedian supracerebellar–transtentorial approach for selective amygdalohippocampectomy. Neurosurg Focus. 2020;48(4):E4. https://doi.org/10.3171/2020.1.focus19909.
48. Schmeiser B, et al. Surgical treatment of mesiotemporal lobe epilepsy: which approach is favorable? Neurosurgery. 2017;81(6):992–1004. https://doi.org/10.1093/neuros/nyx138.
49. Türe U, et al. The paramedian supracerebellar-transtentorial approach to the entire length of the mediobasal temporal region: an anatomical and clinical study. J Neurosurg. 2012;116(4):773–91. https://doi.org/10.3171/2011.12.jns11791.
50. Berker BB, et al. Preserving the cerebellar hemispheric tentorial bridging veins through a novel tentorial cut technique for supracerebellar approaches. J Neurosurg. 2024;140(1):260–70. https://doi.org/10.3171/2023.5.jns23657.
51. Serra C, Türe H, Fırat Z, et al. Microsurgical management of midbrain gliomas: surgical results and long-term outcome in a large, single-surgeon, consecutive series. J Neurosurg. 2024;140(1):104–15. https://doi.org/10.3171/2023.5.jns222219.
52. Fujita H, et al. Modular output circuits of the fastigial nucleus for diverse motor and nonmotor functions of the cerebellar vermis. elife. 2020;9:e58613. https://doi.org/10.7554/elife.58613.
53. Malbari F, et al. Cerebellar mutism syndrome in pediatric neuro-oncology: a multidisciplinary perspective and call for research priorities. Pediatr

Neurol. 2022;132:4–10. https://doi.org/10.1016/j.pediatrneurol.2022.04.014.
54. Raina GB, et al. Holmes tremor. Neurology. 2016;86(10):931–8. https://doi.org/10.1212/wnl.0000000000002440.
55. Liu H, et al. Wernekink commissure syndrome: a rare midbrain syndrome. Neurol Sci. 2012;33(6):1419–21. https://doi.org/10.1007/s10072-012-0966-4.
56. Tamura R, et al. Suboccipital transhorizontal fissure approach for posterior cranial fossa lesions: a cadaveric study and first clinical experience. Oper Neurosurg. 2021;21(6):E479–87. https://doi.org/10.1093/ons/opab345.
57. Pitskhelauri D, et al. Transsylvian insular glioma surgery: new classification system, clinical outcome in a consecutive series of 79 cases. Oper Neurosurg. 2021;20(6):541–8. https://doi.org/10.1093/ons/opab051.
58. Bricolo A, Turazzi S. Surgery for gliomas and other mass lesions of the brainstem. Adv Tech Stand Neurosurg. 1995;22:261–341. https://doi.org/10.1007/978-3-7091-6898-1_5.
59. Zenner P. Two cases of tumor of the pons. J Nerv Ment Dis. 1910;37:27–36.
60. Krause F. Surgery of the brain and spinal cord based on personal experiences. Translated by H. Haubold and M. Thorek. New York: Rebman Co.; 1909–1912.
61. Cushing H. Experiences with cerebellar astrocytomas. Surg Gynecol Obstet. 1931;52:129–204.
62. Cushing H. Experiences with cerebellar medulloblastomas. Acta Path Microbial Scand. 1930;7:1–86.
63. Matson D. Tumors of the posterior fossa. In: Neurosurgery of infancy and childhood. 2nd ed. Springfield: Charles C Thomas; 1969. p. 469–77.
64. Alvisi C. Considerations on the surgical treatment of bulbo-pontine gliomas. Minerva Neurochir. 1962;6:5–7.
65. Pool JL. Gliomas in the region of the brain stem. J Neurosurg. 1968;29:164–7.
66. Hoffman HJ, et al. A clinically and pathologically distinct group of benign brain stem gliomas. Neurosurgery. 1980;7(3):243–8. https://doi.org/10.1227/00006123-198009000-00007.
67. Albright AL, Sclabassi RJ. Use of the cavitron ultrasonic surgical aspirator and evoked potentials for the treatment of thalamic and brain stem tumors in children. Neurosurgery. 1985;17(4):564–8. https://doi.org/10.1227/00006123-198510000-00005.
68. Epstein F, Larry McCleary E. Intrinsic brainstem tumors of childhood: surgical indications. J Neurosurg. 1986;64(1):11–5. https://doi.org/10.3171/jns.1986.64.1.0011.
69. Berger MS, et al. Pediatric brain stem tumors: radiographic, pathological, and clinical correlations. Neurosurgery. 1983;12(3):298–302. https://doi.org/10.1227/00006123-198303000-00008.
70. Bilaniuk LT, Zimmerman RA, Littman P, et al. Computer tomography of brain stem gliomas in children. Radiology. 1980;134:89–95.
71. Cavalheiro S, et al. Surgical approaches for brainstem tumors in pediatric patients. Childs Nerv Syst. 2015;31(10):1815–40. https://doi.org/10.1007/s00381-015-2799-y.
72. Sabbagh AJ, Alaqeel AM. Focal brainstem gliomas. Neurosciences. 2015;20(2):98–106. https://doi.org/10.17712/nsj.2015.2.20140621.

13 Intraoperative Technology and Tools in Glioma Surgery

Giuseppe Demichele, Daniele Armocida, Mauro Palmieri, Maurizio Salvati, and Alessandro Pesce

13.1 Introduction

In the last two decades, technology has become the key feature of glioma surgery. Surgery to remove intra-axial brain tumors is, today, unequivocally technological. Among the different technologies and advanced approaches, we consider, functional technologies, in which a function, for instance, a cognitive function, is intraoperatively examined in order to be preserved, among these, one above all, the awake surgery approaches and intraoperative neuromonitoring [1–3]. Secondary, a significant mention goes to the visualization technologies, such as intraoperative imaging, for instance intraoperative ultrasound (US) and intraoperative magnetic resonance imaging (MRI), which visualize the lesion, the residual tissue during resection and in case of intraoperative fibertracking (FT), the three-dimensional morphology of the white matter tract, with possible intraoperative correction of brain shift phenomena. In this chapter, the role of each of these advanced technologies and techniques is discussed.

G. Demichele
School of Medicine, University of Rome Campus Bio-Medico, Rome, Italy

D. Armocida
Neurosurgery Unit, Dept. Neuroscience "Rita Levi Montalcini", Università degli studi di Torino, Torino, TO, Italy

M. Palmieri
Neurosurgery Division, Human Neuroscience Department, University of Rome "La Sapienza", Rome, Italy

M. Salvati
Neurosurgery Unit, University di Roma "Tor Vergata", Rome, Italy

A. Pesce (✉)
Neurosurgery Division, Department of System Medicine, University of Rome "Tor Vergata", Rome, Italy
e-mail: ale_pesce83@yahoo.it

13.2 Awake Surgery

The technique of awake craniotomies was originally introduced for epilepsy surgery, but it is now mainly used in neuro-oncology. This technique is conceived to maintain the neuro-oncological balance: namely, to remove as much of the tumor as possible without impairing the neurological functions of the patient. Because of the strong potential psychological impact of this technique, appropriate candidate selection is crucial [1]. A successful Awake craniotomy needs a dense interprofessional, collaborative teamwork. Before the procedure, anesthesiologists, operative theater equip and surgical team need to discuss each surgical detail, including the required equipment and patient positioning. Each aspect of this process relies on good communication between surgeons, technician, nurse anesthetists, and anesthesiologist in ensuring a complication-free experience. To ensure the success of awake surgery (AS), the

D. Armocida et al. (eds.), *Neurosurgery's Frontline Role in Gliomas Treatment*,
https://doi.org/10.1007/978-3-031-81850-9_13

correct execution of anesthesiological techniques plays a crucial role. Monitoring by ASA standards, including temperature, noninvasive blood pressure, pulse oximetry, ECG, and ETCO2 is usually recommended; an intra-arterial line may be used for ABG analysis and continuous blood pressure monitoring. Central venous catheterization is done for administration of vasoactive drugs and fluids, while a precordial Doppler will help in the early detection of venous air embolism in the sitting position during craniotomy. Also, the monitors should be placed on the same side as brain lesions to avoid interference with contralateral sensorimotor monitoring. A processed EEG monitor with bispectral index can easily allow to awaken the patient for intraoperative language testing, and the anesthetic dosing can be managed [1]. The awake surgery will be specifically addressed in Chap. 15.

13.3 Direct Electrical Stimulation and Monitoring

A vital technique used during surgery to assess the functional integrity of the brain, spinal cord, brainstem, and cranial and peripheral nerves is intraoperative electrophysiologic monitoring, frequently referred to as neuromonitoring. It is especially advised for individuals who have a higher risk of experiencing a neurological injury

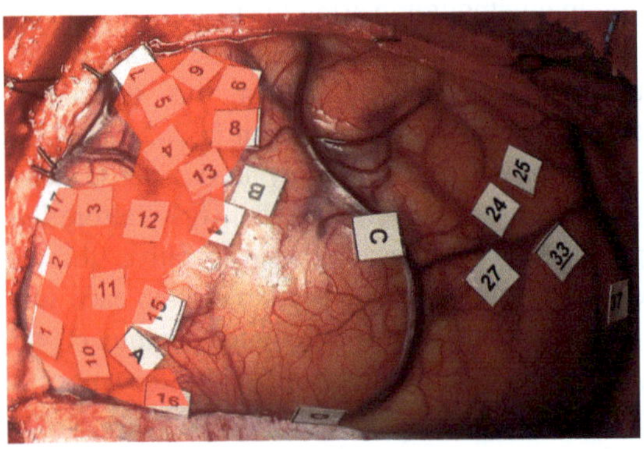

Fig. 13.1 Direct cortical intraoperative stimulation, the red area is the primary motor cortex. Posteriorly areas in which, respectively, an emineglect (27–33) and an optic ataxia (37) were elicitated

during surgery [4] (Fig. 13.1). Monitoring serves to alert surgeons and anesthesiologists to impending injuries so they can modify their treatment plans in time to prevent permanent damage. Electroencephalograms (EEG), spontaneous electromyograms (EMG), visual evoked potentials (VEP), motor-evoked potentials (MEP), triggered electromyography, somatosensory evoked potentials (SSEP), and brainstem auditory evoked potentials (BAEP) are some of the methods that are suitable for recording neuromonitoring [2, 3]. This topic is described with more details in Chap. 14.

13.4 Intraoperative Imaging

As mentioned in previous chapters, gliomas can be challenging to distinguish from surrounding healthy tissue [5, 6], therefore intraoperative imaging techniques were developed to maximize surgical resection extent in patients suffering from low-grade and high-grade gliomas: intraoperative imaging is a useful supplement to glioma surgery because it gathers and displays information in real time throughout the procedure.

T2 weighted or T2w-fluid attenuation inversion recovery magnetic resonance imaging (MRI) is now the accepted standard for resection assistance in non-enhancing gliomas, and T1-weighted MRI with a gadolinium-based contrast agent in enhancing gliomas: it has a clear role in maximizing resection rate, but as main drawbacks has significant costs both in terms of economic and time resources [7]. Intraoperative ultrasound guidance (iUS) is another intraoperative imaging technique: it constantly evolves toward a finer spatial resolution, aiding in the accurate differentiation between pathological and normal tissue, and acting as a real-time topographical orientation guide [8]. Regarding intraoperative CT (iCT), while there is a substantial benefit in terms of acquisition time, cost, maintenance, workflow, and minimization of room logistics such as magnetic shielding, the imaging quality of intra-axial malignant tumors is inferior when compared to iMRI [9].

13.4.1 Intraoperative MRI

In partnership with General Electric (Milwaukee, WI), the Brigham and Women's Hospital created the first intraoperative MRI (iMRI) device for neurosurgery [9]. This first prototype was an open "double donut" style low-field device with a 0.5-T magnet [10]. As a result, the patient could be positioned and secured inside the scanner while the neurosurgeons stood between the coils to reach them [11] (Figs. 13.2 and 13.3). In 1996, the safety and effectiveness of intraoperative magnetic resonance imaging (iMRI) for brain tumor excision was first demonstrated, with one-third of cases revealing residual tumors despite surgical judgment indicating complete resection [12]. Subsequent literature confirmed these findings showing that intraoperative magnetic resonance imaging resolved brain shift issues in traditional navigation systems, making online MR-guided interventional operations easier [13], permitting the direct evaluation of the extent of resection (EOR) and the identification of intraoperative complications [14]. The increase in navigation systems accuracy when coupled to an iMRI system was also reported [15–18]. This early system's primary drawbacks were its low-field strength, which reduced the clarity of the image, and the requirement that all surgical staff members and tools be MRI compatible [15].

Subsequent iMRI systems featured stationary MRIs, requiring patient rotation. Open-configuration iMRIs like Medtronic PoleStar and Siemens had a table that rotated into and out of a 1.5-T closed-bore magnet, requiring less changes to OR suites but having comparatively low-field strength [15, 16].

The modification of diagnostic closed-configuration MRI scanners for intraoperative use was a key advancement in iMRIs. One system, called IMRIS from Deerfield Imaging in Minnetonka, Minnesota, is installed on a rail

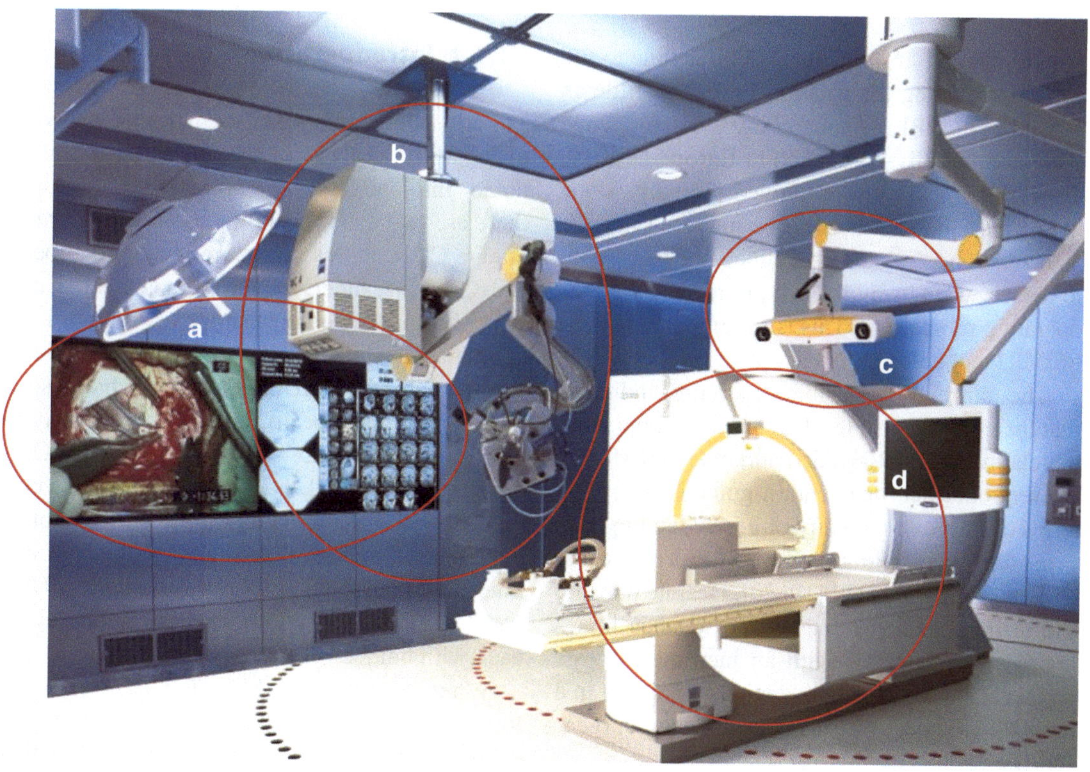

Fig. 13.2 A conventional operating room set up for intraoperative MRI procedures. It highlights the imaging monitor (**a**), the intraoperative microscope (**b**), the neuronavigation system (**c**), and the specialized operative table (**d**)

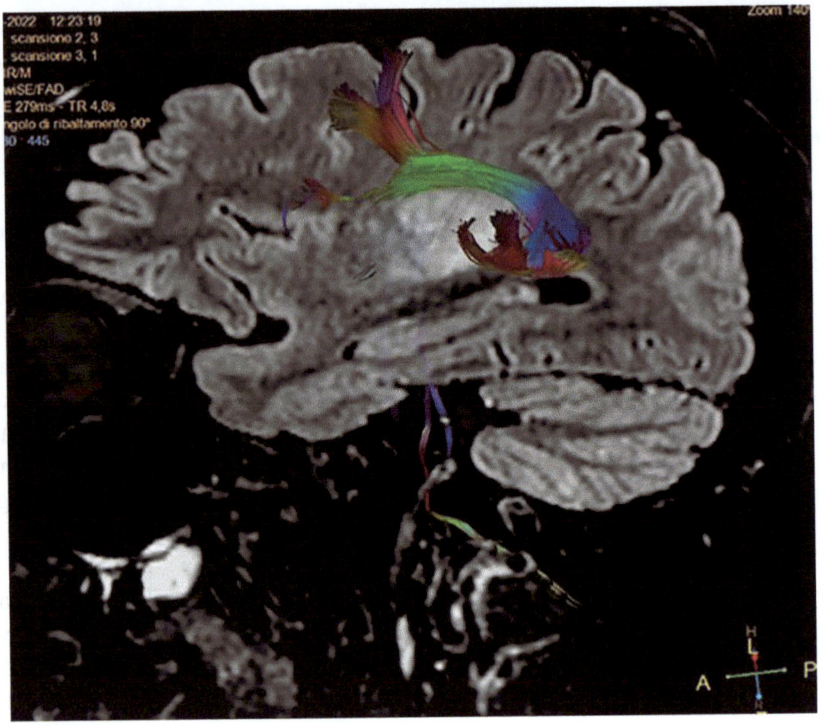

Fig. 13.3 Tractography allows a fine visualization of the white matter bundles and describes their anatomy in respect to the lesion

system which transports the MRI machine to the patient, requiring the patient to move as little as possible [17, 18]. Commercially available since 2005 and initially introduced in Europe in 2010, these systems are now deployed globally. Since the patient does not need to be moved, IV lines, catheters, and endotracheal tubes are less likely to detach when using iMRI equipment in or near operating rooms [15]. This is a significant benefit of iMRI technology.

The currently available literature indicates that there is, at most, level 2 evidence supporting the claim that iMRI-guided surgery outperforms conventional neuronavigation-guided surgery in terms of improving quality of life, extending survival following glioblastoma multiforme resection, or improving EOR [19, 20]. Despite this, the use of intraoperative magnetic resonance imaging is also associated with an increase in costs and times, and is currently a widespread tool in a limited number of advanced neurosurgery centers.

13.4.2 Intraoperative CT

The advent of a number of small, portable devices that may be utilized in the operating room has made intraoperative CT possible. Nowadays, there are two main technologies used by intraoperative CT scanners: the more recent cone-beam CT (CBCT) scanners, which use a conical-shaped X-ray beam detected on a single two-dimensional (2-D) flat panel detector, or the more conventional multidetector CT (MDCT) scanner, which uses a fan-shaped X-ray beam detected by an array of multiple detectors [21–23]. In contrast to MDCT devices, which stack many slices to get a whole picture, CBCT devices just require one rotation of the radiation source to capture the entire region of interest [21]. Because of these variations, MDCT and CBCT are essentially distinct technologies, each with unique benefits and limitations.

When compared to MDCT, CBCT provides lower costs, radiation exposure, and artifact scatter while providing great resolution at high contrast tissue surfaces and sub-millimeter details of bone structures. It helps with perioperative planning for surgeries involving the spine, sinuses, temporal bones, and orthodontics. On the other hand, MDCT scans a wider field of view and yields superior soft tissue resolution [23].

iCT may be used to update neuronavigation systems, adjust for brain shift, and acquire vascular imaging since it allows images to be taken with the patient's head secured in pins [24]. Additionally, this has made it possible to use low-dose CT scan automatic registration approaches that minimize mean target registration errors to less than 1 mm [25].

13.4.3 Intraoperative Ultrasound

Although its usage is not frequently standardized, the recognized applications of intraoperative ultrasound guidance include tumor localization, resection assessment, identification of surrounding arteries and patency of dural sinuses, brain abscess-guided aspiration, and ventriculostomy [8].

2D B-mode was initially used in the development of original ultrasonography methods. This method uses pulsed acoustic waves to show parameters depending on scattering and time and the waves are reflected off the tissue of interest and measured at transducers. The majority of neurosurgical transducers have a frequency range of 1–25 MHz and a depth penetration of up to 10 cm. A fundamental rule of thumb is that the resolution nearer the probe increases with frequency; however, higher frequencies have less penetration and are therefore less able to photograph deeper structures [5, 26]. Transducer type is often dictated by tumor size, craniotomy, anatomy, and surgeon choice.

Intraoperative US can be integrated with the neuronavigation system: navigated US may be used in 2D or 3D, and it interacts with preoperative MRI/CT such that the advantages of both systems work together to compensate for each other's shortcomings when used alone [27, 28]. By combining navigation MRI/CT with a live 2D-US picture, navigated 2D-US (n2DUS) provides improved tumor border delineation, residuum identification, and orientation [29–31]. Nevertheless, for multiplanar views, it needs serial sweeps and is restricted to a single picture plane. Additionally occupying the surgical area, the 2D-US probe restricts access and obscures the positioning of instruments. Comparing serial scans is not always easy [29, 32, 33].

To solve these issues, navigated 3D-US (n3DUS) makes it possible to acquire 3D-US volumes that can be retrospectively manipulated. Manual sweeps of a 2D probe or a matrix-phased array probe can be used to accomplish this. The navigation CT/MRI and the 3D-US volume can be fused, however, once the volume is obtained, the US probe can be removed, enabling the volume to be manipulated and utilized as a guide [29].

Intraoperative ultrasonography can also be helpful in providing up-to-date information regarding brain shift since it provides real-time imaging [34]. Many methods, such as automatic non-rigid registration [35, 36], vessel registration [37, 38], "pseudo-US" methodology [37], and rigid registration employing hyperechoic structures [34] have all been used to correct for brain shift. Since both iUS and iMRI can give updated imaging in the operating room, they are frequently compared.

Current literature shows that glioma surgical excision guided by intraoperative US is a helpful technique for both directing and enhancing the EOR. IoUS can enhance anatomic orientation during surgery when combined with other complimentary technologies and it is a practical, affordable instrument that enhances any current equipment in any neurosurgery operating environment thanks to its real-time imaging, enhanced image quality, compact probe sizes, repeatability, mobility, and relatively low cost [39].

13.5 Navigation and Tractography

Another breakthrough in neuroimaging was made possible by the advent of diffusion MRI tractography toward the end of the 1990s, which allowed for the in vivo observation of white matter fascicular architecture [40]. Diffusion tractography imaging (DTI) is essentially a method of measuring anisotropy, or the intrinsic Brownian motion of water molecules inside axons, by applying multidirectional magnetic resonance sensitizing gradients to brain tissue [41]. Details of methodology are described in the dedicated Chap. 5. Tractography appears to be particularly useful in glioma surgery: the duration of awake neuro-oncological surgery can be decreased using intraoperative guided tractography, which may also aid in the completion of total tumor removal [42–45]. By combining diffusion tensor imaging tractography and neuronavigation, tumor resection can be accomplished more successfully and with less damage, which will improve quality of life and slow the deterioration of functions after surgery (Fig. 13.3). Additionally, tractography may be a helpful preoperative planning technique for more accurate estimation of total tumor removal [46].

Tractography is helpful in identifying displacement, disruption, or infiltration when attempting to see the movement of perilesional white matter. A lesion that shifts white matter pathways without producing damage is referred to as displacement [47]. High-grade gliomas have the potential to produce displacement, disruption, or destruction, whereas metastases and meningiomas, which are non-neural tissue lesions, frequently induce displacement. After a lesion is removed, displaced tracts could go back to their original position, and disrupted tracts might reappear as before a lesion that was pressing on them was removed. Tumor-infiltrated white matter might need to be sacrificed during surgery if it is not essential to function [40]. Despite its utility, tractography has limitations. These include issues related to the acquisition method, the complexity of anatomical structures like crossing fibers, and the presence of brain edema, which can affect the accuracy of the reconstructed images. An early tractography-related randomized controlled study shown definite advantages in terms of improving overall survival, resection extent, and 6-month Karnofsky Performance Scale (KPS) scores in the DTI-assisted high-grade glioma (HGG) group [48]. Patients with low-grade gliomas (LGGs) or high-grade gliomas (HGGs) showed considerably higher average KPS ratings after DTI than after traditional neuronavigational guiding of resection [49].

13.6 Functional Neuroimaging

Functional neuroimaging performed prior to surgery, such as diffusion tensor imaging (DTI) and functional magnetic resonance imaging (fMRI), has become a viable technique for preoperative surgical planning. It shows regional differences in the brain's metabolic rate caused by certain activities. Whenever some of the brain areas get engaged in performing a task, there is an increase in CBF and a change in the concentration of oxygen level. These variations are detected by the BOLD contrast (Blood Oxygen Level Dependent) and can be visualized by MRI.

Among all the approaches, BOLD contrast is the most frequently applied one; it is based on the paramagnetic properties of the deoxygenated hemoglobin, which generates a magnetic field gradient. This method assists in defining the preoperative localization of eloquent brain areas, for instance, the motor, sensory, language, vision, and hearing areas. These are the areas that should be preserved during surgical operations. Also, the imaging data can be merged into the neuronavigation systems, improving the accuracy of the operations and checking the intraoperative findings with direct cortical stimulation (DCS). The combination of functional neuroimaging and advanced surgical techniques ensures better outcomes and minimizes the risks associated with brain surgeries.

13.7 Intraoperative Testing

Through the use of neurocognitive tasks and tests, intraoperative neuropsychological testing enables the assessment of praxis and gnosis functions, visuospatial functions, sensory and motor functions, and language functions in an awake patient.

Building a customized procedure that enables the selection of suitable intraoperative activities based on the patient's lesion location and its association with functional networks is crucial for each intraoperatively tested patient [50, 51]. Patients may be required to do praxic tasks, which involve actions such as picking up things, using tools, or imitating hand gestures, while the surgeon stimulates different brain regions. Changes in the patient's ability to do these tasks following stimulation may indicate a function of certain brain areas in praxis.

Many intraoperative tests utilizing cortical and subcortical mapping have been employed during surgery to assess visuospatial function; each has pros and cons of its own [52]. Despite the lack of a gold standard or a standardized international protocol, the line bisection test is a commonly used technique for mapping visuospatial function in clinical practice [53]. It supports surgeons in making prompt decisions to preserve critical brain functions.

Tests for motor or sensory functions are not well-documented in the literature; nevertheless, some studies report that surgeons monitor these functions by having patients record any movements or sensations. Motor-evoked potentials are a common tool for tracking motor function. Few papers consider the fact that motor and sensory abilities are frequently evaluated during awake brain surgery, define a specific test or paradigm for the evaluation of these domains [54].

The most popular and well-documented in the literature is language function monitoring. To track language functions, a variety of standardized neuropsychological tests are utilized, such as the Boston Naming Test, Pyramid and Palmtree Test, and Test de Dénomination Orale D'Images, in addition to more experimental paradigms [55–57].

13.8 Ultrasonic Aspirator

Ultrasonic aspiration (UA) devices have been a widely utilized in neurosurgery for the past few decades to assist treat a range of intracranial and intraspinal malignancies. The primary benefit of UA is that they enable less invasive surgery by safely debulking big tumors from the inside, protecting nearby brain tissue from injury during the dissection process. The patient's prognosis is improved by the ultrasonic transducer because it reduces tissue selection-related damage to blood arteries and nerve fibers during tumor excision [58–61]. It also shortens surgical times, minimizes blood loss, and enhances the overall standard of the procedure [58, 62, 63]. There are several UA types available today, each made by a separate company. Among the many models available, we can cite three: the CUSA Excel®/Clarity® (Integra®, Plainsboro, NJ, USA), the Sonopet® (Stryker®, Kalamazoo, MI, USA), and the Söring® (Söring GmbH, Quickborn, Germany). Neurosurgeons choose UA kinds based on particular features unique to each instance. Three popular UA varieties seem to have rather similar safety characteristics [58].

The usual frequency range for ultrasonic surgical aspirators is 20–60 kHz. Suction is provided as a vibrating hollow horn presses up on the tissue. As a result of the contact, tissue breaks apart, and the broken material is aspirated. The most widely accepted theory, which likely operates in conjunction with other processes such as the direct jack-hammer effect, shock-induced stress, acoustic microstreaming, and shearing stress, links the interaction to cavitation. Nevertheless, the exact mechanism of interaction remains unclear [64].

13.9 Thulium Laser

Infrared lasers, such as the thulium laser emitting at 1940-nm wavelength, have proven useful for coagulation in neurosurgery because of wavelength-specific water absorption. Following laser application, blood vessels undergo a photothermal tissue change that results in crusting and whitening of the tissue for the selected laser parameter. In a roughly circular region, the laser causes a specific photothermal tissue change (coagulation, ablation). While thulium lasers can provide a tissue-gentle hemostasis by non-contact coagulation, bipolar forceps, which are frequently employed for intraoperative hemostasis, can harm tissue mechanically and thermally [65].

The lack of established use of lasers in neurosurgery can be attributed to uncontrolled tissue interactions caused by inappropriate laser wavelengths. These can result in either photoevaporative effect and inadequate coagulation (CO_2 laser) [65, 66] or deep tissue penetration depth (ND-YAG laser) and associated vascular injury [67–69].

13.10 Conclusions

We wish to conclude making a long story short: today, the only possible, safe and effective glioma surgery is *multitechnological*. This term summarizes the evidence that to safely increase the extent of tumor resection, and thus prolonging survival, surgeons should always rely on a multiplicity of combined technologies aiding the preoperative planning, intraoperative visualization, testing, and resection of such complex lesions.

References

1. Singh K, Dua A. Anesthesia for awake craniotomy. 2023 Jul 6. In: StatPearls [Internet]. Treasure Island: StatPearls Publishing; 2024. PMID: 34283419.
2. Weinzierl MR, Reinacher P, Gilsbach JM, Rohde V. Combined motor and somatosensory evoked potentials for intraoperative monitoring: intra- and postoperative data in a series of 69 operations. Neurosurg Rev. 2007;30(2):109–16; discussion 116. https://doi.org/10.1007/s10143-006-0061-5. Epub 2007 Jan 13. PMID: 17221265.
3. Lall RR, Lall RR, Hauptman JS, Munoz C, Cybulski GR, Koski T, Ganju A, Fessler RG, Smith ZA. Intraoperative neurophysiological monitoring in spine surgery: indications, efficacy, and role of the preoperative checklist. Neurosurg Focus. 2012;33(5):E10. https://doi.org/10.3171/2012.9.FOCUS12235. PMID: 23116090.
4. Ghatol D, Widrich J. Intraoperative neurophysiological monitoring. 2023 Jul 24. In: StatPearls [Internet]. Treasure Island: StatPearls Publishing; 2024. PMID: 33085350.
5. Noh T, Mustroph M, Golby AJ. Intraoperative imaging for high-grade glioma surgery. Neurosurg Clin N Am. 2021;32(1):47–54. https://doi.org/10.1016/j.nec.2020.09.003. Epub 2020 Nov 5.
6. Garzon-Muvdi T, Kut C, Li X, Chaichana KL. Intraoperative imaging techniques for glioma surgery. Future Oncol. 2017;13(19):1731–45. https://doi.org/10.2217/fon-2017-0092. Epub 2017 Aug 10.
7. Verburg N, de Witt Hamer PC. State-of-the-art imaging for glioma surgery. Neurosurg Rev. 2021;44(3):1331–43. https://doi.org/10.1007/s10143-020-01337-9. Epub 2020 Jun 30.
8. Méndez GEF, et al. Utility of intraoperative ultrasound in neurosurgery. Arq Bras Neurocir. 2021;40(2):e113–9.
9. Mislow JM, Golby AJ, Black PM. Origins of intraoperative MRI. Neurosurg Clin N Am. 2009;20(2):137–46. https://doi.org/10.1016/j.nec.2009.04.002.
10. Schenck JF, Jolesz FA, Roemer PB, Cline HE, Lorensen WE, Kikinis R, Silverman SG, Hardy CJ, Barber WD, Laskaris ET, et al. Superconducting open-configuration MR imaging system for image-guided therapy. Radiology. 1995;195(3):805–14. https://doi.org/10.1148/radiology.195.3.7754014. PMID: 7754014.
11. Liang D, Schulder M. The role of intraoperative magnetic resonance imaging in glioma surgery. Surg Neurol Int. 2012;3(Suppl 4):S320–7. https://doi.org/10.4103/2152-7806.103029. Epub 2012 Oct 31.
12. Black PM, Alexander E 3rd, Martin C, Moriarty T, Nabavi A, Wong TZ, Schwartz RB, Jolesz F. Craniotomy for tumor treatment in an intraoperative magnetic resonance imaging unit. Neurosurgery. 1999;45(3):423–31; discussion 431-3. https://doi.org/10.1097/00006123-199909000-00001. PMID: 10493363.
13. Tronnier VM, Wirtz CR, Knauth M, Lenz G, Pastyr O, Bonsanto MM, Albert FK, Kuth R, Staubert A, Schlegel W, Sartor K, Kunze S. Intraoperative diagnostic and interventional magnetic resonance imaging in neurosurgery. Neurosurgery. 1997;40(5):891–900; discussion 900-2. https://doi.org/10.1097/00006123-199705000-00001. PMID: 9149246.
14. Wirtz CR, Bonsanto MM, Knauth M, Tronnier VM, Albert FK, Staubert A, Kunze S. Intraoperative magnetic resonance imaging to update interactive navigation in neurosurgery: method and preliminary experience. Comput Aided Surg. 1997;2(3–4):172–9. PMID: 9377718.
15. Feigl GC, Heckl S, Kullmann M, Filip Z, Decker K, Klein J, Ernemann U, Tatagiba M, Velnar T, Ritz R. Review of first clinical experiences with a 1.5 Tesla ceiling-mounted moveable intraoperative MRI system in Europe. Bosn J Basic Med Sci. 2019;19(1):24–30. https://doi.org/10.17305/bjbms.2018.3777.
16. Nimsky C, Ganslandt O, von Keller B, Fahlbusch R. Preliminary experience in glioma surgery with intraoperative high-field MRI. Acta Neurochir Suppl. 2003;88:21–9. https://doi.org/10.1007/978-3-7091-6090-9_5. PMID: 14531557.
17. Sutherland GR, Louw DF. Intraoperative MRI: a moving magnet. CMAJ. 1999;161(10):1293.
18. Sutherland GR, Kaibara T, Louw D, Hoult DI, Tomanek B, Saunders J. A mobile high-field mag-

netic resonance system for neurosurgery. J Neurosurg. 1999;91(5):804–13. https://doi.org/10.3171/jns.1999.91.5.0804. PMID: 10541238.

19. Kubben PL, ter Meulen KJ, Schijns OE, ter Laak-Poort MP, van Overbeeke JJ, van Santbrink H. Intraoperative MRI-guided resection of glioblastoma multiforme: a systematic review. Lancet Oncol. 2011;12(11):1062–70. https://doi.org/10.1016/S1470-2045(11)70130-9. Epub 2011 Aug 23. PMID: 21868286.
20. Senft C, Bink A, Franz K, Vatter H, Gasser T, Seifert V. Intraoperative MRI guidance and extent of resection in glioma surgery: a randomised, controlled trial. Lancet Oncol. 2011;12(11):997–1003. https://doi.org/10.1016/S1470-2045(11)70196-6. Epub 2011 Aug 23. PMID: 21868284.
21. Miracle AC, Mukherji SK. Conebeam CT of the head and neck, part 1: physical principles. AJNR Am J Neuroradiol. 2009;30(6):1088–95. https://doi.org/10.3174/ajnr.A1653. Epub 2009 May 13.
22. Rumboldt Z, Huda W, All JW. Review of portable CT with assessment of a dedicated head CT scanner. AJNR Am J Neuroradiol. 2009;30(9):1630–6. https://doi.org/10.3174/ajnr.A1603. Epub 2009 Aug 6.
23. Conley DB, Tan B, Bendok BR, Batjer HH, Chandra R, Sidle D, Rahme RJ, Adel JG, Fishman AJ. Comparison of intraoperative portable CT scanners in skull base and endoscopic sinus surgery: single center case series. Skull Base. 2011;21(4):261–70. https://doi.org/10.1055/s-0031-1280681.
24. Barbagallo GM, Maione M, Peschillo S, Signorelli F, Visocchi M, Sortino G, Fiumanò G, Certo F. Intraoperative computed tomography, navigated ultrasound, 5-amino-levulinic acid fluorescence and neuromonitoring in brain tumor surgery: overtreatment or useful tool combination? J Neurosurg Sci. 2024;68(1):31–43. https://doi.org/10.23736/S0390-5616.19.04735-0. Epub 2019 Jul 11. PMID: 31298506.
25. Carl B, Bopp M, Saß B, Pojskic M, Gjorgjevski M, Voellger B, Nimsky C. Reliable navigation registration in cranial and spine surgery based on intraoperative computed tomography. Neurosurg Focus. 2019;47(6):E11. https://doi.org/10.3171/2019.8.FOCUS19621. PMID: 31786552.
26. Serra C, Stauffer A, Actor B, Burkhardt JK, Ulrich NH, Bernays RL, Bozinov O. Intraoperative high frequency ultrasound in intracerebral high-grade tumors. Ultraschall Med. 2012;33(7):E306–12. https://doi.org/10.1055/s-0032-1325369. Epub 2012 Nov 5. PMID: 23129521.
27. Dixon L, Lim A, Grech-Sollars M, Nandi D, Camp S. Intraoperative ultrasound in brain tumor surgery: a review and implementation guide. Neurosurg Rev. 2022;45(4):2503–15. https://doi.org/10.1007/s10143-022-01778-4. Epub 2022 Mar 30.
28. de Quintana-Schmidt C, Salgado-Lopez L, Aibar-Duran JA, Alvarez Holzapfel MJ, Cortes CA, Alvarado JDP, Rodriguez RR, Teixidó JM. Neuronavigated ultrasound in neuro-oncology: a true real-time intraoperative image. World Neurosurg. 2022;157:e316–26. https://doi.org/10.1016/j.wneu.2021.10.082. Epub 2021 Oct 13. PMID: 34655818.
29. Yeole U, Singh V, Mishra A, Shaikh S, Shetty P, Moiyadi A. Navigated intraoperative ultrasonography for brain tumors: a pictorial essay on the technique, its utility, and its benefits in neuro-oncology. Ultrasonography. 2020;39(4):394–406. https://doi.org/10.14366/usg.20044. Epub 2020 Jun 17.
30. Miller D, Heinze S, Tirakotai W, Bozinov O, Sürücü O, Benes L, Bertalanffy H, Sure U. Is the image guidance of ultrasonography beneficial for neurosurgical routine? Surg Neurol. 2007;67(6):579–87; discussion 587-8. https://doi.org/10.1016/j.surneu.2006.07.021. PMID: 17512324.
31. Renovanz M, Hickmann AK, Henkel C, Nadji-Ohl M, Hopf NJ. Navigated versus non-navigated intraoperative ultrasound: is there any impact on the extent of resection of high-grade gliomas? A retrospective clinical analysis. J Neurol Surg A Cent Eur Neurosurg. 2014;75(3):224–30. https://doi.org/10.1055/s--0033-1356486. Epub 2014 Mar 12. PMID: 24622999.
32. Ivanov M, Wilkins S, Poeata I, Brodbelt A. Intraoperative ultrasound in neurosurgery—a practical guide. Br J Neurosurg. 2010;24(5):510–7. https://doi.org/10.3109/02688697.2010.495165. PMID: 20868239.
33. Bal J, Camp SJ, Nandi D. The use of ultrasound in intracranial tumor surgery. Acta Neurochir. 2016;158(6):1179–85. https://doi.org/10.1007/s00701-016-2803-7. Epub 2016 Apr 22. PMID: 27106844.
34. Coupé P, Hellier P, Morandi X, Barillot C. 3D rigid registration of intraoperative ultrasound and preoperative MR brain images based on hyperechogenic structures. Int J Biomed Imaging. 2012;2012:531319. https://doi.org/10.1155/2012/531319. Epub 2012 Jan 19.
35. Machado I, Toews M, Luo J, Unadkat P, Essayed W, George E, Teodoro P, Carvalho H, Martins J, Golland P, Pieper S, Frisken S, Golby A, Wells W 3rd. Non-rigid registration of 3D ultrasound for neurosurgery using automatic feature detection and matching. Int J Comput Assist Radiol Surg. 2018;13(10):1525–38. https://doi.org/10.1007/s11548-018-1786-7. Epub 2018 Jun 4.
36. Machado I, Toews M, George E, Unadkat P, Essayed W, Luo J, Teodoro P, Carvalho H, Martins J, Golland P, Pieper S, Frisken S, Golby A, Wells Iii W, Ou Y. Deformable MRI-ultrasound registration using correlation-based attribute matching for brain shift correction: accuracy and generality in multi-site data. NeuroImage. 2019;202:116094. https://doi.org/10.1016/j.neuroimage.2019.116094. Epub 2019 Aug 22.
37. Mercier L, Fonov V, Haegelen C, Del Maestro RF, Petrecca K, Collins DL. Comparing two approaches to rigid registration of three-dimensional ultrasound and magnetic resonance images for neurosurgery. Int J Comput Assist Radiol Surg. 2012;7(1):125–36.

https://doi.org/10.1007/s11548-011-0620-2. Epub 2011 Jun 2. PMID: 21633799.

38. Reinertsen I, Lindseth F, Unsgaard G, Collins DL. Clinical validation of vessel-based registration for correction of brain-shift. Med Image Anal. 2007;11(6):673–84. https://doi.org/10.1016/j.media.2007.06.008. Epub 2007 Jun 30. PMID: 17681484.
39. Mahboob S, McPhillips R, Qiu Z, Jiang Y, Meggs C, Schiavone G, Button T, Desmulliez M, Demore C, Cochran S, Eljamel S. Intraoperative ultrasound-guided resection of gliomas: a meta-analysis and review of the literature. World Neurosurg. 2016;92:255–63. https://doi.org/10.1016/j.wneu.2016.05.007. Epub 2016 May 10. PMID: 27178235.
40. Panesar SS, Abhinav K, Yeh FC, Jacquesson T, Collins M, Fernandez-Miranda J. Tractography for surgical neuro-oncology planning: towards a gold standard. Neurotherapeutics. 2019;16(1):36–51. https://doi.org/10.1007/s13311-018-00697-x.
41. Stejskal EO, Tanner JE. Spin diffusion measurements: spin echoes in the presence of a time-dependent field gradient. J Chem Phys. 1965;42(1):288–92.
42. Paglia F, Caporlingua A, Armocida D, Rizzo F, Santoro A, D'angelo L. Preoperative 3D volume reconstruction of the posterior wall of the sphenoid sinus with Horos: a free, simple and reliable tool in endoscopic endonasal trans-sphenoidal surgery. Neurocirugia (Astur: Engl Ed). 2022;33(5):219–26. https://doi.org/10.1016/j.neucie.2021.04.008.
43. Abhinav K, Yeh FC, Pathak S, Suski V, Lacomis D, Friedlander RM, Fernandez-Miranda JC. Advanced diffusion MRI fiber tracking in neurosurgical and neurodegenerative disorders and neuroanatomical studies: a review. Biochim Biophys Acta. 2014;1842(11):2286–97. https://doi.org/10.1016/j.bbadis.2014.08.002. Epub 2014 Aug 12. PMID: 25127851.
44. Abhinav K, Yeh FC, Mansouri A, Zadeh G, Fernandez-Miranda JC. High-definition fiber tractography for the evaluation of perilesional white matter tracts in high-grade glioma surgery. Neuro-Oncology. 2015;17(9):1199–209. https://doi.org/10.1093/neuonc/nov113. Epub 2015 Jun 27.
45. Celtikci P, Fernandes-Cabral DT, Yeh FC, Panesar SS, Fernandez-Miranda JC. Generalized q-sampling imaging fiber tractography reveals displacement and infiltration of fiber tracts in low-grade gliomas. Neuroradiology. 2018;60(3):267–80. https://doi.org/10.1007/s00234-018-1985-5. Epub 2018 Jan 25. PMID: 29372286.
46. Aibar-Durán JÁ, de Quintana-Schmidt C, Álvarez Holzpafel MJ, Hernández FM, Cortés CA, Martínez GV, Bertrán GC. Intraoperative use and benefits of tractography in awake surgery patients. World Neurosurg. 2020;137:e347–53. https://doi.org/10.1016/j.wneu.2020.01.210. Epub 2020 Feb 4. PMID: 32032793.
47. Price SJ, Burnet NG, Donovan T, Green HA, Peña A, Antoun NM, Pickard JD, Carpenter TA, Gillard JH. Diffusion tensor imaging of brain tumours at 3T: a potential tool for assessing white matter tract invasion? Clin Radiol. 2003;58(6):455–62. https://doi.org/10.1016/s0009-9260(03)00115-6. PMID: 12788314.
48. Wu JS, Zhou LF, Tang WJ, Mao Y, Hu J, Song YY, Hong XN, Du GH. Clinical evaluation and follow-up outcome of diffusion tensor imaging-based functional neuronavigation: a prospective, controlled study in patients with gliomas involving pyramidal tracts. Neurosurgery. 2007;61(5):935–48; discussion 948-9. https://doi.org/10.1227/01.neu.0000303189.80049.ab. PMID: 18091270.
49. Henderson F, Abdullah KG, Verma R, Brem S. Tractography and the connectome in neurosurgical treatment of gliomas: the premise, the progress, and the potential. Neurosurg Focus. 2020;48(2):E6. https://doi.org/10.3171/2019.11.FOCUS19785.
50. Shi J, Lu D, Pan R, Chen H, Teng H, Xu Y, Bo F, Zhou Q, Zhang Y. Applications of diffusion tensor imaging integrated with neuronavigation to prevent visual damage during tumor resection in the optic radiation area. Front Oncol. 2022;12:955418. https://doi.org/10.3389/fonc.2022.955418.
51. Fernández Coello A, Moritz-Gasser S, Martino J, Martinoni M, Matsuda R, Duffau H. Selection of intraoperative tasks for awake mapping based on relationships between tumor location and functional networks. J Neurosurg. 2013;119(6):1380–94. https://doi.org/10.3171/2013.6.JNS122470. Epub 2013 Sep 20. PMID: 24053503.
52. Conner AK, Glenn C, Burks JD, McCoy T, Bonney PA, Chema AA, Case JL, Brunner S, Baker C, Sughrue M. The use of the target cancellation task to identify eloquent visuospatial regions in awake craniotomies: technical note. Cureus. 2016;8(11):e883. https://doi.org/10.7759/cureus.883.
53. Vallar G, Bello L, Bricolo E, Castellano A, Casarotti A, Falini A, Riva M, Fava E, Papagno C. Cerebral correlates of visuospatial neglect: a direct cerebral stimulation study. Hum Brain Mapp. 2014;35(4):1334–50. https://doi.org/10.1002/hbm.22257. Epub 2013 Feb 18.
54. Ruis C. Monitoring cognition during awake brain surgery in adults: a systematic review. J Clin Exp Neuropsychol. 2018;40(10):1081–104. https://doi.org/10.1080/13803395.2018.1469602. Epub 2018 Aug 1. PMID: 30067443.
55. Deloche G, Hannequin D. Test de dénomination orale d'images: DO 80. ECPA: Les éditions du Centre de psychologie appliquée; 1997.
56. Kaplan E, Goodglass H, Weintraub S. Boston naming test. 2nd ed. Lippincott Williams & Wilkins; 2001.
57. Howard D, Patterson KE. The pyramids and palm trees test. Pearson; 1992.
58. Henzi S, Krayenbühl N, Bozinov O, Regli L, Stienen MN. Ultrasonic aspiration in neurosurgery: comparative analysis of complications and outcome for three commonly used models. Acta Neurochir. 2019;161(10):2073–82. https://doi.org/10.1007/s00701-019-04021-0. Epub 2019 Aug 3.

59. Tang H, Zhang H, Xie Q, Gong Y, Zheng M, Wang D, Zhu H, Chen X, Zhou L. Application of CUSA Excel ultrasonic aspiration system in resection of skull base meningiomas. Chin J Cancer Res. 2014;26(6):653–7. https://doi.org/10.3978/j.issn.1000-9604.2014.12.10.
60. Ramazanov R, Dreval ON, Akatov OV, Zaretsky AA. Ultrasound microneurosurgery. Neurol Res. 1999;21(1):73–6. https://doi.org/10.1080/01616412.1999.11740896. PMID: 10048059.
61. Jallo GI. CUSA EXcel ultrasonic aspiration system. Neurosurgery. 2001;48(3):695–7. https://doi.org/10.1097/00006123-200103000-00054. PMID: 11270564.
62. Baddour HM, Lupa MD, Patel ZM. Comparing use of the Sonopet(®) ultrasonic bone aspirator to traditional instrumentation during the endoscopic transsphenoidal approach in pituitary tumor resection. Int Forum Allergy Rhinol. 2013;3(7):588–91. https://doi.org/10.1002/alr.21143. Epub 2013 Jan 7. PMID: 23292661.
63. Brock M, Ingwersen I, Roggendorf W. Ultrasonic aspiration in neurosurgery. Neurosurg Rev. 1984;7(2–3):173–7. https://doi.org/10.1007/BF01780701. PMID: 6493516.
64. Bond LJ, Cimino WW. Physics of ultrasonic surgery using tissue fragmentation: part II. Ultrasound Med Biol. 1996;22(1):101–17. https://doi.org/10.1016/0301-5629(95)02022-5. PMID: 8928307.
65. Hutfilz A, Theisen-Kunde D, Bonsanto MM, Brinkmann R. Pulsed thulium laser blood vessel haemostasis as an alternative to bipolar forceps during neurosurgical tumour resection. Lasers Med Sci. 2023;38(1):94. https://doi.org/10.1007/s10103-023-03747-9.
66. Ascher PW, Heppner F. CO2-Laser in neurosurgery. Neurosurg Rev. 1984;7(2–3):123–33. https://doi.org/10.1007/BF01780695. PMID: 6436735.
67. Beck OJ. The use of the Nd-YAG and the CO_2 laser in neurosurgery. Neurosurg Rev. 1980;3(4):261–6. https://doi.org/10.1007/BF01650032. PMID: 7279232.
68. Devaux BC, Joly LM, Page P, Nataf F, Turak B, Beuvon F, Trystram D, Roux FX. Laser-assisted endoscopic third ventriculostomy for obstructive hydrocephalus: technique and results in a series of 40 consecutive cases. Lasers Surg Med. 2004;34(5):368–78. https://doi.org/10.1002/lsm.20045. PMID: 15216529.
69. Armocida D, Pesce A, Palmieri M, D'Andrea G, Salvati M, Santoro A, Frati A. Periventricular zone involvement as a predictor of survival in glioblastoma patients: a single centre cohort-comparison investigation concerning a distinct clinical entity. Interdiscip Neurosurg. 2021;25:101185. https://doi.org/10.1016/j.inat.2021.101185.

14 A Primer on Intraoperative Neurophysiological Monitoring (IONM) and Brain Mapping in Neurooncological Surgery

Leonardo Tariciotti, Youssef Zohdy, Beatrice C. Bono, Marco Riva, and Federico Pessina

14.1 Introduction

When operating on supratentorial intra-axial tumours, surgeons must balance oncological radicality with preserving function and quality of life [1–3]. While complete resection may offer the best outcome, damaging essential cortico-subcortical networks can cause permanent neurological deficits, impacting quality of life and reducing survival [4, 5].

The recent reassessment of the traditional localisationist paradigm, pioneered by figures such as Sherrington [6], Broca [7], and Penfield [8] has renewed interest in brain functions. This has led to the development of "hodology," which posits that brain functions arise from spatially distributed dynamic networks of subcortical pathways connecting distinct cortical nodes. These networks may change in patients with brain tumours or post-surgery (i.e., "metaplasticity") [9–11]. In this context, the terms "dominant" and "non-dominant" hemispheres and "eloquent" and "non-eloquent" areas seem outdated and simplistic. The study of brain networks, their interactions ("meta-network"), and the overall human connectome introduces complex data that challenge our understanding of the neural substrates underlying motor control, language, and cognitive functions [12–14]. Choosing the best intraoperative monitoring and mapping protocol is crucial. Awake surgery is generally preferred for preserving neurological functions that require a testable awake patient. However, various factors may necessitate an asleep procedure in oncological and epilepsy surgeries. Intraoperative neurophysiological monitoring (IONM) is a reliable and well-established protocol that includes monitoring and mapping techniques to predict and prevent intraoperative neurological injuries. It is the gold standard for motor function and used for different sensory modalities and cognitive domains [15, 16]. This chapter provides an overview of monitoring and mapping techniques, focusing on their use in

L. Tariciotti (✉)
Department of Neurosurgery, Emory University School of Medicine, Atlanta, GA, USA

Department of Oncology and Hemato-Oncology, University of Milan, Milan, Italy
e-mail: leonardo.tariciotti@emory.edu

Y. Zohdy
Department of Neurosurgery, Emory University School of Medicine, Atlanta, GA, USA

B. C. Bono
Department of Neurosurgery, IRCCS Humanitas Research Hospital, Milan, Italy

M. Riva · F. Pessina
Department of Neurosurgery, IRCCS Humanitas Research Hospital, Milan, Italy

Department of Biomedical Sciences, Humanitas University, Milan, Italy

D. Armocida et al. (eds.), *Neurosurgery's Frontline Role in Gliomas Treatment*,
https://doi.org/10.1007/978-3-031-81850-9_14

awake and asleep surgeries for supratentorial intra-axial brain tumours, from well-established methods to more advanced paradigms and experimental protocols.

14.2 IONM Techniques and Neurophysiological Implications

The selection of a specific modality is based on the need to monitor distinct neural pathways according to the location and nature of the lesion. This tailored approach ensures that the appropriate neural structures are effectively monitored during surgery. In the following section, we will discuss the practical implications of the most commonly used IONM techniques in supratentorial surgeries, including the physiology behind each technique and setup procedures.

14.2.1 Motor Evoked Potential (MEP)

A primary goal of surgery for intra-axial brain lesions is the preservation of motor pathways. The motor evoked potential (MEP) is the action potential signal elicited in peripheral muscles, measured by electromyography (EMG), via motor cortex stimulation [17–19]. While MEP monitors the motor pyramidal tracts, depending on the stimulation intensity and the electrodes' placement, MEPs can be generated at different levels of the brain, including superficial white matter, deep white matter of the internal capsule, and pyramidal decussation.

MEP monitoring of the motor tracts begins with electrical stimulation of the axons of the large Betz cells located in the motor cortex rather than the cell bodies. This can be achieved either transcranially using corkscrew needles inserted into the scalp or by directly stimulating the brain cortex using an electrode strip [20]. The stimulus is transmitted along the corticospinal tract through the spinal cord to the nerve root, then through the peripheral nerve before terminating in the corresponding skeletal muscles.

14.2.1.1 Stimulation Electrodes

Corkscrew electrodes are commonly used for transcranial stimulation, while multi-contact strip electrodes are employed for stimulating an exposed brain. These strip electrodes are placed under the dura, overlapping the precentral gyrus. The latter can be identified directly with cortical probe stimulation (described later in the chapter) or indirectly using the phase-reversal technique to localise the central sulcus (see Fig. 14.1).

Regarding transcranial stimulation, the electrodes are placed using the international 10–20 system [18, 20]. The system's main landmarks are the nasion, inion, and preauricular points, and electrodes are placed at 10% or 20% intervals of the total distance between these landmarks. When monitoring MEPs in the upper limbs, stimulating electrodes are placed at scalp positions C1/C2 or

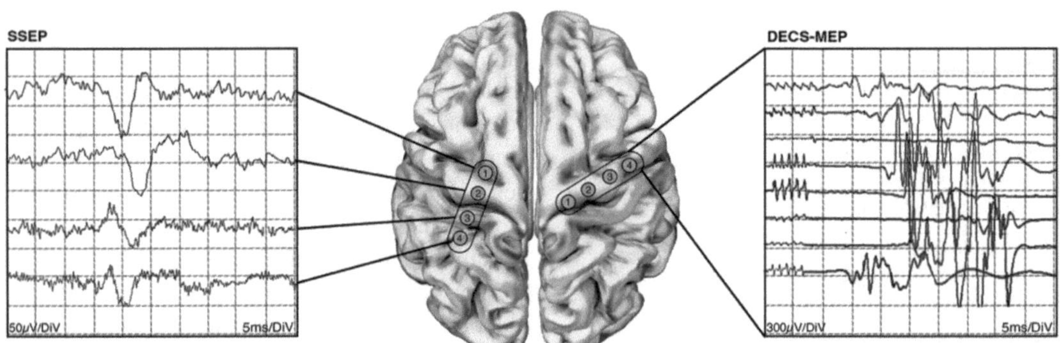

Fig. 14.1 Cortical grid placement for M1-S1 phase reversal identification and direct cortical stimulation for EMPs recording

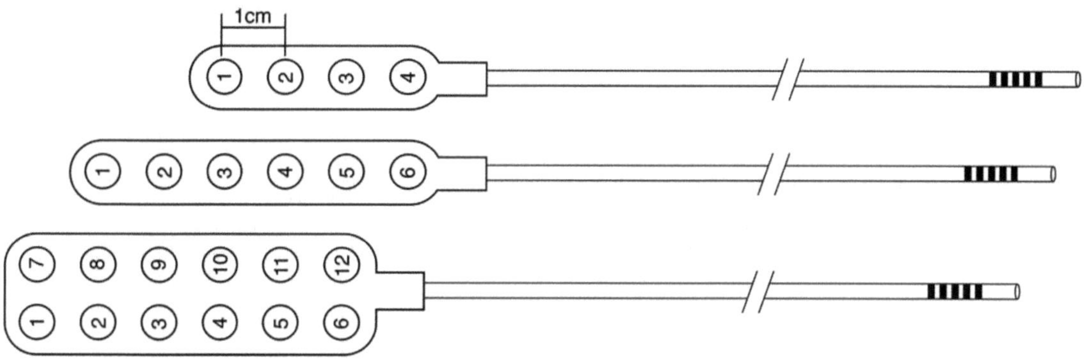

Fig. 14.2 Cortical stimulation grid for electrocorticography and subdural MEP monitoring

C3/C4. External switching of the stimulating positive electrode (anode) and the negative reference electrode (cathode) then allows stimulation of the left or right hemisphere using the same electrode pair. It is worth noting that since the C3/C4 electrodes are closer to the facial motor cortex, jaw muscles, and trigeminal nerves compared to the C1/C2 electrodes, stimulation at C3/C4 can result in stronger biting movements. Thus, C1/C2 electrodes are often preferred unless C3/C4 electrodes are necessary to elicit MEPs. Several stimulating electrode arrangements can elicit MEPs in the lower limbs. Paired electrodes at C1/C2 or C3/C4 can be utilised with external polarity switching. Although these montages often produce bilateral leg MEPs, the responses are typically most robust on the side opposite the anode. Another setup involves placing an anode at Cz and a cathode at Fz. The C1/C2 and C3/C4 montages have the advantage of stimulating motor pathways for both upper and lower limbs with a single stimulus, allowing simultaneous recording of MEPs from both regions. On the other hand, the Cz/Fz montage may more specifically stimulate motor pathways for the lower limbs bilaterally with a single stimulus. The optimal electrode arrangement for stimulation can differ based on the patient and the surgical conditions; therefore, various stimulation montages should be tested to identify the most effective one for each patient.

On the other hand, the placement of stimulating electrodes for direct cortical stimulation (DCS) and MEP elicitation is more straightforward. Depending on the location of the tumour and the surgical exposure, an electrode strip, ranging from 1 × 4 up to 8 × 8, is placed directly on the cortical surface (see Figs. 14.1 and 14.2). This allows for cortical mapping at the beginning of the surgery and continuous DCS MEP monitoring throughout the tumour resection, in addition to Electrocorticography, which can be carried out using the same grid.

14.2.1.2 Stimulation Parameters

To elicit an MEP response, multiple pulse electrical stimulation is used, which is termed stimulation train pulse, given that a single stimulus is often insufficient to elicit a reliable action potential under general anaesthesia. The duration of the inter-pulse interval (the time between stimulus pulses in a train) is critical. If the interval is too long, the postsynaptic potentials do not overlap, losing the benefit of temporal summation. Conversely, if the interval is too short, the stimuli following the first spoke are less effective in activating the corticospinal tract axons due to their refractory periods. Inter-pulse intervals of 2–4 ms or a pulse frequency of 5–10 Hz are generally preferred [18, 20]. A train of 3–5 pulses is sufficient for most patients, while others may need more, with each pulse lasting between 100 and 300 μsec. It is advisable to begin with a standard set of stimulus parameters for initial recordings under anaesthesia and then adjust these parameters as needed to achieve adequate MEPs for IONM for each patient.

14.2.1.3 Response Waves

Corticospinal tract activity induced by cortical stimulation generates "D-waves," which reflect the direct activation of pyramidal cell axons, and multiple "I-waves," which reflect the indirect activation of these pyramidal neurons by cortico-cortical interneurons [21]. Because I-waves are mediated by cortical synaptic activity, they are significantly suppressed by surgical levels of anaesthesia. However, D-waves persist and can be recorded along the spinal cord. Cortical stimulation eventually leads to muscle contraction, producing a compound muscle action potential known as the "M-wave" (myogenic MEP) [22]. As discussed, train stimulation is required to elicit M-waves reliably, especially under anaesthesia. Within the context of supratentorial glioma surgery, M-waves are of choice for reliable cortical mapping and monitoring through the course of surgery.

14.2.1.4 Recording Electrodes and Sites

For accurate MEP monitoring, M-waves should be captured from limb muscles bilaterally. Needle electrodes generally provide stronger signals than surface electrodes, and either type should be securely attached to the skin to avoid displacement during surgery [18, 20]. In the upper limb, M-waves are best recorded from hand muscles such as the thenar or abductor digiti minimi, as these are primarily controlled by the corticospinal tract. Proximal muscles, including those in the forearm and arm, can also be used (see Table 14.1). In the lower limb, the tibialis anterior and abductor hallucis are typically chosen for M-wave monitoring; though more proximal muscles may be used, they usually offer less reliable MEPs.

Additionally, facial muscles like the orbicularis oculi and mentalis can be used. It is important to note that contralateral monitoring is recommended. This serves as an internal reference and is helpful for troubleshooting during signal loss. The balance between cortical monitoring and anaesthesia is critical for effective stimulus recording. Paralytic agents should be avoided during surgery, except for short-acting ones to facilitate intubation, as they interfere with monitoring EMG activity by blocking the neuromuscular junction. Cortical evoked potentials, such as SSEP and MEP, are highly sensitive to many anaesthetic agents, necessitating careful adjustment of anaesthesia levels during their use. For example, halogenated inhalation agents tend to suppress MEP M-waves, especially at high concentrations, while intravenous anaesthetics such as propofol and dexmetatomidine have a lower effect [23, 24].

Notably, a suboptimal anaesthetic regimen sometimes requires higher current intensity to elicit a monitorable EMP through transcranial stimulation under general anaesthesia; tumour-related cortical excitability alterations might also occur. However, MEP elicitation is current-dependent: higher intensities can produce electric volleys deeper underneath the motor cortex and excite the corticospinal tract distal to the surgical field of interest, returning a positive signal regardless of the proximal integrity of the tract (see Fig. 14.3). This should be considered when interpreting MEP recording, and adequate current parameters should be selected and verified for reliable intraoperative monitoring.

Table 14.1 Topographical checklists for EMG recording in upper and lower limbs

Anatomical site	Muscle
Upper limb	Thenar
	Abductor digiti minimi
	Biceps
	Triceps
Lower limb	Abductor hallucis
	Extensor digitorum brevis muscles
	Tibialis anterior
	Gastrocnemius
	Quadriceps
Face	Frontalis
	Orbicularis oculi
	Nasalis
	Orbicularis Oris
	Mentalis

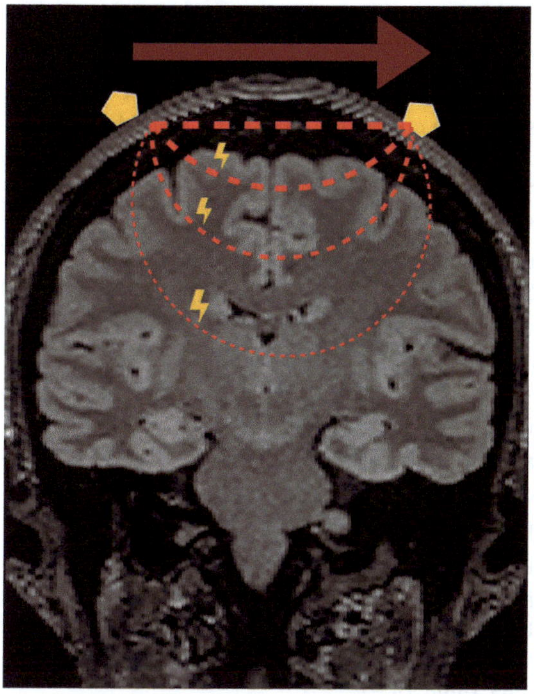

Fig. 14.3 Subcortical current-related volleys during transcranial MEP monitoring. The figure shows the spreading of the transcranial stimulation brain into the white matter (the dotted red lines represent the current). During MEP IONM, more than 80% of the delivered current is spread and lost within the skin and skull, with only a small proportion delivered to the brain tissue. As the current intensity increases, the activation of corticofugal motor fibres becomes deeper, with a preference for axon bending, which is more susceptible to external electric stimulation. When the IOM setup is not optimised, and a deeper-than-expected activation is obtained, no reliable monitoring is provided on the integrity of the proximal corticospinal tract, providing a false safe response. Should corticospinal tract damage occur due to a vascular injury or heating, a warning would be delayed, leading to more severe irreversible damage

14.2.1.5 Workflow and Alarming Criteria

Within the context of supratentorial tumour resection, a standard IONM workflow typically uses a combination of both mapping and monitoring techniques. Depending on the location of the tumours, corkscrew electrodes were initially placed to obtain preoperative baselines bilaterally and continuous stimulation of non-exposed cortical tissue after that. Upon opening the dura and exposing the cortex, direct cortical surface stimulation (DCS) is performed using an electrode strip or a stimulator to identify the central sulcus and the pre- and postcentral gyri (see Fig. 14.1).

Early identification of the motor and sensory cortex is crucial as it helps establish a safe entry zone and provides an electrophysiological baseline for monitoring and predicting postoperative outcomes. The primary EMG measurements during MEP monitoring are response amplitude, latency, and stimulus threshold [25]. Preservation of MEPs at the end of the procedure, with parameters comparable to baseline recordings, typically indicates good motor outcomes with no or transient postoperative deficits. MEP amplitude is usually the parameter of choice, measured from one wave's peak to the opposite polarity's peak. Since transient alterations occur in up to 60% of monitored cases and permanent alterations are defined retrospectively, the surgeon must carefully consider these episodes [26]. One approach is to evaluate the subcortical distance to the corticospinal tract (CST). A more complex scenario is the occurrence of a significant and persistent drop in MEP amplitude. In this case, a drop greater than 50% may indicate injury to the CST. However, it is crucial to rule out reversible causes of MEP alterations, such as hypotension or anaesthesia effects. Other alarm criteria used during MEP monitoring include an increased stimulation threshold required to elicit an MEP and a reduction in the duration and/or complexity of the M-wave [26].

14.2.2 Somatosensory Evoked Potential (SSEP)

While MEP has the ability to assess efferent functions of the brain, SSEP has the unique ability to assess afferent functionality. SSEP monitors the dorsal column–medial lemniscus pathway, which mediates mechanoreception and proprioception, however, they do not monitor the spinothalamic tracts [27]. From a neurophysiological perspective, stimulation of sensory receptors in the skin initiates peripheral sensory nerves, which extend through the nerve root to the ipsilateral dorsal root ganglia at spinal levels [28]. The projections from these first-order neurons form fasciculi gracilis and cuneatus, which carry impulses from the lower and upper extremities, respectively. The first synapse occurs in the lower medulla, then the impulses cross over at the level of the brainstem and form the medial lemniscus. The impulse then ascends to the contralateral thalamus and relays information to the primary somatosensory cortex.

14.2.2.1 Stimulation Electrodes

SSEPs are recorded from the somatosensory cortex after stimulation of an upper or lower extremity nerve. In the upper extremities, the median and ulnar nerve are stimulated, whereas, in the lower extremities, the posterior tibial and peroneal nerve are stimulated. Needle or surface stimulation electrodes are placed distally along the afferent nerve fibre course. For example, when stimulating the median nerve, the cathode is placed between the tendons of the palmaris longus and flexor carpi radialis muscles, 2 cm proximal to the wrist crease, while the anode is placed 2–3 cm distal to the cathode [29–31].

14.2.2.2 Stimulation Parameters

Afferent nerves are stimulated with monophasic pulses with a duration of 0.1–0.3 ms using either a constant voltage or constant current [32]. To minimise electrical stimulus artefacts in the recorded data, it is essential to keep the contact impedances of the stimulating electrodes low. The stimulus intensity is adjusted to produce a consistent muscle twitch, which should be tolerable for the patient. Rapid stimulus delivery rates should be avoided, as they can degrade SEP waveforms; typically, a rate of 2–8 stimuli per second is used. Frequencies that are multiples of the line current frequency (60 Hz) should be avoided to reduce line noise.

SSEPs recorded from the cortical surface are larger (20–500 μV) and have a high signal-to-noise ratio. Accordingly, signal averaging helps reduce random noise while preserving signals that are time-locked to stimulus delivery [32]. Usually, 25–50 repetitions are sufficient to obtain a reproducible response, and at least two trials should be conducted to confirm reproducibility.

14.2.2.3 Response Wave

When reviewing SSEP recordings, it is crucial to understand how they are reported and to have a knowledge of the anatomic origin of commonly used waves [28, 33]. A SSEP waveform reports as N or P followed by a number; N or P corresponds to "negative" upwards deflection or "positive" downwards deflection (the wave polarity), and the number represents the expected latency of the wave in ms, as determined from a healthy population. Each spot monitored along a sensory pathway has a typical recording value; for example, an electrode placed at Erb's point during median nerve monitoring would result in a negative wave with a latency of 9 ms; "N9" waves (see Table 14.2).

The N20/P30 waveforms are recorded over the somatosensory cortex whereas waveforms of the opposite polarity, P20/N30, are recorded over the primary motor cortex. Referential recordings from adjacent electrodes over the pre- and post-central gyri produce a "phase reversal" between the N20 and the P20 [34, 35]. The phase reversal marks the site of the central sulcus. If a clear phase reversal is not identified, the site of the highest amplitude of the N20 and P20 waveforms marks the vicinity of the central sulcus. The central sulcus is localised directly underneath or a few millimetres anterior to the area of highest amplitude. The point at which the N20 and P20 waveforms are the highest amplitude also marks the hand area of the sensory and motor cortices. SSEPs should be obtained from multiple sites on the exposed cortex to map the central sulcus as it is often not linear, especially in the presence of lesions.

14.2.2.4 Recording Electrodes and Site

SSEPs are recording either using corkscrew electrodes places using the 10–20 system or standard subdural electrode grid placed on the cortical sur-

Table 14.2 Reference recording points for SSEPs in upper and lower limbs

Wave name	Polarity	Latency	Description
Upper limb (median nerve stimulation)			
N9	Negative	9 ms	Reflects the response as the sensory signal reaches the brachial plexus
N13	Negative	13 ms	Generated in the cervical spinal cord, representing conduction through the dorsal columns
P14	Positive	14 ms	Reflects conduction through the brainstem, specifically the medial lemniscus or thalamus
N20	Negative	20 ms	Represents the arrival of the sensory signal at the somatosensory cortex in the parietal lobe
Lower limb (posterior tibial nerve stimulation)			
N22	Negative	22 ms	Reflects the response as the sensory signal reaches the popliteal fossa
N34	Negative	34 ms	Generated in the lumbar spinal cord, representing conduction through the dorsal columns
P37	Positive	37 ms	Reflects conduction through the brainstem and arrival at the primary somatosensory cortex in the parietal lobe
N45	Negative	45 ms	Represents further processing in the somatosensory cortex

face. Cranial electrode CP3 is midway between C3 and P3, and electrode CP4 is midway between C4 and P4 [29–31, 36]. And in the context of a specific procedure, CPi denotes either ipsilateral CP3 or CP4, while CPc is the contralateral centroparietal scalp electrode. Recording montages for cortical SSEP components are either cephalic bipolar, in which both electrodes are placed over the head, or referential, in which a reference electrode is placed at a non-cephalic site. Cephalic bipolar montages yield signals with less noise contamination and are usually preferred. For upper limb SSEP studies, electrodes are placed over Erbs point, both ipsilateral and contralateral to the stimulus (labelled EPi and EPc, respectively). Subcortical derivations may be unnecessary in cranial surgery, especially under total intravenous anaesthesia (TIVA) due to robust cortical responses with higher signal-to-noise ratios, allowing faster acquisition of cortical responses and potentially reducing averaging time. Nonetheless, whenever feasible, including subcortical channels is recommended for redundancy and comprehensive recording. Based on recommendations from the ACNS, a standard multichannel EEG montage is advised that incorporates cortical near-field and subcortical far-field signals. For instance:

- Channel 1: CPc—Cpi
- Channel 2: CPc—EPc
- Channel 3: CPi—EPc
- Channel 4: EPi—EPc

14.2.2.5 Measurements and Alarm Criteria

Several characteristics of SSEPs can be measured, including peak latencies, amplitudes, and waveform morphology. Peak latencies are generally consistent across subjects, whereas amplitudes exhibit considerable variability between individuals. Therefore, SSEP latency interpretation relies on more defined values, including absolute latency, interpeak intervals, and right-left differences. Amplitude assessment is based on a comparison with baseline recordings taken for each patient at the beginning of surgery prior to any neuronal manipulation. During surgery, if neural tissue is compromised (i.e., a vascular injury or global hypoperfusion), SSEP components may experience significant amplitude attenuation before latency increases are observed. Consequently, both amplitude and latency should be monitored throughout the procedure. A 50% decrease in SSEP component amplitude or a 10% increase in latency are commonly used as alarm thresholds.

14.2.3 Electroencephalography (EEG)

The electrical activity measured by EEG is generated by groups of pyramidal neurons, whose cell bodies are located in the third and fifth layers of the cerebral cortex. This electrical activity represents the summation of inhibitory and excitatory postsynaptic potentials from pyramidal cells near each recording electrode. It can be measured using scalp electrodes or invasively with subdural grid electrodes or depth electrodes. One of the most important uses of EEG in the context of supratentorial tumour resection is monitoring anaesthesia levels using the observed EEG waves; Delta (1–4 Hz), Theta (4–8 Hz), Alpha (8–12 Hz), and Beta (12–30 Hz) [37, 38]. Alpha and Beta waves are dominant when the patient is awake, but as anaesthesia takes effect, higher frequency activity is replaced by lower frequency activity, a phenomenon known as "slowing." Critical iatrogenic-induced changes in the EEG include a reduction in overall amplitude and a shift to low-frequency activity, possibly progressing to electrocerebral silence due to decreased synaptic activity [37, 38]. Accordingly, analysing EEG waves is crucial for ruling out the anesthetic effects of cortical stimulation suppression, and in the context of awake surgery.

14.2.4 Visual Evoked Potential (VEP)

Visual evoked potentials (VEPs) measure the functional integrity of the optic pathways from the retina to the brain's visual cortex in response to light stimuli. This process begins with the conversion of visual stimuli into nerve signals in the retina, which are then transmitted through the optic nerve, optic chiasma, optic tract, lateral geniculate body, optic radiation, and finally to the visual cortex in the occipital lobe. Currently, VEPs are obtained from the visual cortex by applying a photo-stimulus to the retina, with recordings taken from electrodes on the occipital scalp or a strip electrode gride positioned over the occipital cortex. During surgical resection, warning criteria include a decrease in amplitude of more than 50% for hemianopia and 20% for quadrantanopia. Caution is advised for patients with preexisting visual deficits, as the reliability of VEPs in these cases might be cumbersome [39, 40].

However, implementing neurophysiological techniques for posterior visual pathway mapping is anecdotal and still of limited use, mostly in experimental protocols, compared to awake cortical and subcortical visual mapping [41–44].

14.3 Electrophysiological Principles in Brain Mapping Techniques

To prevent the onset of new postoperative neurological deficits, meticulous intra-operative neurophysiological paradigms must be applied using direct electrical stimulation (DES) at both cortical and subcortical levels. This approach delineates the tumour from surrounding essential cortical sites and white matter bundles while continuous intraoperative neurophysiological monitoring (IONM) verifies the integrity of testable pathways (e.g., somatosensory and motor pathways) [45–49]. This strategy should represent the standard in any function-based oncological resection, maximising the use of available mapping and monitoring techniques. Penfield introduced DES in the early 1900s, translating previous findings from animal models. The method consisted of biphasic (anodal–cathodal), bipolar 50–60 Hz stimulation applied for up to 4 s [8, 50]. This technique has long been used in awake patients for cortical motor and language mapping and was later shown to be effective under general anaesthesia for motor mapping [51]. Widely known as the "Penfield technique" or "Low-frequency technique" (LF), it has been the predominant brain mapping paradigm for decades, particularly in the United States.

In 1993, Taniguchi described a second paradigm, the "high-frequency technique" (HF), which involves monopolar 250–500 Hz multipulse DES (generally a train of five pulses) to elicit motor evoked potentials (MEPs) under general anaesthesia [52]. This method preferentially activates efferent fibres from the primary motor cortex compared to the LF bipolar pulse [53–56]. Since both methods became widely available, surgical practice has evolved, with their use being common in cortical mapping and identifying key white matter bundles (subcortical mapping) [57]. However, the growing literature on their application and the proposed paradigms can lead less experienced surgeons to misconceptions and confusion regarding available strategies for tailoring brain mapping techniques to patients' needs.

A general belief is that the LF technique must use a bipolar probe, as initially proposed by Penfield and later corroborated by Ojemann, while the HF technique relies on a monopolar probe. Despite these common uses, the electrical configuration of the stimulation is independent of the delivering probe, which affects the homogeneity and density of the electrical current rather than the pulse characteristics. Overall, several technical aspects should be considered when planning a function-based resection: the stimulating device, the polarity of the pulse, the stimulation pulse type, width, stimulation frequency (Hz), intensity (mA), and the stimulation probe used to deliver the current. This chapter will comprehensively review these characteristics to better understand how to refine a brain mapping strategy.

14.3.1 Stimulator Device (IONM Console)

Constant-current and constant-voltage stimulating devices have been designed for this purpose. A constant-current stimulator is considered safer and more reliable than a constant-voltage stimulator. The former delivers a predefined current regardless of the impedance of the tissue being stimulated, while the latter relies on the impedance of the surface in contact. Indeed, in case of lowered impedance, the overall current delivery would be unwarrantedly higher than expected, compromising the patient's safety.

14.3.2 Stimulation Polarity

The current direction can be set and modified according to the mapping site (i.e., cortical or subcortical) during the surgical procedure. According to the first animal studies, anodal current (positive) is more effective in direct cortical stimulation, requiring a lower intensity to elicit a recordable effect. When stimulating the motor cortex in primates, selective excitation of fast-conducting corticofugal neurons was achieved with a lower threshold using a positive anodal current [58–61]. Histological investigations on neural tissue also corroborated these findings [59].

Conversely, several studies have demonstrated that nerve fibre activation occurred through depolarisation underneath the cathodal electrode in peripheral nerve fibres. Indirectly, these findings have been translated to subcortical stimulation and myelinated fibres of the corticospinal tract, where cathodal pulses elicited a motor response at a lower intensity than anodal current [62–64]. Despite this being an accepted rule, effective anodal stimulation is also achieved at the cortical and subcortical levels in patients receiving re-surgery after irradiation or with a history of drug-resistant seizures [65, 66]. The neurophysiological bases of this phenomenon are not entirely understood. This concept will be further explored later in this chapter.

14.3.3 Stimulation Parameters

14.3.3.1 Low-Frequency (LF) Technique

The LF paradigm applies a short pulse with a frequency of 50 Hz (Europe) or 60 Hz (North America). The stimulation is a constant pulse (rectangular), monophasic or biphasic, with a duration of up to 1 ms in a sequence lasting 1–4 s. The choice of a biphasic pulse is historically related. When only uncoupled stimulators were available, a monophasic anodal pulse could cause neurotoxic changes confirmed at the histological level, while a biphasic pulse was seen to mitigate those effects. Since the introduction of coupled stimulators and the reduction of stimulation times, the neurotoxic effects of DES have not been reported, and several institutions employ monophasic pulses regularly [59, 67–71].

If a biphasic pulse is chosen for cortical mapping, the first phase should be anodal (for the above reasons), followed by a cathodal phase. The duration of the anodal (stimulating) phase should be between 0.2 and 1 ms. The pulse duration includes the whole delivered pulse (both anodal-positive and cathodal-negative). Accordingly, only half of the pulse stimulates the cortex in a biphasic pulse, while the cathodal phase is used only to avoid cytotoxic effects. This means that a monophasic anodal current of 0.4 ms delivers the same current of a biphasic pulse of 0.8 ms (composed of 0.4 ms of anodal and 0.4 ms of cathodal currents). However, the total charge applied with a biphasic pulse is twofold that of a monophasic pulse (charge = pulse duration x intensity). For this reason, the maximal intensity deliverable is usually set to 20 mA for safety reasons [72, 73].

For example, if a 60-Hz biphasic stimulation is preferred, equivalent to an interstimulus interval (ISI) of 16.7 ms, 1 ms of biphasic current is delivered (0.5 ms for each polarity), followed by 15.7 ms pause (*16.7 ms—stimulus duration*; to facilitate these calculations, it is essential to remember that the *ISI = 1/Frequency* and ISI is the interval between the onset of two stimuli). Then, a single stimulation unit is provided in 16.7 ms and repeated for 1–4 s. This results in 60 biphasic pulse waves delivered in a second (for a 60 Hz setup) (see Fig. 14.4).

A summary of the available parameters for the LF technique is available in Table 14.3.

14.3.3.2 High-Frequency (HF) Technique

The HF paradigm consists of a monophasic wave pulse delivered as a train ranging from 2 to 9 spikes each lasting 0.5 ms (range 0.3–0.8 in advanced settings) with an interstimulus interval (ISI) of 2–4 ms (equivalent to a frequency of 250–500 Hz) delivered every 1–2 s (1 or 0.5 Hz, respectively), either by a monopolar or bipolar probe. As previously described, the polarity of the stimulation (anodal or cathodal) is chosen based on the stimulation's site (cortical or subcortical). This paradigm is optimised to reduce the effects of facilitation of MEP amplitudes and decrement of motor thresholds (MTs) occurring during fast repetition rates of stimulation [54].

For example, suppose a train of 0.5 ms five pulses (To5) is chosen with an ISI equal to 4 ms. In that case, the monophasic current is delivered for 2.5 ms in total (0.5 ms × 5 pulses) within an interval of 16.5 ms (0.5 ms for each monophasic spike plus four intervals between each spike lasting 3.5 ms each) followed by 983.5 ms of absent current, to fulfil a repetition rate of 1 s (or 1 Hz). Following this logic, adjustments in pulse width, frequency of spike stimulation, repetition rate, and number of spikes per train can be easily calculated (see Fig. 14.4).

A summary of the parameters for the HF technique is available in Table 14.3.

14.3.4 Stimulation Probe

Bipolar and monopolar probes are available from different manufacturers, either equipped with spherical or straight tips. For bipolar stimulation, a probe with two tips at a 5–10 mm distance is considered the standard [74]. A straight tip delivering current towards a reference electrode (either located in the frontal region or close to the primary motor cortex according to the use) is used for the monopolar stimulation. The distribution and density of the current delivered and the electric field exerted differ between the two probes.

With any stimulation parameters applied, the monopolar probes deliver a homogeneous radiant spreading electric field resembling a semi-elliptical shape near the stimulation site, with a lower current density on the tissue directing to the reference electrode. The main advantage is the chance of larger spatial stimulation effects during mapping in terms of the activation of fibres at a higher distance from the tip.

In contrast, bipolar probes generate a parallel electric field between the two tips, with homogeneous current density in the surface probed, resulting in more focal tissue stimulation. In addition, a weaker spherical current

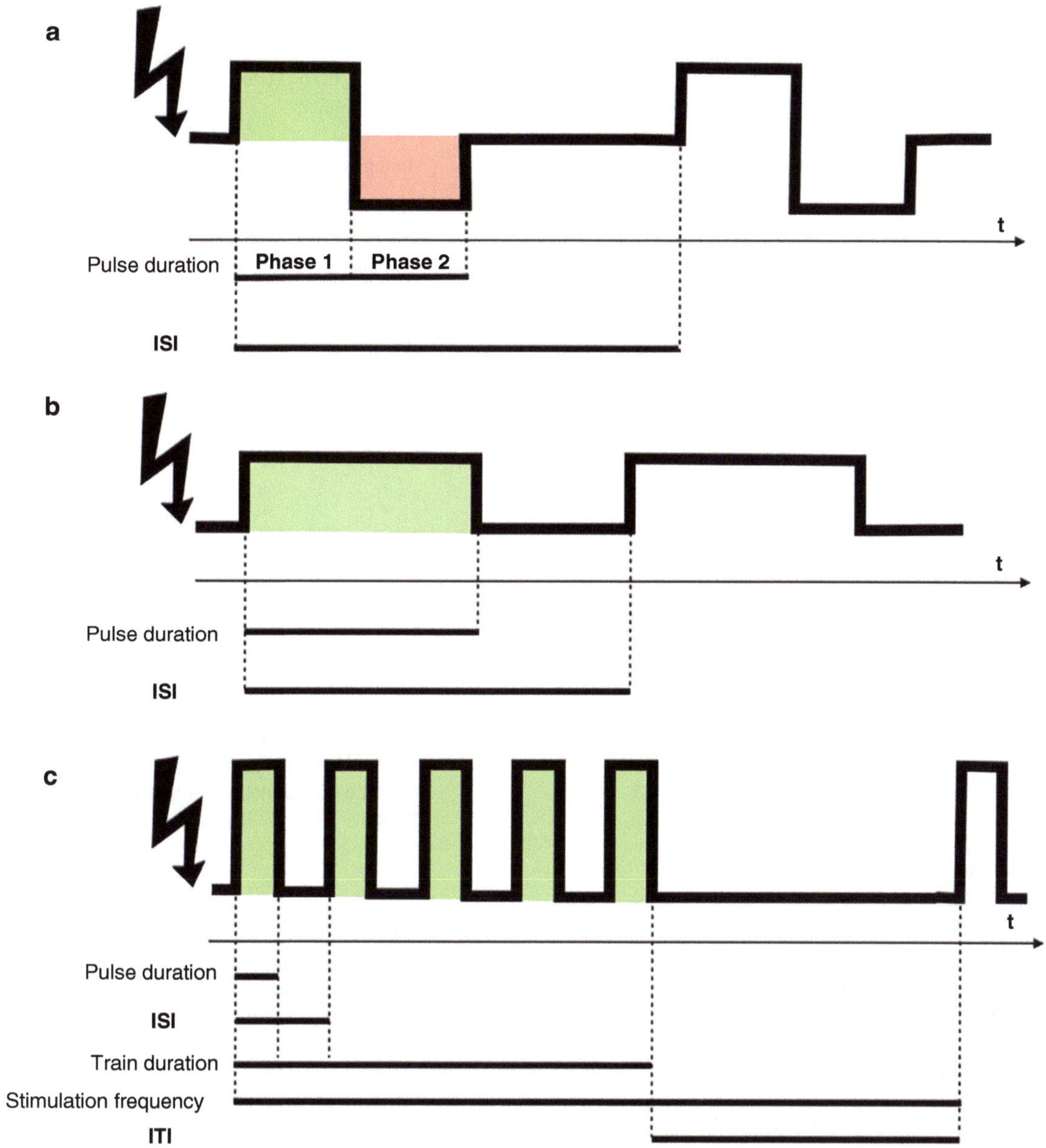

Fig. 14.4 Direct electrical stimulation techniques. Schematic drawing of the 50–60 Hz and the multipulse stimulation techniques. The pulse representation is not scaled between techniques, as is the timeline of stimulation (*t*). (**a**) Depiction of low-frequency (LF) biphasic current delivery for a cortical site stimulation. The anodal (positive) phase is represented in green, while the cathodal (negative) phase is red. On average, the duration of the biphasic pulse is 0.5 ms per phase and 1 ms overall. The interstimulus interval (ISI) represents the interval between the delivery of two consequent stimuli. (**b**) Depiction of low-frequency (LF) monophasic current delivery for a cortical site stimulation. The anodal (positive) phase is represented in green. On average, the duration of the monophasic pulse is 0.5–1 ms. The interstimulus interval (ISI) represents the interval between the delivery of two consequent stimuli. (**c**) Depiction of the high frequency (HF) multipulse stimulation paradigm is represented as a train of five spikes (To5). The anodal current delivered is represented in green to stimulate a cortical site. Single pulse duration lasts usually 0.5 ms, with an interstimulus interval (ISI) of 2–4 ms. With an ISI of 4 ms, the interval between the end of a train's spike and the next is 3.5 ms, with a To5 delivered in 16.5 ms, until the next train is delivered in 983.5 ms (1 Hz) or 314.83 ms (3 Hz; stimulation frequency). The latter is referred to as intertrain interval (ITI)

Table 14.3 Overview of electrophysiological parameters for direct electrical stimulation

Parameters	High frequency (HF)	Low frequency (LF)	
Frequency	250–500 Hz	50 (Europe), 60 (USA) Hz	
Pulse form	Monophasic	Mono/biphasic	
Pulse direction			
Cortical site	Anodal (+)	Monophasic: Anodal (+)	Biphasic: Anodal (first phase); Cathodal (second phase)
Subcortical site	Cathodal (−)	Monophasic: Cathodal (−)	Biphasic: Cathodal (first phase); anodal (second phase)
Duration (individual spike)	0.3–0.5 ms; up to 0.8 ms in high-risk patients	Monophasic: 0.5 ms	Biphasic: 0.5 ms each phase (up to 1 ms per stimulation)
Pulse number	Five (standard To5)	One	
	2–3 (usually To3: In infiltrating tumor within or close to M1)		
	6–9 (usually To9: In high-risk patients)		
Interstimulus interval (ISI)	2–4 ms	16.7–20 ms	
Stimulation duration	To3: 9.5 ms	60 Hz: 0.5–1 ms; 60 biphasic waves per second	
	To5: 18.5 ms	50 Hz: 0.5–1 ms; 50 biphasic waves per second	
	To9: 36.5 ms		
Repetition rate	1 Hz: 1 train per second	0.25 Hz: 1 s (50/60 waves) of stimulation followed by 3 s of pause	
	3 Hz: 3 trains per second	1 Hz: 1 s of stimulation followed by 1 s of pause	
Average use intensity			
Motor mapping			
Asleep	5–15 mA	7–16 mA	
Awake	2–7 mA	2–7 mA	
Language/ cognitive mapping (awake)	1–20 mA (3 Hz To5 setting)	Up to 6 mA (identify working current or 1 mA below afterdischarge occurrence)	
Probe (motor mapping):			
Bipolar	Poorly reported	2.8-fold higher motor threshold; risk of seizure but higher focality	
Monopolar	Lowest motor threhsold (To5)	Poorly reported	
Probe (language and cognitive mapping):			
Bipolar	Poorly reported	Lowest working current; lower but actual risk of ictal events	
Monopolar	Requires a two-fold higher intensity for identifying the working current, but has lower risk of seizure (To5, 500 Hz, ISI 4 ms, 3-Hz repetition rate). Useful in high-risk patients	Poorly reported	

density is also generated around each tip, but its effects are less predictable and probably negligible [75, 76].

The shape of probes' tips has also been investigated as potential confounders for current propagation. However, no difference in thresholds during motor mapping was found when a single-pole tip of bipolar probes was used for monopolar stimulation compared to a standard monopolar probe, excluding an influence of the probes' shape or surfaces on the overall thresholds. These findings are also translated into non-motor mapping, although specific evidence is not currently available [77].

The spatial propagation of current during monopolar and bipolar stimulation affects the sensitivity of the stimulation itself, even though a generalisation encompassing motor and non-motor pathways might oversimply this concept. During subcortical motor mapping, optimal stimulation is obtained when the stimulating current intersects the axons perpendicularly. The radial propagation of monopolar electrical fields simplifies the stimulation technique, increasing the chances of obtaining the optimal orientation between fibres and current. On the other hand, this is less straightforward with bipolar probes: the semi-elliptic electric field residing in between the tips and the larger dimension might require additional trials to obtain the proper orientation for eliciting a corticospinal tract stimulation, increasing mapping timing and exposing the surgeon to false negative results [77]. The characteristics of the bipolar and monopolar probes are depicted in Fig. 14.5.

14.3.5 Recording and Documentation of Stimulation Effects

Using any of stimulation paradigms mentioned above affects the response phenomenon, which can be elicited during an awake or asleep procedure. However, the latter is also influenced by how we investigate the response, namely how we record the stimulation effect. On a more general basis, we can simplify the effect documentation as behavioural (detected by a human operator, usually a neuropsychologist, speech therapist or physical therapist), instrumental (recorded within the IONM platform) and a combination of the two. Some key points for interpreting DES responses in motor and non-motor mapping are summarised below.

14.3.5.1 LF Technique

The LF technique can be used for motor, language, and cognitive mapping, either in awake or asleep (motor only, but this concept is further explored in the last section of this chapter) conditions. When applied over M1, LF DES at an intensity of 2–7 mA elicits a motor response in an awake patient, while 7–16 mA is often required in asleep conditions. The motor response can be detected under visual inspection or by electromyography (EMG) recording. The latter allows a broader range of ipsi- and contralateral muscles to be tested; also, EMG recording facilitates the interpretation of evoked motor responses (especially in behaviourally "negative motor responses) and prompt detection of after discharges before clinical seizures propagate.

LF stimulation typically evokes a progressive intensity-proportional motor unit recruitment during motor cortex stimulation with a prevalent response of extensors over flexors muscle by known somatotopy (see Fig. 14.6). At the subcortical level, motor unit recruitments appear tonic, with more muscles recruited at the same current intensity [66, 71, 78]. Non-motor mapping by means of LF stimulation elicits a disruption of the underlying network involved, causing an identifiable temporary impairment of the function investigated.

14.3.5.2 HF Technique

The HF technique, similar to LF technique, has been proven effective for both motor and "non-motor" mapping. In the context of motor mapping, HF DES on M1 elicits MEPs at EMG recording. The DES intensity required for such response varies in awake (2–7 mA) and asleep (5–15 mA) settings [66]. Although the HF technique can be used in awake patients with behavioural inspection of response, EMG recording

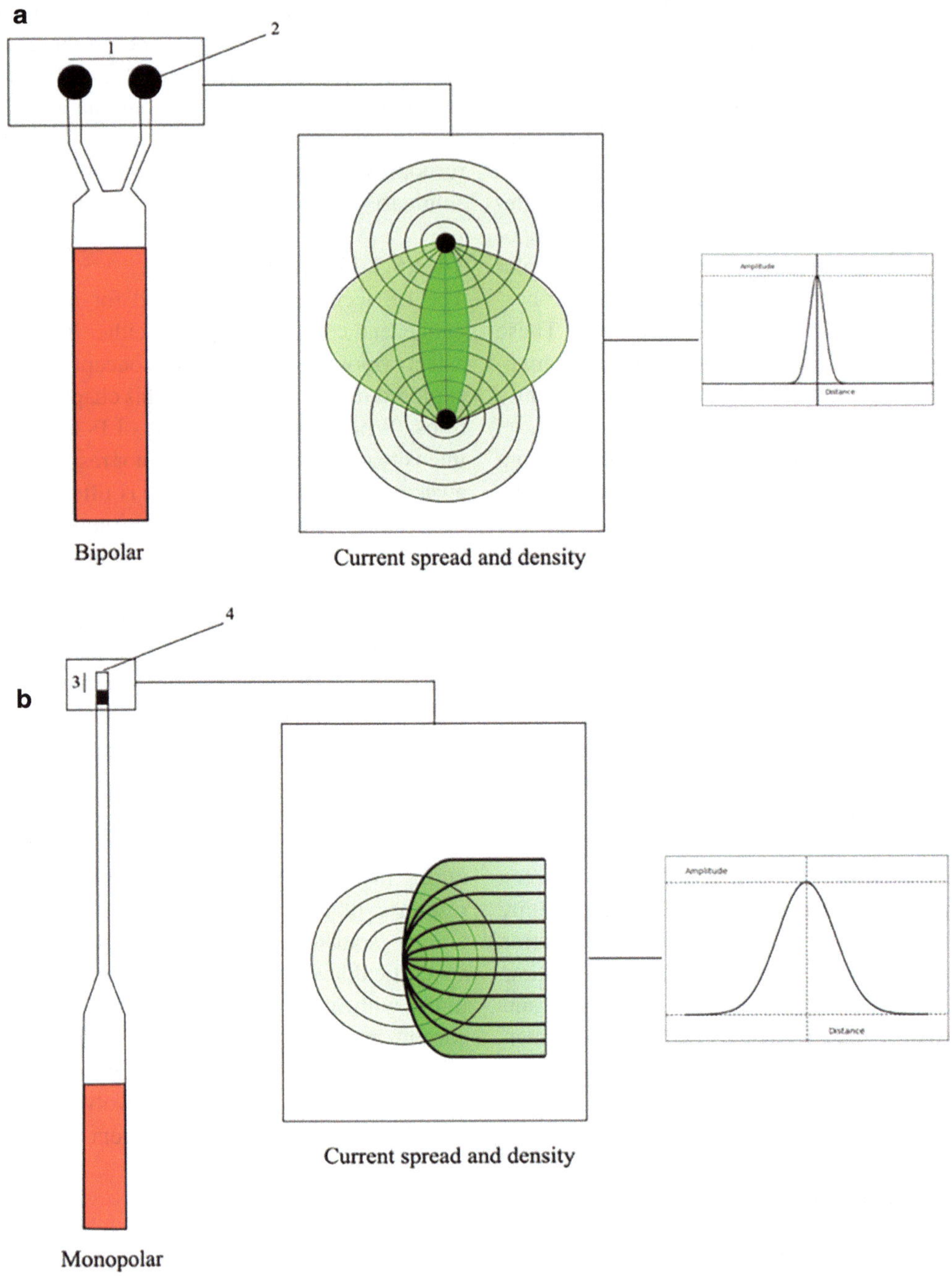

Fig. 14.5 Direct electrical stimulation probes and their characteristics. Stimulation probes. (**a**) Bipolar stimulation probe. (1) Inter-tip distance (average 5–10 mm); (2) tip surface (usually spherical, on average 2 mm diameter, or straight). The central box figure represents the electric field produced using a bipolar probe, with higher current density in the space between the two tips and circumferential spreading around the dipole and each spherical tip. The upper lateral box represents the relation between stimulation amplitude and spatial spreading. (**b**) Monopolar stimulation probe. (3) Active, stimulating probe mounted on a straight or curved handle. The distal segment of the handle close to the tip is usually electrically isolated to avoid unwarranted current spreading when proximal contact with the brain is made during subcortical stimulation. (4) Stimulator tip. The central box depicts the electric field produced when monopolar current is delivered. A weaker electrical field with lower current density is developed radially around the probe, while the highest current is delivered between the probe's tip and the reference electrode, usually placed over the frontal region or in proximity to the motor cortex, according to the use. The lower right box represents the relation between the amplitude of current delivery and its spatial spreading

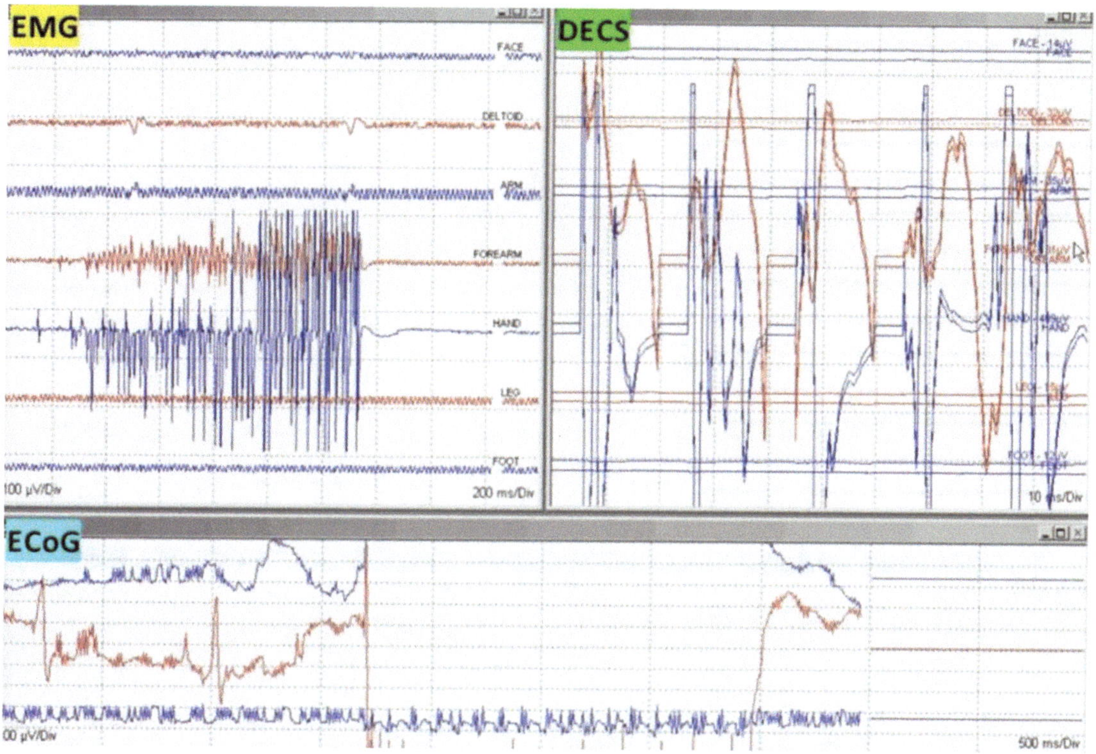

Fig. 14.6 Intraoperative recording of bipolar LF stimulation at the cortical level. Penfield 50 Hz motor mapping evoked responses after bipolar handheld stimulation. Multiple responses are recorded in the forearm and hand muscles. Face: orbicularis oris; deltoid, arm: biceps brachii; forearm: brachioradialis/flexor carpi ulnaris; hand: abductor pollicis brevis/abductor digiti minimi; leg: tibialis anterior; foot: abductor hallucis. *EMG* electromyography, *DECS* Penfield direct electrical cortical stimulation, *ECoG* electrocorticography. (From: Jahangiri FR, Liang M, Kabir SS, Khowash O. Motor mapping of the brain: Taniguchi versus Penfield method. Cureus. 2022 May 11;14(5):e24901. https://doi.org/10.7759/cureus.24901. PMID: 35706721; PMCID: PMC9187213)

and electrocorticography are widely available in several centres [79].

In contrast to the LF technique, HF stimulation elicits a consistent and similar response whether the stimulation site is cortical or subcortical, facilitating the response interpretation. Moreover, real-time MEP analysis can carry out additional information including MEP amplitude, morphology and response latency, other than identifying the muscle recruited (see Fig. 14.7). These data are valuable for a proper interpretation of the evoked responses during cortical and subcortical motor mapping.

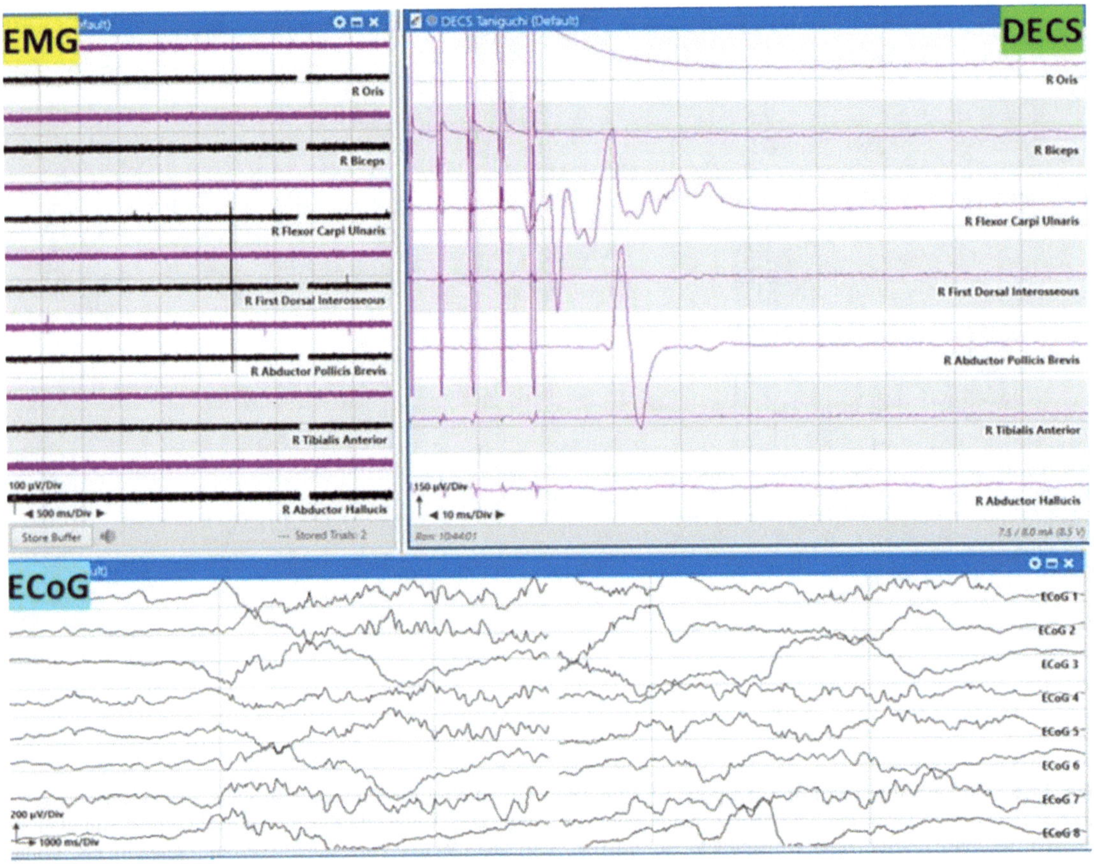

Fig. 14.7 Monopolar HF cortical stimulation record in the forearm (flexor carpi ulnaris) and hand (abductor pollicis brevis) muscles. Oris: orbicularis oris; biceps: biceps brachii; flexor carpi ulnaris, first dorsal interosseous, abductor pollicis brevis, tibialis anterior, and abductor hallucis muscles. *EMG* electromyography, *DECS* Taniguchi direct electrical cortical stimulation, *ECoG* electrocorticography. (From: Jahangiri FR, Liang M, Kabir SS, Khowash O. Motor mapping of the brain: Taniguchi versus Penfield method. Cureus. 2022 May 11;14(5):e24901. https://doi.org/10.7759/cureus.24901. PMID: 35706721; PMCID: PMC9187213)

14.4 Technical Applications and Planning of Brain Mapping Strategies

14.4.1 Motor Mapping

The two paradigms previously described have been widely reported to be effective in eliciting responses in motor cortical areas and subcortical fascicles, with relevant but variable motor function preservation [16, 66, 77, 80, 81]. Independently from the paradigm applied, the first step of motor mapping resides in identifying the motor threshold (MT), which is the lowest current intensity eliciting the lowest reproducible MEP. This threshold provides information about the excitability of the motor cortex and the distance from the stimulated site (particularly at the subcortical level) [16, 71, 77]. Previous findings identified two groups of patients relevant when planning a motor mapping strategy: a "low-risk group," consisting of patients harbouring tumours with limited infiltration of the CST, sharp margins, and no or well-controlled seizures receiving an upfront surgery (no previous irradiation or chemotherapy) and with mild or no preoperative motor deficits; and a "high-risk group," comprehending patients receiving re-operation after other treatments, aedema, CST infiltration, moderate to severe motor deficits preoperatively and long-term uncontrolled seizures [16, 66].

The LF technique—usually delivered through a bipolar probe—is most effective in low-risk patients with a reliable safety profile. However, LF is susceptible to ultrasonic surgical aspirator tools, as the occurrence of false negative responses has been reported [71, 82]. Moreover, LF may still induce intraoperative after-discharge events (range 2–25%) and false negative mapping in some circumstances [83]. False negative mapping should always be suspected when consecutive negative results are obtained in sites (at cortical or subcortical level) where a response was reasonably expected. A common practice is to gradually increase the current in 1–2 mA steps until the limit of 16 mA (asleep) or 8 mA (awake) is reached, confirming the actual "negative mapping."

The use of LF technique in the so-called low-risk patients allowed optimal extent of resection (EOR) rates, above 90% in most series, while in reports on high-risk patients the EOR was less than 50–60%. Moreover, LF motor mapping allowed the identification of positive subcortical sites in more than 40% of stimulation sites, with a risk of postoperative permanent motor deficit in 12% of patients; however, when no true positive site was located subcortically, this risk lowered to less than 3%. Overall, LF can help excite CST fibres only when in very close proximity due to physiological constraints related to the propagation of the current, as previously detailed [84].

The HF paradigm—usually used as a top pulse in combination with a monopolar probe—is highly effective in most patients (both low- and high-risk patients), regardless of preoperative status or anaesthesia regimen; also, so far, no intraoperative tool seems to alter motor current spreading during stimulation. A large body of literature suggests that HF monopolar stimulation is the most efficient technique for reliable M1 stimulation in most excitability conditions and, subcortically, can excite fast-conducting CST fibres with a linear relation between distance and current intensity (with any mA of current required to elicit a subcortical motor response corresponding to an additional millimetre of distance from the CST).

When a subcortical motor site is identified (ex: minimal current intensity required = 10 mA), the resection proceeds with continuous mapping demonstrating a lowering of the threshold required to elicit a motor response until a threshold of 3 mA is reached. This response is interpreted as follows: the initial response corresponds to a 10 mm distance of the probe from the M1-CST fibres; as resection proceeds, additional tumour tissue is resected until the distance from the CST reaches 3 mm, where usually resection is halted to maintain the likelihood of a permanent motor deficit below 2–3%, while the chances of experiencing a temporary motor deficit might be higher and usually resolves within days or weeks.

The recent introduction of ultrasonic aspirators and suction devices mounting a monopolar probe was speculated to be helpful during subcortical resection and mapping, potentially reducing time intervals during resection without active mapping and overall—potentially—reducing surgical duration [83, 85].

Standard HF technique might still fail in some high-risk patients where M1 excitability is altered (i.e., CST or M1 infiltration, oedema, irradiation, etc.). In these tumours, the use of longer pulse trains (7–9 pulses) or longer single pulse width (up to 0.8 ms) provides additional current delivery maintaining the spatial propagation of monopolar stimulation, eliciting cortical, and subcortical motor responses at no expense of additional morbidity, when the standard setup is unsuccessful [65]. Moreover, additional spatial resolution can be obtained using a bipolar probe, especially in tumours growing towards M1 or the SMA [65].

Overall, HF standard paradigm, regardless of the parameter setup, helps achieve EOR > 90%, with a risk of intraoperative seizures or new permanent motor deficits both below 2%, with a negligible false negative rate [16, 65, 86].

However, a different approach is required in tumours within M1, especially when not reaching the cortical surface. Given the advances in intraoperative neurophysiology, these patients once considered inoperable, have recently being offered surgical resection with variable results. The amount of data on LF in these cases is, however, poor, with positive motor cortical and subcortical sites identified in 90% and 73% of cases, respectively, leading to an average gross total resection in half of cases and a 10% chance of permanent motor deficits [16, 66]. LF is mostly useful in awake settings when mapping premotor cortices in tumours invading also M1 as posterior limits of resection. When the tumour is contained within M1 and surrounded by the CST, LF returns multiple cortical positive sites, complicating the identification of an "entry zone." In this scenario, HF provides clearer identification of entry zone and resection boundaries (GTR 73%, morbidity <2%).

For completion, two additional scenarios must be taken into account: high-risk patients and lower grade glioma diffusely infiltrating CST. In the first case, LF and standard HF protocols may fail and return a false negative mapping even at high current intensity. As mentioned before, increasing the number of train spikes to 6–9 or using wider pulses (up to 0.8 ms) may be beneficial. The latter adjustment increases the chances of GTR (>90%) without increasing morbidity [65]. In the second case, positive cortical sites might be identified in most of the explored cortex with a standard technique (HF, To5). By reducing the train to 2–3 pulses, HF allows a discrete mapping of cortical sites with higher (caudal, "new M1") and lower (rostral, "old M1") excitability, providing negative sites in the rostral M1 region as safe entry zone, in accordance with previous studies conducted in primates [65, 66, 87–92]. Similarly, the same approach can be used subcortically once a threshold of 3 mA with an HF To5 is reached to map fast-conducting and highly excitable fibres to be preserved [65].

In these scenarios, an asleep procedure is usually warranted to guarantee a stable cortical excitability and a reliable ongoing evaluation of MEP responses, which might oscillate in awakened patients. This adjustment can enable optimal resection (GTR >88%) without inducing additional permanent deficits (morbidity <2%), despite temporary motor deficits being commonly reported [65, 66].

The aforementioned approach and related modifications cover a large spectrum of possibilities for mapping motor cortical sites and CST fibres to preserve functional integrity. However, in tumours harbouring in the frontal premotor cortex or posterior parietal areas, preoperative global motor performance cannot be preserved entirely just by preserving M1 and its corticofugal fibres. Hand apraxia, which affects the ability to execute refined and tool-oriented motor movements, can severely impact patients' quality of life and, in patients undergoing a standard mapping protocol for tumours within two centimetres from M1, early and 1–3 months postoperative ideomotor apraxia is present in up to 71.1% and 47.4% [93].

Given the interrelation of M1 with non-primary motor areas and an extended frontoparietal subcortical network in planning, performing, and adapting purpose-oriented movements, an awake surgery is required to locate and preserve motor programming and control while the patients perform a reproducible motor task. A continuous and repetitive flexion-extension movement or a more advanced intraoperative test, namely the hand-manipulation-task (hMT), have been proposed [93].

In the latter, the patient performs a rotational movement sequence on a screwdriver-like tool while DES is used to identify relevant cortical (M1, S1, vPM, and dorsal premotor area or dPM and posterior parietal cortex regions or PPC) or subcortical sites (U-fibres, superior longitudinal fasciculus or SLF). Even though the neural correlates related to these mapping strategies are not entirely understood, a potential object-oriented manipulation network—homologue of the lateral grasping network in the monkeys—might be involved and several investigations are still ongoing [92, 94–99]. When this paradigm is applied and tested with bipolar LF technique, the postoperative occurrence of ideomotor apraxia after surgery and 1–3 months reduced dramatically to 28.4% and 8.8%, especially in non-dominant hemispheres. No data is available on the same task mapping with HF technique. However, the following principles reported in the next section might be safely applied accounting for patients' and tumours' characteristics.

Both LF and HF have a role in motor mapping at cortical and subcortical levels, with different applications. However, as previously demonstrated in comparative studies, the effect of the stimulation probe is more pronounced than the frequency applied, with monopolar stimulation being more efficient in activating corticospinal tract fibres than bipolar stimulation. The selection of the appropriate probe and stimulation setting should be tailored to the specific needs of the case, including patient's characteristics, tumour location and features and surgical goal, taking into account that early intraoperative findings might force the surgeon to adjust its mapping paradigm to obtain a complete or maximal safe resection. Advanced adjustments of parameters should be pursued after sufficient experience is gained in standard conditions by the surgical-neurophysiological and anaesthesiologic teams.

It is important also to highlight that subcortical mapping and MEP monitoring work together to enhance the safety of tumour resection. Cortical and subcortical mapping helps prevent direct mechanical or thermal damage to neuronal pathways, but it cannot prevent remote injuries, such as vascular damage from coagulating a perforating artery. Conversely, while MEP monitoring may not prevent mechanical injury—since damage to the corticospinal tract CST may already have occurred by the time MEP changes are detected—it is sensitive to subcortical ischemia.

14.4.2 Mapping of Language and Cognitive Functions

The neuropsychological testing strategy in awake setting is beyond the scope of this chapter and is discussed elsewhere [78, 100, 101]. The bipolar LF technique was the first being introduced by Ojemann to identify cortical language areas, while the monopolar HF paradigm has been more recently refined for cortical (anodal) and subcortical (cathodal) language mapping [45, 102–104]. Despite advancement in the comprehension of cognitive functions and translational findings from clinical neuroscience, there is currently no evidence that mapping cognitive functions requires additional electrophysiological paradigms compared to those used for language functioning, at least in terms of current settings. As such, most leading teams have focused on the selection and combination of neuropsychological tests to be administered, while the stimulation paradigm was directly translated from language mapping studies.

Of interest, recent scientific investigations have focused on stimulation timing during language and cognitive intraoperative testing. Compelling evidence suggests that DES-induced perturbation of network functioning at different stages related to task presentation might unveil different functional impairments and present with different behavioural responses (a pictorial description is available in Fig. 14.8). However, further studies are necessary to support this preliminary data [78, 105]. Although these considerations might change over time, the findings reported in the last part of this chapter relate to the use of DES in awake language mapping and can be cautiously translated to cognitive mapping as well. A detailed approach to cognitive mapping is reported elsewhere [100, 106–109].

Similarly to motor mapping, the first step is to identify the working current for DES, which can be defined with two approaches: the first consists in gradually increasing the current intensity starting from 2 mA on a "potential eloquent site," until a positive site is identified, a limit of 6 mA is reached or after-discharges are identified at the electrocorticography (ECoG); in this last case, the working current is set 1 mA below the current generating after-discharges [110]. The second method consists in stimulating over the ventral premotor (vPM) area increasing the stimulation current until a speech arrest ("anarthria") is elicited, which usually occurs within a 2–6 mA range. It is a good practice to verify the reliability of the working current along the awake procedure as excitability might change after tumour-brain disconnection is started; if so, the stimulation intensity is adjusted to the condition returning anarthria over vPM, accordingly [110]

At the subcortical level, bipolar LF (and monopolar HF stimulation in selected cases) can be used to map the location of the relevant white matter fibres fascicles [ex.: premotor U-fibres, superior longitudinal (SLF I, II, III), arcuate (AF), inferior fronto-occipital (IFOF), and uncinate (UF) fascicles, frontal aslant tract (FAT), fronto-striatal

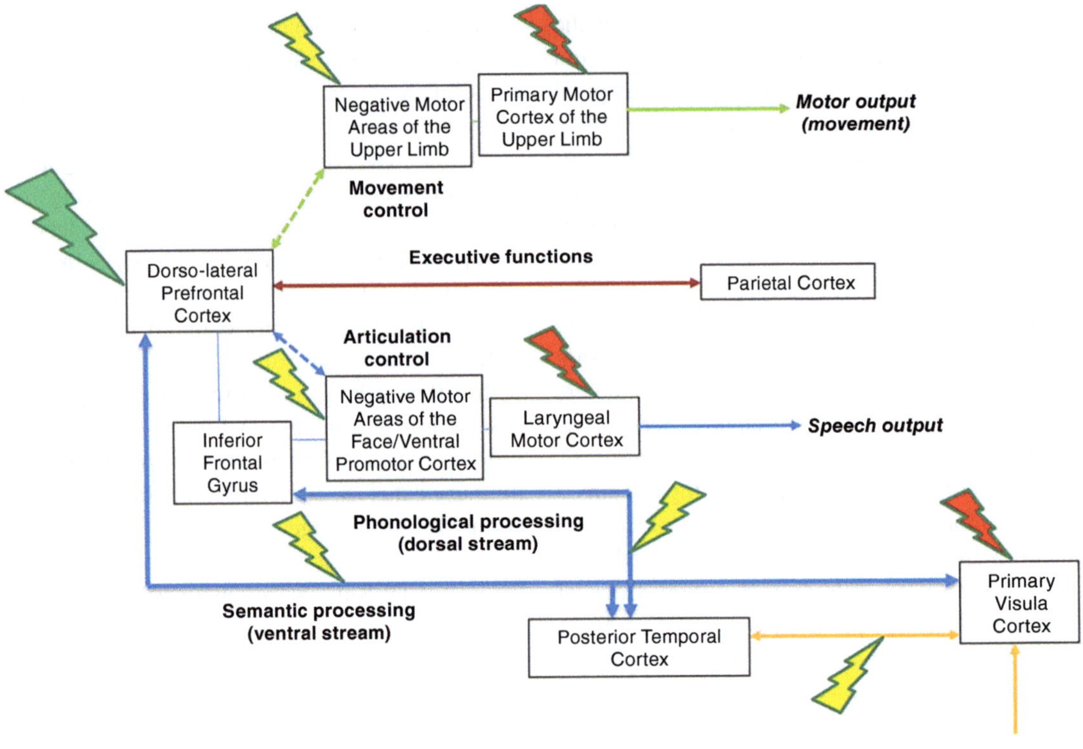

Fig. 14.8 Spatial-time dynamics during DES in awake surgery: Illustration of the three-level model of direct electrostimulation (DES) neural disruption: red lightning bolt symbolises the first level (input/output disruption), yellow lightning bolt symbolises the second level (within-network disruption) and green lightning bolt symbolises the third level (inter-network disruption). This is a schematic representation of the visual system (lower, connectivity in yellow), speech and language system (lower, connectivity in blue), executive functions system (middle, connectivity in brown) and motor system (upper, connectivity in green) in the left hemisphere of an awake patient who performs a dual-task associating picture naming and movement of the right upper limb. DES of the primary visual system induces phosphenes (first level, a red lightning bolt at the level of the optic tracts and/or primary visual cortex), while DES of the occipito-temporal connections induces visual hemiagnosia [second level, a yellow lightning bolt over the posterior inferior longitudinal fasciculus (ILF)]. In parallel, the patient can continue to move the right upper limb. In the speech and language system, DES of the laryngeal motor cortex elicits involuntary vocalisation (first level, red lightning); DES of the ventral premotor cortex and frontoparietal articulatory loop (not shown) elicits speech apraxia/arrest (anarthria); while DES of the dorsal phonological route induces phonemic paraphasia and DES of the ventral semantic route induces semantic paraphasia (second level, red lightning). Of note, stimulating both dorsal and semantic streams may generate complete anomia. In parallel, the patient can continue to move the right upper limb. In the motor system, DES of the primary motor cortex of the upper limb and its corticospinal tracts (motor execution, output) causes an involuntary movement (first level, red lightning); DES of the negative motor cortex (movement control) and its fibres (not shown) generates an arrest of movement (second level, yellow lightning). In parallel, the patient can continue to perform the picture naming task. During DES of the dorsolateral prefrontal cortex (integrative hub), the brain is not able to coordinate its networks (including the frontoparietal connections involved in the executive functions and then the goal maintenance), the patient cannot achieve dual-task anymore: the patient is only capable to perform each task separately, naming or upper limb movement, but not both simultaneously (third level, green lightning). (From: https://doi.org/10.3389/fnhum.2020.00315)

fibres, optic radiation (OR), cingulate fasciculus (CF) among others]. A detailed description of the language testing and anatomo-functional correlates are described elsewhere [78, 100, 111–113].

Although we do not have a technique to precisely estimate the distance from the anatomical structure involved (subcortically), these paradigms allow the elicitation of an "on"/"off" response in most sites, and an intensity-dependent "graded" response has also been reported in a minority of studies [114]. For example, it is known that stimulation current affects language task performance at the cortical level: one study found that at a lower intensity (4 mA), positive naming interference is elicited while increasing the intensity, the type of error changed, and ultimately, speech arrest was obtained [114]. Similarly, the number of positive sites increased by increasing the current intensity. Differences in cortical responses at different sites (frontal, temporal, parietal) when current intensity, duration, or frequency is modified have been poorly investigated. There is also a lack of studies on the relationship between stimulation timing and behavioural effects. With a standard bipolar LF technique, the current is usually applied 1–2 s before task presentation over potentially eloquent areas in the frontal and temporal lobes presenting naming tasks. However, it has been suggested that prolonging the stimulation duration during task presentation and response could elicit a different behavioural response or sensitivity in finding positive sites overall. Potentially, disruption of the tested network through DES might be affected directly by spatio-temporal parameters of stimulation [105]. This concept was also hypothesised for cognitive tasks [12].

14.5 Cortico-Cortical Evoked Potentials (CCEP) for Monitoring Language Function

A detailed description of this technique is beyond the scope of this chapter; however, a brief overview is due. In a recent study, CCEPs were evoked in 95% of attempts and patients later experiencing aphasia after surgery showed delayed N1 and N2 latencies after tumour resection, suggesting that CCEPs might provide an indirect marker for arcuate fasciculus integrity (or at least the dorsal language stream at some extent), or other involved tracts. Preliminary evidence from a few centres suggests that real-time continuous monitoring of CCEPs is feasible (a pictorial representation of CCEP recording is available in Fig. 14.9). However, additional investigations are warranted as additional data from larger cohorts are mandatory to identify potential warning criteria for clinical use.

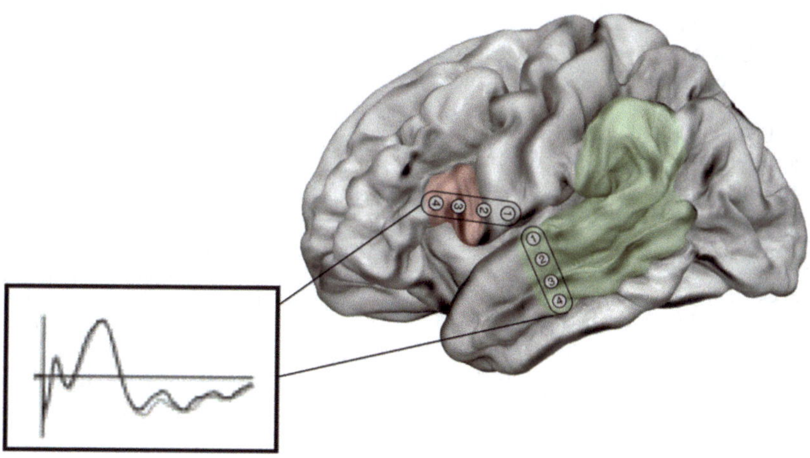

Fig. 14.9 Intraoperative cortico-cortical evoked potential (CCEP) monitoring. "Broca's" motor speech hub is depicted in red. "Wernicke"'s temporoparietal language hub is displayed in green and comprehends regions investigated for CCEP recording in previous studies. The lower left box reports a pictorial representation of a CCEP through bipolar stimulation and recording using a set of two 4-electrodes grids

References

1. Duffau H. Stimulation mapping of white matter tracts to study brain functional connectivity. Nat Rev Neurol. 2015;11:255–65.
2. Herbet G, Maheu M, Costi E, Lafargue G, Duffau H. Mapping neuroplastic potential in brain-damaged patients. Brain. 2016;139:829–44.
3. Sala F, Lanteri P. Brain surgery in motor areas: the invaluable assistance of intraoperative neurophysiological monitoring. J Neurosurg Sci. 2003;47:79–88.
4. Lacroix M, Abi-Said D, Fourney DR, et al. A multivariate analysis of 416 patients with glioblastoma multiforme: prognosis, extent of resection, and survival. J Neurosurg. 2001;95:190–8.
5. Sanai N, Polley M-Y, McDermott MW, Parsa AT, Berger MS. An extent of resection threshold for newly diagnosed glioblastomas. J Neurosurg. 2011;115:3–8.
6. Leyton ASF, Sherrington CS. Observations on the excitable cortex of the chimpanzee, orang-UTAN, and gorilla. Q J Exp Physiol. 1917;11:135–222.
7. Berker EA. Translation of Broca's 1865 report. Arch Neurol. 1986;43:1065.
8. Penfield W, Boldrey E. Somatic motor and sensory representation in the cerebral cortex of man as studied by electrical stimulation. Brain. 1937;60:389–443.
9. Catani M. From hodology to function. Brain. 2007;130:602–5.
10. Duffau H. Functional recovery after surgical resection of low grade gliomas in eloquent brain: hypothesis of brain compensation. J Neurol Neurosurg Psychiatry. 2003;74:901–7.
11. De Benedictis A, Duffau H. Brain hodotopy: from esoteric concept to practical surgical applications. Neurosurgery. 2011;68:1709–23.
12. Herbet G, Duffau H. Revisiting the functional anatomy of the human brain: toward a meta-networking theory of cerebral functions. Physiol Rev. 2020;100:1181–228.
13. Brem S. GLIOMA-06 the GLIOMA CONNECTOME project—update. Neuro-Oncology Adv. 2023;5:iv2.
14. Suero Molina E, Tait MJ, Di Ieva A. Connectomics as a prognostic tool of functional outcome in glioma surgery of the supplementary motor area: illustrative case. J Neurosurg Case Lessons. 2023;6(6):CASE23286. https://doi.org/10.3171/CASE23286.
15. Seidel K, Beck J, Stieglitz L, Schucht P, Raabe A. The warning-sign hierarchy between quantitative subcortical motor mapping and continuous motor evoked potential monitoring during resection of supratentorial brain tumors. J Neurosurg. 2013;118:287–96.
16. Bello L, Riva M, Fava E, Ferpozzi V, Castellano A, Raneri F, Pessina F, Bizzi A, Falini A, Cerri G. Tailoring neurophysiological strategies with clinical context enhances resection and safety and expands indications in gliomas involving motor pathways. Neuro-Oncology. 2014;16:1110–28.
17. Nossek E, Korn A, Shahar T, et al. Intraoperative mapping and monitoring of the corticospinal tracts with neurophysiological assessment and 3-dimensional ultrasonography-based navigation. Clinical article. J Neurosurg. 2011;114:738–46.
18. Legatt AD, Emerson RG, Epstein CM, MacDonald DB, Deletis V, Bravo RJ, López JR. ACNS guideline: transcranial electrical stimulation motor evoked potential monitoring. J Clin Neurophysiol. 2016;33:42–50.
19. Buhl LK, Bastos AB, Pollard RJ, Arle JE, Thomas GP, Song Y, Boone MD. Neurophysiologic intraoperative monitoring for spine surgery: a practical guide from past to present. J Intensive Care Med. 2021;36:1237–49.
20. Macdonald DB, Skinner S, Shils J, Yingling C, American Society of Neurophysiological Monitoring. Intraoperative motor evoked potential monitoring—a position statement by the American Society of Neurophysiological Monitoring. Clin Neurophysiol. 2013;124:2291–316.
21. Deletis V. Intraoperative neurophysiology and methodologies used to monitor the functional integrity of the motor system. In: Deletis V, Shils JL, editors. Neurophysiology in neurosurgery: a modern intraoperative approach. Elsevier; 2020. p. 17–34.
22. Bir M, Gupta U, Jaryal AK, Singh A, Netam R, Kale SS, Chandra SP, Singh M, Rath GP. Predictive value of intraoperative D-wave and m-MEP neurophysiological monitoring in patients with preoperative motor deficits in immediate and late postoperative period. J Craniovertebral Junction Spine. 2021;12:26–32.
23. Kizilay A, Aladag I, Cokkeser Y, Miman MC, Ozturan O, Gulhas N. Effects of partial neuromuscular blockade on facial nerve monitorization in otologic surgery. Acta Otolaryngol. 2003;123:321–4.
24. Lennon RL, Hosking MP, Daube JR, Welna JO. Effect of partial neuromuscular blockade on intraoperative electromyography in patients undergoing resection of acoustic neuromas. Anesth Analg. 1992;75:729–33.
25. Duffau H. Intraoperative neurophysiology during surgery for cerebral tumor. Handb Clin Neurophysiol. 2008;8:491–507.
26. Asimakidou E, Abut PA, Raabe A, Seidel K. Motor evoked potential warning criteria in supratentorial surgery: a scoping review. Cancers (Basel). 2021;13(11):2803. https://doi.org/10.3390/cancers13112803.
27. Garcés-Ambrossi GL, McGirt MJ, Mehta VA, Sciubba DM, Witham TF, Bydon A, Wolinksy J-P, Jallo GI, Gokaslan ZL. Factors associated with progression-free survival and long-term neurological outcome after resection of intramedullary spinal cord tumors: analysis of 101 consecutive cases. J Neurosurg Spine. 2009;11:591–9.

28. Cruccu G, Aminoff MJ, Curio G, Guerit JM, Kakigi R, Mauguiere F, Rossini PM, Treede R-D, Garcia-Larrea L. Recommendations for the clinical use of somatosensory-evoked potentials. Clin Neurophysiol. 2008;119:1705–19.
29. Hu Y, Liu H, Luk KD. Time-frequency analysis of somatosensory evoked potentials for intraoperative spinal cord monitoring. J Clin Neurophysiol. 2011;28:504–11.
30. Emerson RG, Seyal M, Pedley TA. Somatosensory evoked potentials following median nerve stimulation. I. The cervical components. Brain. 1984;107(Pt 1):169–82.
31. Seyal M, Gabor AJ. Generators of human spinal somatosensory evoked potentials. J Clin Neurophysiol. 1987;4:177–87.
32. MacDonald DB. Monitoring somatosensory evoked potentials. In: Deletis V, Shils JL, Sala F, Seidel K, editors. Neurophysiology in neurosurgery : a modern approach. 2nd ed. London: Elsevier, Academic Press; 2020. p. 35–51.
33. Holdefer RN, MacDonald DB, Skinner SA. Somatosensory and motor evoked potentials as biomarkers for post-operative neurological status. Clin Neurophysiol. 2015;126:857–65.
34. Cedzich C, Taniguchi M, Schäfer S, Schramm J. Somatosensory evoked potential phase reversal and direct motor cortex stimulation during surgery in and around the central region. Neurosurgery. 1996;38:962–70.
35. Romstöck J, Fahlbusch R, Ganslandt O, Nimsky C, Strauss C. Localisation of the sensorimotor cortex during surgery for brain tumours: feasibility and waveform patterns of somatosensory evoked potentials. J Neurol Neurosurg Psychiatry. 2002;72:221–9.
36. American Clinical Neurophysiology Society. Guideline 11B. Recommended standards for intraoperative monitoring of somatosensory evoked potentials. Milwaukee: ACNS; 2009.
37. Rajkalyan C, Tewari A, Rao S, Avitsian R. Anesthetic considerations for stereotactic electroencephalography implantation. J Anaesthesiol Clin Pharmacol. 2019;35:434–40.
38. Sun Y, Wei C, Cui V, Xiu M, Wu A. Electroencephalography: clinical applications during the perioperative period. Front Med. 2020;7:251.
39. Kothari R, Bokariya P, Singh S, Singh R. A comprehensive review on methodologies employed for visual evoked potentials. Scientifica (Cairo). 2016;2016:1–9.
40. Soumpasis C, Díaz-Baamonde A, Ghimire P, et al. Intraoperative neuromonitoring of the visual pathway in asleep neuro-oncology surgery. Cancers (Basel). 2023;15:3943.
41. Duffau H, Velut S, Mitchell M-C, Gatignol P, Capelle L. Intra-operative mapping of the subcortical visual pathways using direct electrical stimulations. Acta Neurochir (Wien). 2004;146:265–70.
42. Gummi R, Cho C, Le S, Lee L, Nguyen V, Tippur A, Buch V, Lopez J, Chang F. Direct subcortical stimulation for intraoperative mapping of optic radiations (P1-11.009). Neurology. 2024;102(17_supplement_1):3406. https://doi.org/10.1212/WNL.0000000000205118.
43. Gras-Combe G, Moritz-Gasser S, Herbet G, Duffau H. Intraoperative subcortical electrical mapping of optic radiations in awake surgery for glioma involving visual pathways. J Neurosurg. 2012;117:466–73.
44. Shahar T, Korn A, Barkay G, Biron T, Hadanny A, Gazit T, Nossek E, Ekstein M, Kesler A, Ram Z. Elaborate mapping of the posterior visual pathway in awake craniotomy. J Neurosurg. 2018;128:1503–11.
45. Ojemann GA, Whitaker HA. Language localization and variability. Brain Lang. 1978;6:239–60.
46. Berger MS. Functional mapping-guided resection of low-grade gliomas. Clin Neurosurg. 1995;42:437–52.
47. Bello L, Gambini A, Castellano A, et al. Motor and language DTI fiber tracking combined with intraoperative subcortical mapping for surgical removal of gliomas. NeuroImage. 2008;39:369–82.
48. Bello L, Gallucci M, Fava M, et al. Intraoperative subcortical language tract mapping guides surgical removal of gliomas involving speech areas. Neurosurgery. 2007;60:67–82.
49. Yamaguchi F, Takahashi H, Teramoto A. Navigation-assisted subcortical mapping: intraoperative motor tract detection by bipolar needle electrode in combination with neuronavigation system. J Neuro-Oncol. 2009;93:121–5.
50. Foerster O, Penfield W. The structural basis of traumatic epilepsy and results of radical operation. Brain. 1930;53:99–119.
51. Leroux PD, Berger MS, Haglund MM, Pilcher WH, Ojemann GA. Resection of intrinsic tumors from nondominant face motor cortex using stimulation mapping: report of two cases. Surg Neurol. 1991;36:44–8.
52. Taniguchi M, Cedzich C, Taniguchi M, Cedzich C, Schramm J. Modification of cortical stimulation for motor evoked potentials under general Anesthesia. Neurosurgery. 1993;32:219–26.
53. Deletis V. Intraoperative neurophysiology and methodologies used to monitor the functional integrity of the motor system. In: Deletis V, Shils JL, Sala F, Seidel K, editors. Neurophysiology in neurosurgery : a modern approach. London: Elsevier, Academic Press; 2002. p. 25–51.
54. Deletis V, Camargo AB. Transcranial electrical motor evoked potential monitoring for brain tumor resection. Neurosurgery. 2001;49:1488–9.
55. Deletis V, Isgum V, Amassian VE. Neurophysiological mechanisms underlying motor evoked potentials in anesthetized humans. Clin Neurophysiol. 2001;112:438–44.

56. Kombos T, Suess O, Kern B-C, Funk T, Hoell T, Kopetsch O, Brock M. Comparison between Monopolar and bipolar electrical stimulation of the motor cortex. Acta Neurochir. 1999;141:1295–301.
57. Duffau H, Capelle L, Denvil D, et al. Usefulness of intraoperative electrical subcortical mapping during surgery for low-grade gliomas located within eloquent brain regions: functional results in a consecutive series of 103 patients. J Neurosurg. 2003;98:764–78.
58. Carlson C, Devinsky O. The excitable cerebral cortex. Epilepsy Behav. 2009;15:131–2.
59. Gordon B, Lesser RP, Rance NE, Hart J, Webber R, Uematsu S, Fisher RS. Parameters for direct cortical electrical stimulation in the human: histopathologic confirmation. Electroencephalogr Clin Neurophysiol. 1990;75:371–7.
60. Hern JEC, Landgren S, Phillips CG, Porter R. Selective excitation of corticofugal neurones by surface-anodal stimulation of the baboon's motor cortex. J Physiol. 1962;161:73–90.
61. Patton HD, Amassian VE. Single- and multiple-unit analysis of cortical stage of pyramidal tract activation. J Neurophysiol. 1954;17:345–63.
62. Lorente de No R. A study of nerve physiology. Stud Rockefeller Inst Med Res Repr. 1947;132:1–548.
63. Rudin DO, Eisenman G. The action potential of spinal axons in vitro. J Gen Physiol. 1954;37:505–38.
64. Dreyer SJ, Dumitru D, King JC. Anodal block v anodal stimulation. Am J Phys Med Rehabil. 1993;72:10–8.
65. Rossi M, Conti Nibali M, Viganò L, et al. Resection of tumors within the primary motor cortex using high-frequency stimulation: oncological and functional efficiency of this versatile approach based on clinical conditions. J Neurosurg. 2020;133:642–54.
66. Rossi M, Sciortino T, Conti Nibali M, et al. Clinical pearls and methods for intraoperative motor mapping. Neurosurgery. 2021;88:457–67.
67. Pudenz RH, Bullara LA, Jacques S, Hambrecht FT. Electrical stimulation of the brain. III. The neural damage model. Surg Neurol. 1975;4:389–400.
68. Agnew WF, Yuen TG, Pudenz RH, Bullara LA. Electrical stimulation of the brain. IV. Ultrastructural studies. Surg Neurol. 1975;4:438–48.
69. Merrill DR, Bikson M, Jefferys JGR. Electrical stimulation of excitable tissue: design of efficacious and safe protocols. J Neurosci Methods. 2005;141:171–98.
70. Pudenz RH, Bullara LA, Talalla A. Electrical stimulation of the brain. I. Electrodes and electrode arrays. Surg Neurol. 1975;4:37–42.
71. Szelényi A, Bello L, Duffau H, Fava E, Feigl GC, Galanda M, Neuloh G, Signorelli F, Sala F. Intraoperative electrical stimulation in awake craniotomy: methodological aspects of current practice. Neurosurg Focus. 2010;28:E7.
72. Agnew WF, McCreery DB. Considerations for safety in the use of extracranial stimulation for motor evoked potentials. Neurosurgery. 1987;20:143–7.
73. Kombos T, Süss O. Neurophysiological basis of direct cortical stimulation and applied neuroanatomy of the motor cortex: a review. Neurosurg Focus. 2009;27:E3.
74. Katayama Y, Tsubokawa T, Maejima S, Hirayama T, Yamamoto T. Corticospinal direct response in humans: identification of the motor cortex during intracranial surgery under general anaesthesia. J Neurol Neurosurg Psychiatry. 1988;51:50–9.
75. Nathan SS, Sinha SR, Gordon B, Lesser RP, Thakor NV. Determination of current density distributions generated by electrical stimulation of the human cerebral cortex. Electroencephalogr Clin Neurophysiol. 1993;86:183–92.
76. Phillips CG, Porter R. Unifocal and bifocal stimulation of the motor cortex. J Physiol. 1962;162:532–8.
77. Szelényi A, Senft C, Jardan M, Forster MT, Franz K, Seifert V, Vatter H. Intra-operative subcortical electrical stimulation: a comparison of two methods. Clin Neurophysiol. 2011;122:1470–5.
78. Morshed RA, Young JS, Lee AT, Berger MS, Hervey-Jumper SL. Clinical pearls and methods for intraoperative awake language mapping. Neurosurgery. 2021;89:143–53.
79. Bello L, Fava E, Carrabba G, Bertani G. Combined use of DES, EMG and MEP monitoring, ECoG and EEG for surgical resection of gliomas. Eur Neurol Rev. 2008;3:70.
80. Hervey-Jumper SL, Berger MS. Maximizing safe resection of low- and high-grade glioma. J Neuro-Oncol. 2016;130:269–82.
81. Duffau H, Mandonnet E. The "onco-functional balance" in surgery for diffuse low-grade glioma: integrating the extent of resection with quality of life. Acta Neurochir. 2013;155:951–7.
82. Carrabba G, Mandonnet E, Fava E, Capelle L, Gaini SM, Duffau H, Bello L. Transient inhibition of motor function induced by the cavitron ultrasonic surgical aspirator during brain mapping. Neurosurgery. 2008;63:E178–9.
83. Han SJ, Morshed RA, Troncon I, Jordan KM, Henry RG, Hervey-Jumper SL, Berger MS. Subcortical stimulation mapping of descending motor pathways for perirolandic gliomas: assessment of morbidity and functional outcome in 702 cases. J Neurosurg. 2019;131:201–8.
84. Shiban E, Krieg SM, Haller B, Buchmann N, Obermueller T, Boeckh-Behrens T, Wostrack M, Meyer B, Ringel F. Intraoperative subcortical motor evoked potential stimulation: how close is the corticospinal tract? J Neurosurg. 2015;123:711–20.
85. Schucht P, Seidel K, Jilch A, Beck J, Raabe A. A review of monopolar motor mapping and a comprehensive guide to continuous dynamic motor mapping for resection of motor eloquent brain tumors. Neurochirurgie. 2017;63:175–80.

86. Magill ST, Han SJ, Li J, Berger MS. Resection of primary motor cortex tumors: feasibility and surgical outcomes. J Neurosurg. 2018;129:961–72.
87. Viganò L, Fornia L, Rossi M, et al. Anatomo-functional characterisation of the human "hand-knob": a direct electrophysiological study. Cortex. 2019;113:239–54.
88. Rossi M, Puglisi G, Conti Nibali M, Viganò L, Sciortino T, Gay L, Leonetti A, Zito P, Riva M, Bello L. Asleep or awake motor mapping for resection of perirolandic glioma in the nondominant hemisphere? Development and validation of a multimodal score to tailor the surgical strategy. J Neurosurg. 2022;136:16–29.
89. Rathelot J-A, Strick PL. Subdivisions of primary motor cortex based on cortico-motoneuronal cells. Proc Natl Acad Sci. 2009;106:918–23.
90. Menz VK, Schaffelhofer S, Scherberger H. Representation of continuous hand and arm movements in macaque areas M1, F5, and AIP: a comparative decoding study. J Neural Eng. 2015;12(5):056016. https://doi.org/10.1088/1741-2560/12/5/056016. LK—https://unimi.primo.exlibrisgroup.com/openurl/39UMI_INST/39UMI_INST:VU1?sid=EMBASE&issn=17412552&id=doi:10.1088%2F1741-2560%2F12%2F5%2F056016&atitle=Representation+of+continuous+hand+and+arm+movements+in+macaque+areas+M1%2C+F5%2C+and+AIP%3A+A+comparative+decoding+study&stitle=J.+Neural+Eng.&title=Journal+of+Neural+Engineering&volume=12&issue=5&spage=&epage=&aulast=Menz&aufirst=Veera+Katharina&auinit=V.K.&aufull=Menz+V.K.&coden=&isbn=&pages=-&date=2015&auinit1=
91. Battaglia-Mayer A, Babicola L, Satta E. Parieto-frontal gradients and domains underlying eye and hand operations in the action space. Neuroscience. 2016;334:76–92.
92. Tariciotti L, Mattioli L, Viganò L, et al. Object-oriented hand dexterity and grasping abilities, from the animal quarters to the neurosurgical OR: a systematic review of the underlying neural correlates in non-human, human primate and recent findings in awake brain surgery. Front Integr Neurosci. 2024;18:1324581. https://doi.org/10.3389/fnint.2024.1324581.
93. Rossi M, Fornia L, Puglisi G, et al. Assessment of the praxis circuit in glioma surgery to reduce the incidence of postoperative and long-term apraxia: a new intraoperative test. J Neurosurg. 2018;130:17–27.
94. Fornia L, Rossi M, Rabuffetti M, et al. Direct electrical stimulation of premotor areas: different effects on hand muscle activity during object manipulation. Cereb Cortex. 2020;30:391–405.
95. Fornia L, Rossi M, Rabuffetti M, et al. Motor impairment evoked by direct electrical stimulation of human parietal cortex during object manipulation. NeuroImage. 2022;248:118839.
96. Viganò L, Howells H, Rossi M, et al. Stimulation of frontal pathways disrupts hand muscle control during object manipulation. Brain. 2022;145:1535–50.
97. Fornia L, Ferpozzi V, Montagna M, et al. Functional characterization of the left Ventrolateral premotor cortex in humans: a direct electrophysiological approach. Cereb Cortex. 2018;28:167–83.
98. Fornia L, Leonetti A, Puglisi G, Rossi M, Viganò L, Della Santa B, Simone L, Bello L, Cerri G. The parietal architecture binding cognition to sensorimotor integration: a multimodal causal study. Brain. 2023;147(1):297–310. https://doi.org/10.1093/brain/awad316.
99. Fornia L, Puglisi G, Leonetti A, Bello L, Berti A, Cerri G, Garbarini F. Direct electrical stimulation of the premotor cortex shuts down awareness of voluntary actions. Nat Commun. 2020;11:705.
100. Rossi M, Nibali MC, Torregrossa F, Bello L, Grasso G. Innovation in neurosurgery: the concept of cognitive mapping. World Neurosurg. 2019;131:364–70.
101. Lemaitre A-L, Herbet G, Ng S, Moritz-Gasser S, Duffau H. Cognitive preservation following awake mapping-based neurosurgery for low-grade gliomas: a longitudinal, within-patient design study. Neuro-Oncology. 2022;24:781–93.
102. Ojemann G. Cortical organization of language. J Neurosci. 1991;11:2281–7.
103. Verst SM, de Aguiar PHP, Joaquim MAS, Vieira VG, Sucena ABC, Maldaun MVC. Monopolar 250–500 Hz language mapping: results of 41 patients. Clin Neurophysiol Pract. 2019;4:1–8.
104. Riva M, Fava E, Gallucci M, Comi A, Casarotti A, Alfiero T, Raneri FA, Pessina F, Bello L. Monopolar high-frequency language mapping: can it help in the surgical management of gliomas? A comparative clinical study. J Neurosurg. 2016;124:1479–89.
105. Nakai Y, Sugiura A, Brown EC, Sonoda M, Jeong J, Rothermel R, Luat AF, Sood S, Asano E. Four-dimensional functional cortical maps of visual and auditory language: intracranial recording. Epilepsia. 2019;60:255–67.
106. Bu L, Lu J, Zhang J, Wu J. Intraoperative cognitive mapping tasks for direct electrical stimulation in clinical and neuroscientific contexts. Front Hum Neurosci. 2021;15:612891. https://doi.org/10.3389/fnhum.2021.612891.
107. Prat-Acín R, Galeano-Senabre I, López-Ruiz P, Ayuso-Sacido A, Espert-Tortajada R. Intraoperative brain mapping of language, cognitive functions, and social cognition in awake surgery of low-grade gliomas located in the right non-dominant hemisphere. Clin Neurol Neurosurg. 2021;200:106363.
108. Ng S, Herbet G, Lemaitre A-L, Moritz-Gasser S, Duffau H. Disrupting self-evaluative processing with electrostimulation mapping during awake brain surgery. Sci Rep. 2021;11:9386.
109. Moritz-Gasser S, Herbet G, Duffau H. Mapping the connectivity underlying multimodal (verbal

and non-verbal) semantic processing: a brain electrostimulation study. Neuropsychologia. 2013;51:1814–22.
110. Hervey-Jumper SL, Li J, Lau D, Molinaro AM, Perry DW, Meng L, Berger MS. Awake craniotomy to maximize glioma resection: methods and technical nuances over a 27-year period. J Neurosurg. 2015;123:325–39.
111. Martín-Monzón I, Rivero Ballagas Y, Arias-Sánchez S. Language mapping: a systematic review of protocols that evaluate linguistic functions in awake surgery. Appl Neuropsychol Adult. 2022;29:845–54.
112. Landers MJF, Sitskoorn MM, Rutten G-JM, Mandonnet E, De Baene W. A systematic review of the use of subcortical intraoperative electrical stimulation mapping for monitoring of executive deficits and neglect: what is the evidence so far? Acta Neurochir. 2022;164:177–91.
113. Martín-Monzón I, Amores-Carrera L, Sabsevitz D, Herbet G. Intraoperative mapping of the right hemisphere: a systematic review of protocols that evaluate cognitive and social cognitive functions. Front Psychol. 2024;15:1415523. https://doi.org/10.3389/fpsyg.2024.1415523.
114. Roux F-E, Durand J-B, Djidjeli I, Moyse E, Giussani C. Variability of intraoperative electrostimulation parameters in conscious individuals: language cortex. J Neurosurg. 2017;126:1641–52.

15 Advancements in Awake Glioma Surgery

Alessandro Pesce, Giuseppe Dimichele, Federica Novegno, Daniele Armocida, Alessandro Frati, and Maurizio Salvati

15.1 History of Awake Craniotomy

The term "awake craniotomy" refers to neurosurgical procedures that are performed while the patient is conscious to preserve specific functions (such as movement, vision, speech, writing, etc.) during neurosurgical interventions. These procedures are usually performed with the help of electrophysiological brain stimulation techniques [1].

The conception of "awake surgery" is anything but new; indeed, 12,000 years ago, the Kisii tribe in the southwest of Kenya was already performing neurosurgery procedures under awake conditions, to prevent or alleviate headaches following head trauma. About 1 per 1000 people had these procedures each year, and they entailed the removal of a portion of the skull close to the site of injury. The operations, which used crude instruments and took around 45 min on average, were performed without anesthesia. The operations were well regarded and appeared to have few consequences despite the absence of modern medical resources [2].

According to ancient archeological documents, prior to the development of general anesthesia, awake skull trephinations were effectively performed: 55% of the 214 individuals whose skulls were found in Peru, probably dating back to 2000 years ago, had fully healed. It has been suggested that coca leaves might have made trephination possible following cocaine-induced local anesthesia [3].

Early in the seventeenth century, awake craniotomy was first recorded in "modern" times for the treatment of epilepsy [4]. The poor results of trepanation prompted scientists and physicians to look inside the brain to determine the cause of seizures. Hughlings Jackson's extensive research on focal epilepsy between 1864 and 1870 made him predict that isolated movements would originate from a particular region in the cerebral cortex [5, 6]. This prediction was verified in 1870 when Fritsch and Hitzig were the first people to record the successful induction of limb movements in animals by electrical stimulation of the cerebral cortex [6, 7].

A. Pesce (✉) · F. Novegno
Neurosurgery Division, Department of System Medicine, University of Rome "Tor Vergata", Rome, Italy
e-mail: ale_pesce83@yahoo.it

G. Dimichele
School of Medicine—University of Rome Campus Bio-Medico, Rome, Italy

D. Armocida
Neurosurgery Unit, Dept. Neuroscience "Rita Levi Montalcini", Università degli studi di Torino, Torino, TO, Italy

A. Frati
IRCCS "Neuromed", Pozzilli, IS, Italy

Neurosurgery Division, Human Neurosciences Department, IRCCS "Neuromed", Pozzilli, IS, Italy

M. Salvati
Neurosurgery Unit, University di Roma "Tor Vergata", Rome, Italy

D. Armocida et al. (eds.), *Neurosurgery's Frontline Role in Gliomas Treatment*,
https://doi.org/10.1007/978-3-031-81850-9_15

Bartholow was the first to create the concept of using electrical stimulation to map the human brain in 1874. Using an electrode, he took advantage of a defect in the skull brought on by an epithelioma's invasion to activate the cerebral cortex [6, 8].

In 1886, Hughlings Jackson and his colleague Victor Horsley, whose research on animals had given him an in-depth comprehension of the human cortex, applied electrical stimulation to identify the thumb area and made the decision to remove it since it was the cause of the seizure [6, 9].

In that moment, Jackson demonstrated that in focal seizures, there was a correlation between the seizure and a specific area of the cerebral cortex. This meant that the abnormal electrical activity that triggered the seizure originated from and was localized within a particular region of the brain's cortex. The symptoms experienced during a focal seizure were likely to depend on the function of the specific area affected by the abnormal electrical activity. Electrical stimulation to locate the motor cortex and seizure foci gained a lot of popularity after that.

Attempting to treat individuals with uncontrollable seizures in the late 1920s was Wilder Penfield [6]. To map the brain, he also used a small amount of electric current. He was aware that patients had auras, which are precursors to epileptic seizures and serve as warning signs. He reasoned that by applying a small amount of electric current to the brain to cause this aura, he could find the source of the seizure activity and possibly even damage or remove the affected tissue. During craniotomy, the patients were fully awake, so they could communicate to the surgeon motor and sensory alterations, and the presence of aura. A thyratron stimulator was utilized, along with unilateral or bipolar electrodes made of a platinum wire enclosed in a glass holder [10]. During this period, he meticulously recorded what he discovered during surgery [10–13].

On December 1, 1937, Wilder Penfield and Edwin Boldrey published a 55-page paper in "Brain" titled "Somatic motor and sensory representation in the cerebral cortex of man as studied by electrical stimulation" [13], which marked the homunculus's first appearance in the field of neurological science. The paper is chock-full of meticulously constructed summaries of information obtained from the cortical stimulation of 126 patients who were operated by Penfield in local anesthesia, in a regimen of awake surgery, between 1928 and 1936. To create the first thorough map of motor and somatosensory localization in the human brain, all patient recordings were combined. The homunculus, a distorted humanoid figure, was used to depict this map. Its form represents the amount of cortical region devoted to each body part's motor or somatosensory activities [14].

The study had a significant influence on scientific research as well as neurosurgical practice for a long time. Scientifically, it supported cortical localization as a viable model to explain motor cognition, somatosensory perception, and higher cognitive functions more broadly. Clinically, it helped establish direct cortical stimulation as a significant tool for functional mapping in neurosurgery [14].

Moving to more recent times, in his pioneering study including 117 patients [15], George Ojemann, in 1983, provided a thorough demonstration of the heterogeneity in speech and language mapping. He created a probabilistic map of the speech and language domains using Direct Electrical Stimulation (DES), which accounts for both positive and negative sites of stimulation [16]. Many individuals had many 1–2 cm^2 language center mosaics, often one in the frontal and one or more in the temporoparietal lobe. These mosaics were highly localized. Compared to the classic Broca-Wernicke areas, the area devoted to individual mosaics and the overall language-related area were typically substantially smaller. Notably, significant individual variation existed in the precise site of language function, some of which was associated with the verbal intelligence and sex of the patient. Moreover, George Ojemann introduced the Ojemann Cortical Stimulator (OCS), an electrical stimulator that improved Penfield's technique of motor mapping [17]. Still today, Ojemann cortical stimulators are used by neurosurgeons to map and localize the brain's cortical and subcortical regions to map functional areas intraoperatively and prevent the resection or damage of functional tissue (Fig. 15.1).

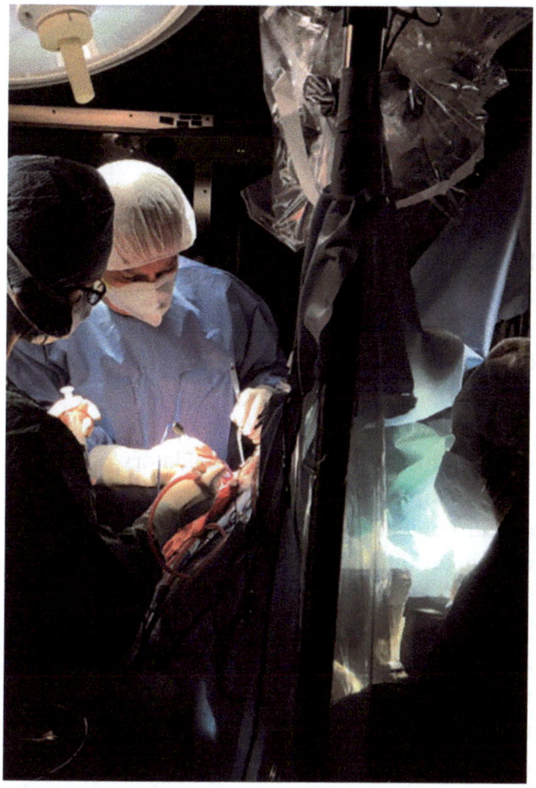

Fig. 15.1 Intraoperative bipolar cortical stimulator. The surgeon is stimulating the temporal cortex during surgery to rule out Language phenomena as speech arrest, paraphasias or anomias

15.2 Setting and Team

Originally used to surgically treat epilepsy, awake craniotomies are now most frequently employed to remove malignancies: the neurosurgeon can maximize tumor removal while maintaining neurological function via an awake craniotomy. The idea of an awake craniotomy may be disturbing for the patient; therefore, the surgical team's job is crucial in choosing the right patient and educating him or her on what to expect throughout the procedure [18].

An effective awake craniotomy requires the use of interprofessional team-based techniques. Before a patient enters the operating room, the anesthesiologist and the surgical team should consult and make plans for the procedure and talk to the operating room nurse about the equipment required for the procedure and the patient's position. Successful procedures are achieved by minimizing complications and fostering effective communication among all team members, including the surgeon, technician, nurse anesthetists, and anesthesiologist/nurse.

Commonly the usage of standard ASA monitoring is recommended, including parameters such as temperature, non-invasive blood pressure, pulse oximeter, ECG, and capnometry monitor. The intra-arterial line is commonly utilized for both arterial blood gas (ABG) analysis and beat-to-beat blood pressure monitoring. It is possible to do a central venous catheterization to provide vasoactive drugs and fluids. Precordial Doppler aids in the detection of venous air embolism in craniotomy patients who are seated. It is recommended that monitors are positioned on the same side as brain lesions to prevent contralateral sensorimotor monitoring interference. The bispectral index, a processed electroencephalography (EEG) monitor, can be utilized to quickly awaken patients for intraoperative language testing and to control the dosage of anesthetic medications [18].

15.3 Techniques of Anesthesia

During the more painful or surgically stimulating moments of the operation, such as applying the Mayfield Pins, performing skin incision, removing the bone flap and opening dura mater, the patient is typically given sedation or anesthesia. The patient may be completely awake during the mapping technique, which involves lesion excision, because brain tissue is not sensitive to pain.

The surgeon, the pathology, the length of the surgery, and the patient's characteristics all affect the anesthesia strategy. Usually, the choice is between conscious sedation and general anesthesia with intraoperative awakening.

15.3.1 Conscious Sedation

Conscious sedation, also known as the "awake-awake-awake" or "full-awake" technique, involves giving moderate sedation at the start of a procedure to help calm the patient and then adjusting the sedation levels as necessary. The goal is to keep the patient awake and able to respond to verbal or tactile cues while maintaining an open airway [19]. It is important to avoid giving too much sedation, as this can lead to complications like airway obstruction, low blood pressure, slowed breathing, and temporary cessation of breathing. Typically, low doses of propofol and/or remifentanil are used for moderate sedation. Dexmedetomidine is another option because of its ability to keep breathing stable and not interfere much with brain wave monitoring.

15.3.2 General Anesthesia with Intraoperative Awakening

The technique known as the "asleep-awake-asleep" technique involves starting the procedure with general anesthesia, maintaining it during stimulating initial parts, and then waking up the patient during critical phases like cortical mapping. Airways management is usually done through endotracheal intubation or a supraglottic airway device. Using a laryngeal mask airway (LMA) is preferred over endotracheal intubation to reduce stimulation during the awake period. Total intravenous anesthesia with propofol and remifentanil infusion is commonly used, with the option of adding dexmedetomidine for extra sedation. Quick-acting inhalation agents like sevoflurane may be used during the sleeping phase.

15.3.3 Regional Scalp Block

Prior to using Mayfield Pins to secure the head during awake craniotomy, a bilateral scalp block is typically done to offer effective pain relief. This block focuses on multiple nerves on both sides of the scalp to reduce the body's reaction to pain, ensuring the patient's comfort while mapping the cortex [20]. The nerves targeted in this block are the supraorbital nerve, supratrochlear nerve, zygomaticotemporal nerve, auriculotemporal nerve, lesser occipital nerve, greater occipital nerve, and greater auricular nerve.

15.4 Intraoperative Neuromonitoring

Electrophysiologic monitoring, also known as neuromonitoring, is used during surgery to evaluate the functional integrity of the brain, spinal cord, brainstem, and cranial and peripheral nerves.

Apart from awake surgery, during which a neuromonitoring is always mandatory, as a general principle, if a patient is more likely to suffer a neurological injury during surgery, intraoperative neurophysiologic monitoring (IONM), is advised [21].

The purpose of monitoring is to notify the anesthesiologist and surgeon of an approaching injury so that they can adjust the course of treatment in time to avoid irreversible harm. Given the significant importance of this tool and the intricacy of the subject matter, we have made the decision to dedicate an entire chapter (Chap. 14) to the topic of neurophysiological monitoring.

15.4.1 Direct Electrical Stimulation

For more than 50 years, direct electrical stimulation (DES), has been a commonly used clinical technique. Clinical uses for DES include mapping sensory, motor, and cognitive functions in real time during awake surgery; determining functional pathways; suppressing epileptiform activity using long-term closed loop devices implanted; and minimizing tremor in motor diseases [22].

Direct current applied locally to brain tissue at 5–15 milliamperes (mA) is the current method of using DES to map brain function [23–25].

Application of DES can be done with a handheld bipolar or monopolar stimulator, or with implanted grids or strips; awake craniotomies are more commonly performed with the former technique, while extra-operative mapping and long-term monitoring of the margins separating epileptogenic from eloquent tissue are more common with the latter technique [22].

When mapping eloquent cortex, direct cortical electrical stimulation is frequently regarded as the gold standard approach, especially when there is overlap with the margins of intended surgical resection. The brain regions known as the eloquent cortex are those that, if eliminated, would result in a notable and severe neurologic impairment. Primary somatosensory cortex (S1, parietal lobe—postcentral gyrus), primary motor cortex (M1, frontal lobe—precentral gyrus), primary visual cortex (V1, occipital pole), and several key language regions, including Broca's and Wernicke's areas, are examples of eloquent cortices [26].

Cortical stimulation mapping (CSM) is a technique for assessing the brain's eloquent cortex. Once a patient has been found to be a good surgical candidate for tumor resection or epilepsy surgery, this is done. Observing a positive or negative phenomenon directly completes the cortical stimulation needed to assess eloquent motor function. Movements that are tonic or clonic are the result of motor activation in positive events. Loss of muscle tone or motor activity as a result of a disruption in motor function is a negative phenomenon.

The primary sensory cortex, also known as the postcentral gyrus, the secondary sensorimotor region in the parietal operculum, and the supplementary sensorimotor area in the mesial frontal cortex are instead all potential locations for mapping somatosensory function [26, 27].

15.4.2 Is Intraoperative Neuromonitoring Infallible?

Despite the great benefits it brings to clinical practice, several studies have highlighted the limits of neurophysiological monitoring, documenting up to 17% of clinical worsening in less than 7 days after surgery in patients with stable intraoperative monitoring [27], up to 21% of false positives after brain metastasis resection [28], a sensitivity of 17.5% and a negative predictive value of 69.4% [29]. This data should be always taken into account: a part of patients undergoing surgery with IONM will undergo a predictable or unpredictable worsening of their functions, even in cases of intraoperative neuromonitoring stability.

15.5 Neuropsychological Testing

Neuropsychology is crucial aspect of Awake Surgery. In neuro-oncological surgery, it is composed of three fundamental moments: preoperative, intraoperative and postoperative [30]. The preoperative neuropsychological evaluation aims at describing the baseline residual functioning of the cognition of the patient. Similarly to what happens postoperatively, this evaluation focuses on "focal aspects," or better defined, on the functional evaluation of language, executive, praxis and visuospatial networks. Several investigations [31] reported detailed batteries of tests used, but still there is no univocal consensus on what test should or should not be employed in surgical setting. Intraoperatively, the surgeon stimulates with cortical and subcortical probes, while the neurophysiologist records the potentials and at the same time the neuropsychologist administers the stimuli. For what strictly the language function is concerned, naming of actions and objects, counting, reading of words and non-words are the most performed tasks. Alteration of the language function in the form of anomia, semantic or phonetic paraphasia or even increased latencies [32], are regarded as confirmatory of eloquence of stimulation point. Although any kind of cognitive or motor task was described, from playing musical instruments to cooking regional recipes [33], the tasks should be carefully selected to be easy fulfilled, demonstrative of the function's integrity and reproducible in the somehow difficult intraoperative conditions [34–36]. The fine neuropsychological evaluation is one the pillars of awake surgery, together with neuromonitoring: and tough a well-trained speech therapist could theoretically replace a neuropsychologist for the language function only, no awake surgery should be performed when either one of the aforementioned two (neuropsychology and neuromonitoring) is unavailable (Fig. 15.2).

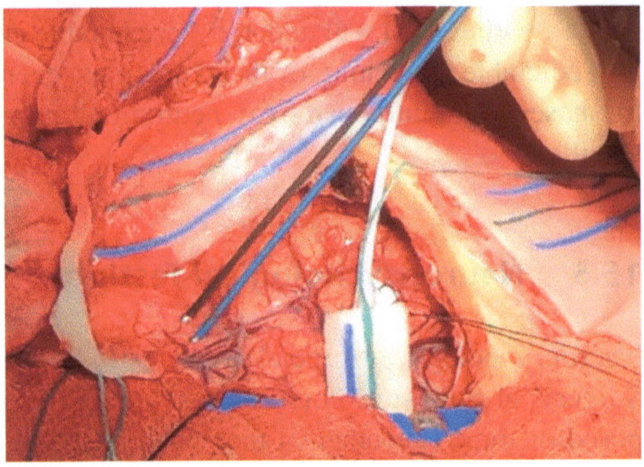

Fig. 15.2 The operative setting. A trasparent drapes facilitates the intraoperative communication between surgeons, nurses, anesthesiologists, and neurophisiologists

15.6 Conclusions

Awake surgery offers the unique possibility to intraoperatively investigate highly complex eloquent networks such as those exerting motor and language functions, and possibly, through appropriate stimulation and testing executive and praxis functions either. It stands as the definitive approach to maintain the neuro-oncologic balance, namely preserving the function while maximizing the extent of resection, in lesions located in eloquent cortical and subcortical structures. The slow, and still constant progress in "connectome science" will, in the upcoming future, furtherly improve the safety of awake surgeries, possibly increasing the awareness of the underlying physiological mechanisms of language, praxis, motor, visuospatial, and executive functions. Awake surgery has nevertheless some recognized limitations. For instance, it is hard to perform awake surgery in intraventricularly located lesions and in prone positions. Furthermore, the indication should be carefully considered in patients suffering from major psychiatric comorbidities and was previously associated to the development of postoperative post-traumatic stress symptoms, especially in vulnerable patients. Such symptoms should be regarded as a potential complication seriously affecting the postoperative course and the quality of life in patients who are already aware of their overall oncologic prognosis. Moreover, a deep and reliable intraoperative neuropsychological testing has its "times," affecting the overall duration of the surgery. Several authors argued that a transcranial magnetic stimulation (TMS) mapping could provide a "functional map," which could be then intraoperatively "neuronavigated". In future, these maps could potentially overcome the necessity of awake approaches: this could be especially true for lesion involving the motor pathways. It is our opinion that, still, at present, awake surgery preserves its undeniable value, and a careful patient and "lesion" selection stands as the foundation to achieve excellent results while performing these complex resections.

References

1. Kobyakov GL, Lubnin AY, Kulikov AS, Gavrilov AG, Goryaynov SA, Poddubskiy AA, Lodygina KS. Awake craniotomy. Zh Vopr Neirokhir Im N N Burdenko. 2016;80(1):107–16. https://doi.org/10.17116/neiro2016801107-116. English, Russian. PMID: 27186613.
2. van den Hombergh P, Froeling FM. Craniotomie; een springlevende traditie bij de Kisii (Kenia) [Craniotomy; a, much-alive tradition with the Kisii (Kenya)]. Ned Tijdschr Geneeskd. 1994;138(52):2621–5. Dutch. PMID: 7808537.
3. Bulsara KR, Johnson J, Villavicencio AT. Improvements in brain tumor surgery: the modern history of awake craniotomies. Neurosurg Focus. 2005;18(4):e5. https://doi.org/10.3171/foc.2005.18.4.6. PMID: 15844868.
4. Marshall C. Surgery of epilepsy and motor disorders. In: A history of neurological surgery. New York: Hafner Publishing Co; 1967. p. 288–305.
5. Jackson JH. Selected writings of John Hughlings Jackson, vol. 1. Staples; 1958.
6. July J, Manninen P, Lai J, Yao Z, Bernstein M. The history of awake craniotomy for brain tumor and its spread into Asia. Surg Neurol. 2009;71(5):621–4; discussion 624-5. https://doi.org/10.1016/j.surneu.2007.12.022. Epub 2008 May 2. PMID: 18452979.
7. Fritsch GT. Uber die elektrische Erregbarkeit des Grosshirns. Arch Anat Physiol. 1870;37:300–32.
8. Bartholow R. Experiments on the functions of the human brain. Br Med J. 1874;1(700):727. PMCID: PMC2302912.
9. Horsley V. Remarks on ten consecutive cases of operations upon the brain and cranial cavity to illustrate the details and safety of the method employed. Br Med J. 1887;1(1373):863.

10. Penfield W, Erickson TC. Epilepsy and cerebral localization. Oxford: Charles C. Thomas; 1941.
11. Penfield W, Jasper H. Epilepsy and the functional anatomy of the human brain. Little, Brown & Co; 1954.
12. Penfield W, Rasmussen T. The cerebral cortex of man; a clinical study of localization of function. Macmillan; 1950.
13. Penfield W, Boldrey E. Somatic motor and sensory representation in the cerebral cortex of man as studied by electrical stimulation. Brain. 1937;60(4):389–443.
14. Catani M. A little man of some importance. Brain. 2017;140(11):3055–61. https://doi.org/10.1093/brain/awx270. PMID: 29088352; PMCID: PMC5841206.
15. Ojemann G, Ojemann J, Lettich E, Berger M. Cortical language localization in left, dominant hemisphere. An electrical stimulation mapping investigation in 117 patients. J Neurosurg. 1989;71(3):316–26. https://doi.org/10.3171/jns.1989.71.3.0316. PMID: 2769383.
16. Rahimpour S, Haglund MM, Friedman AH, Duffau H. History of awake mapping and speech and language localization: from modules to networks. Neurosurg Focus. 2019;47(3):E4. https://doi.org/10.3171/2019.7.FOCUS19347. PMID: 31473677.
17. Jahangiri FR, Dobariya A, Kruse A, Kalyta O, Moorman JD. Mapping of the motor cortex. Cureus. 2020;12(9):e10645. https://doi.org/10.7759/cureus.10645. PMID: 33133815; PMCID: PMC7586383.
18. Singh K, Dua A. Anesthesia for awake craniotomy. 2023 Jul 6. In: StatPearls [internet]. Treasure Island: StatPearls Publishing; 2024. PMID: 34283419.
19. Weinzierl MR, Reinacher P, Gilsbach JM, Rohde V. Combined motor and somatosensory evoked potentials for intraoperative monitoring: intra- and postoperative data in a series of 69 operations. Neurosurg Rev. 2007;30(2):109–16; discussion 116. https://doi.org/10.1007/s10143-006-0061-5. Epub 2007 Jan 13. PMID: 17221265.
20. Lall RR, Lall RR, Hauptman JS, Munoz C, Cybulski GR, Koski T, Ganju A, Fessler RG, Smith ZA. Intraoperative neurophysiological monitoring in spine surgery: indications, efficacy, and role of the preoperative checklist. Neurosurg Focus. 2012;33(5):E10. https://doi.org/10.3171/2012.9.FOCUS12235. PMID: 23116090
21. Ghatol D, Widrich J. Intraoperative neurophysiological monitoring. 2023 Jul 24. In: StatPearls [internet]. Treasure Island: StatPearls Publishing; 2024. PMID: 33085350.
22. Mahon BZ, Miozzo M, Pilcher WH. Direct electrical stimulation mapping of cognitive functions in the human brain. Cogn Neuropsychol. 2019;36(3–4):97–102. https://doi.org/10.1080/02643294.2019.1630375. PMID: 31514643.
23. Szelényi A, Bello L, Duffau H, Fava E, Feigl GC, Galanda M, Neuloh G, Signorelli F, Sala F. Workgroup for Intraoperative Management in Low-Grade Glioma Surgery within the European Low-Grade Glioma Network. Intraoperative electrical stimulation in awake craniotomy: methodological aspects of current practice. Neurosurg Focus. 2010;28(2):E7. https://doi.org/10.3171/2009.12.FOCUS09237. PMID: 20121442.
24. Sanai N, Mirzadeh Z, Berger MS. Functional outcome after language mapping for glioma resection. N Engl J Med. 2008;358(1):18–27. https://doi.org/10.1056/NEJMoa067819. PMID: 18172171.
25. Kayama T. Guidelines committee of the Japan awake surgery conference. The guidelines for awake craniotomy guidelines committee of the Japan awake surgery conference. Neurol Med Chir (Tokyo). 2012;52(3):119–41. https://doi.org/10.2176/nmc.52.119. PMID: 22450477.
26. Vakani R, Nair DR. Electrocorticography and functional mapping. Handb Clin Neurol. 2019;160:313–27. https://doi.org/10.1016/B978-0-444-64032-1.00020-5. PMID: 31277857.
27. Raco A, Pesce A, Fraschetti F, Frati A, D'Andrea G, Cimatti M, Acqui M. Motor outcomes after surgical resection of lesions involving the motor pathway: a prognostic evaluation scale. World Neurosurg. 2017;103:748–56. https://doi.org/10.1016/j.wneu.2017.04.063. Epub 2017 Apr 19. PMID: 28434952.
28. Obermueller T, Schaeffner M, Shiban E, Droese D, Negwer C, Meyer B, Ringel F, Krieg SM. Intraoperative neuromonitoring for function-guided resection differs for supratentorial motor eloquent gliomas and metastases. BMC Neurol. 2015;15:211. https://doi.org/10.1186/s12883-015-0476-0. PMID: 26487091; PMCID: PMC4618356.
29. Silverstein JW, Shah HA, Unadkat P, Vilaysom S, Boockvar JA, Langer DJ, Ellis JA, D'Amico RS. Short and long-term prognostic value of intraoperative motor evoked potentials in brain tumor patients: a case series of 121 brain tumor patients. J Neuro-Oncol. 2023;161(1):127–33. https://doi.org/10.1007/s11060-022-04229-8. Epub 2023 Jan 11. PMID: 36629962.
30. Herbet G, Duffau H. Neuropsychological assessment before, during and after "awake" brain surgery for a slow-growing tumor. In: The SAGE handbook of clinical neuropsychology: clinical neuropsychological assessment and diagnosis. SAGE Publications Ltd; 2023. p. 650–67. https://doi.org/10.4135/9781529789539.
31. Skrap M, Marin D, Ius T, Fabbro F, Tomasino B. Brain mapping: a novel intraoperative neuropsychological approach. J Neurosurg. 2016;125(4):877–87.
32. Moritz-Gasser S, Herbet G, Maldonado IL, Duffau H. Lexical access speed is significantly correlated with the return to professional activities after awake surgery for low-grade gliomas. J Neuro-Oncol. 2012;107:633–41.
33. https://youtu.be/F6Pqd1YEXpY?si=2E6ofPTiSG7uwnHe.
34. Milian M, Luerding R, Ploppa A, Decker K, Psaras T, Tatagiba M, et al. "Imagine your neighbor mows the lawn": a pilot study of psychologi-

cal sequelae due to awake craniotomy. J Neurosurg. 2013;118(6):1288–95.

35. Sollmann N, Krieg SM, Säisänen L, Julkunen P. Mapping of motor function with neuronavigated transcranial magnetic stimulation: a review on clinical application in brain tumors and methods for ensuring feasible accuracy. Brain Sci. 2021;11(7):897.
36. Sondergaard RE, Martino D, Kiss ZH, Condliffe EG. TMS motor mapping methodology and reliability: a structured review. Front Neurosci. 2021;15:709368.

Part IV

Part IV

Updated Therapeutic Protocols for Glioblastomas

16

Francesco Bruno, Alessia Pellerino, Edoardo Pronello, and Roberta Rudà

16.1 Introduction

16.1.1 Current Standard Treatment

16.1.1.1 Radiotherapy and Concomitant Temozolomide

Radiotherapy (RT) retains a major role in the standard treatment of glioblastoma (GBM), as it is useful for tumor control and improvement of both progression-free and overall survival (OS). Conventional standard RT is indicated after surgery (ideally within 2 months from resection) and should be associated with concurrent temozolomide (TMZ) [1]. The most employed RT schedule delivers 60 Gy in 2-Gy daily fractions over 6 weeks. TMZ is given orally (75 mg/m^2 daily) during all the radiation treatment period [2, 3]. Other dose schedules have been investigated but without clear benefit. In particular, there is no indication for doses >60 Gy [4].

The association with radiotherapy and concurrent TMZ is a milestone of GBM treatment, which was established as a standard after the publication of a phase III trial of the European Organization for Research and Treatment of Cancer (EORTC) and National Cancer Institute of Canada Clinical Trials Group (NCIC) in 2005. This trial compared the association of RT and TMZ to RT alone, and results clearly favored the combination modality [2]. In the long-term 5-year analysis, OS was 27.2% (95% CI 22.2–32.5) at 2 years, 16.0% (12.0–20.6) at 3 years, 12.1% (8.5–16.4) at 4 years, and 9.8% (6.4–14.0) at 5 years with RT and TMZ, versus 10.9% (7.6–14.8), 4.4% (2.4–7.2), 3.0% (1.4–5.7), and 1.9% (0.6–4.4) with RT alone (hazard ratio 0.6, 95% CI 0.5–0.7; $p < 0.001$). A benefit of combined therapy was observed in all prognostic subgroups, including patients aged 60–70 years. *MGMT* promoter methylation was the strongest predictor of outcome and benefit from TMZ chemotherapy, even if the advantage of the combined modality was significant is higher in methylated patients (OS 23.4 versus 15.3 months for combined RT/TMZ versus RT alone, $p = 0.004$) as compared to unmethylated patients (OS 12.6 versus 11.8 months for combined RT/TMZ versus RT alone, $p = 0.035$) [3].

RT employs ionizing radiations that induce double-strand DNA damage and tumor cell death. However, endothelial cells of the neovasculature of the tumors are also vulnerable to radiation-

F. Bruno · A. Pellerino · E. Pronello · R. Rudà (✉)
Division of Neuro-Oncology, Department of Neuroscience "Rita Levi Montalcini", University and City of Health and Science Hospital, Turin, Italy
e-mail: roberta.ruda@unito.it

D. Armocida et al. (eds.), *Neurosurgery's Frontline Role in Gliomas Treatment*,
https://doi.org/10.1007/978-3-031-81850-9_16

induced damage [5], and their disruption may lead to radiation-induced MRI changes, known as pseudoprogression and radionecrosis [6]. These conditions are common pitfall in GBM management and should be carefully considered after RT shortly.

The so-called pseudoprogression occurs most commonly within the first 3 months from RT. It is usually characterized by increased contrast enhancement peritumoural edema and necrosis [6] which mimic tumor regrowth However, patients with pseudoprogression typically do not experience neurological deterioration [7]. Furthermore, pseudoprogression prevails among patients with *MGMT*p methylated tumors, and in some studies, it has been associated to increased survival advantage. Even if timing of MRI changes and clinical correlates may help to distinguish pseudoprogression from radionecrosis and disease progression, advanced MRI (such as diffusion and perfusion studies) and positron emission tomography (PET) may be useful in the differential diagnosis [6, 8, 9].

16.1.1.2 Adjuvant Chemotherapy with Temozolomide

Standard first-line chemotherapy agent for GBM is represented by TMZ. TMZ is an alkylating agent, which causes DNA damage and interferes with tumor proliferation. One mechanism of TMZ action is the depletion of the repair enzyme O6-methylguanine-DNA methyltransferase (MGMT), which explains why TMZ is especially effective against tumors with methylation of the *MGMT* promoter, where the enzyme activity is silenced [10, 11]. There are different reasons supporting the use of TMZ as a standard chemotherapy treatment in GBM: penetration through the blood–brain barrier is good, oral formulation improves patient's compliance and toxicity profile is more favorable (no cumulative myelotoxicity) than other commonly used oral chemotherapies, such as lomustine and procarbazine. Moreover, TMZ it does not induce or inhibit significantly the liver cytochrome system, which translate in a low risk of interactions with other drugs, such as steroids or antiseizure medications (ASMs) [12].

Common adverse events include nausea and/or vomiting, fatigue, dose-dependent myelosuppression (especially thrombocytopenia and leukopenia). Other rarer adverse events are dose-independent pancytopenia, increase of liver enzymes, skin rash, photosensitivity. Very rare adverse events include hair loss, fragility of cutaneous appendages, and periodontitis. Second hematological tumors are uncommon as potential complication of long-term treatment with TMZ [13]. The standard schedule of adjuvant TMZ is 150–200 mg/m^2 on days 1–5 every 28 days [2]. Dose should be reduced in case of poor tolerability and/or hematologic toxicity. In particular, patients undergoing treatment with TMZ should be carefully monitored with monthly blood tests to rule out thrombocytopenia <100,000/mm^3 and neutropenia <1500/mm^3; similarly, occurrence of any drug-related adverse events must be promptly recognized with careful periodic clinical evaluations.

TMZ may also be administered with intensified schedules, which include metronomic and dose-dense TMZ [14]. The metronomic schedule consists in a lower dose of TMZ (50 mg/m^2), which is given daily without interruptions. Metronomic TMZ seems to have a direct toxic effect on tumor endothelial cells, which would result also in an antiangiogenic activity [15]. Moreover, continuous exposition to TMZ seems to increase methylation and inhibition of the *MGMT* promoter, thus enhancing antitumor activity especially in *MGMT*p methylated tumors. Dose-dense chemotherapy is given at the dose of 150 mg/m^2 days 1–7 and 15–21 of a 28-day cycle. With dose-dense TMZ, the interval between doses is reduced, whereas the dose density is boosted. Thus, tumor cells should be more likely to be damaged between cycles, with higher treatment efficacy [16]. In a phase II trial investigating the activity and tolerability of dose-dense versus metronomic TMZ, both regimens appeared to be feasible and quite well-tolerated. Dose-dense TMZ was associated with a median OS of 17.1 months and 1-year survival of 80%, while in case of metronomic TMZ OS was 15.1 months and 1-year survival 69%. Main toxicities were leukopenia and elevation of liver enzymes (in the latter case, especially in the metronomic subgroup) [14]. However, a significant benefit from dose-dense regimens of TMZ was not confirmed by other studies, where higher doses were associated with greater toxicity and deterioration in function and quality of life [17, 18]. Moreover, in a phase II randomized, multicentre, open-label trial of continuing adjuvant TMZ beyond six cycles (GEINO 14–01), patients exposed to 12 months of adjuvant TMZ did not seem to benefit in terms 6-month PFS and OS as compared to those undergoing only 6 cycles (median PFS 9.5 months versus 7.7 months, $p = 0.95$; median OS 18.2 months versus 23.3 months, $p = 0.16$). In addition, 12 cycles of TMZ were associated to higher adverse effects (thrombocytopenia, lymphopenia, nausea, and vomiting) [19]. However, it is unclear whether an extended duration of TMZ treatment is useful in some certain subgroups of patients, such as incompletely resected or MGMT methylated tumors.

Ultimately, the development of resistance to TMZ acts as the limiting factor in GBM treatment, one of the major factors is the presence of tumor stem cells, which are intrinsically TMZ-resistant. Furthermore, many other molecular mechanisms are emerging, including the involvement of other DNA repair systems, aberrant signaling pathways, autophagy, epigenetic modifications, microRNAs, and extracellular vesicle production [20].

The addition of other chemotherapy agents to adjuvant TMZ has been the object of several investigations. In an open-label, phase III trial on newly diagnosed GBM patients with *MGMT*p methylation, the addition of lomustine (CCNU) to TMZ versus standard TMZ was associated with better OS (48.1 versus 31.4 months, respectively), and the occurrence of significant adverse events (grade 3 according to Common Terminology Criteria for Adverse Events—CTCAE) was similar in the two groups (51% versus 59% in TMZ and TMZ/CCNU groups, respectively). However, the limitation of this trial is the small sample size. The association of TMZ with antiangiogenic agents, such as bevacizumab, has also been explored. Bevacizumab is a humanized monoclonal antibody that inhibits vascular endothelial growth factor (VEGF). A combination of bevacizumab with has been investigated in two large, randomized phase III trials. However, despite prolonging PFS in both trials, the addition of bevacizumab did not translate in an OS advantage [21, 22].

16.1.2 New Perspectives

16.1.2.1 Targeted Therapy

Targeted therapies employ drugs that are specifically engineered to interact with molecular pathways involved in the proliferation and survival of cancer cells. Such an approach provides a more accurate and less toxic alternative to conventional chemotherapy. Additionally, the combination of TMZ with targeted agents not only may enhance the treatment effectiveness for brain tumors but also minimize chemotherapy side effects, ultimately leading to improved patient outcome and progress in cancer treatment.

Epidermal Growth Factor Receptor (EGFR)

The epidermal growth factor receptor (EGFR) gene has been extensively studied in GBM due to an overexpression in approximately 60% of tumors and amplification in over 40% [23]. Nearly 50% of GBM tumors with EGFR amplification have a deletion mutation known as EGFRvIII, which leads to disrupted gene regulation [24]. In recent years, various clinical trials have explored therapies targeting EGFR or EGFRvIII.

Rindopepimut, a vaccine targeting EGFRvIII conjugated with keyhole limpet hemocyanin, was evaluated in the Phase III ACT IV trial (NCT01480479). This trial assessed the efficacy of adding rindopepimut to standard chemoradiation but found no significant survival benefit for patients with newly diagnosed GBM [25].

The antibody-drug conjugate depatuxizumab mafodotin (Depatux-M), which targets cells with EGFR amplification, was studied in GBM patients [26]. Depatuxizumab mafodotin internalizes and releases the antimicrotubule agent monomethyl auristatin F. However, when used with concurrent TMZ, it did not improve survival outcomes compared to TMZ alone in patients with recurrent *EGFR*-amplified GBM [27]. Additionally, in a study involving newly diagnosed GBM patients (NCT02573324), it did not significantly enhance progression-free survival compared to standard therapy [28].

The monoclonal antibody GC118, which has strong inhibitory effects against high-affinity EGFR ligands, was tested in patients with *EGFR*-amplified recurrent GBM in an open-label, single-arm phase II trial (NCT03618667). Unfortunately, the primary outcome of a 6-month progression-free survival rate was only 5.6% (95% CI 0.3–25.8%), with a median overall survival of 5.7 months (range 2–22.0 months) [29]. Another approach involved AMG 596, a bispecific T cell engager targeting EGFRvIII-positive tumor antigens. In its initial trial (NCT03296696), among the eight evaluable patients, one experienced a partial response and two had stable disease at initial follow-up [30].

Inhibitors of the EGFR tyrosine kinase have also been largely investigated. Erlotinib, a reversible *EGFR* tyrosine kinase inhibitor, failed to demonstrate improved OS when combined with small molecules bevacizumab and TMZ in newly diagnosed patients in two phase 2 studies [31, 32]. Similar outcomes were observed in a phase 2 study evaluating erlotinib in combination with sorafenib [33]. Gefitinib, a reversible and specific EGFR tyrosine kinase inhibitor, did not improve OS when concurrent with RT in newly diagnosed patients [34], or as adjuvant therapy after RT. Afatinib, an irreversible pan-inhibitor of the ErbB family (including *EGFR* and EGFRvIII), did not outperform TMZ in a phase 2 study (NCT00727506). However, it showed increased PFS in patients with tumors expressing EGFRvIII or *EGFR* amplification [35]. Dacomitinib, a pan-HER family inhibitor approved for *EGFR*-mutant NSCLC, provided minimal benefits in GBM when tested as monotherapy in tumors with *EGFR* amplification or the common *EGFR* mutation EGFRvIII [36].

ERAS-801, a newly developed EGFR inhibitor with better CNS penetration, is under evaluation in patients with recurrent GBM (NCT05222802). In preclinical models, ERAS-801 demonstrated a survival benefit in 93% of EGFR mutant and/or amplified cases, showing significant brain penetration and prolonged survival compared to erlotinib [37]. Another EGFR inhibitor, WSD0922-Fu, is being studied for its potential to prolong stable disease in patients with EGFRvIII-mutant high-grade astrocytoma (NCT04197934) [38].

BRAF

BRAF, part of the Raf kinase family, facilitates cellular proliferation via the MAP kinase/ERK signaling pathway. The *BRAF* V600E mutation is present in several tumor types, including a minority of GBM patients. This mutation is prevalent in epithelioid GBM, where it occurs in 50–93% of cases [39]. Vemurafenib, an early BRAF inhibitor, was tested in patients with *BRAF* V600-mutated glioma (NCT01524978). Among 11 patients with *BRAF*-mutant malignant diffuse glioma, one showed a partial response, and five had stable disease for 6 months [40].

Further investigations have explored the concurrent use of BRAF and MEK inhibitors for treating low-grade and high-grade glioma, showing promising results. A phase 2 clinical trial (NCT02684058) involving 110 pediatric patients with *BRAF* V600-mutated low-grade glioma randomly assigned participants to receive either dabrafenib plus trametinib or standard chemotherapy. At a median follow-up of 18.9 months, an overall response rate of 47% was observed in the combination therapy group, compared to 11% in the standard chemotherapy group (risk ratio, 4.31; 95% CI 1.7–11.2; $p < 0.001$). Additionally, significant improvements were seen in clinical benefit (risk ratio 1.88; 95% CI 1.3–2.7) and median progression-free survival (hazard ratio 0.31; 95% CI 0.17–0.55; $p < 0.001$) in the combination group [41]. Another study (NTC02034110) evaluated dabrafenib and trametinib in 45 adult patients with recurrent or refractory *BRAF* V600E-mutated high-grade glioma, reporting an objective response in 33% of patients, including three complete responses and 12 partial responses [42]. This combination has been recently approved by registration authorities for any type of solid tumors with *BRAF* V600 mutation or fusion (Fig. 16.1). More recently, a study examined a new combination of BRAF and MEK inhibitors in patients with *BRAF*-mutant GBM (NCT03973918). In a small series, concurrent use of encorafenib (BRAF inhibitor) and binimetinib (MEK inhibitor) led to sustained responses in all GBM patients and in 50% of those with anaplastic pleomorphic xanthoastrocytoma, though the study closed early due to enrollment challenges [43]. Despite the rarity of *BRAF* V600E-mutated GBM these studies highlight the potential benefits of combination therapy using BRAF and MEK inhibitors in gliomas harboring the *BRAF* V600E mutation. An open issue is whether to search for BRAF alterations in all GBM patients or only in some subgroups (longer patients at recurrence?)

PI3K/AKT/mTOR Pathway

The loss of the tumor suppressor gene phosphatase and tensin homolog (*PTEN*) on chromosome ten occurs in up to 60% of GBM patients [44]. This loss leads to activating mutations in the PIK3CA and PI3K/mTOR pathways, promoting uncontrolled cell proliferation [23]. Consequently, mTOR-targeted compounds, like temsirolimus (CCI-779) and everolimus, have been explored in GBM treatment. Both everolimus and temsirolimus have been evaluated in newly diagnosed GBM setting. When combined with radiotherapy (RT) and temozolomide (TMZ), everolimus did not significantly improve survival compared to

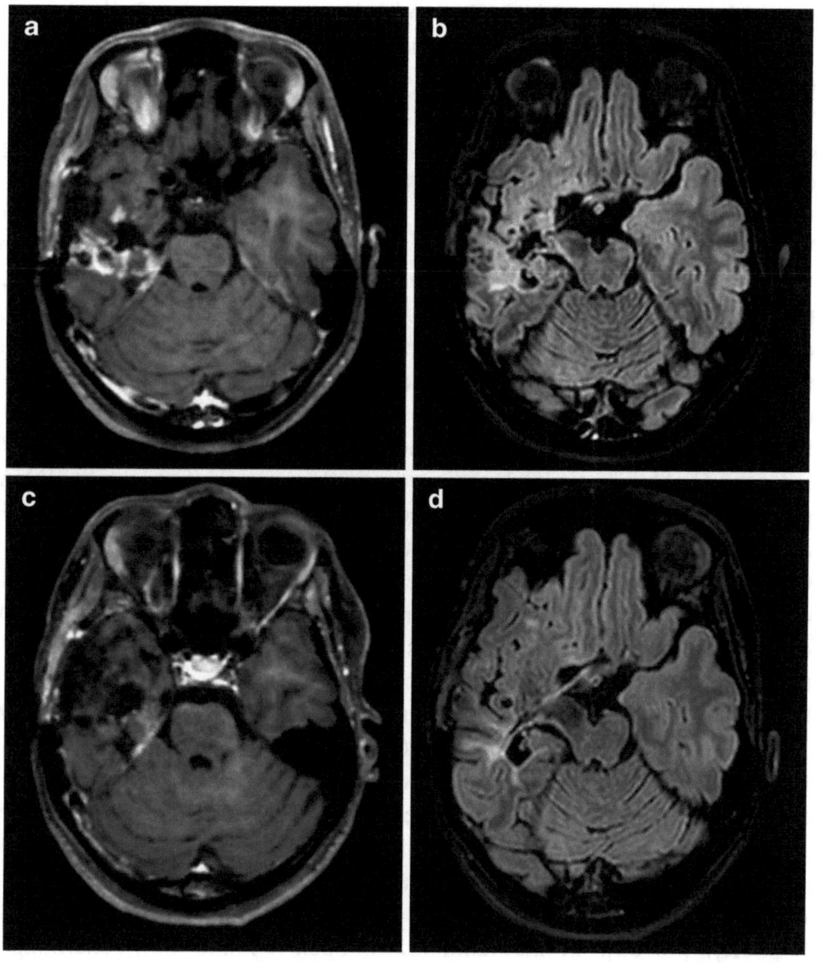

Fig. 16.1 In this figure, we present the case of a 20-year-old woman diagnose with an epithelioid GBM, BRAF V600E mutant, who was treated with dabrafenib 300 mg daily and trametinib 2 mg daily at recurrence after first-line radiotherapy and temozolomide. (**a**) Axial post-contrast T1 sequence at recurrence (before receiving dabrafenib and trametinib); (**b**) axial FLAIR sequence at recurrence (before receiving dabrafenib and trametinib); (**c**) axial post-contrast T1 sequence after two cycles of dabrafenib and trametinib; (**d**) axial FLAIR sequence after two cycles of dabrafenib and trametinib. Overall, the patient presented a near complete response (CR) of the contrast-enhanced target lesion according to RANO criteria

standard therapy [45], and the same was true for temsirolimus [46]. Additionally, mTOR inhibitors have been poorly tolerated in these clinical trials. Paxalisib, a brain-penetrant small molecule inhibitor of PI3K and mTOR, initially showed promise by prolonging progression-free survival and overall survival at maximum tolerated dose [47], but subsequent studies did not meet the criteria to advance to a major GBM trial.

Cyclin-Dependent Kinase (CDK)

The retinoblastoma (Rb) cell cycle control pathway is commonly altered in GBM due to homozygous deletions of CDKN2A/B, amplifications of CDK4 or CDK6, or alterations in the RB1 gene. Abemaciclib, a potent CDK4/6 inhibitor with good brain penetration, was investigated in newly diagnosed GBM patients in the INSIGHT trial. Patients were randomized to receive either standard radiotherapy and TMZ or radiochemotherapy followed by adjuvant abemaciclib. While abemaciclib was well-tolerated and associated with longer progression-free survival, it did not demonstrate an improvement in overall survival compared to standard radiochemotherapy [48].

Vascular Endothelial Growth Factor (VEGF)

VEGF is a critical mediator of angiogenesis in GBM. Bevacizumab, a VEGF inhibitor, has been extensively studied in GBM. It has been already reported in a previous section that the association of bevacizumab with chemoradiation as first-line therapy was ineffective. Also, in one study of recurrent GBM, bevacizumab achieved a median progression-free survival of 16 weeks and a radiographic response in 71% of patients [49]. Other VEGF inhibitors have also been tested in GBM. Among those, regorafenib is probably the one that acquired the greater interest in recent times. Regorafenib is an oral inhibitor of several kinases involved in tumor angiogenesis (VEGFR1–3 and TIE2), oncogenesis (KIT, RET, RAF1, and BRAF), and in the interaction between tumor and microenvironment (platelet-derived growth factor receptor [PDGFR] and fibroblast growth factor receptor [FGFR]), and tumor immunity (colony-stimulating factor 1 receptor [CSF1R]) [50–53]. In the randomized, open-label, phase 2 REGOMA trial, regorafenib improved OS (median OS: 7.4 vs 5.6 months, $p = 0.0009$) and PFS (6-month PFS, 16.9% vs 8.3%, $p = 0.022$) of recurrent GBM patients as compared with lomustine [54]. Other subsequent real-life studies showed similar impact on survival, but a higher rate of adverse than in REGOMA [55–60]: interestingly, dose adjustment and an escalation schedule has been proposed to improve tolerability with similar efficacy [61].

Despite these initial promising results, the regorafenib arm of the GBM Adaptive Global Initiative Learning Environment (AGILE) trial was closed because regorafenib failed to demonstrate an improvement in OS in both recurrent and newly diagnosed tumors.

16.1.2.2 Targeting DNA Repair Pathways

Radiation therapy is highly effective for GBM due to the ability to damage tumor DNA. However, tumor cells acquire radioresistance through enhanced DNA damage response mechanisms [62].

There are several mechanisms of DNA damage repair (DDR) in tumor cells and compounds to inhibit. Among these, poly (ADP-ribose) polymerase (PARP) inhibitors, which prevent single-strand DNA repair, are the most studied in GBM [63]. PARP inhibitors are being evaluated in combination with radiotherapy, chemotherapy, or antiangiogenic agents [64, 65].

Unfortunately, DNA damage repair (DDR) inhibitors have generally yielded disappointing results thus far. The myelosuppressive effects of PARP inhibitors also raise concerns about their safety when used in combination with TMZ.

16.1.3 Immunotherapies

16.1.3.1 Immune Checkpoint Inhibitors

Immune checkpoint inhibitors (ICIs) have transformed the treatment landscape for certain solid tumors, such as metastatic melanoma [66], non-small cell lung cancer [67], and renal cell carcinoma [68], generating interest in their potential role in treating GBM [69]. The primary mechanism of ICIs is to reduce tumor-induced immunosuppression, thereby enhancing the immune system's ability to recognize and attack the tumor [70].

The two main checkpoint regulators, currently targeted in immunotherapy, are cytotoxic T-lymphocyte-associated protein 4 (CTLA-4) and programmed cell death protein 1 (PD-1) [71]. T cell receptor activation leads to the expression of CTLA-4, which promotes self-tolerance and prevents autoimmunity [72]. PD-1, an inhibitory receptor on T cells, binds to its ligand PD-L1, which is expressed on tumor cells, thus inhibiting T cell activation [72]. Blocking these pathways with anti-CTLA-4 agents (such as ipilimumab, tremelimumab) or anti-PD-1/PD-L1 agents (such as pembrolizumab, nivolumab, atezolizumab) may trigger a more robust immune response against the tumor.

However, ICIs have not been proven effective in newly diagnosed GBM [69]. The phase III study, CheckMate 498 (NCT02617589), compared the efficacy of nivolumab plus RT with TMZ plus RT in 560 patients with newly diagnosed *MGMT*p unmethylated GBM [73]. The median overall survival was longer in the TMZ plus RT group (14.9 months) compared to the nivolumab plus RT group (13.4 months) ($p = 0.0037$), reaffirming TMZ plus RT as the standard of care [73]. The CheckMate 548 trial (NCT02667587), another phase III study, involved 716 patients with newly diagnosed *MGMT*p methylated GBM [74]. All patients received standard care treatment with RT plus TMZ, with either nivolumab or a placebo. Median progression-free survival was similar between the two groups (10.6 months for nivolumab versus 10.3 months for placebo), and median overall survival was slightly longer in the placebo group (32.1 months) compared to the nivolumab group (28.9 months).

Several hypotheses could explain the limited efficacy of ICIs in GBM in comparison with other cancers. GBM is now considered "immunologically cold," characterized by a low number of infiltrating lymphocytes leading to a loss of effector function [70, 75]. Additionally, GBMs exhibit a low mutational burden resulting in fewer neoantigen development for immune attack [69, 70]. Furthermore, GBMs generally express lower levels of PD-L1 compared to other tumors responsive to ICIs, with PD-L1 expression observed in 61–88% of GBM cases [76].

GBM promotes immune quiescence through the secretion of immunosuppressive paracrine factors such as transforming growth factor-ß (TGF-ß), interleukin-10 (IL-10), and prostaglandin E2 [77]. It also induces an inhibitory phenotype in tumor-associated macrophages and microglia [78]. Moreover, GBM may cause systemic immune dysfunction, evidenced by T cell lymphopenia and sequestration in the bone marrow in treatment-naïve patients with glioblastoma and other intracranial tumors [79]. The use of corticosteroids and TMZ in GBM treatment further enhances immunosuppression.

Tumors with a higher mutational load, which correlates with increased immunogenicity, might be more responsive to ICIs. High tumor mutational burden can result from mutations in mismatch repair genes like MSH2, MLH1, MSH6, and PMS2, suggesting a greater likelihood of response to ICIs. Another factor contributing to high mutational burden is the post-treatment effect of radiation and TMZ [80]. Approximately, 10% of GBM patients develop hypermutated tumors after chemoradiation, indicating that ICIs may be beneficial for recurrent GBM with a high mutation load [80], but this has not been confirmed in the clinical setting. Future research should explore the potential of combining ICIs with other immunotherapies, such as CAR-T cells, oncolytic viruses, vaccines, or integrating them with other treatment modalities to achieve better tumor control [69, 70, 72].

16.1.3.2 Vaccine-Based Therapies

Vaccine-based therapies represent another approach to leveraging the immune system against GBM. These therapies work by exposing patient's antigen-presenting cells to tumor-associated antigens, thereby stimulating an immune response targeting the tumor [70, 72]. Unlike traditional chemotherapy, these vaccines are disease-targeted. The primary mechanisms of vaccine therapy for GBM include peptide vaccines, dendritic cell vaccines, and individualized vaccines.

16.1.3.3 Peptide Vaccines

Peptide vaccines, among the most extensively studied for GBM treatment, consist of amino acids forming either single or multiple peptides [81]. A significant challenge in their development is selecting a target antigen consistently expressed on GBM cells. This was evident in a phase III, randomized clinical trial involving newly diagnosed GBM patients with confirmed EGFRvIII expression, all of whom had undergone standard radiation therapy and concurrent TMZ [25]. In this trial, 371 patients received monthly doses of rindopepimut, an EGFRvIII-targeting peptide vaccine, while 374 received a control treatment. The trial was prematurely halted due to futility, as there was no significant difference in survival between the two groups. Notably, both groups experienced a loss of EGFRvIII expression in 57–59% of patients' tumors [82], suggesting that tumor evolution occurred independently of rindopepimut therapy. This phenomenon, known as "antigen escape," occurs when a targetable mutation loses relevance as the tumor progresses.

Other experimental vaccines have targeted various peptides in GBM. For example, survivin, an intracellular anti-apoptotic protein that regulates cell division, has high expression in GBM cells, being a potential vaccine target [83]. Another peptide vaccine, DSP-7888, targets the Wilm's tumor 1 peptide (WT1), a cell growth transcription factor present in GBM and other solid tumors [84].

To address the heterogeneity and evolving nature of GBM, multipeptide vaccines like IMA950 have been developed. IMA950 includes nine MHC I and II peptides from the GBM surface. In a phase I/II study, newly diagnosed GBM patients treated with IMA950, combined with poly-ICLC, exhibited 63.2% single-peptide CD8+ T cell responses and 36.8% multipeptide CD8+ T cell responses [85]. Furthermore, 84.6% of patients showed tumor-specific CD4+ T cell responses, indicating the immunogenicity of IMA950 against GBM.

The promising initial results for SurVaxM, DSP-7888, and IMA950 are being further explored in combination with other immunotherapies, including pembrolizumab (NCT04013672, NCT03665545) and bevacizumab (NCT03149003).

16.1.3.4 Dendritic Cell Vaccines

Dendritic cells, key antigen-presenting cells, are crucial for establishing both innate and adaptive immunity. In GBM-targeting vaccines, dendritic cells are used to enhance the immune response. The process involves isolating dendritic cells from the patient blood, exposing them to tumor antigens ex vivo, maturing them with cytokines, and then reintroducing them into the patient [86]. After administration, these dendritic cells migrate to lymphoid organs to present antigens to T cells, thereby initiating an immune response [87].

To date, dendritic cell vaccinations have not consistently shown a definitive survival benefit in GBM patients, though there is some encouraging evidence. For instance, a phase III clinical trial (NCT00045968) involving 331 newly diagnosed glioblastoma patients who had undergone surgery and chemoradiotherapy compared TMZ plus DCVax-L to TMZ plus placebo [88]. The primary endpoint was progression-free survival, which was 6.2 months for DCVax-L recipients versus 7.6 months for the placebo group ($p = 0.47$), not meeting the primary endpoint [89]. However, patients could cross over to the vaccine at progression. The median overall survival for newly diagnosed glioblastoma patients receiving DCVax-L was 19.3 months from randomization, compared to 16.5 months in the control group ($p = 0.002$). Additionally, survival was higher at 48 months (15.7% vs. 9.9%) and at 60 months (13% vs. 5.7%) in the DCVax-L group [90]. Patients with *MGMT*p methylation receiving DCVax-L also had better survival (median overall survival of 30.2 months from randomization) compared to controls (21.3 months) ($p = 0.03$) [90].

A phase II randomized trial involving newly diagnosed GBM patients tested a dendritic cell vaccine (ICT-107) [91]. The dendritic cells were exposed to six stem-cell-associated peptides in

GBM. Even if no significant difference in median OS between ICT-107 recipients and controls was seen (17 versus 15 months), patients with HLA-A2 receiving ICT-107 had a stronger immune response and longer median overall survival (33.7 months compared to 23.9 months in the control group). This indicates that patient factors, like HLA status, are crucial for the response to dendritic cell vaccine therapy and potentially other immunotherapies for GBM.

Another dendritic cell vaccine, Audencel, was tested in a randomized phase II trial involving GBM patients who had undergone at least 70% surgical resection. The study found no difference in median OS between those receiving standard care and those receiving standard care plus Audencel [92]. In contrast, a study from China Medical University on 34 newly diagnosed GBM patients showed that an adjuvant dendritic cell vaccine, administered post-operatively and continued for 6 months, resulted in a median OS of 31.9 months, compared to 15 months for the control group receiving standard care [93].

16.1.3.5 Individualized Vaccines

Individualized vaccines leverage data from patients' tumors to tailor treatments. A phase I trial involving glioblastoma patients treated with APVAC1, a personalized vaccine derived from patient transcriptomes and tumor peptides, showed CD8+ T cell responses [94]. APVAC2, targeting neoepitopes, also elicited CD4+ T cell responses against the neoepitopes [94]. Another phase I/Ib trial demonstrated that personalized antigen vaccines could induce neoantigen specific responses in both CD4+ and CD8+ T cells in patients not treated with dexamethasone [95].

16.1.3.6 Viral Oncolytics

Genetically engineered viruses are appealing as antineoplastic agents because they can target tumor cells, replicating within them and causing cell death—a process known as "oncolysis." Additionally, these viruses can deliver beneficial genetic material to the infected tumor cells, thus inducing cytotoxicity and stimulating a more robust and sustained local immune response against the antigens released by the lysing tumor cells [96]. Although viral oncolytics have not yet demonstrated significant efficacy either as standalone treatments or in combination with other therapies for GBM, there is considerable potential to explore various viral vector types, delivery methods, patient subsets, and combinatorial strategies with other immunotherapies.

Adenoviruses are a class of viral oncolytics utilized in the treatment of GBM. One notable adenoviral vector is aglatimagene besadenovec (AdV-tk), which incorporates herpes simplex virus (HSV) thymidine kinase. When AdV-tk is injected into the tumor environment, it preferentially infects tumor cells. Subsequent administration of anti-HSV drugs like valacyclovir results in targeted tumor cell death [97]. In a phase IIa study (NCT00589875), patients with GBM who received AdV-tk followed by valacyclovir had a median post-therapy survival of 16.7 months, compared to 13.7 months in the control group [98]. Another phase II study (NCT00870181) explored intra-arterial infusion of AdV-TK followed by ganciclovir and mannitol to disrupt the blood-brain barrier in patients with recurrent GBM. This approach resulted in significantly longer median progression-free survival (34.9 weeks vs. 7.4 weeks; $p < 0.001$) and OS (45.7 weeks vs. 8.6 weeks; $p < 0.001$) compared to controls [99]. Another adenovirus-based therapy, Ad-RTs-IL-12, contains an interleukin-12 (IL-12) transgene. IL-12 has antineoplastic properties but is highly toxic when administered systemically. The Ad-RTs-IL-12 vector allows for ligand-inducible expression of IL-12 through velemidex, limiting IL-12 effects to the tumor microenvironment [72, 100]. A phase I study (NCT04006119) confirmed the safety of Ad-RTs-IL-12, velemidex, and nivolumab [100].

16.1.4 CAR-T Cell Therapy

CAR-T cell therapy is an innovative approach for treating GBM by targeting tumor-specific antigens. This therapy consists of extracting T cells from a patient's blood, genetically modifying to express chimeric antigen receptors (CARs), that recognize specific antigens on tumor cells, and then reinfusing these engineered cells into the patient [96, 101]. CARs are synthetic proteins that combine an antigen-recognition domain with T cell activating domains, enabling targeted immune responses against tumor cells. While CAR-T therapy has shown success in hematologic cancers and is FDA-approved for some lymphomas and leukemias, its application in GBM is still under investigation [102].

A Phase I/II trial (NCT01454596) with anti-EGFRvIII CAR-T cells in recurrent EGFRvIII-positive GBM patients noted a patient death, possibly due to T cell-induced increased pulmonary vascular permeability, and no significant clinical improvement [103]. Another Phase I study (NCT02209376) reported a median OS of around 8 months, with CAR-T-EGFRvIII cells detectable for up to 30 days post-infusion [104].

IL13Rα2, overexpressed in multiple malignancies and 75% of GBM cases, represents another target. A pilot study of intracranially delivered IL13Rα2-targeted CAR-T cells showed temporary brain inflammation but no survival benefit, despite transient responses [105].

HER2, overexpressed in many cancers including up to 80% of GBMs, was targeted in a Phase I study (NCT01109095) where patients showed a median overall survival of 11.1 months from first T cell infusion [106]. However, presence of HER2 on normal tissues poses toxicity risks [107]. Other targets, including B7-H3, CD147 (EMMPRIN), disialoganglioside GD2, and chlorotoxin (CLTX), are also under investigation.

Cytokine release syndrome (CRS) and immune effector cell-associated neurotoxicity (ICANS) are common complications of CAR-T therapy, with the latter potentially causing fatal cerebral oedema [108]. Due to the immunosuppressive microenvironment and limited leukocyte migration through the blood–brain barrier, direct administration of CAR-T cells into the tumor has been proposed, though the risk of ICANS remains uncertain [109].

CAR-Natural Killer (NK) cells are also being studied for their ability to recognize multiple tumor antigens and potentially avoid CRS [110]. HER2-specific CAR-NK cells have demonstrated anti-GBM activity, leading to a Phase I trial (NCT03383978) [111]. However, NK cells face barriers such as lower numbers in peripheral blood and challenges in crossing the blood–brain barrier [112]. They must be irradiated before infusion to prevent secondary malignancy, which limits their lifespan for antitumor activity [110]. In summary, while CAR-T therapy is a promising treatment for GBM, questions remain about the optimal antigen targets, delivery methods, and therapy duration before it can become an effective treatment for glioblastoma.

16.1.5 Other Approaches in Glioblastoma Treatment

16.1.5.1 Tumor Treating Fields (TTFs)

Tumor treating fields (TTFs) represent an additional treatment for newly diagnosed GBM, in combination with TMZ. TTFs consist of four transducer arrays applied for at least 18 h daily to the shaved scalp and connected to a portable device [113]. In a phase III trial (EF-11) comparing TTFs with physician's-choice chemotherapy in the recurrent setting, TTFs demonstrated efficacy, with an objective response rate of 14% compared with 9.6% of chemotherapy. However, no improvement in overall survival was demonstrated [114]. Conversely, in a phase III trial on 695 newly diagnosed GBM (EF-14), a benefit in progression-free survival and overall survival was seen in the combination TMZ/TTFs group versus TMZ alone (6.7 versus 4.0 months, $p < 0.001$, and 20.9 versus 16.0 months, $p < 0.001$, respectively) [115]. With regard to tolerability, treatment with TTFs was not associated with poorer quality of life, as reported in a dedicated sub-analysis of the EF-14 trial [116].

16.1.5.2 Focused Ultrasound Therapy

Focused ultrasound (FUS) therapy uses sound waves to treat various medical conditions, including GBM. It can operate at high or low intensity, each with distinct mechanisms and applications:

High-Intensity Focused Ultrasound (HIFU): Utilizes thermal effects to cause protein denaturation and DNA fragmentation, leading to coagulative necrosis of tumor cells [117, 118].

Low-Intensity Focused Ultrasound (LIFU): Relies on acoustic cavitation to temporarily open the blood-brain barrier (BBB), enhancing drug delivery to brain tumors. LIFU is being explored in multiple clinical trials for its potential to improve the outcome in GBM [119]. Sonodynamic therapy, which combines LIFU with sonosensitising agents like 5-ALA, is also under investigation for its ability to generate reactive oxygen species and kill tumor cells [120].

16.1.5.3 Magnetic Nanoparticles

Magnetic nanoparticles are being developed for their potential to cross the BBB and deliver therapeutic agents directly to GBM cells:

Biomimetic Therapeutic Nanoparticles: These nanoparticles, mimicking glioma cells, can convert lactate to pyruvic acid and hydrogen peroxide, inducing cell cycle arrest and tumor cell death. They show promise in preclinical models for their stability and targeting efficiency [121].

Gold Nanoparticles: Designed to target the tight junction protein JAM-A, these nanoparticles can temporarily disrupt the BBB, allowing enhanced delivery of chemotherapy drugs like paclitaxel to brain tumors when activated by a laser [122].

16.1.5.4 Carbon Ion Radiotherapy (CIRT)

CIRT involves using carbon ions to deliver high-energy radiation, causing severe double-strand breaks in DNA. This method is particularly attractive against radioresistant tumors like GBM and is being explored in several international clinical trials [123]. CIRT offers the advantage of delivering higher radiation doses precisely to the tumor while sparing surrounding healthy tissue.

16.1.5.5 Surgically Targeted Radiation Therapy

Surgically targeted radiation therapy aims to deliver radiation at the time of surgery, potentially improving local tumor control:

Intraoperative Radiotherapy (IORT): Includes techniques like intraoperative electron radiotherapy (IOERT) and low-energy X-ray IORT (LEX-IORT), which deliver radiation during surgery but have not yet shown significant improvements in overall survival [124, 125].

Interstitial Brachytherapy (IBT): Uses radiation-emitting seeds implanted post-surgery to continue to deliver to the tumor site. GammaTile, a newer form of IBT, uses cesium-131 seeds in a collagen matrix to provide localized radiation therapy, showing promise in extending recurrence-free survival [126].

16.1.6 Convection Enhanced Delivery (CED)

CED is a method of delivering therapeutics directly to brain tumors by creating pressure gradients that force drugs through the interstitial spaces of the brain bypassing the BBB. CED is being explored for delivering various treatments, including conjugated toxins, liposomal carriers, and viral therapies [127].

References

1. Weller M, van den Bent M, Preusser M, et al. EANO guidelines on the diagnosis and treatment of diffuse gliomas of adulthood. Nat Rev Clin Oncol. 2021;18(3):170–86. https://doi.org/10.1038/s41571-020-00447-z.
2. Stupp R, Mason WP, van den Bent MJ, et al. Radiotherapy plus concomitant and adjuvant temozolomide for glioblastoma. N Engl J Med. 2005;352(10):987–96. https://doi.org/10.1056/NEJMoa043330.
3. Stupp R, Hegi ME, Mason WP, et al. Effects of radiotherapy with concomitant and adjuvant temozolomide versus radiotherapy alone on survival in glioblastoma in a randomised phase III study: 5-year analysis of the EORTC-NCIC trial. Lancet Oncol. 2009;10(5):459–66. https://doi.org/10.1016/S1470-2045(09)70025-7.
4. Lawrence YR, Li XA, el Naqa I, et al. Radiation dose–volume effects in the brain. Int J Radiat Oncol Biol Phys. 2010;76(3):S20–7. https://doi.org/10.1016/j.ijrobp.2009.02.091.

5. Mooi WJ. Radiation pathology: Farjado LF, Berthrong M, Anderson RE. Oxford University Press, 2001. ISBN 0 19 511023 4. J Clin Pathol. 2002;55(6):480.
6. Ellingson BM, Chung C, Pope WB, Boxerman JL, Kaufmann TJ. Pseudoprogression, radionecrosis, inflammation or true tumor progression? Challenges associated with glioblastoma response assessment in an evolving therapeutic landscape. J Neuro-Oncol. 2017;134(3):495–504. https://doi.org/10.1007/s11060-017-2375-2.
7. Taal W, Brandsma D, de Bruin HG, et al. Incidence of early pseudo-progression in a cohort of malignant glioma patients treated with chemoirradiation with temozolomide. Cancer. 2008;113(2):405–10. https://doi.org/10.1002/cncr.23562.
8. Galldiks N, Dunkl V, Stoffels G, et al. Diagnosis of pseudoprogression in patients with glioblastoma using O-(2-[18F]fluoroethyl)-l-tyrosine PET. Eur J Nucl Med Mol Imaging. 2015;42(5):685–95. https://doi.org/10.1007/s00259-014-2959-4.
9. Taylor C, Ekert JO, Sefcikova V, Fersht N, Samandouras G. Discriminators of pseudoprogression and true progression in high-grade gliomas: a systematic review and meta-analysis. Sci Rep. 2022;12(1):13258. https://doi.org/10.1038/s41598-022-16726-x.
10. Hegi ME, Diserens AC, Gorlia T, et al. MGMT gene silencing and benefit from temozolomide in glioblastoma. N Engl J Med. 2005;352(10):997–1003. https://doi.org/10.1056/NEJMoa043331.
11. Newlands ES, Stevens MFG, Wedge SR, Wheelhouse RT, Brock C. Temozolomide: a review of its discovery, chemical properties, pre-clinical development and clinical trials. Cancer Treat Rev. 1997;23(1):35–61. https://doi.org/10.1016/S0305-7372(97)90019-0.
12. Agarwala SS, Kirkwood JM. Temozolomide, a novel alkylating agent with activity in the central nervous system, may improve the treatment of advanced metastatic melanoma. Oncologist. 2000;5(2):144–51. https://doi.org/10.1634/theoncologist.5-2-144.
13. Dixit S, Baker L, Walmsley V, Hingorani M. Temozolomide-related idiosyncratic and other uncommon toxicities: a systematic review. Anti-Cancer Drugs. 2012;23(10):1099–106. https://doi.org/10.1097/CAD.0b013e328356f5b0. https://journals.lww.com/anti-cancerdrugs/Fulltext/2012/11000/Temozolomide_related_idiosyncratic_and_other.11.aspx.
14. Clarke JL, Iwamoto FM, Sul J, et al. Randomized phase II trial of chemoradiotherapy followed by either dose-dense or metronomic temozolomide for newly diagnosed glioblastoma. J Clin Oncol. 2009;27(23):3861–7. https://doi.org/10.1200/JCO.2008.20.7944.
15. Kurzen H, Schmitt S, Näher H, Möhler T. Inhibition of angiogenesis by non-toxic doses of temozolomide. Anti-Cancer Drugs. 2003;14(7):515–22. https://doi.org/10.1097/00001813-200308000-00003. https://journals.lww.com/anti-cancerdrugs/Fulltext/2003/08000/Inhibition_of_angiogenesis_by_non_toxic_doses_of.3.aspx.
16. Wick A, Felsberg J, Steinbach JP, et al. Efficacy and tolerability of temozolomide in an alternating weekly regimen in patients with recurrent glioma. J Clin Oncol. 2007;25(22):3357–61. https://doi.org/10.1200/JCO.2007.10.7722.
17. Balana C, Mesia Barroso C, Berron SDB, et al. Randomized phase IIb clinical trial of continuation or non-continuation with six cycles of temozolomide after the first six cycles of standard first-line treatment in patients with glioblastoma: a Spanish research group in neuro-oncology (GEINO) trial. JCO. 2019;37(15_suppl):2001. https://doi.org/10.1200/JCO.2019.37.15_suppl.2001.
18. Gilbert MR, Wang M, Aldape KD, et al. Dose-dense temozolomide for newly diagnosed glioblastoma: a randomized phase III clinical trial. J Clin Oncol. 2013;31(32):4085–91. https://doi.org/10.1200/JCO.2013.49.6968.
19. Balana C, Vaz MA, Manuel Sepúlveda J, et al. A phase II randomized, multicenter, open-label trial of continuing adjuvant temozolomide beyond 6 cycles in patients with glioblastoma (GEINO 14-01). Neuro-Oncology. 2020;22(12):1851–61. https://doi.org/10.1093/neuonc/noaa107.
20. Singh N, Miner A, Hennis L, Mittal S. Mechanisms of temozolomide resistance in glioblastoma—a comprehensive review. Cancer Drug Resist. 2021;4(1):17–43. https://doi.org/10.20517/cdr.2020.79.
21. Chinot OL, Wick W, Mason W, et al. Bevacizumab plus radiotherapy–temozolomide for newly diagnosed glioblastoma. N Engl J Med. 2014;370(8):709–22. https://doi.org/10.1056/NEJMoa1308345.
22. Gilbert MR, Dignam JJ, Armstrong TS, et al. A randomized trial of bevacizumab for newly diagnosed glioblastoma. N Engl J Med. 2014;370(8):699–708. https://doi.org/10.1056/NEJMoa1308573.
23. Le Rhun E, Preusser M, Roth P, et al. Molecular targeted therapy of glioblastoma. Cancer Treat Rev. 2019;80:101896. https://doi.org/10.1016/j.ctrv.2019.101896.
24. Nishikawa R, Ji XD, Harmon RC, et al. A mutant epidermal growth factor receptor common in human glioma confers enhanced tumorigenicity. Proc Natl Acad Sci. 1994;91(16):7727–31. https://doi.org/10.1073/pnas.91.16.7727.
25. Weller M, Butowski N, Tran DD, et al. Rindopepimut with temozolomide for patients with newly diagnosed, EGFRvIII-expressing glioblastoma (ACT IV): a randomised, double-blind, international phase 3 trial. Lancet Oncol. 2017;18(10):1373–85.
26. van Den Bent M, Gan HK, Lassman AB, et al. Efficacy of depatuxizumab mafodotin (ABT-414) monotherapy in patients with EGFR-amplified, recurrent glioblastoma: results from a multi-center,

international study. Cancer Chemother Pharmacol. 2017;80(6):1209–17.
27. Van Den Bent M, Eoli M, Sepulveda JM, et al. INTELLANCE 2/EORTC 1410 randomized phase II study of Depatux-M alone and with temozolomide vs temozolomide or lomustine in recurrent EGFR amplified glioblastoma. Neuro-Oncology. 2020;22(5):684–93.
28. Reardon DA, Lassman AB, Van Den Bent M, et al. Efficacy and safety results of ABT-414 in combination with radiation and temozolomide in newly diagnosed glioblastoma. Neuro-Oncology. 2017;19(7):965–75.
29. Choi SW, Jung HA, Cho HJ, et al. A multicenter, phase II trial of GC1118, a novel anti-EGFR antibody, for recurrent glioblastoma patients with amplification. Cancer Med. 2023;12(15):15788–96. https://doi.org/10.1002/cam4.6213.
30. Rosenthal MA, Balana C, van Linde ME, et al. ATIM-49 (LTBK-01). AMG 596, A NOVEL ANTI-EGFRVIII BISPECIFIC T CELL ENGAGER (BITE®) MOLECULE FOR THE TREATMENT OF GLIOBLASTOMA (GBM): PLANNED INTERIM ANALYSIS IN RECURRENT GBM (RGBM). Neuro-Oncology. 2019;21(Supplement_6):vi283. https://doi.org/10.1093/neuonc/noz219.1195.
31. Clarke JL, Molinaro AM, Phillips JJ, et al. A single-institution phase II trial of radiation, temozolomide, erlotinib, and bevacizumab for initial treatment of glioblastoma. Neuro-Oncology. 2014;16(7):984–90. https://doi.org/10.1093/neuonc/nou029.
32. Raizer JJ, Giglio P, Hu J, et al. A phase II study of bevacizumab and erlotinib after radiation and temozolomide in MGMT unmethylated GBM patients. J Neuro-Oncol. 2016;126(1):185–92. https://doi.org/10.1007/s11060-015-1958-z.
33. Peereboom DM, Ahluwalia MS, Ye X, et al. NABTT 0502: a phase II and pharmacokinetic study of erlotinib and sorafenib for patients with progressive or recurrent glioblastoma multiforme. Neuro-Oncology. 2013;15(4):490–6. https://doi.org/10.1093/neuonc/nos322.
34. Chakravarti A, Wang M, Robins HI, et al. RTOG 0211: a phase 1/2 study of radiation therapy with concurrent gefitinib for newly diagnosed glioblastoma patients. Int J Radiat Oncol Biol Phys. 2013;85(5):1206–11. https://doi.org/10.1016/j.ijrobp.2012.10.008.
35. Reardon DA, Nabors LB, Mason WP, et al. Phase I/randomized phase II study of afatinib, an irreversible ErbB family blocker, with or without protracted temozolomide in adults with recurrent glioblastoma. Neuro-Oncology. 2015;17(3):430–9. https://doi.org/10.1093/neuonc/nou160.
36. Sepúlveda-Sánchez JM, Vaz MÁ, Balañá C, et al. Phase II trial of dacomitinib, a pan–human EGFR tyrosine kinase inhibitor, in recurrent glioblastoma patients with EGFR amplification. Neuro-Oncology. 2017;19(11):1522–31. https://doi.org/10.1093/neuonc/nox105.
37. Froelich W. A new drug targeting EGFR in glioblastoma tumors. Oncol Times. 2021;43(24):21–2. https://journals.lww.com/oncology-times/fulltext/2021/12200/a_new_drug_targeting_egfr_in_glioblastoma_tumors.8.aspx.
38. Kizilbash SH, Jaeckle KA, Mrugala MM, et al. First-in-human phase 1 trial of the safety, tolerability, pharmacokinetics, and preliminary antitumor activity of WSD0922-Fu: initial report from dose escalation cohort. J Clin Oncol. 2023;41(16_suppl):3109. https://doi.org/10.1200/JCO.2023.41.16_suppl.3109.
39. Nakajima N, Nobusawa S, Nakata S, et al. BRAF V600E, TERT promoter mutations and CDKN2A/B homozygous deletions are frequent in epithelioid glioblastomas: a histological and molecular analysis focusing on intratumoral heterogeneity. Brain Pathol. 2018;28(5):663–73. https://doi.org/10.1111/bpa.12572.
40. Kaley T, Touat M, Subbiah V, et al. BRAF inhibition in BRAF(V600)-mutant gliomas: results from the VE-BASKET study. J Clin Oncol. 2018;36(35):3477–84. https://doi.org/10.1200/JCO.2018.78.9990.
41. Eric B, Hansford JR, Luisa GM, et al. Dabrafenib plus trametinib in pediatric glioma with BRAF V600 mutations. N Engl J Med. 2023;389(12):1108–20. https://doi.org/10.1056/NEJMoa2303815.
42. Wen PY, Stein A, van den Bent M, et al. Dabrafenib plus trametinib in patients with BRAFV600E-mutant low-grade and high-grade glioma (ROAR): a multicentre, open-label, single-arm, phase 2, basket trial. Lancet Oncol. 2022;23(1):53–64. https://doi.org/10.1016/S1470-2045(21)00578-7.
43. Schreck K, Strowd R, Nabors LB, et al. CTNI-60. PRELIMINARY RESULTS OF BINIMETINIB AND ENCORAFENIB IN ADULTS WITH RECURRENT BRAF V600E-MUTATED HIGH-GRADE GLIOMA. Neuro-Oncology. 2022;24(Supplement_7):vii86. https://doi.org/10.1093/neuonc/noac209.325.
44. Chen C, Zhu S, Zhang X, et al. Targeting the synthetic vulnerability of PTEN-deficient glioblastoma cells with MCL1 inhibitors. Mol Cancer Ther. 2020;19(10):2001–11. https://doi.org/10.1158/1535-7163.MCT-20-0099.
45. Ma DJ, Galanis E, Anderson SK, et al. A phase II trial of everolimus, temozolomide, and radiotherapy in patients with newly diagnosed glioblastoma: NCCTG N057K. Neuro-Oncology. 2015;17(9):1261–9. https://doi.org/10.1093/neuonc/nou328.
46. Wick W, Gorlia T, Bady P, et al. Phase II study of radiotherapy and temsirolimus versus radiochemotherapy with temozolomide in patients with newly diagnosed glioblastoma without MGMT promoter hypermethylation (EORTC 26082). Clin Cancer Res. 2016;22(19):4797–806. https://doi.org/10.1158/1078-0432.CCR-15-3153.

47. Wen PY, de Groot JF, Battiste J, et al. Paxalisib in patients with newly diagnosed glioblastoma with unmethylated MGMT promoter status: final phase 2 study results. J Clin Oncol. 2022;40(16_suppl):2047. https://doi.org/10.1200/JCO.2022.40.16_suppl.2047.
48. Lee EQ, Trippa L, Fell G, et al. Preliminary results of the abemaciclib arm in the individualized screening trial of innovative glioblastoma therapy (INSIGhT): a phase II platform trial using Bayesian adaptive randomization. J Clin Oncol. 2021;39(15_suppl):2014. https://doi.org/10.1200/JCO.2021.39.15_suppl.2014.
49. Kreisl TN, Kim L, Moore K, et al. Phase II trial of single-agent bevacizumab followed by bevacizumab plus irinotecan at tumor progression in recurrent glioblastoma. J Clin Oncol. 2009;27(5):740–5. https://doi.org/10.1200/JCO.2008.16.3055.
50. Schmieder R, Hoffmann J, Becker M, et al. Regorafenib (BAY 73-4506): antitumor and antimetastatic activities in preclinical models of colorectal cancer. Int J Cancer. 2014;135(6):1487–96.
51. Abou-Elkacem L, Arns S, Brix G, et al. Regorafenib inhibits growth, angiogenesis, and metastasis in a highly aggressive, orthotopic colon cancer model. Mol Cancer Ther. 2013;12(7):1322–31.
52. Wilhelm S, Dumas J, Adnane L, et al. A new oral multikinase inhibitor of angiogenic, stromal and oncogenic receptor tyrosine kinases with potent preclinical antitumor activity. Int J Cancer. 2011;129(1):245–55.
53. Zopf D, Fichtner I, Bhargava A, et al. Pharmacologic activity and pharmacokinetics of metabolites of regorafenib in preclinical models. Cancer Med. 2016;5(11):3176–85.
54. Lombardi G, De Salvo GL, Brandes AA, et al. Regorafenib compared with lomustine in patients with relapsed glioblastoma (REGOMA): a multicentre, open-label, randomised, controlled, phase 2 trial. Lancet Oncol. 2019;20(1):110–9. https://doi.org/10.1016/S1470-2045(18)30675-2.
55. Lombardi G, Caccese M, Padovan M, et al. Regorafenib in recurrent glioblastoma patients: a large and monocentric real-life study. Cancers (Basel). 2021;13(18):4731. https://doi.org/10.3390/cancers13184731.
56. Kebir S, Rauschenbach L, Radbruch A, et al. Regorafenib in patients with recurrent high-grade astrocytoma. J Cancer Res Clin Oncol. 2019;145(4):1037–42. https://doi.org/10.1007/s00432-019-02868-5.
57. Zeiner PS, Kinzig M, Divé I, et al. Regorafenib CSF penetration, efficacy, and MRI patterns in recurrent malignant glioma patients. J Clin Med. 2019;8(12):2031. https://doi.org/10.3390/jcm8122031.
58. Tzaridis T, Gepfner-Tuma I, Hirsch S, et al. Regorafenib in advanced high-grade glioma: a retrospective bicentric analysis. Neuro-Oncology. 2019;21(7):954–5. https://doi.org/10.1093/neuonc/noz071.
59. Treiber H, von der Brelie C, Malinova V, Mielke D, Rohde V, Chapuy CI. Regorafenib for recurrent high-grade glioma: a unicentric retrospective analysis of feasibility, efficacy, and toxicity. Neurosurg Rev. 2022;45(5):3201–8. https://doi.org/10.1007/s10143-022-01826-z.
60. Werner JM, Wolf L, Tscherpel C, et al. Efficacy and tolerability of regorafenib in pretreated patients with progressive CNS grade 3 or 4 gliomas. J Neurooncol. 2022;159(2):309–17. https://doi.org/10.1007/s11060-022-04066-9.
61. Rudà R, Bruno F, Pellerino A, et al. Observational real-life study on regorafenib in recurrent glioblastoma: does dose reduction reduce toxicity while maintaining the efficacy? J Neuro-Oncol. 2022;160(2):389–402. https://doi.org/10.1007/s11060-022-04155-9.
62. Bao S, Wu Q, McLendon RE, et al. Glioma stem cells promote radioresistance by preferential activation of the DNA damage response. Nature. 2006;444(7120):756–60. https://doi.org/10.1038/nature05236.
63. Rose M, Burgess JT, O'Byrne K, Richard DJ, Bolderson E. PARP inhibitors: clinical relevance, mechanisms of action and tumor resistance. Front Cell Dev Biol. 2020;8:564601. https://www.frontiersin.org/journals/cell-and-developmental-biology/articles/10.3389/fcell.2020.564601.
64. Sim HW, Galanis E, Khasraw M. PARP inhibitors in Glioma: a review of therapeutic opportunities. Cancers (Basel). 2022;14(4):1003. https://doi.org/10.3390/cancers14041003.
65. Sim HW, McDonald KL, Lwin Z, et al. A randomized phase II trial of veliparib, radiotherapy, and temozolomide in patients with unmethylated MGMT glioblastoma: the VERTU study. Neuro-Oncology. 2021;23(10):1736–49. https://doi.org/10.1093/neuonc/noab111.
66. James L, Vanna C-S, Rene G, et al. Combined nivolumab and ipilimumab or monotherapy in untreated melanoma. N Engl J Med. 2015;373(1):23–34. https://doi.org/10.1056/NEJMoa1504030.
67. Brahmer J, Reckamp KL, Baas P, et al. Nivolumab versus docetaxel in advanced squamous-cell non–small-cell lung cancer. N Engl J Med. 2015;373(2):123–35. https://doi.org/10.1056/NEJMoa1504627.
68. Motzer RJ, Escudier B, McDermott DF, et al. Nivolumab versus everolimus in advanced renal-cell carcinoma. N Engl J Med. 2015;373(19):1803–13. https://doi.org/10.1056/NEJMoa1510665.
69. van den Bent MJ, Geurts M, French PJ, et al. Primary brain tumours in adults. Lancet. 2023;402(10412):1564–79. https://doi.org/10.1016/S0140-6736(23)01054-1.
70. Wen PY, Weller M, Lee EQ, et al. Glioblastoma in adults: a Society for Neuro-Oncology (SNO) and European Society of Neuro-Oncology (EANO) consensus review on current management and future

directions. Neuro-Oncology. 2020;22(8):1073–113. https://doi.org/10.1093/neuonc/noaa106.
71. Robert C. A decade of immune-checkpoint inhibitors in cancer therapy. Nat Commun. 2020;11(1):3801. https://doi.org/10.1038/s41467-020-17670-y.
72. Sener U, Ruff MW, Campian JL. Immunotherapy in glioblastoma: current approaches and future perspectives. Int J Mol Sci. 2022;23(13):7046. https://doi.org/10.3390/ijms23137046.
73. Omuro A, Brandes AA, Carpentier AF, et al. Radiotherapy combined with nivolumab or temozolomide for newly diagnosed glioblastoma with unmethylated MGMT promoter: an international randomized phase III trial. Neuro-Oncology. 2023;25(1):123–34. https://doi.org/10.1093/neuonc/noac099.
74. Lim M, Weller M, Idbaih A, et al. Phase III trial of chemoradiotherapy with temozolomide plus nivolumab or placebo for newly diagnosed glioblastoma with methylated MGMT promoter. Neuro-Oncology. 2022;24(11):1935–49. https://doi.org/10.1093/neuonc/noac116.
75. Woroniecka K, Chongsathidkiet P, Rhodin K, et al. T-cell exhaustion signatures vary with tumor type and are severe in glioblastoma. Clin Cancer Res. 2018;24(17):4175–86. https://doi.org/10.1158/1078-0432.CCR-17-1846.
76. Nduom EK, Wei J, Yaghi NK, et al. PD-L1 expression and prognostic impact in glioblastoma. Neuro-Oncology. 2016;18(2):195–205. https://doi.org/10.1093/neuonc/nov172.
77. Jackson CM, Choi J, Lim M. Mechanisms of immunotherapy resistance: lessons from glioblastoma. Nat Immunol. 2019;20(9):1100–9. https://doi.org/10.1038/s41590-019-0433-y.
78. Lee EQ. Immune checkpoint inhibitors in GBM. J Neuro-Oncol. 2021;155(1):1–11. https://doi.org/10.1007/s11060-021-03859-8.
79. Chongsathidkiet P, Jackson C, Koyama S, et al. Sequestration of T cells in bone marrow in the setting of glioblastoma and other intracranial tumors. Nat Med. 2018;24(9):1459–68. https://doi.org/10.1038/s41591-018-0135-2.
80. Touat M, Li YY, Boynton AN, et al. Mechanisms and therapeutic implications of hypermutation in gliomas. Nature. 2020;580(7804):517–23. https://doi.org/10.1038/s41586-020-2209-9.
81. Saxena M, van der Burg SH, Melief CJM, Bhardwaj N. Therapeutic cancer vaccines. Nat Rev Cancer. 2021;21(6):360–78. https://doi.org/10.1038/s41568-021-00346-0.
82. Binder DC, Ladomersky E, Lenzen A, et al. Lessons learned from rindopepimut treatment in patients with EGFRvIII-expressing glioblastoma. Transl Cancer Res. 2018;7(Suppl 4):S510–3. https://tcr.amegroups.org/article/view/20301. Accessed 1 Jan 2018.
83. Fenstermaker RA, Ciesielski MJ, Qiu J, et al. Clinical study of a survivin long peptide vaccine (SurVaxM) in patients with recurrent malignant glioma. Cancer Immunol Immunother. 2016;65(11):1339–52. https://doi.org/10.1007/s00262-016-1890-x.
84. Spira A, Hansen AR, Harb WA, et al. Multicenter, open-label, phase I study of DSP-7888 dosing emulsion in patients with advanced malignancies. Target Oncol. 2021;16(4):461–9. https://doi.org/10.1007/s11523-021-00813-6.
85. Migliorini D, Dutoit V, Allard M, et al. Phase I/II trial testing safety and immunogenicity of the multipeptide IMA950/poly-ICLC vaccine in newly diagnosed adult malignant astrocytoma patients. Neuro-Oncology. 2019;21(7):923–33. https://doi.org/10.1093/neuonc/noz040.
86. Palucka K, Banchereau J. Cancer immunotherapy via dendritic cells. Nat Rev Cancer. 2012;12(4):265–77. https://doi.org/10.1038/nrc3258.
87. Neth BJ, Webb MJ, Parney IF, Sener UT. The current status, challenges, and future potential of therapeutic vaccination in glioblastoma. Pharmaceutics. 2023;15(4):1134. https://doi.org/10.3390/pharmaceutics15041134.
88. Liau LM, Ashkan K, Tran DD, et al. First results on survival from a large phase 3 clinical trial of an autologous dendritic cell vaccine in newly diagnosed glioblastoma. J Transl Med. 2018;16(1):142. https://doi.org/10.1186/s12967-018-1507-6.
89. Preusser M, van den Bent MJ. Autologous tumor lysate-loaded dendritic cell vaccination (DCVax-L) in glioblastoma: breakthrough or fata morgana? Neuro-Oncology. 2023;25(4):631–4. https://doi.org/10.1093/neuonc/noac281.
90. Liau LM, Ashkan K, Brem S, et al. Association of autologous tumor lysate-loaded dendritic cell vaccination with extension of survival among patients with newly diagnosed and recurrent glioblastoma: a phase 3 prospective externally controlled cohort trial. JAMA Oncol. 2023;9(1):112–21. https://doi.org/10.1001/jamaoncol.2022.5370.
91. Wen PY, Reardon DA, Armstrong TS, et al. A randomized double-blind placebo-controlled phase II trial of dendritic cell vaccine ICT-107 in newly diagnosed patients with glioblastoma. Clin Cancer Res. 2019;25(19):5799–807. https://doi.org/10.1158/1078-0432.CCR-19-0261.
92. Buchroithner J, Erhart F, Pichler J, et al. Audencel immunotherapy based on dendritic cells has no effect on overall and progression-free survival in newly diagnosed glioblastoma: a phase II randomized trial. Cancers (Basel). 2018;10(10):372. https://doi.org/10.3390/cancers10100372.
93. Cho DY, Yang WK, Lee HC, et al. Adjuvant immunotherapy with whole-cell lysate dendritic cells vaccine for glioblastoma multiforme: a phase II clinical trial. World Neurosurg. 2012;77(5):736–44. https://doi.org/10.1016/j.wneu.2011.08.020.
94. Hilf N, Kuttruff-Coqui S, Frenzel K, et al. Actively personalized vaccination trial for newly diagnosed glioblastoma. Nature. 2019;565(7738):240–5. https://doi.org/10.1038/s41586-018-0810-y.

95. Keskin DB, Anandappa AJ, Sun J, et al. Neoantigen vaccine generates intratumoral T cell responses in phase Ib glioblastoma trial. Nature. 2019;565(7738):234–9. https://doi.org/10.1038/s41586-018-0792-9.
96. Webb MJ, Sener U, Vile RG. Current status and challenges of oncolytic virotherapy for the treatment of glioblastoma. Pharmaceuticals (Basel). 2023;16(6):793. https://doi.org/10.3390/ph16060793.
97. Eastham JA, Chen SH, Sehgal I, et al. Prostate cancer gene therapy: herpes simplex virus thymidine kinase gene transduction followed by ganciclovir in mouse and human prostate cancer models. Hum Gene Ther. 1996;7(4):515–23. https://doi.org/10.1089/hum.1996.7.4-515.
98. Wheeler LA, Manzanera AG, Bell SD, et al. Phase II multicenter study of gene-mediated cytotoxic immunotherapy as adjuvant to surgical resection for newly diagnosed malignant glioma. Neuro-Oncology. 2016;18(8):1137–45. https://doi.org/10.1093/neuonc/now002.
99. Ji N, Weng D, Liu C, et al. Adenovirus-mediated delivery of herpes simplex virus thymidine kinase administration improves outcome of recurrent high-grade glioma. Oncotarget. 2016;7(4):4369–78. https://www.oncotarget.com/article/6737/text/. Accessed 1 Jan 2015.
100. Chiocca EA, Gelb AB, Chen CC, et al. Combined immunotherapy with controlled interleukin-12 gene therapy and immune checkpoint blockade in recurrent glioblastoma: an open-label, multi-institutional phase I trial. Neuro-Oncology. 2022;24(6):951–63. https://doi.org/10.1093/neuonc/noab271.
101. Sterner RC, Sterner RM. CAR-T cell therapy: current limitations and potential strategies. Blood Cancer J. 2021;11(4):69. https://doi.org/10.1038/s41408-021-00459-7.
102. Bagley SJ, Desai AS, Linette GP, June CH, O'Rourke DM. CAR T-cell therapy for glioblastoma: recent clinical advances and future challenges. Neuro-Oncology. 2018;20(11):1429–38. https://doi.org/10.1093/neuonc/noy032.
103. Goff SL, Morgan RA, Yang JC, et al. Pilot trial of adoptive transfer of chimeric antigen receptor–transduced T cells targeting EGFRvIII in patients with glioblastoma. J Immunother. 2019;42(4):126–35. https://journals.lww.com/immunotherapy-journal/fulltext/2019/05000/pilot_trial_of_adoptive_transfer_of_chimeric.4.aspx.
104. O'Rourke DM, Nasrallah MP, Desai A, et al. A single dose of peripherally infused EGFRvIII-directed CAR T cells mediates antigen loss and induces adaptive resistance in patients with recurrent glioblastoma. Sci Transl Med. 2017;9(399):eaaa0984. https://doi.org/10.1126/scitranslmed.aaa0984.
105. Brown CE, Badie B, Barish ME, et al. Bioactivity and safety of IL13Rα2-redirected chimeric antigen receptor CD8+ T cells in patients with recurrent glioblastoma. Clin Cancer Res. 2015;21(18):4062–72. https://doi.org/10.1158/1078-0432.CCR-15-0428.
106. Ahmed N, Brawley V, Hegde M, et al. HER2-specific chimeric antigen receptor–modified virus-specific T cells for progressive glioblastoma: a phase 1 dose-escalation trial. JAMA Oncol. 2017;3(8):1094–101. https://doi.org/10.1001/jamaoncol.2017.0184.
107. Morgan RA, Yang JC, Kitano M, Dudley ME, Laurencot CM, Rosenberg SA. Case report of a serious adverse event following the administration of T cells transduced with a chimeric antigen receptor recognizing ERBB2. Mol Ther. 2010;18(4):843–51. https://doi.org/10.1038/mt.2010.24.
108. Grant SJ, Grimshaw AA, Silberstein J, et al. Clinical presentation, risk factors, and outcomes of immune effector cell-associated neurotoxicity syndrome following chimeric antigen receptor T cell therapy: a systematic review. Transplant Cell Ther. 2022;28(6):294–302. https://doi.org/10.1016/j.jtct.2022.03.006.
109. Brown CE, Alizadeh D, Starr R, et al. Regression of glioblastoma after chimeric antigen receptor T-cell therapy. N Engl J Med. 2016;375(26):2561–9. https://doi.org/10.1056/NEJMoa1610497.
110. Maggs L, Cattaneo G, Dal AE, Moghaddam AS, Ferrone S. CAR T cell-based immunotherapy for the treatment of glioblastoma. Front Neurosci. 2021;15:662064. https://www.frontiersin.org/journals/neuroscience/articles/10.3389/fnins.2021.662064.
111. Zhang C, Burger MC, Jennewein L, et al. ErbB2/HER2-specific NK cells for targeted therapy of glioblastoma. JNCI J Natl Cancer Inst. 2016;108(5):djv375. https://doi.org/10.1093/jnci/djv375.
112. Alkins R, Burgess A, Ganguly M, et al. Focused ultrasound delivers targeted immune cells to metastatic brain tumors. Cancer Res. 2013;73(6):1892–9. https://doi.org/10.1158/0008-5472.CAN-12-2609.
113. Hottinger AF, Pacheco P, Stupp R. Tumor treating fields: a novel treatment modality and its use in brain tumors. Neuro-Oncology. 2016;18(10):1338–49. https://doi.org/10.1093/neuonc/now182.
114. Stupp R, Wong ET, Kanner AA, et al. NovoTTF-100A versus physician's choice chemotherapy in recurrent glioblastoma: a randomised phase III trial of a novel treatment modality. Eur J Cancer. 2012;48(14):2192–202. https://doi.org/10.1016/j.ejca.2012.04.011.
115. Stupp R, Taillibert S, Kanner A, et al. Effect of tumor-treating fields plus maintenance temozolomide vs maintenance temozolomide alone on survival in patients with glioblastoma: a randomized clinical trial. JAMA. 2017;318(23):2306–16. https://doi.org/10.1001/jama.2017.18718.
116. Taphoorn MJB, Dirven L, Kanner AA, et al. Influence of treatment with tumor-treating fields on health-related quality of life of patients with newly diagnosed glioblastoma: a secondary analysis of a randomized clinical trial. JAMA Oncol.

2018;4(4):495–504. https://doi.org/10.1001/jamaoncol.2017.5082.

117. Hersh AM, Bhimreddy M, Weber-Levine C, et al. Applications of focused ultrasound for the treatment of glioblastoma: a new frontier. Cancers (Basel). 2022;14(19):4920. https://doi.org/10.3390/cancers14194920.

118. Elhelf IAS, Albahar H, Shah U, Oto A, Cressman E, Almekkawy M. High intensity focused ultrasound: the fundamentals, clinical applications and research trends. Diagn Interv Imaging. 2018;99(6):349–59. https://doi.org/10.1016/j.diii.2018.03.001.

119. Roberts JW, Powlovich L, Sheybani N, LeBlang S. Focused ultrasound for the treatment of glioblastoma. J Neuro-Oncol. 2022;157(2):237–47. https://doi.org/10.1007/s11060-022-03974-0.

120. D'Ammando A, Raspagliesi L, Gionso M, et al. Sonodynamic therapy for the treatment of intracranial gliomas. J Clin Med. 2021;10(5):1101. https://doi.org/10.3390/jcm10051101.

121. Lu G, Wang X, Li F, et al. Engineered biomimetic nanoparticles achieve targeted delivery and efficient metabolism-based synergistic therapy against glioblastoma. Nat Commun. 2022;13(1):4214. https://doi.org/10.1038/s41467-022-31799-y.

122. Noorani I, de la Rosa J. Breaking barriers for glioblastoma with a path to enhanced drug delivery. Nat Commun. 2023;14(1):5909. https://doi.org/10.1038/s41467-023-41694-9.

123. Malouff TD, Peterson JL, Mahajan A, Trifiletti DM. Carbon ion radiotherapy in the treatment of gliomas: a review. J Neuro-Oncol. 2019;145(2):191–9. https://doi.org/10.1007/s11060-019-03303-y.

124. van Solinge TS, Nieland L, Chiocca EA, Broekman MLD. Advances in local therapy for glioblastoma—taking the fight to the tumour. Nat Rev Neurol. 2022;18(4):221–36. https://doi.org/10.1038/s41582-022-00621-0.

125. Cifarelli CP, Jacobson GM. Intraoperative radiotherapy in brain malignancies: indications and outcomes in primary and metastatic brain tumors. Front Oncol. 2021;11:768168. https://www.frontiersin.org/journals/oncology/articles/10.3389/fonc.2021.768168.

126. Budnick HC, Richardson AM, Shiue K, et al. GammaTile for gliomas: a single-center case series. Cureus. 2021;13(11):e19390. https://doi.org/10.7759/cureus.19390.

127. Jahangiri A, Chin AT, Flanigan PM, Chen R, Bankiewicz K, Aghi MK. Convection-enhanced delivery in glioblastoma: a review of preclinical and clinical studies. J Neurosurg JNS. 2017;126(1):191–200. https://doi.org/10.3171/2016.1.JNS151591.

17 Radiation Oncology Treatments in Glioma Patients: From Standard Protocols to New Directions

Giuseppe Minniti, Raffaella De Pietro, Daniele Armocida, and Lucy Zaccaro

17.1 Introduction

The World Health Organization (WHO) 2021 classification of central nervous system (CNS) tumors (CNS5) [1] introduced significant updates, incorporating molecular markers alongside histopathological features to refine tumor classification, achieve the correct diagnosis and guide treatment. This, together with clinical features, has helped to distinguish between those diffuse gliomas that primarily occur in adults (*adult-type*) and those that occur primarily in children (*pediatric-type*), considering that these tumor groups are also prognostically distinct [2].

Radiotherapy is a crucial modality in the treatment of various cancers, including brain tumors such as gliomas [1–3]. Traditional radiation delivers beams of photons to destroy cancer cells and reduce tumor size. The treatment is delivered to the patient through linear accelerators (LINACs) that, accelerating electrons to very high speeds through electromagnetic waves, generate high-energy X-rays (photons). These photons are directed at the tumor while sparing the surrounding healthy tissue, even though a small amount of it will also get irradiated at lower doses. Advances in imaging and technology have enabled more precise tumor localization and dose delivery, thus reducing the volume of health nearby tissue exposed to high radiation doses [3].

Radiation techniques have evolved throughout the years, from three-dimensional conformal RT (3D-CRT) to more precise techniques. Among these, intensity-modulated radiation therapy (IMRT) reduces the exposure to healthy tissue modulating the beam intensity. Volumetric arc therapy (VMAT) is an advanced form of IMRT that delivers radiation in a continuous arc around the patient, further enhancing precision and treatment efficiency. Furthermore, the use of appropriate image guided RT (IGRT) systems, using either orthogonal X-rays or cone beam computed tomography (CBCT), allows to achieve high-precise patient positioning during treatment and, thus, to reduce set-up margins [4]. In recent years, proton therapy centers have increased in

G. Minniti (✉)
Department of Radiological Sciences, Oncology and Anatomical Pathology, "Sapienza" University of Rome, Rome, RM, Italy

IRCCS Neuromed, Pozzilli, Isernia (IS), Italy
e-mail: giuseppe.minniti@uniroma1.it

R. De Pietro · L. Zaccaro
Department of Radiological Sciences, Oncology and Anatomical Pathology, "Sapienza" University of Rome, Rome, RM, Italy

D. Armocida
Neurosurgery Unit, Dept. Neuroscience "Rita Levi Montalcini", Università degli studi di Torino, Torino, TO, Italy

D. Armocida et al. (eds.), *Neurosurgery's Frontline Role in Gliomas Treatment*,
https://doi.org/10.1007/978-3-031-81850-9_17

numbers. Proton beam therapy offers superior precision of dose delivery, reducing the exposure to surrounding healthy tissues and potentially lowering the risk of side effects. This makes it particularly beneficial for treating tumors in sensitive or hard-to-reach areas and for pediatric patients. However, due to its higher cost and limited availability, proton therapy is used less frequently than conventional photon therapy. The adaptive radiotherapy (ART or 4D-RT) exploits IGRT systems to modify the treatment plan in response to changes in the patient's anatomy or tumor size during treatment. This ensures that the radiation dose continues to be accurately targeted at the tumor while sparing healthy tissues as much as possible.

17.2 Fundamentals of Radiation Oncology

Among the radiotherapy target volume concepts, three major definitions are identified, as illustrated in Fig. 17.1:

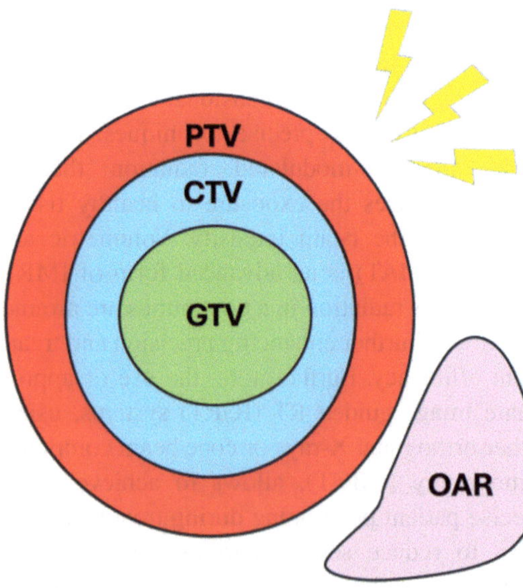

Fig. 17.1 Schematic representation of target volumes for gliomas radiotherapy

- *GTV* (Gross Tumor Volume), the visible macroscopic tumor;
- *CTV* (Clinical Target Volume), an expansion of GTV, which accounts for microscopical extension of the tumor beyond the GTV;
- *PTV* (Planning Target Volume), an expansion of CTV, which accounts for daily set-up uncertainties and organ motion.

The organs at risk (OARs) are the healthy tissues near the target, whose irradiation could cause damages; while treating brain cancer is important to delineate critical structures such as the brainstem, optic nerves, chiasm, and cochleae. Constraints are dose limit values for OARs to take into consideration while making a treatment plan, based on clinical evidence and guidelines to minimize the risk of both acute and long-term radiation-induced damage. For example, the maximum dose (Dmax) received by any point in the brainstem should generally not exceed 54 Gy, while the mean dose (Dmean) should be kept below 45 Gy [5].

A fractionation scheme refers to how the total dose of radiation—measured in Gray (Gy)—is divided into smaller fractions (treatment sessions), over a specific period. There are different fractionation schemes, according to tumor location, size and radio-sensibility:

- *Conventional Fractionation (cFRT)*: the total dose is delivered in 1.8–2.0 Gy per fraction, 5 days a week over several weeks (e.g., 60 Gy delivered in 30 fractions of 2 Gy each).
- *Hypofractionation (HFRT)*: uses larger doses per fraction, reducing the number of treatment sessions (e.g., 40 Gy delivered in 15 fractions of 2.67 Gy each).
- *Hyperfractionation*: delivers smaller doses per fraction but increases the number of fractions and sometimes the frequency (e.g., twice daily).
- *Accelerated Fractionation*: delivers the total dose in a shorter overall time, often by increasing the number of fractions per week by treating twice on some days.
- *Stereotactic Radiotherapy (SRT) and Stereotactic Radiosurgery (SRS)*: SRT deliv-

ers very high doses per fraction in a small number of fractions (e.g., 54 Gy delivered in 3 fractions of 18 Gy each); SRS delivers a high dose in a single fraction (e.g., 24 Gy in 1 fraction).

When it comes to brain tumors, IMRT and VMAT represent the most used techniques, with treatment dose delivered using cFRT or HFRT schemes. SRT and SRS are mostly chosen in case of small tumors (e.g., schwannoma, brain metastasis) or for re-irradiation purposes.

17.3 Radiation Therapy in Grade 2 Adult-Type Diffuse Gliomas, IDH-Mutant

Grade 2 astrocytomas and oligodendrogliomas are treated with surgery in the first instance and maximal surgical resection, if safely feasible, is the best approach [6].

Younger patients (~40–45 years) who are asymptomatic or with pre-operative seizures only (managed with drug therapy), can go through observation alone after gross total resection (GTR). Adjuvant treatment is often used in low-grade gliomas (LGGs) patients with high-risk characteristics: post-surgical residual tumor, more than 40 years of age, large pre-operative tumor size (>5 cm), tumor crossing the midline [7].

In this adjuvant setting, the standard of care (SoC) consists of radiation treatment, given usually within 3 months after surgery, followed by chemotherapy. The use of chemotherapy alone is controversial and could be an option to reduce the risk of neurocognitive decline in patients with large tumor volumes [8].

Following the indications given by RTOG 9802 [9], RT followed by six cycles of PCV is considered the SoC for patients with grade 2 gliomas deemed to require post-surgical management (high-risk group). In this subgroup, better overall survival (OS) and progression-free survival (PFS) were observed after 3 years since randomization.

The PCV regimen consist in the administration of procarbazine (60 mg/m^2/day orally, days 8–21 of each cycle), lomustine (CCNU) (110 mg/m^2 orally, day 1 of each cycle), vincristine (1.4 mg/m^2 intravenously, days 8 and 29 of each cycle).

Adjuvant RT plus temozolomide (TMZ) given for 12 cycles (for 5 days every 28 days) is also a valid and less toxic alternative. In RTOG 0424 [10], the 3-year OS of patients treated with adjuvant TMZ was superior to the one of the historical control group treated with RT alone.

According to a recent study conducted on 103 patients [11], TMZ-based chemoradiation has been associated with survival benefit in patients with grade 2 IDH-mutant astrocytoma. However, it is suggested to defer chemoradiation until time of progression in younger asymptomatic patients receiving extensive resection, while early postoperative treatment should be recommended in high-risk patients. It remains to be established more clearly which features describe better the high-risk group; for example, in this study, age cut off of 40 years was not related to improved OS or PFS.

The phase III IWOT study (Wait or Treat?) [12] enrolls patients with clinically favorable IDH-mutant astrocytoma that do not need immediate postoperative treatment. It will establish whether early adjuvant treatment with RT and adjuvant TMZ in resected IDH-mutated astrocytoma will improve outcome, and whether benefits of early treatment outweigh the potential side effects.

When adjuvant radiotherapy can be delayed, new therapies like *vorasidenib* should be considered. Vorasidenib is an oral inhibitor of IDH1 and IDH2, which increases PFS and time to second treatment in IDH1 or IDH2-mutated LGGs [13].

17.3.1 Radiotherapy Doses, Volumes and Techniques

The purpose of radiotherapy in gliomas is to improve local control without inducing neurotoxicity. To do so, the recommended prescribed dose is of 45–54 Gy given in 1.8 Gy daily fractions, with IMRT or VMAT technique, whose dose distribution in the brain parenchyma allows reduced acute and late toxicity. A dose between 50.4 and 54 Gy is the most widely used radiation regimen for the adjuvant treatment in LGGs, with no benefit with higher doses [14, 15].

Proton radiation therapy is conditionally recommended as an option, especially for tumors located near critical OARs responsible for neurocognitive function (NCF) (e.g., hippocampus) [16].

Usually, target volumes were based on patterns of failure studies demonstrating that 80% to 90% of recurrences occur within 20 mm of the cavity for LGGs [17]. However, it has been proven that the use of large RT fields is implicated in the onset of late neurocognitive decline [18]. A retrospective analysis of 113 patients with IDH-mutant low-grade glioma [19] assessed that most of the recurrences fell into the hypothetical 5 mm CTV (at the center, inside or at the edge of it). In detail, the recurrence outside the 5-mm CTV was 10% versus 8% of the original CTV.

In light of these findings, recent trials have reduced the GTV-CTV expansion to 10 mm (*NRG BN005*, *NCT03180502*) or 5 mm (*EORTC 1635, NCT03763422*); however, the effect of these smaller fields on pattern of failure is not yet known. Thus, a GTV to CTV margin of 10–15 mm is recommended for target volumes defined by MRI-based planning for patients with IDH-mutant grade 2 glioma.

For tumors that have undergone GTR or subtotal resection (STR), the GTV is generated by contouring the residual T2/FLAIR-weighted hyperintense volume, resection cavity, and T1-weighted residual contrast-enhancing tissue (if present) on a postoperative MRI that is fused to the planning CT scan. For tumors that have undergone biopsy only, the GTV is generated by contouring the T2/FLAIR-weighted hyperintense volume and T1-weighted contrast-enhancing tissue on an MRI [20]. In either case, to account for subclinical extension of tumor, a CTV is created by uniformly expanding the GTV by 10–15 mm while respecting anatomic boundaries (e.g., the osseous skull, ventricles, falx, and tentorium). When the CTV involves routes of spread along white matter tracts (e.g., the corpus callosum or brainstem), the CTV should not be cropped in these structures, even when it crosses midline.

Finally, an expansion of CTV by 3–5 mm is recommended to generate the PTV, to account for set-up uncertainties (e.g., MRI fusion accuracy, mask immobilization, beam characteristics). Daily image guidance allows to reduce PTV margins to 3 mm and achieve greater conformality within dose/volume constraints [21].

17.4 Radiation Therapy in Grade 3 and 4 Adult-Type Diffuse Gliomas, IDH-Mutant

17.4.1 Oligodendroglioma, IDH-Mutant and 1p/19q-Codeleted, Grade 3

Both grade 2 and grade 3 oligodendrogliomas have relatively favorable long-term outcomes. For IDH-mutant, 1p/19q-codeleted oligodendroglioma, grade 3, the extent of resection is an important prognostic factor [22]. As for grade 2, a “watch-and-wait” strategy can be applied to grade 3 young patients (less than 40 years of age) with a good KPS (Karnofsky Performance Status) score, after GTR and in absence of neurological deficits.

In case of adjuvant treatment, radiotherapy should follow between 3 and 5 weeks after surgery [23], followed by 6 cycle of chemotherapy (PCV schedule). EORTC 26951 proved that oligodendroglioma patients treated with RT and PCV had better OS and PFS than those treated with RT alone.

The modified CODEL trial [24] will address whether temozolomide-based chemoradiotherapy is similarly effective as radiotherapy followed by PCV in grade 3 oligodendroglioma patients. Recently, Kacimi et al. [25] reported a better OS outcome in 207 patients treated with RT/PCV compared to 98 treated with RT/TMZ (median OS not reached versus 140 months, respectively). This data suggests that the improved safety profile of TMZ comes at the cost of inferior efficacy in this population.

17.4.2 Astrocytoma, IDH-Mutant and 1p19q Intact, Grade 3 and Grade 4

For grade 3, IDH-mutant, 1p19q non-codeleted astrocytomas adjuvant RT-chemotherapy is recommended, as this histology is proven to be more aggressive.

The phase III CATNON trial (EORTC 26053–22,054) [26] randomized patients with anaplastic astrocytoma to RT alone, RT with concomitant TMZ, RT with adjuvant TMZ, and RT with concomitant followed by adjuvant TMZ. At the second interim analysis, OS was improved with RT and adjuvant TMZ. To be noted, this trial included grade 3 IDH-mutant astrocytoma, but also IDH-wildtype astrocytoma (considered glioblastoma in the 2021 WHO classification). In general, either RT with sequential chemotherapy or RT with concurrent/sequential chemotherapy is recommended for patients with IDH-mutant, CNS5 WHO grade 3 astrocytoma.

In both high-grade oligodendrogliomas and high-grade astrocytomas, radiotherapy is the primary treatment for unresectable tumors, associated or not with chemotherapy.

17.4.3 Radiotherapy Doses, Volumes, and Techniques

Among patients with grade 3 adult-type diffuse glioma, the recommended dose ranges from 50 to 60 Gy given in 1.8–2 Gy daily fractions, with IMRT or VMAT technique. This difference in dose range is based upon subtypes.

For patients with grade 3 IDH-mutant astrocytoma, the recommended dose range is 59.4–60 Gy delivered in 1.8 or 2 Gy daily fractions. Multiple randomized trials recommend the same dose of 59.4 Gy (1.8 Gy daily fractions) for patients with grade 3 oligodendroglioma, IDH-mutant and 1p/19q-codeleted. However, a conditional recommendation over lower doses is also taken into consideration, based on expert opinions and data highlighting how IDH and 1p/19q status are associated with less aggressive tumor despite the grade 3 designation [20]. Thus, a dose of 54 Gy—the upper range of dose used for low-grade gliomas—may be considered.

In both grade 3 histologies, a hypo-fractionated schedule of 40,05 Gy in 15 fractions (2.67 Gy/fr) is appropriated for older patients (more than 70 years of age) or for those with unfavorable prognosis defined by a low KPS score (<70) [23].

The target delineation of grade 3 diffuse gliomas is similar to those grade 2, but usually with slightly larger CTV margins [7].

In high-grade gliomas (HGGs), the GTV is contoured on a postoperative MRI fused to the planning CT scan. It should include the surgical resection cavity with any residual enhancement, identified in T2/FLAIR-weighted and T1-weighted images, respectively. Then, a volumetric expansion of 1–2 cm is applied to the GTV to generate the CTV. A final expansion of 0.3–0.5 cm is required to create the PTV. Alternatively, a two-phase approach may be considered including a boost to any residual enhancement on T1 postcontrast imaging [20].

17.5 Radiation Therapy in Grade 4 Adult-Type Diffuse Gliomas, IDH-Wildtype

Glioblastoma (GBM), IDH-wildtype, grade 4, is the most aggressive form of adult-type diffuse glioma, carrying a poor prognosis and the necessity of a multimodal approach.

Whenever feasible, surgery is the first-line treatment, and it should involve gross total resection. The SoC is surgery followed by radio-chemotherapy according to the Stupp protocol [27]: concomitant temozolomide (75 mg/m^2 daily throughout radiotherapy, including weekends) plus at least six cycles of maintenance TMZ (150–200 mg/m^2, once a day for 5 consecutive days every 28 days), up to 12 cycles.

The advantage in terms of survival of temozolomide has been linked to patients with *MGMT* promoter-methylated [28], thus its testing has become standard practice.

A new approach combining temozolomide with lomustine in the newly diagnosed GBM might extend OS in patients with *MGMT* promoter-methylated glioblastoma [29].

However, this approach also deprives patients from lomustine, the standard of care at recurrence. A phase 3 trial did not show OS benefit adding bevacizumab to TMZ based chemoradiotherapy [30], leading bevacizumab to not be approved for the treatment of newly diagnosed GBMs.

17.5.1 Radiotherapy Doses, Volumes and Techniques

For patients less than 70 years old of age, in good general and neurological condition, RT treatment is given in a conventional fractionation of 60 Gy in 30 fractions. In patients with more than 70 years of age and/or frail (KPS score < 70), a hypo-fractionated regimen is considered, consisting of 40 Gy in 15 fractions (2.67 Gy/fr), which has similar activity to irradiation with 60 Gy [31] and the advantage of being less a toll on the elderly's health.

The current ESTRO-EANO guideline reports the standard for target delineation of glioblastoma [32] (Fig. 17.2):

- GTV: defined on MRI as T1 contrast-enhancing tumor (for biopsy only patients) or resection cavity plus residual contrast-

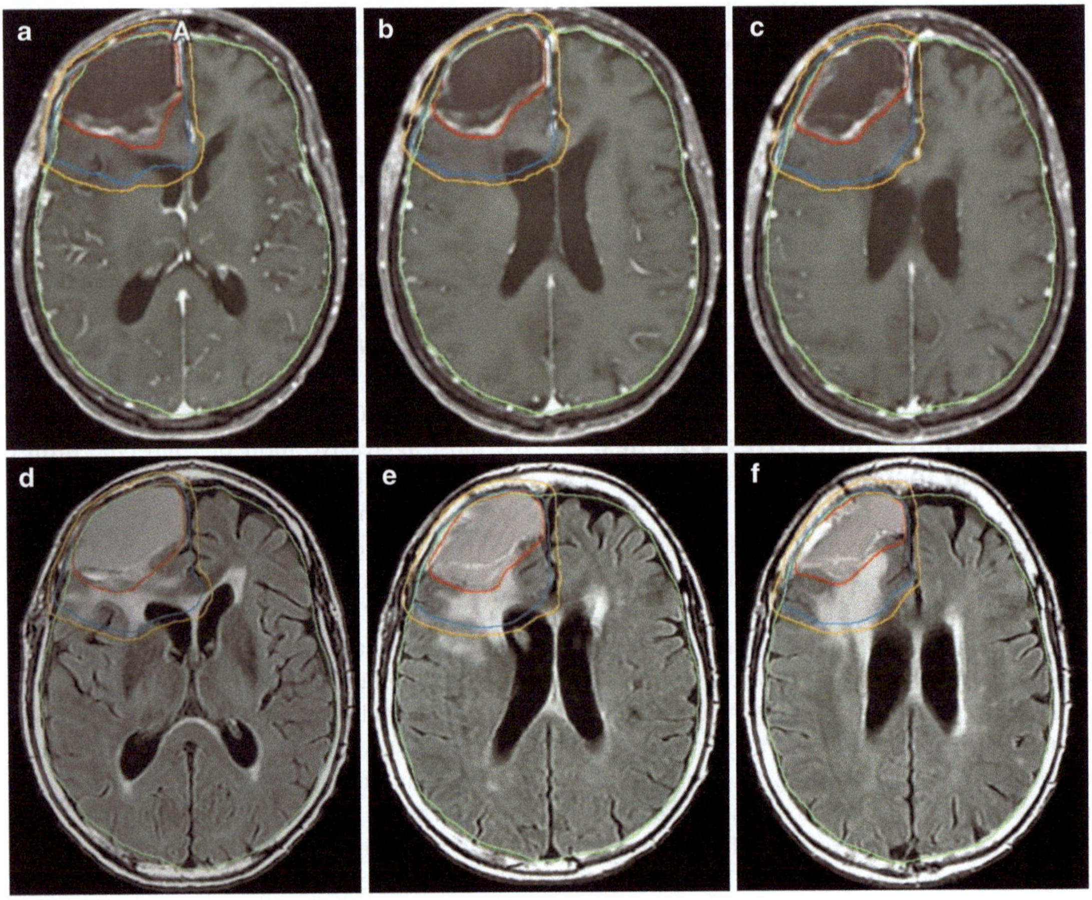

Fig. 17.2 (**a**–**f**) 65-year-old patient with a right frontal glioblastoma. The GTV (red contour) was expanded by 1.5 cm to generate the CTV (blue contour) and constrained at anatomical barriers (bone, falx), whereas no correction was applied at the genu corporis callosi. No further CTV expansion was applied and the FLAIR abnormalities visible in the right frontal lobe were not included (panels **e**, **f**). The PTV (orange) was generated by a 3-mm geometric expansion of the CTV (orange) [32]

enhancing tumor (if present), not including peri-tumoral edema.
- CTV: a 15 mm margin around the GTV should be applied in all directions, edited to take account of anatomical barriers to tumor spread (skull, ventricles, falx, tentorium, optic chiasm, brainstem). Inclusion of edema within CTV is not advised, whereas T2/FLAIR signal abnormalities may represent non-enhancing tumor and should be considered for inclusion within the CTV. In 'molecularly defined' glioblastomas, similar margins of 10–15 mm should be applied; however, the optimal GTV-to-CTV strategy needs to be better defined in future studies.
- PTV: CTV-PTV margin should be based on the institutional fixation technique and local quality assurance measurements. Modern LINACs with daily IGRT enable PTV margin reduction to spare surrounding normal tissue. A PTV margin of 3 mm is recommended, but 2–5 mm is acceptable.

Minniti et al. [33] evaluated 207 GBM patients who recurred after standard chemoradiation. In these patients the CTV was generated by adding a 2 cm margin to the GTV, according to the previous guidelines. For each patient, a theoretical plan consisting of reduced 1 cm GTV-to-CTV margin was created to compare patterns of failure and radiation doses to normal brain. Following replanning with 1 cm reduced margin, dosimetric analysis showed similar patterns of failure.

This result provides the basis for evaluating GTV-to-CTV margin reduction in future clinical trials, also aided by integration of PET images in the diagnosis and target delineation of tumor extent [34].

17.6 Diffuse Midline Glioma, H3 K27-Altered, Grade 4

Diffuse midline gliomas (in the previous classification called 'diffuse intrinsic pontine gliomas'—DIPGs) are tumors arising in the midline structures of the brain (brainstem, thalamus, or spinal cord) and harboring the H3 K27 mutation. They are highly aggressive WHO grade 4 tumors, often presenting a diffuse infiltrative growth, which causes 90% of children dying within 2 years from the initial diagnosis [35].

Diffuse midline gliomas (DMGs) are inoperable tumors and radiotherapy treatment remains the SoC, even though it provides only temporary clinical relief [36]. The radiation treatment is typically given at a dose of 54–60 Gy in 1.8–2.0 Gy fractions [37] over 6 weeks. The most common delivery method is photon beam radiotherapy; however, proton therapy is a valid alternative, minimizing exposure to critical near anatomical structures.

Since DMGs often recur within the area of treatment, according to SIOPE (European Society for Paediatric Oncology) recommendations re-irradiation is an option if at least 3–6 months between the two treatments have passed and if radio-necrosis is excluded after uprofont radiotherapy [38]. Different schemes have been investigated, with no severe neurotoxicity associated with re-irradiation doses <24 Gy administered over 10–12 fractions [39]; whereas an improvement in median survival times has been demonstrated.

17.7 Research Trials, Innovations and Modern Treatments in Glioma Patients

In recent years, the field of glioma treatment has seen significant advancements, driven by innovations in research and technology. A number of groundbreaking clinical trials are reshaping the treatment landscape for gliomas. For instance, studies like RTOG1205 [40] have explored novel combinations of therapies, such as the integration of radiotherapy with bevacizumab (BEV). While these trials have demonstrated some success in extending PFS, the impact on overall survival has been less pronounced, underscoring the ongoing need for research to find more effective and enduring treatment strategies. Furthermore, the identification of molecular markers has led to the development of promising new therapies, such as vorasidenib, that allow the postponement of radiation treatment. This represents a significant shift toward treatments tailored to the genetic profile of tumors.

Modern advancements in radiotherapy techniques, such as proton therapy (PT), are also transforming the glioma management. Proton therapy provides a more precise targeting of tumor tissue, reducing the dose delivered to surrounding healthy brain structures. This helps minimizing neurocognitive decline and other long-term side effects commonly associated with conventional radiation therapy. Additionally, the integration of advanced imaging technologies, like MR-LINAC systems, enables real-time treatment adjustments, further enhancing the precision and effectiveness of radiotherapy.

17.7.1 Low-Grade Gliomas

As previously mentioned, adjuvant RT in low-grade gliomas can be postponed in low-risk patients. In this setting, new drug therapies are being evaluated in order to increase time to second treatment.

Vorasidenib is an oral inhibitor able to penetrate the blood-brain barrier and target IDH1 and IDH2 enzymes, which are mutated in LGGs. A randomized double-blind phase 3 trial compared the efficacy and safety outcomes of vorasidenib versus placebo in IDH-mutant low-grade glioma patients (INDIGO Trial) [13]. Three hundred and thirty-one patients who had undergone surgery only were randomized to receive vorasidenib ($n = 168$) (40 mg once daily) or matched placebo ($n = 163$) in 28-day cycles. Treatment with either drug continued until neuroimaging-confirmed disease progression (DP) or unacceptable toxicity; patients in the placebo group developing DP crossed over to the vorasidenib group.

At the neuroimaging assessment, 47 of 168 patients in the vorasidenib group and 88 of 163 patients in the placebo group showed DP. After a median follow-up of 14.2 months, PFS was 27.7 months and 11.1 months in the vorasidenib group and in the control group, respectively. The secondary endpoint was time to next intervention: the probability of being alive and receiving no treatment at 18 months was 85.6% in the vorasidenib group compared to 47.4% in the placebo group. Vorasidenib has demonstrated a good safety and tolerability profile; most of the reported adverse events (AEs) are low-grade, with the most common being an increase in transaminases. These results indicate that vorasidenib can effectively delay the need for RT and other subsequent treatments. Extending the period prior to radiotherapy means reducing the cumulative exposure to radiation and its long-term side effects, maintaining a better quality of life for a longer time.

17.7.2 Glioblastoma

Recurrence in GBM patients is an almost inevitable event that necessitates undergoing new lines of treatment, such as repeated surgery, radiation, and chemotherapy [41].

REGOMA is an Italian randomized multicenter open-label phase 2 trial. One hundred and nineteen patients suffering from recurrent GBM (already treated with surgery and radiotherapy plus chemotherapy as first-line treatment) were randomized to receive regorafenib ($n = 59$) (160 mg daily for 21 days every 28 days) or lomustine ($n = 60$) (110 mg/m^2 every 6 weeks) until disease progression, death, unacceptable toxicity or withdrawal of consent [42]. The primary endpoint of the study was the comparison in OS: after a median follow-up of 15.4 months, the median OS were 7.4 and 5.6 months in the regorafenib and in the lomustine group, respectively. PFS was also described between the two groups: 2 months for regorafenib (16.9% at 6 months) and 1.9 months for lomustine (8.3% at 6 months).

The improvement in OS in patients treated with regorafenib defined, for the first time, the efficacy and safety of this drug in monotherapy. REGOMA-OSS, a large, multicenter, prospective, observational study, confirmed the REGOMA data in a real-world setting. The survival was very similar to the REGOMA trial with a better-controlled toxicity profile [43]. These trials represent a valuable approach considering the lack of clear guidelines in the treatment of recurrent glioblastoma. They are particularly important for understanding the potential integration of new drug therapies with existing radiotherapy treatments. Regorafenib could potentially be used to control tumor growth before, during, or after RT, optimizing the therapeutic window and improving patient outcomes.

An extensive literature review conducted by De Pietro et al. [44] underlines how reirradiation is increasingly used as treatment option in patients with recurrent glioblastoma after first-line chemoradiation, although the debate is still open regarding the clinical benefit of combining systemic therapies with re-irradiation.

In this regard, the *RTOG1205*—a randomized phase 2 study—investigated the role of bevacizumab, a recombinant humanized monoclonal IgG1 antibody that inhibits vascular endothelial growth factor (VEGF), reducing the growth of new blood vessels. Patients were randomized to receive BEV alone (10 mg/kg once every 2 weeks until DP) [control arm] or BEV plus re-RT (35 Gy/10 fr) [experimental arm] [40]. The primary and secondary endpoints were OS and PFS, respectively. The median OS in the experimental arm was 10.1 months versus 9.7 months in the control arm. The median PFS was 7.1 months (54.3% at 6 months) in the experimental arm and 3.8 months (29.1% at 6 months) in the control arm. Although RTOG1205 demonstrated an improvement in PFS at 6 months in patients receiving re-RT and bevacizumab, the study failed to prove a real benefit in OS.

Christ et al. [45] investigated the benefit of re-irradiation when associated with other systemic therapies (e.g., bevacizumab, pembrolizumab, nivolumab, temozolomide). The retrospective study involved 117 patients who underwent a total of 129 re-irradiation sessions, receiving chemotherapy before or during the radiation treatment. Most patients underwent concomitant treatment with RT (>59.4 Gy) and TMZ; 70 of 129 patients had fractionated RT and 38 of 129 patients had SRS or SRT (1–5 fractions). The median time to relapse was 14.5 months; the median PFS was 3.6 months, while the median OS was 7.3 months. Treatments with bevacizumab before re-RT showed a higher percentage of relapses compared to those who did not receive prior BEV. The OS in the two groups corroborates this data, being 7.2 months in the BEV group and 8.5 months in the other. Other systemic treatments concomitant with re-RT did not show significant differences in terms of OS and PFS.

In conclusion, re-irradiation combined with chemotherapy seems promising in managing glioma recurrences by improving progression-free survival. However, these strategies do not significantly enhance overall survival. Future research should focus on optimizing these combinations to increase both PFS and OS while minimizing adverse effects, as well as exploring novel therapies that might offer more substantial survival benefits.

One of the most promising ongoing trial is the LEGATO trial, a randomized phase 3 study involving several European countries that compares lomustine plus re-irradiation with lomustine alone for treatment of patients with first progression of glioblastoma [46]. Lomustine is considered the SoC for glioblastoma progression, but its concomitant administration with radiotherapy has never been investigated. This trial will enroll patients from 43 centers in 11 countries, for a total of 411 participants who will be randomized 1:1 to receive either lomustine (110 mg/m^2 every 6 weeks) or lomustine with radiotherapy (35 Gy in 10 fractions).

The primary endpoint is overall survival; secondary endpoints are PFS, response rate, neurocognitive function, health-related QoL, and health economic parameters. The study is scheduled for completion in 2028, and its results hold the promise of advancing the treatment of glioblastoma recurrence. A novel approach to glioblastoma patients explored the use of Tumor Treating Fields (TTF) (Optune©, Novocure, Switzerland), alternating electric fields that disrupt tumour cell mitosis. In the final analysis of a randomized clinical trial [47], the addition of TTF to maintenance temozolomide after standard chemo-radiotherapy showed a statistically significant improvement in PFS and OS. After these promising results, the role of TFF is under further investigation in ongoing clinical trials.

17.7.3 Diffuse Midline Glioma

Despite numerous clinical trials exploring various treatments, including radiotherapy and chemotherapy, significant progress in managing DMGs has been limited. In a recent review by Lo Greco et al. [48], the authors discuss various approaches, including a combination of nimotuzumab (anti-EGFR drug) and vinorelbine (a semisynthetic vinca alkaloid) with multiple courses of radiation (2 or 3 courses) on 3 children. In all children, both neurological improvements after each radiotherapy course and radiological response were observed.

Fleischhack et al. also reported the results of a phase 3 clinical trial evaluating the efficacy of concomitant nimotuzumab and radiotherapy [49]. By binding to EGFR, nimotuzumab interferes with the receptor's signaling pathways, which are crucial for tumor cell proliferation and survival.

This study enrolled 42 patients, aged 3–20 years, with newly diagnosed DMG, confirmed clinically and radiologically. The primary endpoint was PFS at 6 months following the administration of nimotuzumab (150 mg/m^2 weekly for 12 weeks) alongside RT between weeks 3 and 9. Following the initial 12 cycles, patients continued to receive nimotuzumab every other week until disease progression or unacceptable toxicity. Of the 42 patients, 2 (4.8%) achieved a partial response, 27 (64.3%) experienced stable disease, 10 (23.8%) showed DP; 3 patients were not evaluable. The median PFS was 5.8 months; the median OS was 9.4 months. AEs associated with the treatment included alopecia, vomiting, headache, and dermatological issues related to radiotherapy. Overall, the combination of radiotherapy and nimotuzumab was deemed feasible and tolerable, however, further research is needed to optimize treatment strategies and improve patient outcomes.

17.8 Modern and Advanced Treatments in Glioma Patients

17.8.1 Proton Therapy

Particle therapy with protons has become increasingly available due to the expansion of proton therapy centers across Europe over the last decade [50]. Proton therapy's advantage lies in its ability to spare normal tissue through the Bragg peak effect [51], offering potential benefits in different scenarios, from first-line treatments to re-irradiations. The effectiveness of PT in treating gliomas is attributed to the unique properties of protons, which deposit energy more precisely within neoplastic tissue compared to photons (Fig. 17.3). This precision can mitigate side

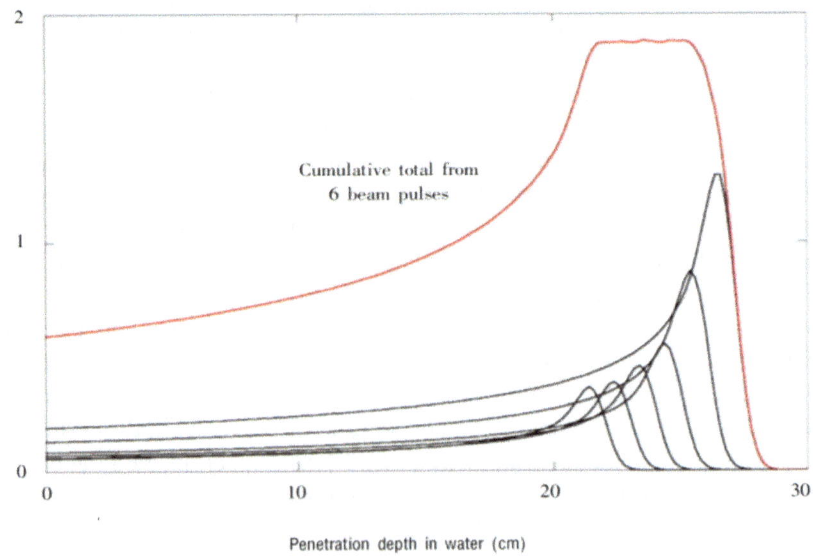

Fig. 17.3 Once the desired proton beam energy has been produced, it still needs to be "spread out" to cover the entire tumor, as a mono-energetic proton beam would only cover a small portion of the tumor with its Bragg peak. The figure represents multiple Bragg peaks at various depths that form the spread out Bragg peak (SOBP), displayed as a red line [51]

effects associated with traditional radiation therapy, such as neurocognitive disorders.

Various publications suggest that proton therapy decreases the risk of neurocognitive decline, providing at the same time local control and overall survival rates comparable to photon therapy [52–55]. Goff et al. published a review on the use of proton therapy (PT) for gliomas, detailing dose escalation studies in GBMs, re-irradiation and cognitive sparing [53]. In 2024, Eekers et al. [54] critically reviewed a series of studies published between 2001 and 2022 on PT in adult glioma patients. All the recent publications reported lower rates of symptomatic toxicity following PT for LGGs; however, only few studies included patients with glioblastoma. In the absence of high-quality evidence, the superiority of PT remains controversial.

Currently, an ongoing German prospective phase 3 trial (GRIPS trial) [55] is evaluating cumulative toxicity and survivals in patients with newly diagnosed GBM treated with photon (standard arm) or proton (experimental arm) radiation. The primary endpoint is toxicity of grade 2 or greater, assessed by CTCAE criteria, with secondary endpoints including PFS, OS, late and acute toxicity, neurocognitive status, and quality of life. GRIPS is the first study to investigate the differences in toxicity between proton therapy and traditional photon-based radiotherapy.

The results of a multicentric Dutch in silico ROCOCO trial [52] demonstrated how intensity-modulated proton therapy (IMPT) decreases dose to brain OARs compared to photon RT. One-hundred treatment plans for 25 LGG patients were generated and analyzed comparing different treatment modalities (VMAT, IMRT, Tomotherapy, IMPT) (Fig. 17.4). Overall, all techniques showed an excellent coverage, but IMPT was the best one to reduce dose to the OARs (brain, hippocampus, and cerebellum), especially the contralateral ones.

Proton therapy is also applied in the treatment of diffuse midline gliomas. A 2019 retrospective study by Muroi et al. [57] included 12 pediatric patients with newly diagnosed DMGs treated with PT (54 Gy in 30 fractions). This study also reviewed the medical records of ten patients who underwent conventional photon therapy. The analysis indicated no significant survival differences between the two groups, but despite its potential benefits, proton beam therapy remains a challenging and costly treatment option due to its limited availability.

17.8.2 Adaptive Radiotherapy

Among the latest advancements in the field of radiation oncology, adaptive radiotherapy (ART) is currently one of the most investigated. ART involves continuously adjusting treatment to account for changes in size, shape or location of the tumor or of the nearby organs.

MRI-guided radiotherapy (MRgRT) is a form of ART. It has emerged as a transformative technology, particularly exemplified by the MRI-linear accelerator (MR-LINAC) systems, such as the Unity MR-LINAC (Elekta Instruments AB, Stockholm, Sweden). This technology allows for real-time visualization and adjustment of the treatment plan based on daily MRI scans, offering enhanced precision in targeting tumors and sparing healthy tissues. This capability is particularly beneficial in the treatment of brain tumors, including gliomas, where tumor dynamics can change rapidly.

Recent literature, including a review by Guerini et al. [58], highlights the two primary adaptive radiotherapy workflows utilized with MR-LINAC systems: adapt-to-position (ATP) and adapt-to-shape (ATS). ATP involves re-optimizing the treatment plan based on isocenter shifts determined from rigid translations, while ATS allows for comprehensive plan adaptation based on updated patient anatomy visible on daily MRI scans. The adaptive nature of these workflows ensures that radiotherapy plans can be adjusted to reflect changes in tumor volume and position, potentially improving dose distribution to the tumor and reducing exposure to surrounding OARs [59].

The MOMENTUM study [56], which evaluated patients with high-grade gliomas undergoing radiotherapy on the Unity MR-LINAC, demonstrated that daily MRI could reveal significant changes in tumor volume and characteristics. Notably, detectable changes in the GTV and apparent diffusion coefficient (ADC) were

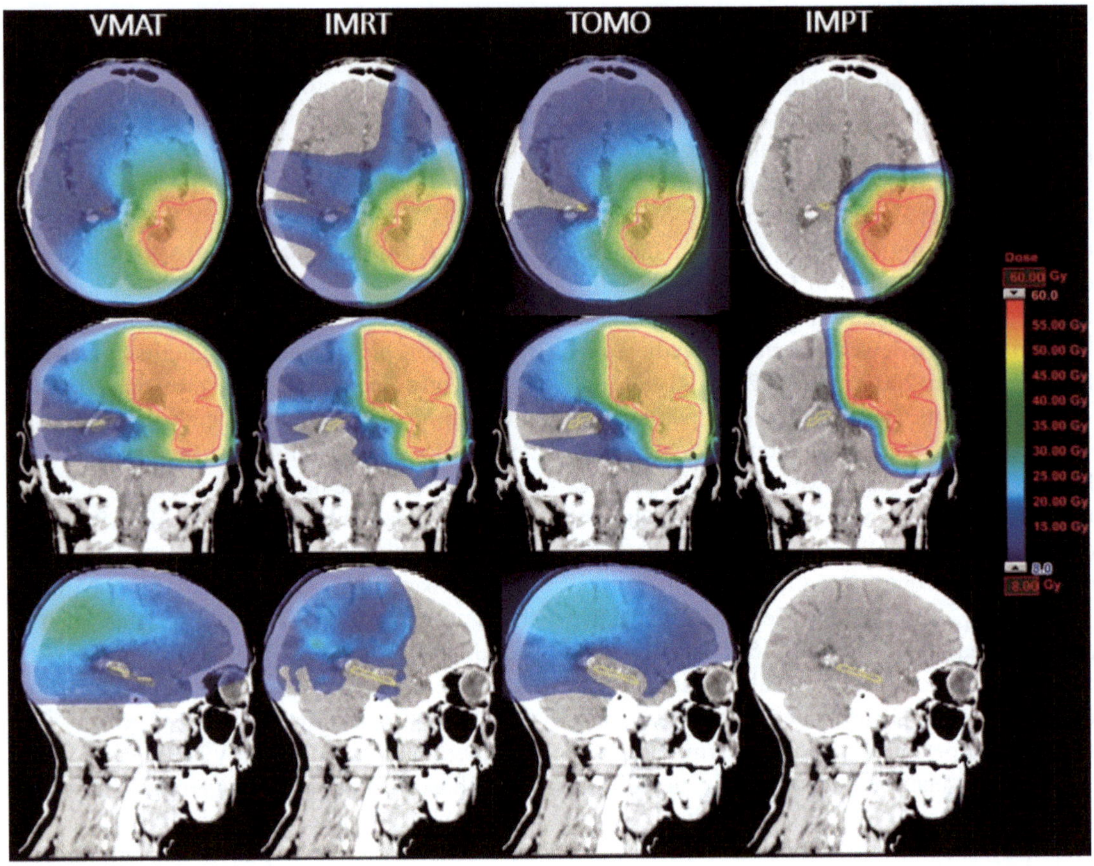

Fig. 17.4 Example of a radiation treatment plans for a patient with a left parieto-occipital LGG. The CTV (pink), hippocampus (yellow) and dose distribution (ranging from low dose depicted in blue to high dose in red) are given for the VMAT, TOMO (tomotherapy), IMRT, and IMPT treatment plans, in the axial (upper row), coronal (middle row), and sagittal (lower row) view. A large low-dose bath (in blue) can be noted when using either of the photon techniques (VMAT, IMRT, TOMO) [56]

observed in a substantial number of cases, with variations in ADC values potentially indicating alterations in tumor cellularity or treatment response [60]. Similarly, Tseng et al. [61] reported the initial experience of ten high-grade glioma patients (4 GBMs) that completed chemoradiotherapy on Unity MR-LINAC at a median dose of 60 Gy in 30 fractions. They observed that volume changes in high-grade gliomas necessitated replanning in several patients due to significant increases in tumor or edema size during the course of treatment. For each of the four patients who exhibited PD during follow-up, the region of recurrence included most of the low-ADC region measured during treatment (Fig. 17.5).

These findings underscore the potential of MR-LINAC systems to enhance treatment precision by enabling real-time adaptation of radiotherapy plans. However, challenges remain, such as determining the optimal timing and frequency for adaptive interventions and balancing the benefits of real-time imaging with the need for efficient treatment time.

Future research will explore how diffusion-weighted imaging (DWI) on MR-LINACs can be used to guide dose escalation strategies. Initial studies suggest that low-ADC regions, identified through MR-LINAC DWI, may serve as valuable targets for dose escalation in glioblastomas. The prognostic value of changes in DWI metrics, as compared to traditional contrast-enhancing GTV

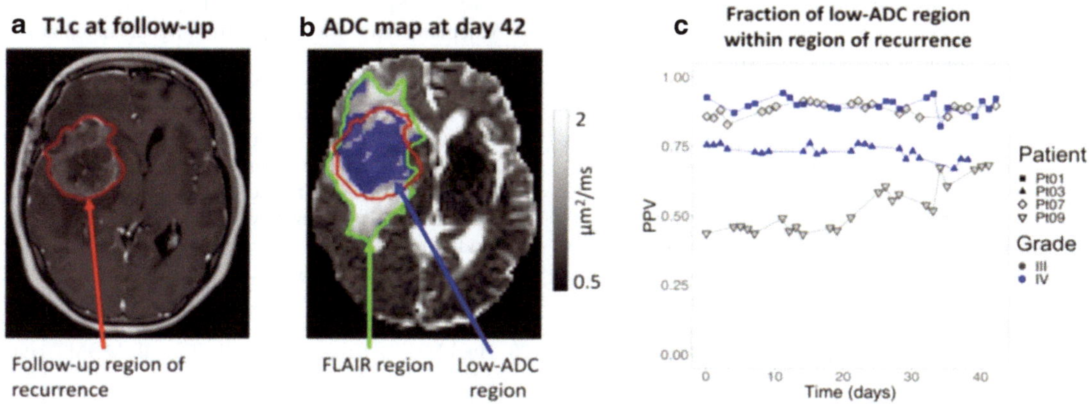

Fig. 17.5 Overlap between intra-treatment low-ADC regions and recurrent tumor [61]. (**a**): The postcontrast T1-weighted image (T1c) with the region of recurrence indicated by the red contour. Note that the recurrence region was taken as the enhancing tumor for the Grade 4 patients and the FLAIR hyperintensity for the Grade 3 patients. (**b**): The ADC map from the MR-Linac for Day 42 from first fraction of radiotherapy, corresponding to the last day of radiation, with the future recurrence region (red contour), FLAIR region (green contour), and low-ADC region (blue colorwash). The low-ADC region is mostly contained in the recurrence region. (**c**): The positive predictive value (PPV) over time for the voxel-wise prediction of the recurrence region by the low-ADC region. By the end of treatment, most of the low-ADC region is contained within the recurrence region for all patients

metrics, appears promising. For example, MR-LINAC DWI changes between weeks 2 and 5 seem to correlate more strongly with overall survival and PFS than changes in the GTV [62]. This could potentially lead to more effective treatment regimens that better address treatment-resistant tumor regions while minimizing adverse effects on healthy brain tissue.

Significant advancements in the radiotherapy are offering both new opportunities and challenges. Photon treatment with conventional LINACs (e.g., ELEKTA Versa HD®) remains the most common radiation delivery method. However, photon treatment with MR-LINACs and proton beam radiation has the potential to improve treatment outcomes for patients with brain tumors. Ongoing development in this field will be crucial for optimizing radiotherapy strategies and translating these advancements into clinical practice.

References

1. Louis DN, Perry A, Wesseling P, et al. The 2021 WHO classification of tumors of the central nervous system: a summary. Neuro-Oncology. 2021;23(8):1231–51. https://doi.org/10.1093/neuonc/noab106.
2. Śledzińska P, Furtak J, Pasternak A. The new WHO classification of central nervous system tumors 2021—key points and practical applications. Clin Neuropathol. 2021;40(1):29–38.
3. Brat DJ, Aldape K, Colman H, et al. cIMPACT-NOW update 3: recommended diagnostic criteria for "diffuse astrocytic glioma, IDH-wildtype, with molecular features of glioblastoma, WHO grade IV". Acta Neuropathol. 2018;136(5):805–10. https://doi.org/10.1007/s00401-018-1913-0.
4. Scaringi C, Agolli L, Minniti G. Technical advances in radiation therapy for brain tumors. Anticancer Res. 2018;38(11):6041–5. https://doi.org/10.21873/anticanres.12954.
5. Scoccianti S, Detti B, Gadda D, et al. Organs at risk in the brain and their dose-constraints in adults and in children: a radiation oncologist's guide for delineation in everyday practice. Radiother Oncol. 2015;114(2):230–8. https://doi.org/10.1016/j.radonc.2015.01.016.
6. Jakola AS, Myrmel KS, Kloster R, et al. Comparison of a strategy favoring early surgical resection vs a strategy favoring watchful waiting in low-grade gliomas. JAMA Oncol. 2017;3(3):198–205. https://doi.org/10.1093/annonc/mdx230.
7. Weller M, van den Bent M, Hopkins K, et al. EANO guideline for the diagnosis and treatment of adult astrocytic and oligodendroglial gliomas. Lancet Oncol. 2017;18(6):e315–29.
8. Rudà R, Soffietti R. Is the use of temozolomide alone in the treatment of low-grade gliomas justified? Expert Rev Neurother. 2017;17(8):693–6.
9. Bell EH, Zhang P, Shaw EG, et al. Comprehensive genomic analysis in NRG oncology/RTOG 9802:

a phase III trial of radiation therapy (RT) with or without procarbazine, CCNU, and vincristine (PCV) chemotherapy in high-risk low-grade glioma. J Clin Oncol. 2020;38(29):3407–17.
10. Fisher BJ, Hu C, Macdonald DR, et al. Phase 2 study of radiation therapy with concurrent and adjuvant temozolomide for pure and mixed anaplastic oligodendroglioma: NRG oncology/RTOG 0424. Int J Radiat Oncol Biol Phys. 2020;106(4):791–800.
11. Minniti G, Amelio D, Amichetti M, et al. Hypofractionated radiation therapy and chemotherapy for patients with high-risk low-grade gliomas: a multicenter study. Neuro-Oncology. 2023;25(4):644–52. https://doi.org/10.1007/s11060-023-04418-z.
12. https://clinicaltrials.gov/study/NCT03763422.
13. Mellinghoff IK, van den Bent MJ, Roth P, et al. Vorasidenib in IDH1- or IDH2-mutant low-grade glioma. N Engl J Med. 2023;388(4):199–208. https://doi.org/10.1056/NEJMoa2304194.
14. Byrne E, Davies AM, Rundle S, et al. Adjuvant radiotherapy for WHO grade 2 gliomas. Cochrane Database Syst Rev. 2022;2(1):CD012716.
15. Breen WG, Brown PD, Ballman KV, et al. Does higher radiation dose improve outcomes for low-grade gliomas? Int J Radiat Oncol Biol Phys. 2021;110(4):1034–41.
16. van der Weide HL, Vulto IM, Kroese MC, et al. Proton therapy in the treatment of low-grade gliomas: a systematic review. Radiother Oncol. 2020;150:109–15. https://doi.org/10.1016/j.radonc.2020.11.004.
17. Fukuya Y, Ikuta S, Maruyama T, et al. Tumor recurrence patterns after surgical resection of intracranial low-grade gliomas. J Neuro-Oncol. 2019;144(3):519–28. https://doi.org/10.1007/s11060-019-03250-8.
18. Douw L, Klein M, Fagel SS, et al. Cognitive and radiological effects of radiotherapy in patients with low-grade glioma: long-term follow-up. Lancet Neurol. 2009;8(9):810–8.
19. Jaspers JPM, Ijzerman-Korevaar M, Dirven L, et al. Patterns of recurrence in IDH-mutant low-grade glioma patients: retrospective analysis and implications for radiotherapy field design. Radiother Oncol. 2021;159:78–85. https://doi.org/10.1016/j.radonc.2021.05.013.
20. Halasz LM, Attia A, Bradfield L, et al. Radiation therapy for IDH-mutant grade 2 and grade 3 diffuse glioma: an ASTRO clinical practice guideline. Pract Radiat Oncol. 2022;12(5):370–86. https://doi.org/10.1016/j.prro.2022.05.004.
21. Halasz LM, Catalano PJ, Dunn IF, et al. Improved survival with reduced radiation treatment volume in low-grade glioma. Neuro-Oncology. 2022;24(4):656–63.
22. Wick W, Osswald M, Wick A. Oligodendrogliomas in adults. J Clin Oncol. 2020;38(15):1783–91.
23. Press RH, Shu HG, Shim H, et al. Outcomes and patterns of care in anaplastic oligodendrogliomas: an analysis of the national cancer data base. Cancer. 2019;125(24):4374–84. https://doi.org/10.1002/cncr.32797.
24. https://clinicaltrials.gov/ct2/show/NCT00887146.
25. Kacimi SE, Psimaras D, Boukhari A, et al. Chemotherapy for anaplastic oligodendrogliomas: analysis of the French national network. Neuro-Oncology. 2022;24(3):431–42.
26. van den Bent MJ, Erridge SC, Vogelbaum MA, et al. Adjuvant and concomitant temozolomide in newly diagnosed anaplastic glioma: long-term results of the CATNON trial. J Clin Oncol. 2021;39(23):2563–73.
27. Stupp R, Mason WP, van den Bent MJ, et al. Radiotherapy plus concomitant and adjuvant temozolomide for glioblastoma. N Engl J Med. 2005;352(10):987–96. https://doi.org/10.1056/NEJMoa043330.
28. Hegi ME, Diserens AC, Gorlia T, et al. MGMT gene silencing and benefit from temozolomide in glioblastoma. N Engl J Med. 2005;352(10):997–1003.
29. Herrlinger U, Tzaridis T, Mack F, et al. Lomustine-temozolomide combination therapy versus standard temozolomide therapy in newly diagnosed glioblastoma with methylated MGMT promoter: a randomized, double-blind, phase 3 trial. Lancet. 2019;393(10172):678–88.
30. Gilbert MR, Dignam JJ, Armstrong TS, et al. A randomized trial of bevacizumab for newly diagnosed glioblastoma. N Engl J Med. 2014;370(8):699–708. https://doi.org/10.1056/NEJMc1403303.
31. Roa W, Kepka L, Kumar N, et al. International randomized phase III trial of short-course versus standard radiation therapy in elderly patients with newly diagnosed glioblastoma. J Clin Oncol. 2015;33(35):4145–50.
32. Niyazi M, Wrensch M, Berger MS, et al. Current standards and advances in radiotherapy for glioblastoma. Neuro-Oncology. 2016;18(4):477–86.
33. Minniti G, Amelio D, Amichetti M, et al. Patterns of failure and dose-limiting normal tissue complications in glioblastoma patients treated with reduced-margin radiation fields. Radiother Oncol. 2023;179:43–50. https://doi.org/10.1016/j.radonc.2022.11.024.
34. Galldiks N, Albert NL, Sommerauer M, et al. PET imaging in patients with gliomas: a report of the RANO/PET working group. J Nucl Med. 2023;64(1):52–60. https://doi.org/10.2967/jnumed.122.264859.
35. Di Ruscio V, Del Baldo G, Fabozzi F, et al. Pediatric diffuse midline gliomas: an unfinished puzzle. Diagnostics (Basel). 2022;12(9):2064. https://doi.org/10.3390/diagnostics12092064.
36. Hargrave D, Bartels U, Bouffet E. Diffuse brainstem gliomas in children: critical review of clinical trials. Lancet Oncol. 2006;7(3):241–8. https://doi.org/10.1016/S1470-2045(06)70615-5.
37. Robison NJ, Kieran MW. Diffuse intrinsic pontine glioma: a reassessment. J Neuro-Oncol. 2014;119(1):7–15. https://doi.org/10.1007/s11060-014-1448-8.
38. Janssens GO, Gandola L, Bolle S, et al. Survival benefit for patients with diffuse intrinsic pontine glioma (DIPG) undergoing re-irradiation at first progression: A matched-cohort analysis on behalf

of the SIOP-E-HGG/DIPG working group. Eur J Cancer. 2017;73:38–47. https://doi.org/10.1016/j.ejca.2016.12.007.
39. Amsbaugh MJ, Mahajan A, Grosshans DR, et al. Reirradiation of large-volume recurrent pediatric brain tumors with proton therapy. Int J Radiat Oncol Biol Phys. 2020;106(1):104–12. https://doi.org/10.1016/j.ijrobp.2019.10.006.
40. Tsien CI, Pugh SL, Dicker AP, et al. NRG oncology/RTOG1205: a randomized phase II trial of concurrent bevacizumab and reirradiation versus bevacizumab alone as treatment for recurrent glioblastoma. J Clin Oncol. 2023;41(6):1285–95. https://doi.org/10.1200/jco.22.00164.
41. Schaff LR, Mellinghoff IK. Glioblastoma and other primary brain malignancies in adults. JAMA. 2023;329(7):574. https://doi.org/10.1001/jama.2023.0023.
42. Lombardi G, De Salvo GL, Brandes AA, et al. Regorafenib compared with lomustine in patients with relapsed glioblastoma (REGOMA): a multicentre, open-label, randomised, controlled, phase 2 trial. Lancet Oncol. 2019;20(1):110–9. https://doi.org/10.1016/s1470-2045(18)30675-2.
43. Caccese M, Desideri I, Villani V, et al. REGOMA-OSS: a large, Italian, multicenter, prospective, observational study evaluating the efficacy and safety of regorafenib in patients with recurrent glioblastoma. ESMO Open. 2024;9(4):102943. https://doi.org/10.1016/j.esmoop.2024.102943.
44. De Pietro R, Zaccaro L, Marampon F, Tini P, De Felice F, Minniti G. The evolving role of reirradiation in the management of recurrent brain tumors. J Neurooncol. 2023;164(2):271–86. https://doi.org/10.1007/s11060-023-04407-2.
45. Christ SM, Youssef G, Tanguturi SK, et al. Re-irradiation of recurrent IDH-wildtype glioblastoma in the bevacizumab and immunotherapy era: target delineation, outcomes and patterns of recurrence. Clin Trans Radiat Oncol. 2024;44:100697. https://doi.org/10.1016/j.ctro.2023.100697.
46. Preusser M, Kazda T, Rhun EL, et al. Lomustine with or without reirradiation for first progression of glioblastoma, LEGATO, EORTC-2227-BTG: study protocol for a randomized phase III study. Trials. 2024;25(1):366. https://doi.org/10.1186/s13063-024-08213-7.
47. Stupp R, Taillibert S, Kanner A, et al. Effect of Tumor-Treating Fields Plus Maintenance Temozolomide vs Maintenance Temozolomide Alone on Survival in Patients With Glioblastoma: A Randomized Clinical Trial. JAMA. 2018;1;319(17):1824. https://doi.org/10.1001/jama.2018.3431.
48. Lo Greco MC, Marano G, La Rocca M, et al. Latest Advancements in the Management of H3K27M-Mutant Diffuse Intrinsic Pontine Glioma: A Narrative Review. Cancers (Basel). 2025;17(3):420. https://doi.org/10.3390/cancers17030420.
49. Fleischhack G, Massimino M, Warmuth-Metz M, et al. Nimotuzumab and radiotherapy for treatment of newly diagnosed diffuse intrinsic pontine glioma (DIPG): a phase III clinical study. J Neuro-Oncol. 2019;143(1):107–13. https://doi.org/10.1007/s11060-019-03140-z.
50. Grau C, Durante M, Georg D, Langendijk JA, Weber DC. Particle therapy in Europe. Mol Oncol. 2020;14(7):1492–9. https://doi.org/10.1002/1878-0261.12677.
51. Liu H, Chang JY. Proton therapy in clinical practice. Chin J Cancer. 2011;30(5):315–26. https://doi.org/10.5732/cjc.010.10529.
52. Eekers DBP, Roelofs E, Cubillos-Mesías M, et al. Intensity-modulated proton therapy decreases dose to organs at risk in low-grade glioma patients: results of a multicentric in silico ROCOCO trial. Acta Oncol. 2019;58(1):57–65. https://doi.org/10.1080/0284186X.2018.1529424.
53. Goff KM, Zheng C, Alonso-Basanta M. Proton radiotherapy for glioma and glioblastoma. Chin Clin Oncol. 2022;11(6):46. https://doi.org/10.21037/cco-22-92.
54. Eekers DBP, Zegers CML, Ahmed KA, Amelio D, Gupta T, Harrabi SB, Kazda T, Scartoni D, Seidel C, Shih HA, Minniti G. Controversies in neuro-oncology: focal proton versus photon radiation therapy for adult brain tumors. Neurooncol Pract. 2024;11(4):369–82. https://doi.org/10.1093/nop/npae040.
55. König L, Jäkel C, Von Knebel Doeberitz N, et al. Glioblastoma radiotherapy using intensity modulated radiotherapy (IMRT) or proton radiotherapy—GRIPS trial (glioblastoma radiotherapy via IMRT or proton BeamS): a study protocol for a multicenter, prospective, open-label, randomized, two-arm, phase III study. Radiat Oncol. 2021;16(1):240. https://doi.org/10.1186/s13014-021-01962-8.
56. de Mol van Otterloo SR, Christodouleas JP, Blezer ELA, et al. The MOMENTUM study: an international registry for the evidence-based introduction of MR-guided adaptive therapy. Front Oncol. 2020;10:1328. https://doi.org/10.3389/fonc.2020.01328.
57. Muroi A, Mizumoto M, Ishikawa E, et al. Proton therapy for newly diagnosed pediatric diffuse intrinsic pontine glioma. Childs Nerv Syst. 2019;36(3):507–12. https://doi.org/10.1007/s00381-019-04420-9.
58. Guerini AE, Nici S, Magrini SM, et al. Adoption of hybrid MRI-linac systems for the treatment of brain tumors: a systematic review of the current literature regarding clinical and technical features. Technol Cancer Res Treat. 2023;22:15330338231199286. https://doi.org/10.1177/15330338231199286.
59. Powers M, Baines J, Crane R, et al. Commissioning measurements on an Elekta Unity MR-Linac. Phys Eng Sci Med. 2022;45(2):457–73. https://doi.org/10.1007/s13246-022-01113-7.
60. Lawrence LSP, Chan RW, Chen H, et al. Accuracy and precision of apparent diffusion coefficient measurements on a 1.5 T MR-Linac in central nervous system tumor patients. Radiother Oncol. 2021;164:155–62. https://doi.org/10.1016/j.radonc.2021.09.020.

61. Tseng CL, Chen H, Stewart J, et al. High grade glioma radiation therapy on a high field 1.5 Tesla MR-Linac—workflow and initial experience with daily adapt-to-position (ATP) MR guidance: a first report. Front Oncol. 2022;12:1060098. https://doi.org/10.3389/fonc.2022.1060098.
62. Lawrence LSP, Chan RW, Chen H, et al. Diffusion-weighted imaging on an MRI-linear accelerator to identify adversely prognostic tumor regions in glioblastoma during chemoradiation. Radiother Oncol. 2023;188:109873. https://doi.org/10.1016/j.radonc.2023.109873.

Management of Recurrent Gliomas: An Update of Strategies and Treatment Options

18

Fabio Cofano, Alberto Morello, Francesca Rizzo, Raffaele De Marco, and Diego Garbossa

18.1 Introduction

Gliomas are notorious for having high recurrence rates, which makes patient care and prognosis more difficult even with advancements in treatment. The goal of this update is to present a comprehensive analysis of many approaches including surgery, chemotherapy, radiation therapy, and laser interstitial thermotherapy (LITT). The recurrence of gliomas is mainly detected by imaging studies, particularly magnetic resonance imaging (MRI). The gold standard in order to differentiate between treatment-related alterations like radiation necrosis and tumor recurrence is still magnetic resonance imaging (MRI) with gadolinium contrast. Advanced imaging techniques, including magnetic resonance spectroscopy (MRS), perfusion MRI, and positron emission tomography (PET), can offer additional metabolic and functional data to distinguish true tumor progression from pseudoprogression or radiation necrosis.

F. Cofano (✉) · A. Morello · F. Rizzo · R. De Marco
Neurosurgery Unit, Department of Neuroscience "Rita Levi Montalcini", AOU Città della Salute e della Scienza di Torino, University Hospital, University of Turin, Turin, Italy
e-mail: fabio.cofano@unito.it

D. Garbossa
Neurosurgery Unit, Dept. Neuroscience "Rita Levi Montalcini", Università degli studi di Torino, Torino, TO, Italy

We present an update on the management of recurrent gliomas, examining the various strategies that can be used in low- and high-grade gliomas (LGG and HGG).

18.2 Recurrence in High-Grade Gliomas

Grade 3 and grade 4 gliomas are defined as "high-grade" gliomas, which have a 2-year survival rate of less than 20% [1].

The disease progression is described by Response Assessment in Neuro-Oncology (RANO) Criteria as a ≥25% increase in the sum of the products of perpendicular diameters of enhancing lesions or the presence of new lesions or substantial worsening in T2/FLAIR sequences or substantial clinical decline [2].

Despite recent advancements in the understanding of the molecular heterogeneity, tumor phenotype, and tumor microenvironment, which provides insight for potential targets of targeted therapies, the treatment of recurrent HGG (rHGG) is challenging. To date, there is no consensus on the protocol for treating rHGG due to discordant results. We review the evaluation of currently applied treatment strategies for patients with rHGG to gain more information on their potential benefits and optimal approach.

D. Armocida et al. (eds.), *Neurosurgery's Frontline Role in Gliomas Treatment*, https://doi.org/10.1007/978-3-031-81850-9_18

18.3 Surgical Management

Surgery plays an important role in the management of rHGG, especially in the presence of symptomatic mass effect or diagnostic uncertainty. Surgery for rHGG aims to decrease tumor burden to increase the effectiveness of adjuvant therapies, relieve symptoms caused by the mass effect, and obtain tissue for histological confirmation to provide personalized therapeutic strategies. Research has indicated that for some patients, surgery can increase survival and quality of life [3]. Park et al. [4] found that a second surgery in recurrent glioblastoma (GBM) patients could extend survival, especially in those with a good functional status and a long interval since the initial surgery. Intraoperative neurophysiologic monitoring (IONM) and awake craniotomy help maximize the extent of resection (EOR) of rHGG located in eloquent areas of the brain and minimize the postoperative deficits [5]. EOR is a recognized prognostic factor, and a greater EOR at both the first and the second (i.e., for recurrent tumors) surgery is associated with higher survival rates [6]. The median overall survival (OS) is found to be superior after re-surgery (11.9 months) as compared with the second-line chemotherapy (4.5–10.8 months) [7]. There is then evidence that re-resection is associated with favorable outcomes when a postoperative volume of less than 1 cm^3 residual contrast enhancement (CE) tumor can be surgically achieved [8]. Furthermore, Karschnia et al. excluded that the prognostic associations of re-resection were induced by the presence of clinical or molecular confounders including MGMT promotor methylation status [8]. In contrast to newly diagnosed GBM [9], Karschnia et al. found no evidence of benefit from "supramaximal" resection of non-CE tumor [8].

One factor to be evaluated is the proximity of the tumor to the ventricle. Indeed, in an evaluation between complications and distance of tumor from the ventricle, the multifocal/multicentric tumor progression emerged statistically significant [10]. Consequently, a close tumor–ventricle distance requires a more aggressive surgical intervention, impacting the outcome (Fig. 18.1).

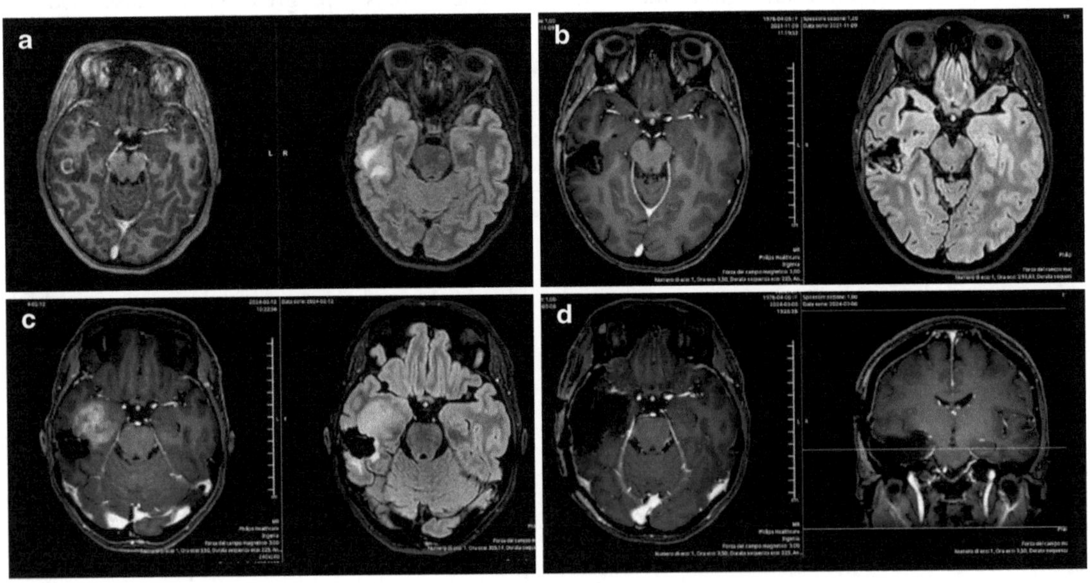

Fig. 18.1 Illustration of radiological patterns of temporal HGG progression. (**a**) Pre-operative MR images. (**b**) Postoperative MR images at 48 h after the first surgery without residual tumor. (**c**) MR images obtained in the same patient with a pattern of infiltrative recurrence involving white matter tracts. (**d**) Postoperative MR images at 48 h after the second surgery with total resection

Surgery for recurrent glioma aiming at molecularly informed treatment is associated with a reasonable surgical morbidity and an acceptable risk of neurological deficits, which does not appear to be significantly higher than in primary surgery. Given that most patients receive gross total resection (GTR) and drugs targets, a multimodal approach for patients with recurrent gliomas may include targeted therapy [11].

All the possible advantages of surgery must be carefully balanced against the potential risks, particularly in eloquent brain regions. This is especially true for patients with a high extent of resection, with a reasonable rate of permanent neurological deficits, ranging from 4% to 8%, and surgical complication rates of 9–22% [12, 13]. The decision to re-operate a recurrent glioma is complex and depends on various factors, rather than a strict numerical limit. The following are the main factors that could influence the choice to proceed with reoperation:

- Patient's Functional Status.
  - The patient's overall health, neurological function, and surgical tolerance are critical factors to consider. Reoperation is more likely to be beneficial for patients with good performance status [e.g., Karnofsky Performance Status (KPS)].
- Tumor Characteristics.
  - Location: During surgery, there is an increased risk of tumors in eloquent brain areas (regions responsible for critical functions like speech or movement).
  - Extent of Recurrence: The possibility of achieving a significant resection is influenced by the size and invasiveness of the recurrent tumo, then when the disease is localized and does not affect eloquent brain regions, deep structures, or both hemispheres.
  - Histology: Aggressive or high-grade tumors, such as GBM, may recur more rapidly and frequently.
- Previous Treatments.
  - Prior Surgeries: Because of scar tissue and anatomical changes, every surgery increases the complexity of following procedures.
  - Radiation Therapy: Tissue alterations induced on by prior radiation may make surgery more difficult.
  - Chemotherapy: Surgical decisions, especially those related to wound healing and infection risk, may be influenced by the kind and degree of previous chemotherapy.
- Surgical Goals.
  - Symptom Relief: Alleviating symptoms like headaches, seizures, or neurological deficits can justify reoperation.
  - Reduction of Tumor Burden: Reducing the tumor bulk may increase the effectiveness of adjuvant therapies and potentially extend survival.
- Risks vs. Benefits.
  - The potential benefits of reoperation must balance the risks, which increase with each additional procedure. Risks include neurological deficits, infections, bleeding, and prolonged recovery times.

18.4 Radiotherapy

Re-irradiation is an option for selected patients with rHGG, particularly those who have a long interval since initial radiotherapy and have tumors located in regions that can tolerate further radiation. Stereotactic radiosurgery (SRS) and fractionated stereotactic radiotherapy (FSRT) are commonly used techniques. SRS has the ability to deliver a single high dose of radiation to a tumor with the capacity to spare surrounding normal tissue due to very steep dose gradient generated by conformal treatment [14]. FSRT offers the ability to reduce treatment margins and volume with more conformal treatment compared with even primary treatment and allow for higher dose per fraction treatment. There is less concern for potential severe side effects than may be with SRS alone. These modalities allow the delivery of high doses of radiation to the tumor while sparing surrounding normal brain tissue. Although standards of re-irradiation are not yet defined for rHGG mainly due to paucity of high-level prospective or randomized control studies, re-irradiation of various techniques is an established salvage option for selected patients, especially in case of a good performance status (KPS >60), localized/unifocal disease, and with a time interval between initial radiation and re-irradiation of at least 6 months [15]. The review of Marwah et al. found that combination therapy may improve OS and progression-free survival (PFS) with acceptable toxicity in select patients with rHGG compared to re-irradiation or systemic therapy alone [16].

Re-irradiation of rHGG is a viable option but comes with limitations and risks that must be carefully considered. Here are the primary factors that influence the decision to proceed with re-irradiation:

- Cumulative Dose and Interval.
  - Cumulative Radiation Dose: The total amount of radiation a patient has received is critical. There is a maximum lifetime dose that tissues can tolerate without severe damage. Previous radiation doses are taken into account to avoid exceeding this threshold.
  - Interval Since Last Radiation: The length of time since the last radiation treatment affects tissue recovery and tolerance. Longer intervals generally allow for better tissue recovery, making re-irradiation more feasible.
- Tumor Location and Size.
  - Location: Tumors located near critical structures or in previously irradiated areas require careful planning to minimize the risk of damage to healthy tissues.
- Radiation Technique and Modality:
  - SRS: Delivers high doses of radiation to a precise area, minimizing exposure to surrounding healthy tissue. Suitable for small, localized recurrences.
  - FSRT: Administers smaller doses over several sessions, reducing the risk of radiation-induced toxicity.
- Patient's Clinical Status:
  - Performance Status: The patient's overall health and neurological function are crucial. Those with better performance status are more likely to tolerate re-irradiation and benefit from it.
  - Symptoms: Symptom control and quality of life considerations often guide decisions about re-irradiation, especially if the intent is palliative.
- Risks and Side Effects:
  - Radiation Necrosis: A serious complication where irradiated brain tissue becomes necrotic, leading to significant neurological deficits. The risk increases with higher cumulative doses.
  - Neurocognitive Decline: Repeated radiation exposure can affect cognitive function, necessitating a careful balance between tumor control and quality of life.

There is no absolute limit to re-irradiation for recurrent gliomas, but careful considerations of cumulative doses, interval since previous irradiation, tumor characteristics, and patient's clinical status are needed. Multidisciplinary evaluation involving neuro-oncologists, radiation oncologists, and other specialists is essential to tailor re-irradiation plans that maximize benefits while minimizing risks.

18.5 Chemotherapy

Chemotherapy remains a cornerstone in the management of recurrent gliomas, with temozolomide (TMZ) being the most commonly used agent. In patients with recurrent GBM (rGBM), the use of TMZ with different dosing schedules than the standard one (150–200 mg/m^2, for 5 days every 28 days) should not be considered as a first-choice treatment option [17].

In patients with good performance status, the use of regorafenib at the time of relapse after standard first-line radio-chemotherapy treatment with temozolomide may be considered. The RE-GOMA study, a multicenter, Italian, randomized phase II trial, showed statistically significant longer survival in regorafenib-treated patients than in lomustine-treated patients; same superiority also for PFS, which appear superior in the regorafenib arm [18].

Bevacizumab (BEV), an anti-angiogenic agent targeting vascular endothelial growth factor (VEGF), has shown promise in recurrent gliomas by reducing peritumoral edema and enhancing quality of life. However, its impact on OS is limited. Patients with rGBM could gain benefits in PFS, palliative, and cognitive advantages from BEV treatment, although the OS benefits cannot be verified with high-quality evidence. Furthermore, BEV combined therapy (especially with lomustine and radiotherapy) showed higher efficacy than BEV monotherapy in the survival of patients with rGBM [19]. However, the literature is unclear, in fact in the results of Wick et al., the treatment with lomustine plus BEV did not confer a survival advantage over treatment with lomustine alone in patients with progressive GBM [20].

18.6 Targeted Therapy and Immunotherapy

The molecular heterogeneity of gliomas stimulated the research for targeted therapies. Numerous studies have shown that glioma has an immunosuppressive nature, and the crosstalk between tumor cells and tumor immune microenvironment can lead to resistance and recurrence. Agents targeting specific mutations, such as EGFRvIII and IDH1/2, are under investigation. Despite initial enthusiasm, results have been modest, and effective biomarkers for patient selection remain elusive at present. Immunotherapy, including checkpoint inhibitors (CI) and vaccines, represents a rapidly expanding area of research [21, 22]. These issues are addressed in more detail in Chap. 16.

18.7 Tumor Treating Fields Therapy (TTFields)

TTFields are low intensity, intermediate frequency (150–200 kHz), alternating electric fields that cause mitotic arrest and apoptosis, resulting in the suppression of tumor growth and spread. TTFields therapy is locoregional, rather than systemic, since the electric fields are continuously generated by a wearable device and delivered via arrays placed directly on the scalp surface at the site of the tumor. In a randomized phase 3 trial involving 237 patients with rGBM whose several lines of prior therapy had failed, TTFields monotherapy was compared with the treating physician's best choice of salvage chemotherapy. Although no survival difference was observed, the response rate to treatment was 14% in the TTFields arm vs. 9.6% (IC95% 3.9–18.8%) in the control arm ($p = 0.19$) [23]. Well-designed prospective trials will be needed to establish with certainty the role of TTFields in the treatment of recurrent glioma.

18.8 Laser Interstitial Thermotherapy (LITT)

Laser Interstitial Thermotherapy (LITT; also known as stereotactic laser ablation or SLA) is a minimally invasive treatment modality that has recently gained prominence in the treatment of malignant brain tumor. LITT acts as a stereotaxically guided laser probe to precisely deliver heat to surrounding brain tissue using magnetic resonance MR thermometry which enables real-time thermal imaging and greater control of laser energy delivery, allowing to carefully monitor the ablation of diseased tissue, sparing the surrounding brain tissue, so as to reduce iatrogenic damage [24]. When patients are not eligible for re-resection due to the number of prior recurrences, lack of trial options, poor KPS, or other eligibility criteria, LITT remains an important treatment option, particularly when LITT can be followed with chemotherapy as also shown in prior reports [25]. LITT is particularly useful for recurrent gliomas in deep or eloquent brain areas where conventional surgery poses high risks.

18.9 Supportive Care and Palliative Therapy

Supportive care is an integral part of rHGG management, addressing symptoms such as seizures, headaches, cognitive deficits, and psychological distress. Multidisciplinary care involving neurooncologists, neurosurgeons, radiation oncologists, and palliative care specialists is essential to optimize quality of life and provide holistic care.

Palliative therapy for patients with rHGG is indicated when the primary goal shifts from prolonging survival to improving quality of life and managing symptoms. The decision to move to palliative care involves several considerations:

- Advanced Disease Stage.
  - Extensive Tumor Burden: When the tumor has progressed significantly despite multiple lines of treatment, leading to a large tumor burden.
  - Multifocal or Diffuse Disease: Tumors that are widespread and not amenable to localized treatments.
- Functional Decline.
  - Poor Performance Status: Patients with a low KPS or Eastern Cooperative Oncology Group (ECOG) performance status, indicating significant impairment in daily activities and self-care.
  - Neurological Deterioration: Progressive neurological deficits that impair essential functions such as mobility, speech, and cognitive abilities.
- Limited Treatment Options.
  - Treatment-Resistant Disease: Tumors that have become resistant to conventional therapies, including surgery, chemotherapy, and radiation.
  - Cumulative Toxicity: Patients who have experienced significant toxicity from previous treatments, making further aggressive therapy impractical.
- Patient and Family Preferences.
  - Quality of Life Priorities: Patients who prioritize quality of life and symptom control over aggressive treatments that offer limited survival benefits.
  - Informed Decision-Making: Discussions with patients and families about the prognosis, potential benefits, and risks of further treatment.
- Components of Palliative Therapy.
  - Pain Control: Use of analgesics, including opioids, to manage pain.
  - Seizure Management: Antiepileptic drugs to control seizures.
  - Edema Control: Steroids such as dexamethasone to reduce cerebral edema and alleviate symptoms like headaches and nausea.
  - Nutritional Support: Assistance with maintaining adequate nutrition, including dietary counseling and supplements.
  - Psychological Support: Counseling and mental health services to address anxiety, depression, and emotional distress.
  - Physical Therapy: Rehabilitation services to maintain mobility and function as much as possible.
- Hospice Care and Caregiver Support:
  - End-of-Life Planning: Comprehensive care that focuses on comfort, dignity, and support during the final stages of life. Hospice care can be provided at home, in hospice facilities, or in hospitals.
  - Education and Counseling: Helping families understand the disease trajectory and prepare for changes.
  - Respite Care: Temporary relief for primary caregivers to prevent burnout and ensure continuous care for the patient.
- Timing of Palliative Therapy.
- The transition to palliative therapy should be considered in case of:
  - Disease Progression: The glioma continues to progress despite aggressive treatment.
  - Patient Wishes: The patient expresses a desire to focus on comfort rather than extending life.
  - Medical Team Recommendation: The healthcare team assesses that further curative treatment is unlikely to provide significant benefit and may cause harm.

18.10 Recurrence in Low-Grade Gliomas

As mentioned in Chap. 7, early and maximal surgical resection is the standard initial treatment for LGGs because it reduces tumor volume, which delays MT and extends OS [26–31].

However, because of the high recurrence rate and the propensity for MT, LGG poses a formidable challenge in neuro-oncology. Treatment of recurrences is subject to wide variation in clinical practice. There is no consensus on the optimal threshold for or timing of retreatment. In essentially all cases, repeat surgery is considered, and depending on the opinions of the treatment team members, some centers utilize repeat surgery more than others. Re-irradiation with conventional beam therapy is usually not recommended at first recurrence due to concern for side effects and radiation necrosis [32]. Although it is necessary to reconsider all treatment options when evaluating a patient with tumor recurrence, currently the practice mainly uses surgery or chemotherapy in the treatment of rLGG. Re-irradiation is reserved for patients not eligible for surgery, further chemotherapy, or clinical trials.

18.11 Diagnosis of Recurrence

Radiological diagnosis of tumor recurrence was generally based on criteria of Response Assessment in Neuro-Oncology (RANO) working group [33] and included ≥25% increase of the product of perpendicular diameters of the lesion or appearance of new hyperintense area(s) on T2-weigthed and/or FLAIR images not attributable to effects of adjuvant therapy, or appearance or expansion of the contrast-enhanced areas on T1-weighted images, in association with "tumor pattern" on MRS and definite radio-isotope uptake on positron emission tomography with ^{11}C-methionine (MET-PET). Appearance of a new area of contrast enhancement on T1-weighted MRI was considered as a sign of MT [33]. Differentiation of tumor recurrence and radiation-induced necrosis was mainly based on MET-PET. Compared to the gold standard MRI, MET-PET offers complementary information comparable to standard methods and appears to be a critical tool for differentiating tumor recurrence from other entities such as pseudoprogression, radiation necrosis, and pseudoregression.

18.12 The Pattern of "Migratory" Recurrence

Recurrence typically occurs within years of the initial surgery, even in cases of GTR. MT represents a critical and irreversible event in the course of LGGs, and the inability to predict its occurrence on a linear timeline makes the timing of therapeutic interventions uncertain. Satar et al. showed the prognostic factors on MT in LGGs: presentation with epileptic seizures, velocity of diametric expansion (VDE) >8 mm/y, VDE >4 mm/y, rCBV >1.75, preoperative tumor volume (PTV) ≥5 cm (65 ml), PTV ≥100 ml, cortical involvement, IDH-wildtype, TP53 mutation, and TMZ monotherapy [34].

Glioma regrowth also allows massive brain reorganization with a reassignment of peritumoral functional areas identified during the first surgery. This neuroplastic potential may result from several factors (e.g., initial resection, postoperative functional rehabilitation, and speed of tumor expansion) and opens the door for a multistep surgical approach to optimize both EOR and OS. In fact, although glioma relapse usually arises locally, around the previous surgical cavity, LGG also has the propensity to migrate along associative white matter tracts or even commissural fibers to reach the contralateral hemisphere [35]. The "migratory" pattern of recurrence in the context of LGGs refers to a pattern of tumor regrowth that spreads primarily along white matter tracts, rather than remaining in a cortical area. If LGGs recurring after initial surgery show a more migratory pattern, with a prominent spread along the white matter tracts, then the EOR has a high risk of being lower at the time of reoperation [36]. This connectomal constraint plays an important role in the decision to re-operate, because the plastic potential is low at the level of the axonal fibers -as opposed to a high plastic potential at the level of the cortex, which argues in favor of iterative surgeries for tumor recurrence with a more bulky pattern and that mainly involves the cortical areas [37].

Slow tumor growth over time allows the brain to reorganize, creating opportunities for further surgical resections based on these connectome changes. However, rapid tumor progression, as in the case of MT, may limit the potential for plasticity and EOR. Therefore, when considering reoperation for rLGG, it is critical to carefully evaluate the pattern of recurrence, taking into account both spatial and temporal aspects of tumor regrowth. The challenge is to anticipate what type of migration the cancer cells will adopt and whether they will allow reintervention.

An interesting work studied patients undergoing iterative awake surgeries for LGG and classified patients into two groups based on a high or low level of plasticity investigated by means of longitudinal cortico-subcortical direct electrostimulation mapping (DEM) [36]. Interestingly, cortical tumors with sharper borders generated more efficient reactional plastic potential than wide infiltrative tumors with less distinct borders. In addition, the subgroup showing preponderant cortical regrowth had greater EOR and earlier functional recovery after reoperation. These results support the hypothesis that a cortical regrowth with a limited infiltration of white matter pathways may open the window for more extensive resection at reoperation and that patients with such a nonmigratory relcurrence pattern are ideal candidates for a second surgery [38].

Because of frequent functional remodeling between the first and second surgery, or even between the second and third surgery, it is highly recommended to awake the patient to benefit not only from an accurate electrical mapping but also from an extensive cognitive and emotional monitoring performed in real time throughout the resection [39]. In order to improve the sensitivity of such neuropsychological assessment in the operating room, which should also take into consideration the spatial relationships between the lesion and surrounding eloquent pathways according to the tumor location, the use of a multitasking protocol has been suggested, because it requires recruiting multiple neural circuits by increasing the cognitive demand, as a mirror of the meta-network [39].

18.13 Repeat Surgery

Repeat operations should be integrated into a more comprehensive multimodal therapeutic attitude, including chemotherapy and radiotherapy. In case of rapid postoperative regrowth of LGGS, early reoperation should be considered if functionally feasible, with adjuvant treatment to be performed immediately after the last surgery. On the contrary, if the regrowth is slow after the initial resection, it may be proposed to postpone adjuvant therapies, especially radiotherapy. Indeed, irradiation of the white matter tracts has a risk to generate delayed cognitive deteriorations [40]. Moreover, radiotherapy-induced alterations in the brain microenvironment may contribute to recurrent glioma aggressiveness [41]. Therefore, in case of a slow LGG re-progression after the first surgery, particularly in case of large resection, a simple surveillance based on regular MRI monitoring with volumetric measurement and growth rate calculation can be considered, even in LGGs with MT foci in the center of the tumor [42].

However, although reoperation should be preferred at recurrence, when the LGGs relapse exhibits a more migratory pattern along the white matter tracts, because EOR has a high risk to be less, chemotherapy may be discussed [43]. Studies have shown that reoperation to address tumor recurrence is a safe and effective therapeutic approach, resulting in increased survival and preservation of quality of life [44]. Beyond the fact that overall quality of life is usually preserved, chemotherapy may induce a tumor shrinkage with a lesser degree of infiltration of the subcortical fibers, then reopening the window to a reoperation with improvement of the EOR [45]. The same principle can be applied after a second or even a third surgery, allowing to reach an OS close to 18 years [46].

In deciding whether to re-operate, there are several factors to consider. Patients who benefit from a second surgery typically have a larger EOR and lower residual tumor volume at the time of their first surgery, longer time interval between surgeries, better functional status (KPS score) and young age.

In selected patients with rLGG, reoperation with awake DEM was associated with favorable oncological outcomes, a low postsurgical morbidity, a high rate of return to work postoperatively and seizure control [38]. To optimize outcomes, it is best to re-operate before symptom onset (e.g., seizures and cognitive or behavioral changes) and before MT. This positive result is probably due to the cytoreduction effect of repeat resections, which may delay LGGs malignant transformation. The ability to perform repeat resections with low risk of morbidity is largely due to the use of intraoperative mapping in awake patients. In fact, neurocognitive abilities are often preserved after surgery. Awake mapping is critical because the slow regrowth of the LGGs allows for functional reorganization of the brain over time, enabling neurosurgeons to adapt the resection and preserve eloquent areas.

18.14 Oncological Considerations

The mostly widely accepted prognostic factors are age at diagnosis, KPS score, and neurological status before primary surgery, maximum diameter, eloquent location, and bi-hemispheric extension of the tumor, EOR and residual lesion volume, histological type of the neoplasm, and presence of IDH1/IDH2 mutations and 1p/19q co-deletion [47, 48].

Current guidelines, although based on studies that are not recent, suggest a benefit from chemotherapy treatment with nitrosoureas or temozolomide in patients with rLGG with the appearance of enhancement [49, 50].

On the other hand, IDH1-mutant tumors much more often show non-early onset and slow progression recurrence, whereas 1p/19q co-deletion has been associated with non-early onset of relapse and its regional or marginal location. Therefore, it can be hypothesized that realization of the positive prognostic impact of IDH1/IDH2 mutations and 1p/19q co-deletion may be in part related to more favorable characteristics of relapse at the time of its development [30]. In particular, mutations in IDH1 or IDH2 are frequently observed in gliomas, as discovered through whole-exome sequencing over 15 years ago [51]. Gliomas with IDH1 or IDH2 mutations were consistently found to be less aggressive than IDH1-wild-type and IDH2-wild-type infiltrative gliomas, so screening for these mutations, through sequencing or use of an antibody specific for the most common variant, IDH1 R132H, soon became the standard of care for prognostication in people with glioma [52]. Mutant IDH produces the oncometabolite d-2-hydroxyglutarate (D-2-HG), which induces DNA and histone hypermethylation and interferes with immunity, thereby stimulating tumor growth. Selective inhibitors of mutant IDH, such as ivosidenib and vorasidenib, have been shown to reduce D-2-HG levels and induce cell differentiation in preclinical models and induce MRI-detectable responses in early clinical trials [53]. The phase III INDIGO trial demonstrated the superiority of vorasidenib over placebo in residual or recurrent non-enhancing grade 2 gliomas after surgery, thus raising the prospect of delaying of chemoradiotherapy [54]. The results of the INDIGO trial tend to be practice-changing: given the magnitude of improvement in primary and secondary end points compared with placebo, it is expected that vorasidenib will be approved by authorities such as the FDA and the European Medicines Agency and become a standard first-line treatment, at least for non-enhancing grade 2 IDH1-mutant and IDH2-mutant gliomas with residual or progressive tumor following surgery.

18.15 Radiomic: Emerging Role of Artificial Intelligence in Recurrence

Recently, the use of artificial intelligence (AI) has already changed our behaviors and our society and it will increasingly impact the healthcare world as well. Application of AI has been extended to the processing of MRI in glioma. Radiomics, a recent method that aims at extracting features from medical images using data-characterization algorithms, not only has the potential to reflect the underlying characteristics of tumor but is also easier to predict glioma recurrence [55]. Although some models are not suitable for clinical use at this point, the different areas of AI application in the field of recurrence glioma with refined pre-operative diagnostics and outcome predictions will significantly influence the future of neurosurgery [56–58]. Therefore, neurosurgeons will continue to make the decisions on the indications for surgery but an optimized statement on diagnosis, treatment options and on the risk of surgery will be made by neurosurgeons with the help of AI in the future.

References

1. Marra JS, Mendes GP, Yoshinari GHJ, da Silva GF, Mazin SC, de Oliveira HF. Survival after radiation therapy for high-grade glioma. Rep Pract Oncol Radiother. 2019;24(1):35–40.
2. Wen PY, Macdonald DR, Reardon DA, Cloughesy TF, Sorensen AG, Galanis E, et al. Updated response assessment criteria for high-grade gliomas: response assessment in neuro-oncology working group. J Clin Oncol Off J Am Soc Clin Oncol. 2010;28(11):1963–72.
3. Suchorska B, Weller M, Tabatabai G, Senft C, Hau P, Sabel MC, et al. Complete resection of contrast-enhancing tumor volume is associated with improved survival in recurrent glioblastoma-results from the DIRECTOR trial. Neuro Oncol. 2016;18(4):549–56.
4. Park JK, Hodges T, Arko L, Shen M, Dello Iacono D, McNabb A, et al. Scale to predict survival after surgery for recurrent glioblastoma multiforme. J Clin Oncol Off J Am Soc Clin Oncol. 2010;28(24):3838–43.
5. Barbagallo GMV, Certo F, Di Gregorio S, Maione M, Garozzo M, Peschillo S, et al. Recurrent high-grade glioma surgery: a multimodal intraoperative protocol to safely increase extent of tumor resection and analysis of its impact on patient outcome. Neurosurg Focus. 2021;50(1):E20.
6. Oppenlander ME, Wolf AB, Snyder LA, Bina R, Wilson JR, Coons SW, et al. An extent of resection threshold for recurrent glioblastoma and its risk for neurological morbidity. J Neurosurg. 2014;120(4):846–53.
7. Ringel F, Pape H, Sabel M, Krex D, Bock HC, Misch M, et al. Clinical benefit from resection of recurrent glioblastomas: results of a multicenter study including 503 patients with recurrent glioblastomas undergoing surgical resection. Neuro Oncol. 2016;18(1):96–104.
8. Karschnia P, Dono A, Young JS, Juenger ST, Teske N, Häni L, et al. Prognostic evaluation of re-resection for recurrent glioblastoma using the novel RANO classification for extent of resection: a report of the RANO resect group. Neuro Oncol. 2023;25(9):1672–85.
9. Incekara F, Smits M, van der Voort SR, Dubbink HJ, Atmodimedjo PN, Kros JM, et al. The association between the extent of glioblastoma resection and survival in light of MGMT promoter methylation in 326 patients with newly diagnosed IDH-wildtype glioblastoma. Front Oncol. 2020;10:1087.
10. Cofano F, Bianconi A, De Marco R, Consoli E, Zeppa P, Bruno F, et al. The impact of lateral ventricular opening in the resection of newly diagnosed high-grade gliomas: a single center experience. Cancers (Basel). 2024;16(8):1574. https://doi.org/10.3390/cancers16081574.
11. Alhalabi OT, Dao Trong P, Kaes M, Jakobs M, Kessler T, Oehler H, et al. Repeat surgery of recurrent glioma for molecularly informed treatment in the age of precision oncology: a risk-benefit analysis. J Neurooncol. 2024;167(2):245–55.
12. Bloch O, Han SJ, Cha S, Sun MZ, Aghi MK, McDermott MW, et al. Impact of extent of resection for recurrent glioblastoma on overall survival: clinical article. J Neurosurg. 2012;117(6):1032–8.
13. Chaichana KL, Zadnik P, Weingart JD, Olivi A, Gallia GL, Blakeley J, et al. Multiple resections for patients with glioblastoma: prolonging survival. J Neurosurg. 2013;118(4):812–20.
14. Barnett GH, Linskey ME, Adler JR, Cozzens JW, Friedman WA, Heilbrun MP, et al. Stereotactic radiosurgery—an organized neurosurgery-sanctioned definition. J Neurosurg. 2007;106(1):1–5.
15. Minniti G, Niyazi M, Alongi F, Navarria P, Belka C. Current status and recent advances in reirradiation of glioblastoma. Radiat Oncol. 2021;16(1):36.
16. Marwah R, Xing D, Squire T, Soon YY, Gan HK, Ng SP. Reirradiation versus systemic therapy versus combination therapy for recurrent high-grade glioma: a systematic review and meta-analysis of survival and toxicity. J Neurooncol. 2023;164(3):505–24.
17. Gilbert MR, Wang M, Aldape KD, Stupp R, Hegi ME, Jaeckle KA, et al. Dose-dense temozolomide for newly diagnosed glioblastoma: a randomized phase III clinical trial. J Clin Oncol Off J Am Soc Clin Oncol. 2013;31(32):4085–91.
18. Lombardi G, De Salvo GL, Brandes AA, Eoli M, Rudà R, Faedi M, et al. Regorafenib compared with lomustine in patients with relapsed glioblastoma (REGOMA): a multicentre, open-label, randomised, controlled, phase 2 trial. Lancet Oncol. 2019;20(1):110–9.
19. Fu M, Zhou Z, Huang X, Chen Z, Zhang L, Zhang J, et al. Use of bevacizumab in recurrent glioblastoma: a scoping review and evidence map. BMC Cancer. 2023;23(1):544.
20. Wick W, Gorlia T, Bendszus M, Taphoorn M, Sahm F, Harting I, et al. Lomustine and bevacizumab in progressive glioblastoma. N Engl J Med. 2017;377(20):1954–63.
21. Pu Y, Zhou G, Zhao K, Chen Y, Shen S. Immunotherapy for recurrent glioma-from bench to bedside. Cancers (Basel). 2023;15(13):3421. https://doi.org/10.3390/cancers15133421.

22. Bianconi A, Palmieri G, Aruta G, Monticelli M, Zeppa P, Tartara F, et al. Updates in glioblastoma immunotherapy: an overview of the current clinical and translational scenario. Biomedicines. 2023;11(6):1520. https://doi.org/10.3390/biomedicines11061520.
23. Stupp R, Wong ET, Kanner AA, Steinberg D, Engelhard H, Heidecke V, et al. NovoTTF-100A versus physician's choice chemotherapy in recurrent glioblastoma: a randomised phase III trial of a novel treatment modality. Eur J Cancer. 2012;48(14):2192–202.
24. Lee I, Kalkanis S, Hadjipanayis CG. Stereotactic laser interstitial thermal therapy for recurrent high-grade gliomas. Neurosurgery. 2016;79(Suppl 1):S24–34.
25. Morello A, Bianconi A, Rizzo F, Bellomo J, Meyer AC, Garbossa D, et al. Laser interstitial thermotherapy (LITT) in recurrent glioblastoma: what window of opportunity for this treatment? Technol Cancer Res Treat. 2024;23:15330338241249026.
26. Ostrom QT, Cioffi G, Waite K, Kruchko C, Barnholtz-Sloan JS. CBTRUS statistical report: primary brain and other central nervous system tumors diagnosed in the United States in 2014-2018. Neuro Oncol. 2021;23(12 Suppl 2):iii1–iii105. https://doi.org/10.1093/neuonc/noab200.
27. Louis DN, Perry A, Wesseling P, Brat DJ, Cree IA, Figarella-Branger D, et al. The 2021 WHO classification of tumors of the central nervous system: a summary. Neuro Oncol. 2021;23(8):1231–51.
28. Han S, Liu Y, Cai SJ, Qian M, Ding J, Larion M, et al. IDH mutation in glioma: molecular mechanisms and potential therapeutic targets. Br J Cancer. 2020;122(11):1580–9.
29. McGirt MJ, Chaichana KL, Attenello FJ, Weingart JD, Than K, Burger PC, et al. Extent of surgical resection is independently associated with survival in patients with hemispheric infiltrating low-grade gliomas. Neurosurgery. 2008;63(4):700–8.
30. Fukuya Y, Ikuta S, Maruyama T, Nitta M, Saito T, Tsuzuki S, et al. Tumor recurrence patterns after surgical resection of intracranial low-grade gliomas. J Neurooncol. 2019;144(3):519–28.
31. Murphy ES, Leyrer CM, Parsons M, Suh JH, Chao ST, Yu JS, et al. Risk factors for malignant transformation of low-grade glioma. Int J Radiat Oncol Biol Phys. 2018;100(4):965–71.
32. Carabenciov ID, Buckner JC. Controversies in the therapy of low-grade gliomas. Curr Treat Options Oncol. 2019;20(4):25.
33. van den Bent MJ, Wefel JS, Schiff D, Taphoorn MJB, Jaeckle K, Junck L, et al. Response assessment in neuro-oncology (a report of the RANO group): assessment of outcome in trials of diffuse low-grade gliomas. Lancet Oncol. 2011;12(6):583–93.
34. Satar Z, Hotton G, Samandouras G. Systematic review-time to malignant transformation in low-grade gliomas: predicting a catastrophic event with clinical, neuroimaging, and molecular markers. Neurooncol Adv. 2021;3(1):vdab101.
35. Ferracci F-X, Michaud K, Duffau H. The landscape of postsurgical recurrence patterns in diffuse low-grade gliomas. Crit Rev Oncol Hematol. 2019;138:148–55.
36. Picart T, Herbet G, Moritz-Gasser S, Duffau H. Iterative surgical resections of diffuse glioma with awake mapping: how to deal with cortical plasticity and connectomal constraints? Neurosurgery. 2019;85(1):105–16.
37. Duffau H. White matter tracts and diffuse lower-grade gliomas: the pivotal role of myelin plasticity in the tumor pathogenesis, infiltration patterns, functional consequences and therapeutic management. Front Oncol. 2022;12:855587.
38. Ribeiro L, Ng S, Duffau H. Recurrent insular low-grade gliomas: factors guiding the decision to reoperate. J Neurosurg. 2023;138(5):1216–26.
39. Duffau H, Ng S, Lemaitre A-L, Moritz-Gasser S, Herbet G. Constant multi-tasking with time constraint to preserve across-network dynamics throughout awake surgery for low-grade glioma: a necessary step to enable patients resuming an active life. Front Oncol. 2022;12:924762.
40. Blonski M, Obara T, Brzenczek C, Pouget C, Dillier C, Meyer M, et al. Initial PCV chemotherapy followed by radiotherapy is associated with a prolonged response but late neurotoxicity in 20 diffuse low-grade glioma patients. Front Oncol. 2022;12:827897.
41. Gupta K, Burns TC. Radiation-induced alterations in the recurrent glioblastoma microenvironment: therapeutic implications. Front Oncol. 2018;8:503.
42. Pallud J, Blonski M, Mandonnet E, Audureau E, Fontaine D, Sanai N, et al. Velocity of tumor spontaneous expansion predicts long-term outcomes for diffuse low-grade gliomas. Neuro Oncol. 2013;15(5):595–606.
43. Duffau H. Dynamic interplay between lower-grade glioma instability and brain metaplasticity: proposal of an original model to guide the therapeutic strategy. Cancers (Basel). 2021;13(19):4759. https://doi.org/10.3390/cancers13194759.
44. Blonski M, Taillandier L, Herbet G, Maldonado IL, Beauchesne P, Fabbro M, et al. Combination of neoadjuvant chemotherapy followed by surgical resection as a new strategy for WHO grade II gliomas: a study of cognitive status and quality of life. J Neurooncol. 2012;106(2):353–66.
45. Spena G, Garbossa D, Barletta L, Prevost C, Versari P. Preoperative chemotherapy for infiltrative low-grade oligoastrocytoma: a useful strategy to maximize surgical resection -case report. Neurol Med Chir (Tokyo). 2010;50(5):410–3.
46. Hamdan N, Duffau H. Extending the multistage surgical strategy for recurrent initially low-grade gliomas: functional and oncological outcomes in 31 consecutive patients who underwent a third resection under awake mapping. J Neurosurg. 2022;136(4):1035–44.
47. Daniels TB, Brown PD, Felten SJ, Wu W, Buckner JC, Arusell RM, et al. Validation of EORTC prognostic factors for adults with low-grade glioma: a report

using intergroup 86-72-51. Int J Radiat Oncol Biol Phys. 2011;81(1):218–24.
48. Chang EF, Smith JS, Chang SM, Lamborn KR, Prados MD, Butowski N, et al. Preoperative prognostic classification system for hemispheric low-grade gliomas in adults. J Neurosurg. 2008;109(5):817–24.
49. Buckner JC, Gesme DJ, O'Fallon JR, Hammack JE, Stafford S, Brown PD, et al. Phase II trial of procarbazine, lomustine, and vincristine as initial therapy for patients with low-grade oligodendroglioma or oligoastrocytoma: efficacy and associations with chromosomal abnormalities. J Clin Oncol Off J Am Soc Clin Oncol. 2003;21(2):251–5.
50. Quinn JA, Reardon DA, Friedman AH, Rich JN, Sampson JH, Provenzale JM, et al. Phase II trial of temozolomide in patients with progressive low-grade glioma. J Clin Oncol. 2003;21(4):646–51. https://doi.org/10.1200/JCO.2003.01.009.
51. Yan H, Parsons DW, Jin G, McLendon R, Rasheed BA, Yuan W, et al. IDH1 and IDH2 mutations in gliomas. N Engl J Med. 2009;360(8):765–73.
52. Horbinski C, Kofler J, Kelly LM, Murdoch GH, Nikiforova MN. Diagnostic use of IDH1/2 mutation analysis in routine clinical testing of formalin-fixed, paraffin-embedded glioma tissues. J Neuropathol Exp Neurol. 2009;68(12):1319–25.
53. Rudà R, Horbinski C, van den Bent M, Preusser M, Soffietti R. IDH inhibition in gliomas: from preclinical models to clinical trials. Nat Rev Neurol. 2024;20(7):395–407. https://doi.org/10.1038/s41582-024-00967-7.
54. Wen P, Mellinghoff I, van den Bent M, Blumenthal D, Touat M, Peters K, et al. LTBK-06. Impact of vorasidenib treatment on mutant IDH1 or IDH2 diffuse glioma tumor growth rate: results from the randomized, double-blind, phase 3 indigo study. Neuro Oncol. 2023;25(Supplement_5):v310–1. https://doi.org/10.1093/neuonc/noad179.1202.
55. Zanier O, Da Mutten R, Vieli M, Regli L, Serra C, Staartjes VE. DeepEOR: automated perioperative volumetric assessment of variable grade gliomas using deep learning. Acta Neurochir (Wien). 2023;165(2):555–66. https://doi.org/10.1007/s00701-022-05446-w.
56. Della Pepa GM, Caccavella VM, Menna G, Ius T, Auricchio AM, Sabatino G, et al. Machine learning-based prediction of early recurrence in glioblastoma patients: a glance towards precision medicine. Neurosurgery. 2021;89(5):873–83.
57. Cepeda S, Luppino LT, Pérez-Núñez A, Solheim O, García-García S, Velasco-Casares M, et al. Predicting regions of local recurrence in glioblastomas using voxel-based radiomic features of multiparametric postoperative MRI. Cancers (Basel). 2023;15(6):1894. https://doi.org/10.3390/cancers15061894.
58. Habib A, Jovanovich N, Hoppe M, Ak M, Mamindla P, Colen RR, et al. MRI-based radiomics and radiogenomics in the management of low-grade gliomas: evaluating the evidence for a paradigm shift. J Clin Med. 2021;10(7):1411. https://doi.org/10.3390/jcm10071411.

19 Radionecrosis in Gliomas: The Diagnostic and Therapeutic Challenge: A Narrative Review

Francesco Paglia, Daniele Armocida, and Lorenzo Sgarbanti

19.1 Introduction

Radionecrosis (RN) is a rare side effect of cranial radiotherapy that must always be taken into account when evaluating a patient with a recurrent enhancing lesion, given the appropriate clinical context. This delayed effect of radiation injury can occur in about 3–24% of patients who receive standard radiation therapy. RN typically develops between 3 and 12 months after treatment, most commonly at the site of the highest radiation dose, which is usually close to the original tumor and surrounding the surgical cavity [1].

RN could be a serious complication: it is a reaction of healthy brain tissue to radiotherapy, characterized by necrosis and fibrinous exudate near the edge of an irradiated cerebral glial lesion [2, 3]. It is frequently asymptomatic but, in 8–10% of cases [4], it can cause several symptoms such headaches, focal neurological deficits, neurocognitive dysfunction, and seizures [5].

F. Paglia (✉)
Rome Human Neurosciences Department, AUO "Policlinico Umberto I", Neurosurgery Division, Sapienza University, Rome, Italy

D. Armocida
Neurosurgery Unit, Dept. Neuroscience "Rita Levi Montalcini", Università degli studi di Torino, Torino, TO, Italy

L. Sgarbanti (✉)
Department of Neurosurgery, University Hospital S. Anna of Ferrara, Ferrara, Italy
e-mail: lorenzo.sgarbanti@edu.unife.it

19.2 Epidemiology and Risk Factors

The actual occurrence of RN is challenging to establish and falls between 3 and 50% in all patients who undergo radiotherapy or radiosurgery [3, 5–7]. This wide range is influenced by the fact that histological confirmation is not always required in all studies, so the incidence could be higher in studies that rely primarily on imaging-based diagnosis. Furthermore, improvements in diagnostic imaging quality and frequency have contributed to this range [5, 6]. RN has several risk factors that can impact this range. While many risk factors have been identified, it is difficult to determine the direct cause-and-effect relationship for RN. The main risk factors are as follows:

19.2.1 Dose-Volume Interplay

The risk of developing radionecrosis increases with higher doses of radiation administered in a single session. To reduce or avoid this risk, fractionated stereotactic radiotherapy (SRT) and stereotactic radiosurgery have been suggested as alternatives to single-fraction treatment [3, 5].

D. Armocida et al. (eds.), *Neurosurgery's Frontline Role in Gliomas Treatment*,
https://doi.org/10.1007/978-3-031-81850-9_19

The maximum tolerated doses for single-fraction SRT varied depending on the size of the tumor: 24 Gy for tumors ≤20 mm, 18 Gy for tumors 21–30 mm, and 15 Gy for tumors 31–40 mm in diameter. Consequently, patients with larger lesions are at a higher risk of developing RN compared to those with smaller tumor masses [2].

19.2.2 Planning Target Volume (PTV) Margin

The planning target volume should consider geometric uncertainties in delivery and treatment planning while also compensating for possible deviations in patient positioning and including potential microscopic spread. The latest guidelines indicate expanding up to 3 mm in the treated area, reducing it from 5 mm in the 2016 guidelines [8]. This safety margin becomes 0 mm when lesions are near the brainstem or near another brain structure at radiological risk [5]. The larger the glioma volume, the larger the PTV and consequently the larger the irradiated area [6]. However, it is particularly debated how a larger PTV may be a risk factor of radionecrosis and that this may vary the median survival and progression-free survival, because conflicting results have been found in the literature [6, 8, 9].

19.2.3 Prior Radiation Exposure

Prior radiation exposure increases the risk of RN especially if the patient has previously undergone whole-brain radiotherapy or stereotactic radiosurgery or is currently undergoing the combination of whole-brain radiotherapy and SRT [6]. Reirradiation, in cases of tumor recurrence, submits the patient to additional exposure.

19.2.4 Chemotherapy

In the management of patients with gliomas, the standard treatment after surgery includes radiotherapy with concomitant and maintenance temozolomide adjuvant chemotherapy [10]. The use of this specific drug may produce by itself changes mimicking radiation damage, including cerebral necrosis, but Ruben et al. have demonstrated also how it increase the necrotic risk if associated to radiotherapy [11]. It is suspected it is due to the enhanced susceptibility of brain tissue after administration of anti-cancer drugs [3, 6, 12].

19.2.5 Location

The different structures of the brain have varying sensitivities to radiation, which can affect their risk of RN [2, 13]. Although further research is needed to confirm this, the frontal cortex appears to be the most vulnerable. This uncertainty is likely due to the fact that frontal site is also a common site for gliomas with larger tumor volumes [14]. The depth of the lesion can also impact the likelihood of RN, as superficial cortical lesions are less risky due to the dispersion of radiation doses into extraparenchymal tissues [6]. During radiation therapy, it is important to limit the resection margin and dose near the most radiosensitive organs to avoid complications and neurological deficits. Organs at risk in neuroradiotherapic regimens include the brainstem, hippocampus, pituitary, optic nerve and chiasm, circle of Willis, cochlea, retina, lens, lacrimal glands, salivary glands, thyroid, spinal cord, cauda equina, and brachial plexus [13]. The recommended dose limits for SRT on these organs vary: for the brainstem, it is 12.5 Gy to avoid major neurological deficits; for the optic chiasm, it is 8 Gy; and for the cochlea, it is 4–6 Gy up to a maximum of 12 Gy, especially in cases of inner ear invasion. However, dose limits for the hippocampus are currently unknown. Radiotherapy doses greater than 7.3 Gy delivered to 40% of the bilateral hippocampal area have been linked to long-term memory impairment [2, 13].

19.2.6 Age

Calderon et al. showed statistically that in patients under 65 years of age, the risk of developing radionecrosis after exposure to radiotherapy is higher than in patients over 65 years of age. The main reason for this is not yet clear but it is speculated that it is because younger patients have more immune system activity than older patients, which actively engages in the pathogenesis of RN [9].

19.2.7 Intrinsic Radiosensitivity

Each patient has its own inherent radiosensitivity that is impossible to quantify, but some patients are more susceptible to developing radionecrosis. Some researchers have demonstrated this by exposing skin fibroblasts (in vitro), taken from people who have developed RN, to radiation and evaluated survival curves, confirming the hypotesis [6].

19.3 Symptomatology

Radionecrosis is mainly asymptomatic but in 8–10% [4] of cases, it may provoke symptoms such as headaches, nausea, confusion, or lethargy, which can be caused by increased intracranial pressure, cognitive impairment, personality changes, memory loss, seizures, or focal deficits related to the location of the lesion [3, 6, 15, 16]. Radiation injury can lead to cognitive deterioration, but it may also be related to the volume and amount of irradiated tissue in the hippocampal dentate gyrus, owing to the presence of radiosensitive neural stem cells [13]. These symptoms severely affect the quality of life of patients and can even shorten their survival time. The management of radiation injuries depends primarily on the presence of symptoms.

19.3.1 Physiopathology

Exposure of brain tissue to radiation results in various effects that can be categorized based on the time elapsed since radiation treatment: acute toxicity, which occurs immediately after treatment; early delayed neurotoxicity, which develops within 12 weeks of treatment; and delayed neurotoxicity, which can emerge 3 months to several years after treatment. While the first two are typically reversible and temporary, the latter can lead to irreversible damage, including radiation necrosis and radiation leukoencephalopathy [15]. Although there are two main theories that explain the pathophysiology of RN, it is likely that the true cause is a combination of both or multiple factors.

19.3.2 Vascular Injury Theory

Irradiation of brain tissue can break the blood–brain barrier, producing increased capillary leakiness and vascular permeability, establishing an imbalance in tissue homeostasis. The damage of astrocyte active endothelial apoptosis, mediated by acid sphingomyelinase, especially with radiation in large fraction sizes >8Gy [3, 6, 15, 17]. This endothelial damage produce oxygen free radicals, inflammatory cytokine, such as tumor-necrosis factor and interleukin-1 beta [6], vascular endothelial growth factor (VEGF) upregulation and over-expression, and over-expression of intercellular adhesion molecules (ICAM-1) [6, 15, 17]. Subsequently, as result of the hypoxia signal, linked to increased VEGF production, a dysfunctional proliferation of the endothelial cells is set up, generating more vasogenic edema, increases in blood–brain barrier permeability and fibroblast infiltration. This cascade leads to vessel narrowing, thrombosis, fibrinoid necrosis of small vessels, due to the activation of fibroblasts, resulting in ischemic stroke or hemorrhage and vascular endothelial cells death, which it may occur months to years after radiotherapy [3, 13, 15]. (Fig. 19.1).

19.3.3 Glial Cell Theory

Brain tissue damaged by radiation therapy produces excessive amounts of proinflammatory cytokines such as VEGF, TNF-α, IL-1α, IL-6, and TGF-β, leading to chronic inflammation [3]. This process is enhanced by the direct injury caused by ionizing radiation on brain cells, which increases reactive oxygen species that result in single- and double-stranded DNA damage. This leads to cell swelling and necrosis. Chronic

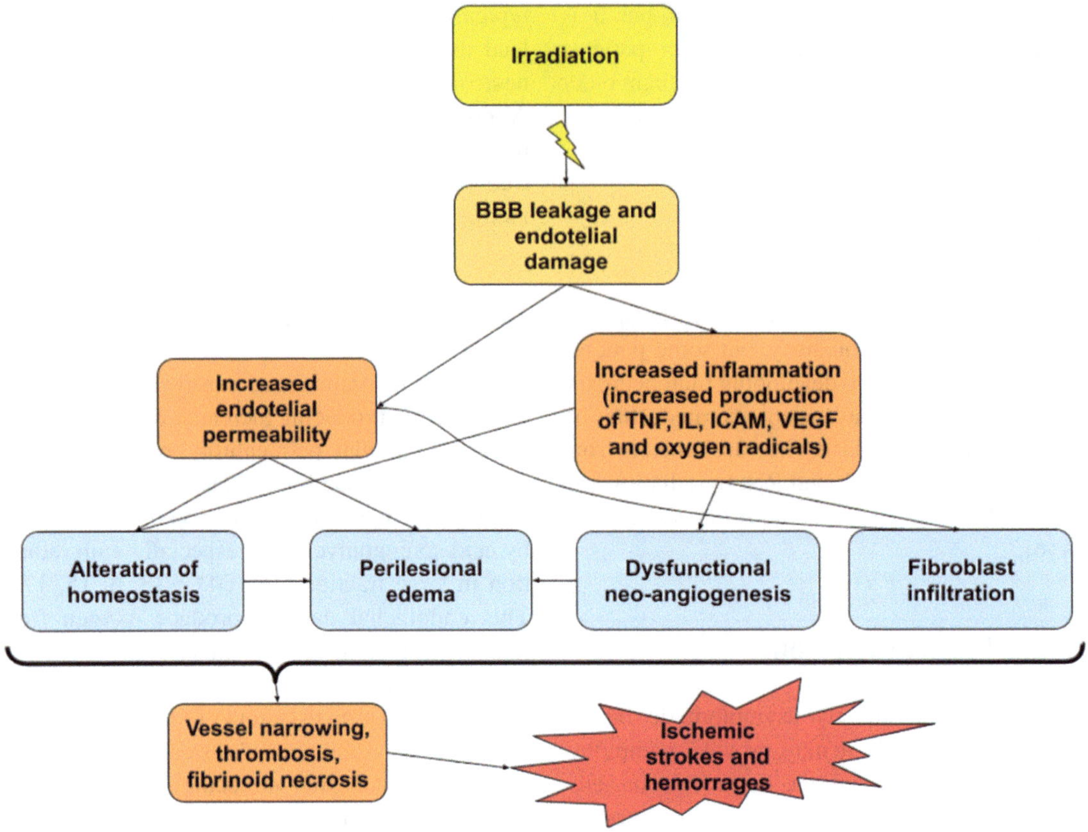

Fig. 19.1 Flowchart of vascular injury theory

inflammation and direct injury harm astrocytes, oligodendrocytes, and neural progenitor cells [3]. As a result, necrotic fragments are formed, which are difficult to remove, initiating a vicious cycle of neuroinflammation and altering cellular composition with an increased number of reactive astrocytes, leading to gliosis [13]. Furthermore, some neuronal stem cells, including O-2A cells, which are precursors of oligodendrocytes, undergo cell death, leading to a decrease in myelin production [3]. This results in a phenomenon of demyelination, named as glial cell theory, whereby the brain tissue most frequently affected by radiotherapy is primarily white matter. Demyelination can also cause a reduction in brain volume after radiation damage, leading to focal brain atrophy, which is clinically linked to cognitive impairment [3]. This phenomenon is most evident in the periventricular white matter due to poor blood supply without collateral vessels, resulting in more vulnerable areas with post-irradiation ischemic effects [13]. Furthermore, at a metabolic level, there is a decrease in glycolysis that can be observed by the lower uptake of radiolabeled glucose in PET exams [3]. On the other hand, chronic inflammation and tissue necrosis lead to hypoxia, which then causes the overproduction and upregulation of VEGF by astrocytes, resulting in angiogenesis. The newly formed blood vessels are delicate and thin, making them sensitive to radiation's effects, such as rupture or thrombosis. This can lead to an increase in cerebral perilesional edema [3]. The disruption of the blood-brain barrier allows more immune cells to pass through, which further increases the expression of proinflammatory factors and chemokines and activates matrix metalloproteinases (MMPs). This leads to a loss of blood–brain barrier integrity and the recruitment of peripheral immune cells to the injured area [3] (Fig. 19.2).

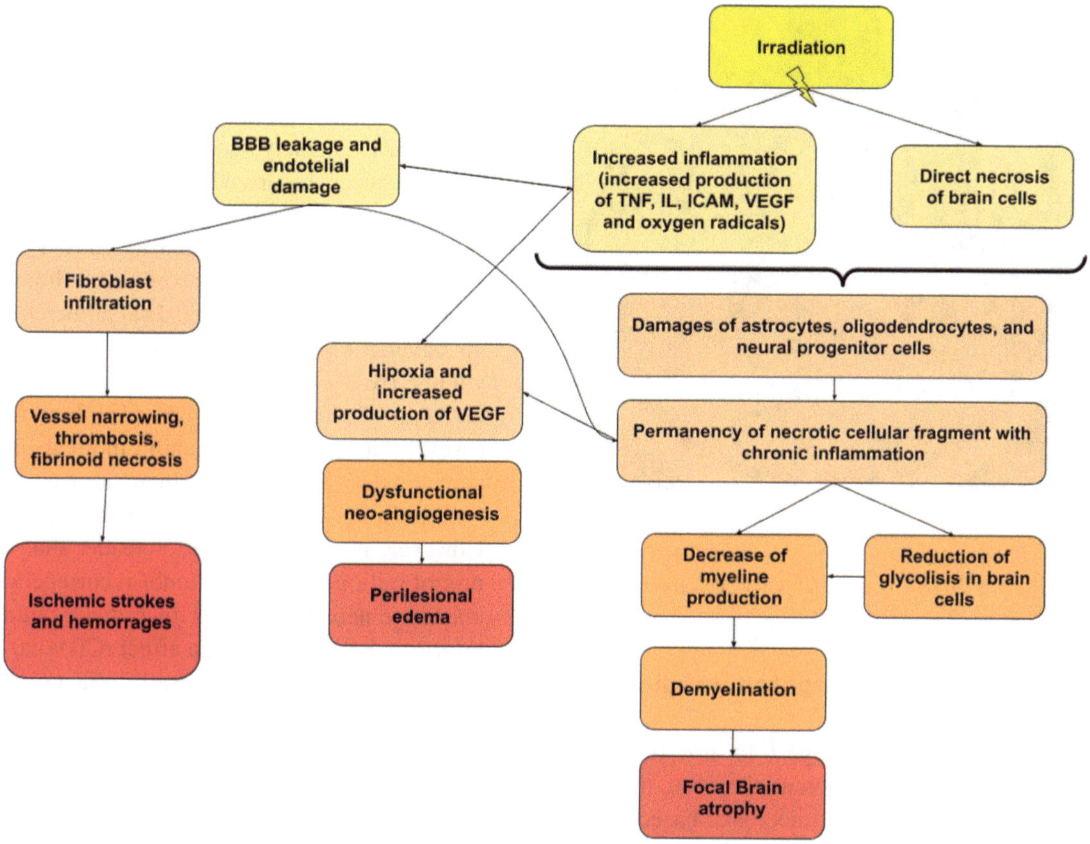

Fig. 19.2 Flowchart of glial cell theory

19.4 Diagnosis and Imaging Study

The primary obstacle in managing radionecrosis is accurately detecting it radiologically and distinguishing it from other types of lesions, especially glioma recurrences [8, 10]. Contrast-enhanced MRI is commonly used to evaluate radiation necrosis and should be performed every 2–3 months for the initial year after completing radiotherapy, with additional scans if clinically necessary [2]. However, both tumor recurrence and radiation brain injury can cause contrast enhancement and perilesional edema, making it difficult to diagnose them correctly [6]. This overlap is due to the increased permeability and leakage of the blood–brain barrier (BBB) [12]. It is also possible for both radionecrosis and tumor recurrence to occur at the same time. Radiation brain injury can demonstrate a morphological pattern described as "Swiss cheese," "soap bubble," or "cut-green pepper" on contrast-enhanced magnetic resonance imaging (MRI), but this pattern has a low positive predictive value of only 25% [6]. If a patient has undergone surgery and has a suspicious lesion after radiation treatment, comparing it with an MRI scan performed within 72 hours postoperatively may help identify any residual pathological tissue early [8]. Overall, conventional T1- or T2-weighted contrast-enhanced scans have a low predictive value in distinguishing RN from other brain lesions. Therefore, various advanced imaging techniques have been developed to aid in the diagnosis, such as MR diffusion, MR perfusion, MR spectroscopy, positron emission tomography (PET), PET-CT, PET-MRI, chemical exchange saturation transfer (CEST), and radiomics (Fig. 19.3).

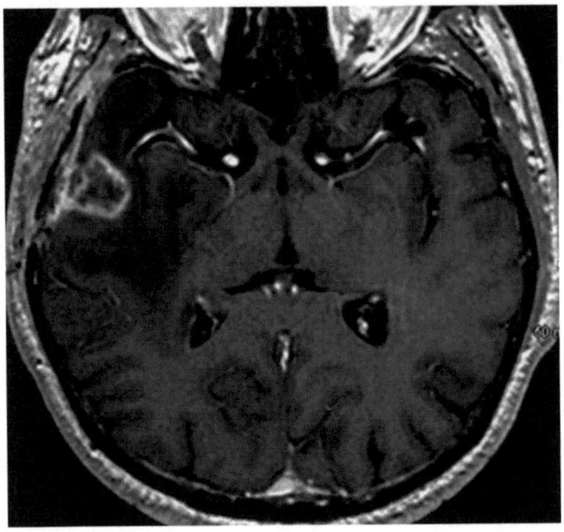

Fig. 19.3 Right temporal radionecrosis with nodular contrast-enhancement and irregular boundaries containing fine internal reticulation giving it a "cut-green pepper" appearance [35]

19.4.1 Diffusion-Weighted Imaging

Nichelli et al. [12] suggest to use diffusion-weighted imaging as a potential tools to differentiate recurrent tumor and necrosis, based on the difference of apparent diffusion coefficient (ADC) between them. A low ADC value suggests increased cellularity, which may indicate the recurrence of glioma. Conversely, low cellularity and a higher ADC value are associated with radiation-induced brain injury. It is also possible for glioma to recur in tissue with radionecrosis, making differentiation challenging. Several factors can affect ADC changes, including coagulative necrosis, calcifications, edema, gliosis, liquefactive necrosis, hemorrhage, fibrosis, and inflammatory infiltrates caused by radiation. Patients who have received bevacizumab during therapy may have a high ADC value that should be considered in the differential diagnosis [12].

19.4.2 MRI Study Perfusion

MRI perfusion is a technique that uses gadolinium-based contrast agents to measure the perfusion of a tissue in relation to surrounding tissues [13]. This images can be captured by the following methods: dynamic susceptibility contrast (DSC), dynamic contrast-enhanced (DCE), or arterial spin labeling (ASL) [13].

(a) DSC–MRI is widely used for detecting suspected cancer recurrence by utilizing T2 weighted contrast-enhanced scans and measuring changes in signal intensity caused by the initial passage of an intravenously administered contrast agent bolus. This allows for the calculation of the relative cerebral blood volume (rCBV), which serves as an indirect indicator of cerebral blood flow [13]. In most cases, tumor recurrences exhibit more abundant and denser vasculature than radionecrosis, resulting in higher rCBV values [12]. However, it is important to consider that a mix of radionecrosis and tumor recurrences, abundant neoangiogenesis in radiant brain injury, or BBB leakage can affect rCBV calculations and the overall diagnosis. Additionally, artifacts caused by petechial hemorrhage or surgical clips, as well as variations in rCBV values among machines, must be taken into account [13]. Two supplementary parameters calculated from DSC-MRI are the relative peak height (rPH) and the percentage of signal recovery (PSR). rPH accounts for the maximum signal intensity during the contrast agent bolus's passage through the capillary vascularization and is highly correlated with rCBV. It has been demonstrated to have good sensitivity and specificity in discriminating between radionecrosis and gliomas. PSR, on the other hand, is calculated from the lowest signal intensity during the passage of gadolinium-based contrast agents and the postcontrast signal intensity [13]. It provides information about contrast agent leakage through the BBB and is higher in radiant brain injury than in tumor recurrence (Figs. 19.4 and 19.5).

(b) The DCE-MRI is based on T1 weighted contrast-enhanced scans obtained over a prolonged period (5 minutes or longer) to gives information about contrast agent leakage through BBB and about vascular per-

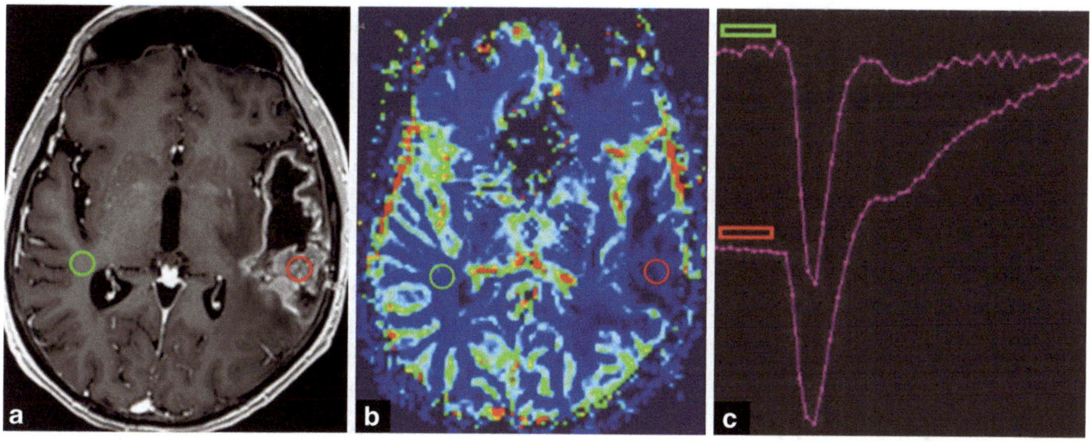

Fig. 19.4 Left temporal glioblastoma treated with RT and temozolomide. The patient repeats MRI after 3 months starting RT. This imaging shows a vast area of necrosis with new contrast-enhancement. The curve parameters (rCBV = 0.9; PSR = 100; rHP = 0.72) suggest radionecrosis which is confirmed by the secondary regression of the contrast-enhancement [35]

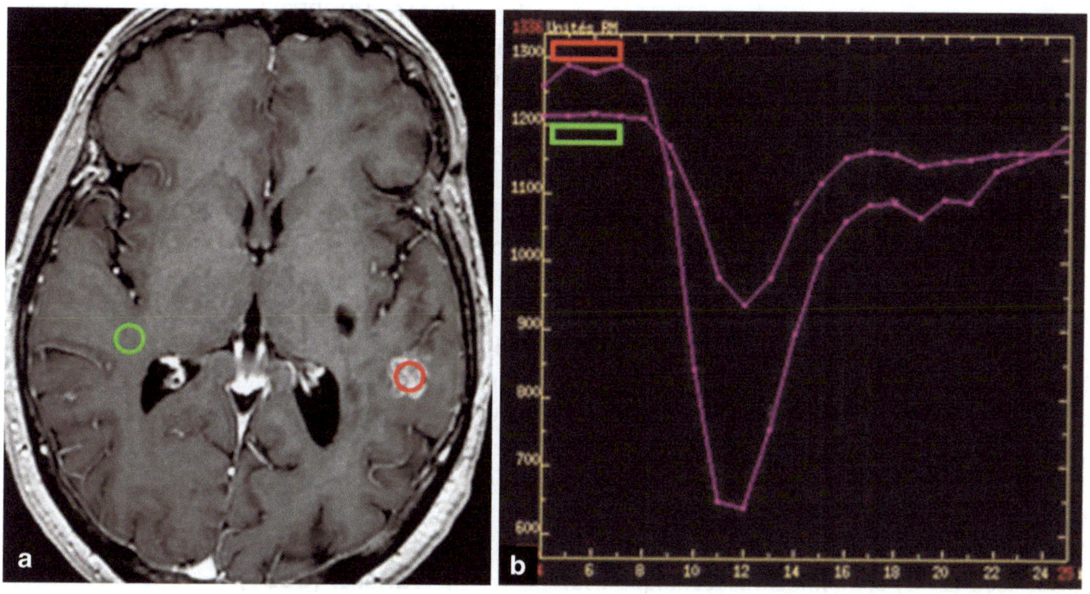

Fig. 19.5 Appearances of nodular contrast-enhancement above the initial surgical site for the glioblastoma. The curve parameters (rCBV = 0.9; PSR = 0.66; rHP = 2.3) showed tumor neoangiogenesis and its recurrence [35]

meability. The latter is parameterized through K_{trans}, which calculates the volume of fluid exchanged between intravascular and extravascular spaces and it is higher in radionecrosis than tumor recurrences [12, 13]. This technique is particularly useful when DSC-MRI present susceptibility artifacts [13].

(c) ASL-MRI is a noninvasive contrast-free perfusion MRI technique, which uses magnetically labeled blood protons as an endogenous tracer. This technique calculates cerebral blood flow (CBF) which has been reported that is higher in lesions with recurrent glioma than radionecrosis [13]. Moreover, it is fewer affected by leakage of

BBB and extravasation of contrast-enhanced agents than DCE-MRI and DSC MRI. This technique presents many advantages over previous perfusion MRI scans, such as fewer susceptibility artifacts with high accuracy results [12], the lack of the need for intravenous injection, especially in patients with renal failure, difficult intravenous access and allergic reaction to gadolinium-based contrast agents [13].

19.4.3 MR Spectroscopy

As previously reported in the dedicated chapter, magnetic resonance spectroscopy (MRS) examines the composition of metabolites and molecules present in individual voxels. Tumor recurrence may show increased choline-creatinine (Cho:Cr) and choline–N-acetyl aspartate (Cho:NAA) levels, which are markers of cell membrane turnover [13] Conversely, radionecrosis is characterized by high lactate and lipids levels and low levels of other metabolites [6, 13]. This technique provides valuable information about the investigated lesion; however, its usefulness is limited by the size of the voxels, which must be larger than 1 cm^3. Therefore, smaller lesions may be subject to sampling errors with heterogeneous signals [6], especially if they are close to the ventricular system, skull, or surgical clips due to signal contamination [13]. Although the use of MRS in the routine examination of these lesions is not yet widely agreed upon in the literature, some studies have shown good diagnostic accuracy by combining this technique with MRI perfusion [13] (Figs. 19.6 and 19.7).

19.4.4 Pet

PET is an imaging technique that typically employs Fluorodeoxyglucose (FDG) as a contrast-enhanced agent, particularly for staging extracranial cancers due to the increased glucose metabolism in tumors. However, brain tumor recurrences may poorly capture the tracer due to their necrotic component, while radionecrosis can manifest with increased uptake caused by high metabolism. Additionally, false positives may arise from the presence of a healthy, hypercaptant cerebral cortex adjacent to the lesion [13]. In contrast, studies have shown that amino acid tracers, such as Carbon-11 methionine (MET), fluoro-l-thymidine (FLT), fluoroethyltyrosine (FET), and 6-[18F]-fluoro-L-3,4-dihydroxyphenylalanine (F-DOPA), offer better specificity and sensitivity [2, 16, 18]. This is because tumor cells consume a high amount of amino acids, leading to increased cell proliferation and extracellular matrix production, and these tracers can easily pass through the BBB. Moreover, cancer tissue has relatively higher amino acid uptake than normal brain tissue, resulting in better contrast and delineation between brain tumors and healthy brain parenchyma [2, 16, 18]. PET images also have better definition than magnetic resonance spectroscopy [2, 6]. However, image acquisition time is longer than that of conventional techniques, and an on-site cyclotron is required due to the short half-life of 11C [19]. False positives related to increased uptake by healthy tissue or inflammation may also be present [13], especially after radiotherapy [19]. Recently, new technologies and machines have enabled the development of mixed PET-CT and PET-MRI techniques, which offer reduced scanning time and less radiation exposure [18]. However, these methods are particularly expensive when combined with MRI and CT [18].

19.4.5 Chemical Exchange Saturation Transfer (CEST)

Chemical exchange saturation transfer (CEST) is a cutting-edge method of contrast-enhanced MRI that utilizes endogenous molecules, such as mobile proteins and peptides, found within a tumor microenvironment [6, 20]. This technique is built upon the molecular phenomenon of "chemical exchange," which involves the exchange of protons between amide groups of a metabolite and the surrounding water. Standard MRI is not well-suited for studying the concentration of protein metabolites that are present in low amounts. To

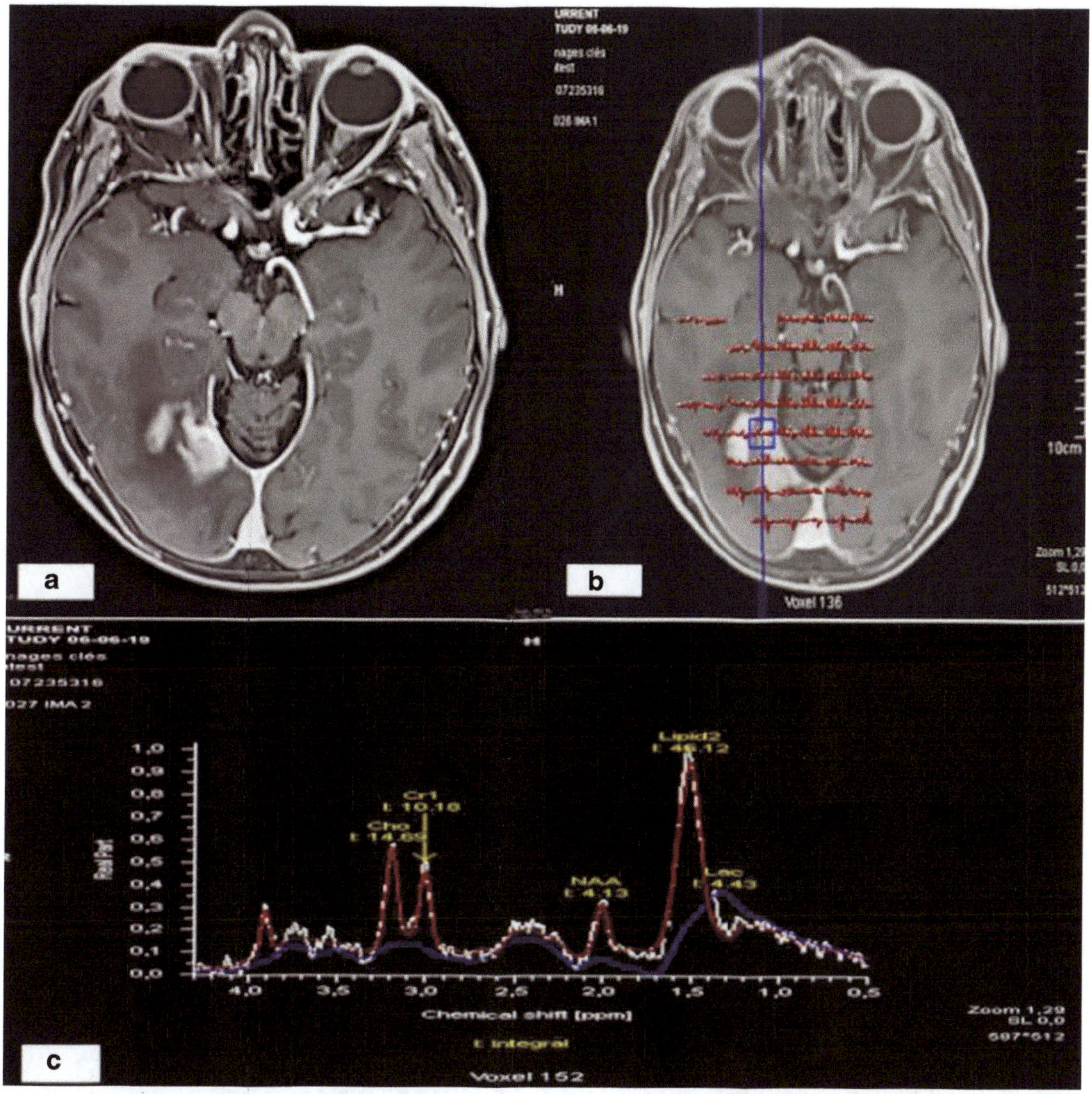

Fig. 19.6 This imaging shows a right temporo-occipital lesion. (**a**) Axial T1 FAT-SAT with Gadolinium showing a contrast enhancement. (**b**) voxel chosen. (**c**) Voxel's spectrum suggesting a radionecrosis (Cho/Cr = 1,44-Cho/NAA = 3,56-Cho/Lip + Lac = 0,29) [36]

overcome this limitation, CEST relies on the emission of a specific radiofrequency pulse at a particular frequency, which "saturates" the protons of the metabolites that are being analyzed. Following this process, the proton exchange process begins, causing the nearby water signal to decrease, and the concentrations of the metabolites can be indirectly identified [20, 21]. The negative peaks in the water spectrum after using certain frequencies are an indication of chemical-specific substances [20]. This technique has shown promising results in differentiating between radionecrosis and tumor recurrence, as the concentration of protein and, therefore, amide groups is much higher in the latter [20, 21]. Additionally, CEST is highly sensitive and specific in differentiating between high-grade and low-grade gliomas, as well as in monitoring early tumor response to chemoradiation therapy, especially when combined with perfusion- and diffusion-weighted imaging [18].

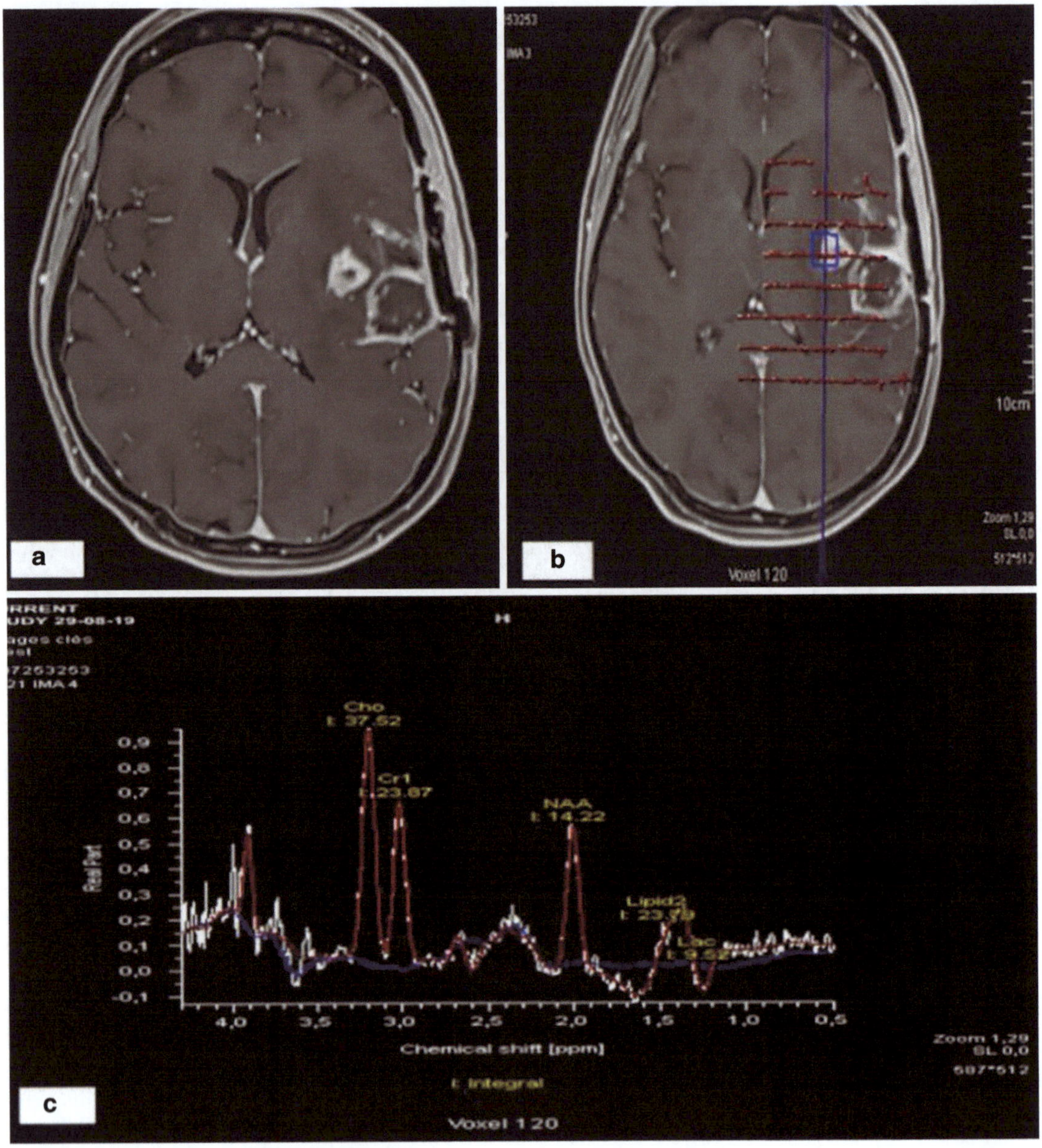

Fig. 19.7 This imaging shows a left insular lesion. (**a**) Axial T1 FAT-SAT with Gadolinium showing a contrast enhancement. (**b**) Voxel chosen. (**c**) Spectrum indicating tumor tissues (Cho/Cr = 1,57-Cho/NAA = 2,64-Cho/Lip + Lac = 1,13) [36]

19.4.6 Radiomics

Radiomics is a sophisticated analysis that leverages advanced computer tools, including deep learning models, to extract data from a patient's radiological images. Depending on the center where it is employed, data are gathered from two or more conventional MR sequences (T1, T2, FLAIR, T1 with gadolinium contrast, DWI) and advanced MR sequences (MR perfusion, CEST) as well as PET (18F-FDG and 11C-MET) [12, 19]. When multiparametric images are utilized, the effectiveness of radiomics surpasses that of a single modality. It is widely believed that the performance of radiomics surpasses traditional radiologist diagnosis [19]. According to reports, it

Table 19.1 Summary table of RN characteristics with the various imaging techniques and their limitations

	How to recognize radionecrosis	Limitations and differential diagnosis
MR diffusion-weighted imaging	It is related to low cellularity and potentially an higher ADC than tumor recurrences.	Coagulative necrosis, calcifications, edema, gliosis, liquefactive necrosis, hemorrhage, fibrosis, and inflammatory infiltrate caused by radiation can influence a variation of ADC.
MR spectroscopy	It exhibits an high rate of lactate and lipid and low rate of the other metabolites.	The signal may be contaminated if the size of the lesion is less than 1 cm^3 and if it is near the ventricles, skull, and surgical metal clips.
MR perfusion		
Dynamic susceptibility contrast	It presents a lower rCBV and rPH with higher PSR than tumor recurrences.	It is possible to find situation where there is a mix of radionecrosis and tumor recurrences, abundant neoangiogenesis in radiant brain injury or a BBB leakage which can influence the correct calculation of r CBV. Furthermore, artifacts could be produced by petechial hemorrhage or surgical clips and rCBV values vary between machines.
Dynamic contrast-enhanced	It presents a higher K_{trans} than tumor recurrences.	
Arterial spin labeling	It presents a lower CBF than tumor recurrences.	
PET	Using tracers with amino acids, radionecrosis has lower uptake respect tumor recurrence.	Increased uptake by healthy tissue or as a result of inflammation may be present, especially after radiotherpy.
Chemical exchange saturation transfer	Radionecrosis results in less protein concentration and therefore amide group, and the resulting signal will be less intense than tumor recurrence.	

has a sensitivity and specificity of 66% and 87%, respectively, in distinguishing tumor progression and radionecrosis [4]. This technique enables the acquisition of additional information without the need for further examinations. It predicts tumor behavior, treatment response, and patient outcomes, including prognosis, survival, and post-treatment evaluation of gliomas and glioblastomas [19]. Although radiomics holds great promise for future use, there is still room for improvement in extracting and processing information using analysis software (Table 19.1).

19.5 Biopsy and Anatomopathological Examination

Based on our analysis, several highly advanced imaging techniques have been developed, each with its own set of limitations. To enhance diagnostic accuracy, a multimodal approach is recommended [6, 13]. However, biopsy remains the gold standard for obtaining a definitive diagnosis. This is especially crucial in cases where patients exhibit worsening symptoms and a worsening radiological picture despite receiving conservative treatment. On anatomopathological examination, it is common to find a combination of radionecrosis and residual or recurrent tumor [13]. Histologically, RN is characterized by an area of coagulative and fibrinoid necrosis with persistent inflammation [3, 7]. The vessel walls appear thickened with fibrinoid aggregates, and thrombized and necrotic capillaries can be identified [3]. The necrotic area is usually paucicellular with a low nucleocytoplasmic ratio, accompanied by focal areas of perivascular lymphocytes [7] or foamy macrophages and hemosiderophages [6], which are associated with inflammation. It is surrounded by a demyelinated and highly gliotic area [6, 13]. In some histological findings of patients who undergo stereotactic radiosurgery, residual tumor cells intercalated in an area of radionecrosis can also be identified [6]. In contrast, recurrent tumor appears as a densely cellularized area with a high nucleocytoplasmic ratio and copious vascularization.

19.5.1 Pseudoprogression

Radiologically and histopathologically, pseudoprogression can be difficult to differentiate from radionecrosis, but it has some distinct characteristics. Generally, pseudoprogression appears within 3 months after completing radiotherapy and chemotherapy, and it is asymptomatic, resolving without treatment modification [10, 14]. On MRI, pseudoprogression mimics tumor recurrence or progression due to contrast enhancement. Physiologically, it is an early delayed brain injury with marked local tissue reaction linked to vasogenic edema, which normally resolves spontaneously, and transient demyelination [22]. Abbasi et al. reported that pseudoprogression occurred in 36% (95% confidence interval, 33–40%) of high-grade glioma patients [22]. In contrast, radionecrosis is considered a late delayed brain injury (occurring 6 months after the end of therapy) and can be symptomatic, requiring drug or surgical treatment in some cases [12, 13]. Additionally, patients with the O6–methylguanine DNA methyltransferase (MGMT) gene promoter, which typically produces a DNA repair enzyme that can induce chemoresistance due to methylation, exhibit more frequent pseudoprogression and increased sensitivity to temozolomide [13].

19.6 Treatment

19.6.1 Wait-and-See Approach

Close observation and clinical follow-up are the main strategy for asymptomatic patients or for small volume radionecrosis. Frequent imaging controls is usually recommended at the beginning, every 6–8 weeks, until the lesion is considered stable/regressed and then the checks are separated by 12–16 weeks [3, 6, 16]. Spontaneous resolution of the lesion can be seen, because it is not always an irreversible progressive process [6]. Some authors propose treatment with pentoxifylline and vitamin E or a short-course of corticosteroids but without high scientific evidenced base [16].

19.6.2 Corticosteroids

Steroids are the first line of treatment to symptomatic radionecrosis in attempt to control the edema and mass effect. Oral corticosteroids (such as dexamethasone at the dose of 4–8 mg per day with a gradual taper of the dose) reduce the inflammatory cascade and cytokines produced in the radiation injury lesion and improving the permeability of blood-brain barrier [3, 15, 16]. With the start of therapy, there is usually a reduction in edema associated with improvement in symptoms. Unfortunately, many patients will require long-term application of glucocorticoids, which it can cause hormonal dependence and steroid-complications, such as myopathy, iatrogenic Cushing's syndrome, gastric ulcers, hyperglycemia, cataracts, osteoporosis, liver damage, and bone aseptic necrosis [3, 16]. Zhou et al. showed that the increased number of infections, related to drug-induced immunodeficiency, is associated more with cycles with high doses of corticosteroids than with cycles with lower dosages, with the equal clinical effect [23]. Moreover, the lack of response to corticosteroids is not infrequent [24]. The International Stereotactic Radiosurgery Society (ISRS) suggest this flowchart (Fig. 19.8) for the management of symptomatic corticosteroid refractory and/or corticosteroid intolerant radionecrosis [16].

19.6.3 Bevacizumab

Bevacizumab is a humanized monoclonal antibody that blocks VEGF. By locking this growth factor, this drug succeeds in normalizing the permeability of the BBB, decreasing vasogenic edema and finally neurological symptomatology [3]. There is no uniformity among studies on the

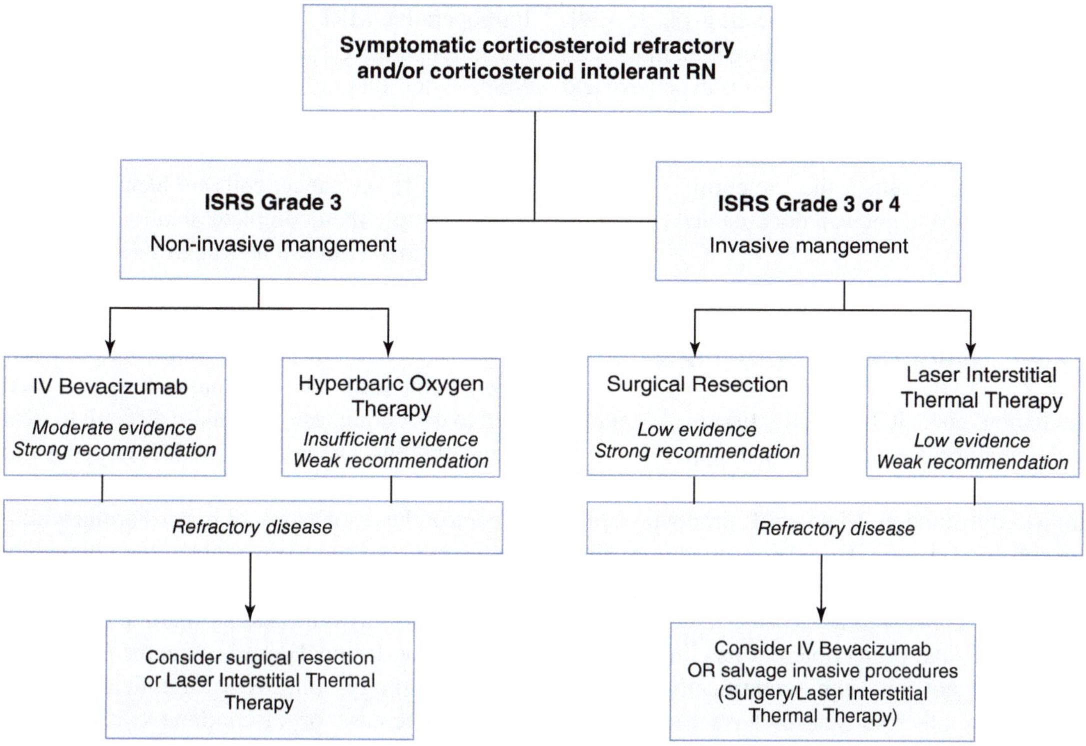

Fig. 19.8 Management flowchart for symptomatic corticosteroid-refractory RN [16]

dosing of this drugs and the range is from 1 mg/kg to 15 mg/kg for up to 8 weeks, which may have included multiple cycles [25]. It has been shown in many studies to be beneficial in improving symptoms, in both adults and children, with the opportunity of decreasing or discontinuing corticosteroids therapy [3, 15, 16, 25–27]. But side effects should be taken into account, such as hypertension, cerebral hemorrhage, deep vein thrombosis, pulmonary embolism, stroke and wound dehiscence [13, 16, 25]. In conclusion, Bevacizumab can be considered a conservative treatment choice in cases of symptomatic radionecrosis refractory to corticosteroid treatment.

19.6.4 Heparin and Warfarin

Heparin and warfarin usually prevent coagulation and inhibit neutrophil chemotaxis and cytokine release so Gantz et al., as the first, used them to block the ischemia caused by the vascular injury to prevent radionecrosis progression [3, 15]. From this study, patients presented improvements in symptomatology and control images. However, the possible side effects of using these drugs such as the risk of bleeding must be considered. Additional clinical trails have been conducted on a limited number of patients so as encouraging as the results are, further confirmation is needed [3, 15].

19.6.5 Hyperbaric Oxygen Therapy (HBOT)

Hyperbaric oxygen therapy is a treatment that is already used for myonecrosis, compromised soft tissue grafts and flaps, crush injuries, necrotizing soft tissue infections, and refractory osteomyelitis [28]. Retrospective studies have shown that some patients with radiation brain damage found benefit from undergoing HBOT in a 100% oxygen chamber for up to 5 times per week which it can be repeated up to 40 times. It helps to increase oxygen concentration, restore perfusion and angiogenesis, and promote healing [3, 15, 29]. The disadvantages of this treatment lie in the fact that many sessions are needed, it is expensive and require specialized facilities [6]. Although the results of these retrospective studies show encouraging results, the scientific evidence remains poor and not well documented [3, 15, 16, 28–30].

19.6.6 Neuroprotective Therapies

Radiation once it hits brain tissue triggers an inflammatory reaction with a major release of free radicals. These lead to cell death and neurological dysfunction. Chan et al. proposed alpha-tocopherol (vitamin E) as a treatment to limit neuronal cell death following radiation exposure. Vitamin E appears to act as free radical scavengers for cellular protection, but its clinical application has not yet been scientifically accepted [24]. Many other substances have been investigated in their possible role as neuroprotectants and biologically active substances for prevention and treatment of radiation-induced brain damage, such as Vitamin C, phytochemicals, immunomodulator, cytoprotectant, but their application remains limited [3, 29, 31].

19.7 Treatment for Medically Refractory Radionecrosis

19.7.1 Laser Interstitial Thermal Ablation (LITT)

Laser interstitial thermal therapy is an increasingly utilized tool in the management of radionecrosis due to its minimally invasive nature, its low complication rate, and its ability to therapeutically intervene for either diagnosis. LITT relies on the transmission of laser electromagnetic radiation to the target tissue, which absorbs photons and releases thermal energy. This heat is distributed in the surrounding tissue, causing coagulative necrosis of the lesion [3]. This procedure is conducted under general anesthesia and the patient is positioned in the high-field Intraoperative MRI. A burr hole is executed and the intraoperative trajectory is then checked by MRI. After that, a stereotactic biopsy is performed to confirm if it is radionecrosis and to make real-time treatment decision based on pathology. If any cancer cells are identified in the biopsy sample then complete ablation should be the main goal, if not, a less aggressive intervention may be sufficient to stop the inflammatory cascade of radionecrosis [32]. Finally, the laser probe is placed and heat is administered to the target point [33]. This technique has also been used to treat brain lesions that are difficult to treat surgically [34]. Using real-time MR imaging and thermometry during the procedure, it is possible to control the distribution of hyperthermia within the target tissue and to maintain a sharp boundary zone between pathological and normal tissue, thus limiting any unnecessary thermal damage to adiacent non-lesional cortex. After the procedure, symptomatology improves significantly, and patients decrease or discontinue corticosteroid therapy [32]. The use of LITT is typically recommended for smaller necrotic lesions [7]. An additional advantage of LITT is that patients do not have to stop chemotherapy and wait for the wound to fully heal before resuming it [32]. The limitations of this technique are related to the fact that it requires specialized equipment and a trained team and the area near the dura and cerebral vessels can be challenging for LITT because of the heat-sink effect [16]. With the increasingly widespread use of this mini-invasive technique, patients can be treated more aggressively with radiosurgery [32]. However, the effectiveness of this procedure is still debated [16, 32].

19.7.2 Surgery

Surgery is recommended for symptomatic patients with easily accessible and located lesions in non-eloquent areas when conservative management has failed or there is diagnostic uncertainty. It is also considered a first-line treatment when there is a mass effect that does not respond to steroid therapy, acute neurologic deficit, steroid dependency or toxicity, bevacizumab intolerance, or a contraindication [7]. Surgical resection has several advantages, including relief of mass effect, edema reduction, and the possibility of weaning off steroids, symptomatic control, and histological confirmation. The removal of the necrotic nidus blocks the inflammatory cascade that generates the lesion, leading to improved symptomatology [16]. However, in some cases, normal brain tissue surrounding the removed necrotic lesions may continue to cause necrosis, leading to continuous progression of symptoms [3]. It is crucial to choose patients carefully by evaluating their surgical accessibility, potential intraoperative complications, overall performance status, and life expectancy, especially for those with a limited prognosis. Extensive surgical resection is recommended, as it is associated with a reduction in the postoperative volumetric T2-FLAIR signal. However, defining the margins of a necrotic tumor intraoperatively can be difficult due to the absence of a clear cleavage plan [7]. Complications such as wound breakdown, poor healing, CSF leaks, and postoperative infection may occur after craniotomy, further delaying the resumption of oncologic therapy. Although surgery is a reliable and useful treatment option for controlling symptomatology and achieving histologic control, it has many limitations, and its potential complications should not be overlooked (Table 19.2). According to the latest recommendations from the International Society of Stereotactic Radiosurgery (December 2022), a clinical classification of these lesions has been compiled with associated treatment based on the latest scientific evidence, as well as a management flowchart for symptomatic corticosteroid-refractory radionecrosis [16]. (Fig. 19.8).

Table 19.2 ISRS grading system based on the severity of RN, diagnosed by radiology or pathology, with the proposed management and follow-up recommendations [16]

ISRS grade	Description of severity	Recommended management and follow-up
1	Asymptomatic and no prior corticosteroid administration	Close surveillance with repeat imaging at 6–12 week intervals Consider a short-course of cortico- steroids (e.g. dexamethasone). Surgical resection can be considered first line if a pathologic diagnosis is urgently required to guide further management.
2	Symptomatic and no prior corticosteroid administration	Dexamethasone can be started as 4–8 mg/d, with or without an initial bolus, and tapered gradually. Generally, a 3–6 week course of steroids may be required. Repeat imaging should be considered at 6–12 week intervals. Surgical resection can be considered first line if a pathologic diagnosis is urgently required to guide further management.
3	Symptomatic and corticosteroid- refractory	Bevacizumab at doses ranging between 5 and 10 mg/kg every 2–3 week for 2–4 cycles Repeat imaging after two cycles and after the 4th cycle for response assessment and to guide corticosteroid tapering as required. Repeat imaging should be considered at 2–3 months intervals to ensure improvement and/or stability.
		LITT/surgery Repeat imaging should be considered at 2–3 months intervals to ensure improvement and/or stability.
		HBOT Repeat imaging should be considered at 2–3 months intervals to ensure improvement and/or stability.
4	Symptomatic with neurologic impairment, progressive RN despite a trial of noninvasive treatments, dependency on high doses of corticosteroid.	Surgical resection Repeat imaging should be considered at 2–3 months intervals to ensure improvement and/or stability.

19.8 Prevention

Prevention to the onset of radionecrosis is mainly based on the reduction of risk factors, especially reducing the volume and the maximum dose of radiation to brain parenchyma. However, some authors suggest the use of bevacizumab and nerve growth factor, as the most effective and cost-effective method to prevent radiation injury, but more clinical studies are needed to confirm it [3]. Other substances, such as Flavonoids, Vitamin C and E, Valproic acid, Memantine, Minocycline, Fingolimod and Melatonin are indicated as promising neuroprotective agents, by Lalkovičová, that are being studied to preventively shield brain tissue from ionizing radiation [31].

19.9 Conclusion

RN is a rare but serious side effect of radiotherapy and radiosurgery. It has some risk factors that can be worked on to prevent its occurrence. The diagnosis is challenging. It is important to differentiate RN especially from tumor recurrence. In this process, traditional and new diagnostic imaging techniques have improved in the recent years, but the gold standard remains the biopsy. Nowadays, many conservative pharmacological treatments have been developed and help in the management of RN, such as corticosteroids and Bevacizumab. However, surgery with total or subtotal resection or minimally invasive techniques, such as LITT, remains the first-line therapy in some cases.

References

1. Rane N, Quaghebeur G. CNS effects following the treatment of malignancy. Clin Radiol. 2012;67(1):61–8. https://doi.org/10.1016/j.crad.2011.01.010.
2. Lupattelli M, Tini P, Nardone V, et al. Stereotactic radiotherapy for brain oligometastases. Rep Pract Oncol Radiother. 2022;27(1):15–22. https://doi.org/10.5603/RPOR.a2021.0133.
3. Yang X, Ren H, Fu J. Treatment of radiation-induced brain necrosis. Ghose J, ed. Oxidative Med Cell Longev. 2021;2021:1–15. https://doi.org/10.1155/2021/4793517.
4. Daisne JF, De Ketelaere C, Jamart J. The individual risk of symptomatic radionecrosis after brain metastasis radiosurgery is predicted by a continuous function of the V12Gy. Clin Transl Radiat Oncol. 2021;27:70–4. https://doi.org/10.1016/j.ctro.2021.01.003.
5. Crouzen JA, Petoukhova AL, Broekman MLD, et al. SAFESTEREO: phase II randomized trial to compare stereotactic radiosurgery with fractionated stereotactic radiosurgery for brain metastases. BMC Cancer. 2023;23(1):273. https://doi.org/10.1186/s12885-023-10761-1.
6. Vellayappan B, Tan CL, Yong C, et al. Diagnosis and Management of Radiation Necrosis in patients with brain metastases. Front Oncol. 2018;8:395. https://doi.org/10.3389/fonc.2018.00395.
7. Newman WC, Goldberg J, Guadix SW, et al. The effect of surgery on radiation necrosis in irradiated brain metastases: extent of resection and long-term clinical and radiographic outcomes. J Neuro-Oncol. 2021;153(3):507–18. https://doi.org/10.1007/s11060-021-03790-y.
8. Cao H, Xiao Z, Zhang Y, et al. Dosimetric comparisons of different hypofractionated stereotactic radiotherapy techniques in treating intracranial tumors > 3 cm in longest diameter. J Neurosurg. 2020;132(4):1024–32. https://doi.org/10.3171/2018.12.JNS181578.
9. Calderon B, Vazquez L, Belkacemi M, Pourel N. Stereotactic radiotherapy for brain metastases: predictive factors of radionecrosis. Eur J Med Res. 2023;28(1):233. https://doi.org/10.1186/s40001-023-01178-4.
10. Minniti G, Niyazi M, Alongi F, Navarria P, Belka C. Current status and recent advances in reirradiation of glioblastoma. Radiat Oncol. 2021;16(1):36. https://doi.org/10.1186/s13014-021-01767-9.
11. Ruben JD, Dally M, Bailey M, Smith R, McLean CA, Fedele P. Cerebral radiation necrosis: incidence, outcomes, and risk factors with emphasis on radiation parameters and chemotherapy. Int J Radiat Oncol Biol Phys. 2006;65(2):499–508. https://doi.org/10.1016/j.ijrobp.2005.12.002.
12. Nichelli L, Casagranda S. Current emerging MRI tools for radionecrosis and pseudoprogression diagnosis. Curr Opin Oncol. 2021;33(6):597–607. https://doi.org/10.1097/CCO.0000000000000793.
13. Katsura M, Sato J, Akahane M, Furuta T, Mori H, Abe O. Recognizing radiation-induced changes in the central nervous system: where to look and what to look for. Radiographics. 2021;41(1):224–48. https://doi.org/10.1148/rg.2021200064.
14. Walker AJ, Ruzevick J, Malayeri AA, et al. Postradiation imaging changes in the CNS: how can we differentiate between treatment effect and disease progression? Future Oncol. 2014;10(7):1277–97. https://doi.org/10.2217/fon.13.271.
15. Rahmathulla G, Marko NF, Weil RJ. Cerebral radiation necrosis: a review of the pathobiology, diagno-

sis and management considerations. J Clin Neurosci. 2013;20(4):485–502. https://doi.org/10.1016/j.jocn.2012.09.011.
16. Vellayappan B, Lim-Fat MJ, Kotecha R, et al. A systematic review informing the management of symptomatic brain radiation necrosis after stereotactic radiosurgery and international stereotactic radiosurgery society recommendations. Int J Radiat Oncol. 2024;118(1):14–28. https://doi.org/10.1016/j.ijrobp.2023.07.015.
17. Nordal RA, Wong CS. Intercellular adhesion Molecule-1 and blood-spinal cord barrier disruption in central nervous system radiation injury. J Neuropathol Exp Neurol. 2004;63(5):474–83. https://doi.org/10.1093/jnen/63.5.474.
18. Niyazi M, Andratschke N, Bendszus M, et al. ESTRO-EANO guideline on target delineation and radiotherapy details for glioblastoma. Radiother Oncol. 2023;184:109663. https://doi.org/10.1016/j.radonc.2023.109663.
19. Alizadeh M, Broomand Lomer N, Azami M, et al. Radiomics: the new promise for differentiating progression, recurrence, Pseudoprogression, and Radionecrosis in glioma and glioblastoma Multiforme. Cancers. 2023;15(18):4429. https://doi.org/10.3390/cancers15184429.
20. Mehrabian H, Desmond KL, Soliman H, Sahgal A, Stanisz GJ. Differentiation between radiation necrosis and tumor progression using chemical exchange saturation transfer. Clin Cancer Res. 2017;23(14):3667–75. https://doi.org/10.1158/1078-0432.CCR-16-2265.
21. Jabehdar Maralani P, Chan RW, Lam WW, et al. Chemical exchange saturation transfer MRI: what neuro-oncology clinicians need to know. Technol Cancer Res Treat. 2023;22:15330338231208613. https://doi.org/10.1177/15330338231208613.
22. Abbasi AW, Westerlaan HE, Holtman GA, Aden KM, van Laar PJ, van der Hoorn A. Incidence of tumour progression and Pseudoprogression in high-grade gliomas: a systematic review and meta-analysis. Clin Neuroradiol. 2018;28(3):401–11. https://doi.org/10.1007/s00062-017-0584-x.
23. Zhuo X, Huang X, Yan M, et al. Comparison between high-dose and low-dose intravenous methylprednisolone therapy in patients with brain necrosis after radiotherapy for nasopharyngeal carcinoma. Radiother Oncol. 2019;137:16–23. https://doi.org/10.1016/j.radonc.2019.04.015.
24. Chan AS, Cheung M, Law SC, Chan JH. Phase II study of alpha-tocopherol in improving the cognitive function of patients with temporal lobe radionecrosis. Cancer. 2004;100(2):398–404. https://doi.org/10.1002/cncr.11885.
25. Hill S, MacDougall D. Bevacizumab for the treatment of patients with brain Radionecrosis. Can. J Health Technol. 2022;2(12):10.51731/cjht.2022.519.
26. Climans SA, Ramos RC, Jablonska PA, Shultz DB, Mason WP. Bevacizumab for cerebral Radionecrosis: a single-center experience. Can J Neurol Sci J Can Sci Neurol. 2023;50(4):573–8. https://doi.org/10.1017/cjn.2022.64.
27. Dahl NA, Liu AK, Foreman NK, Widener M, Fenton LZ, Macy ME. Bevacizumab in the treatment of radiation injury for children with central nervous system tumors. Childs Nerv Syst. 2019;35(11):2043–6. https://doi.org/10.1007/s00381-019-04304-y.
28. Co J, De Moraes MV, Katznelson R, et al. Hyperbaric oxygen for radiation necrosis of the brain. Can J Neurol Sci J Can Sci Neurol. 2020;47(1):92–9. https://doi.org/10.1017/cjn.2019.290.
29. Chung C, Bryant A, Brown PD. Interventions for the treatment of brain radionecrosis after radiotherapy or radiosurgery. Cochrane Database Syst Rev. 2018;7(7):CD011492. https://doi.org/10.1002/14651858.CD011492.pub2.
30. Bennett M, Feldmeier J, Hampson N, Milross C, Smee R. Hyperbaric oxygen therapy for late radiation tissue injury. In: The Cochrane Collaboration, editor. Cochrane database of systematic reviews. Wiley; 2004. p. CD005005. https://doi.org/10.1002/14651858.CD005005.
31. Lalkovičová M. Neuroprotective agents effective against radiation damage of central nervous system. Neural Regen Res. 2022;17(9):1885. https://doi.org/10.4103/1673-5374.335137.
32. Chan M, Tatter S, Chiang V, et al. Efficacy of laser interstitial thermal therapy for biopsy-proven radiation necrosis in radiographically recurrent brain metastases. Neuro-Oncol Adv. 2023;5(1):vdad031. https://doi.org/10.1093/noajnl/vdad031.
33. Rahmathulla G, Recinos PF, Valerio JE, Chao S, Barnett GH. Laser interstitial thermal therapy for focal cerebral radiation necrosis: a case report and literature review. Stereotact Funct Neurosurg. 2012;90(3):192–200. https://doi.org/10.1159/000338251.
34. Rahmathulla G, Recinos PF, Kamian K, Mohammadi AM, Ahluwalia MS, Barnett GH. MRI-guided laser interstitial thermal therapy in neuro-oncology: a review of its current clinical applications. Oncology. 2014;87(2):67–82. https://doi.org/10.1159/000362817.
35. Raimbault A, Cazals X, Lauvin MA, Destrieux C, Chapet S, Cottier JP. Radionecrosis of malignant glioma and cerebral metastasis: a diagnostic challenge in MRI. Diagn Interv Imaging. 2014;95(10):985–1000. https://doi.org/10.1016/j.diii.2014.06.013.
36. De Lucia F, Lefebvre Y, Lemort MP. Interest of routine MR spectroscopic techniques for differential diagnosis between radionecrosis and progression of brain tumor lesions. Eur J Radiol Open. 2022;9:100449. https://doi.org/10.1016/j.ejro.2022.100449.

Part V

Part V

Neurorehabilitation Serves as a Valuable Tool for the Care, Management, and Prognosis of Gliomas

20

Marco Calegari, Daniele Armocida, Veronica Di Palma, and Alessandro Pesce

20.1 Introduction

Gliomas represent the most common type of intracranial tumors, comprising about 70% of all cases. Recent advancements in standard treatment approaches, including surgical removal, radiation therapy, and drug-based treatments, have extended the lifespan of glioma patients [1]. This increased survival rate necessitates more extensive rehabilitative care [2]. The symptoms of glioma vary based on the tumor's specific location, its impact on nearby functional structures, and the stage of treatment (before surgery, after surgery, during therapies) [3]. These symptoms often encompass seizures, headaches, exhaustion, and impairments in motor, sensory, and cognitive functions [4]. Consequently, prompt and comprehensive rehabilitation is crucial for enhancing functional outcomes and improving the quality of life (QoL) of glioma patients [5], as well as their overall survival (OS) [5–7].

Neurorehabilitation for glioma patients aims to address the multifaceted physical, cognitive, and emotional deficits resulting from both the tumor's biology and functional anatomy, as well as its treatment at various stages of the disease [4]. Research has emphasized the significance of customized and multidisciplinary rehabilitation interventions for glioma patients and their caregivers, designed to address their specific neurological conditions and evolving needs [7–9]. While physical rehabilitation focuses on enhancing motor skills, awareness, and psychological well-being in these patients [10, 11], cognitive rehabilitation can lead to improved neurocognitive performance, which appears to be essential for the continually increasing overall survival and functional outcomes of these patients [3, 12, 13]. Furthermore, interventions such as physiotherapy and occupational therapy have been demonstrated to be safe and feasible for glioma patients, yielding significant improvements in health-related quality of life, cognitive function, and physical functioning [14]. This chapter highlights the importance of rehabilitation programs tailored to the specific needs of glioma patients, which can significantly impact their cognitive function, QoL, and overall well-being. These interventions play a vital role in overcoming the

M. Calegari (✉)
Neurorehabilitation Center, Emeis Group, Casa di Cura Madonna dei Boschi, Buttigliera Alta, TO, Italy
e-mail: calegari90@gmail.com

D. Armocida (✉)
Neurosurgery Unit, Dept. Neuroscience "Rita Levi Montalcini", Università degli studi di Torino, Torino, TO, Italy

V. Di Palma
Fondazione "Santa Lucia", Rome, Italy

A. Pesce
Policlinico Tor Vergata (PTV), Neurosurgery Unit, Università degli Studi di Roma (Tor Vergata), Rome, Italy

D. Armocida et al. (eds.), *Neurosurgery's Frontline Role in Gliomas Treatment*,
https://doi.org/10.1007/978-3-031-81850-9_20

numerous challenges faced by glioma patients, ultimately leading to improvements in functional and oncological outcomes within the context of enhanced patient care [15, 16].

20.2 Functional Impact of Gliomas

Gliomas can have a significant effect on a person's life, leading to various physical, cognitive, and emotional impairments. The symptoms will change based on the tumor's location, size, and growth rate and mode of the tumoral lesion [17]. Many of these can be slow growing, such as low-grade gliomas, and the function of the surrounding area can remain intact for a long time [18]. In the nearby area, the tumor may activate progressive functional compensatory remodeling of brain networks [19]. In other cases, with rapid tumor growth, symptoms may appear earlier and improve after tumor resection if the tumor mass has not damaged the surrounding nerve fibers.

These patients often present with a wide range of disorders, including motor, sensory, and cognitive deficits, including speech and psychic disturbances. Motor disorders certainly receive the most attention and are often treated in the early postoperative period. *Motor* disorders can be caused by tumors in the motor cortex or related pathways and can result in hemiparesis, spasticity, ataxia, and general muscle weakness, leading to reduced mobility and difficulty in performing activities of daily living (ADL). These can be associated with *motor-sensory* dysfunction, especially when gliomas affect or involve sensory pathways. The resulting symptoms can include numbness, tingling or loss of proprioception, with indirect effects on movement and coordination [20–22].

Depending on the location of the tumor, patients may also experience problems with memory, executive function, attention, visual perception, and processing speed. These *cognitive* disorders may occur in the pre- or postoperative period and may be exacerbated by adjuvant treatments [23]. A recent review of the literature by Gehrke et al. [24] found that the most common cognitive impairments reported in the existing research, beyond the effects of age, education, and gender, are deficits in memory (working memory), executive functions (cognitive control and flexibility, speed of cognitive processing, visual search, planning, and prediction) and general attention, although the impairments are also specific to the brain circuit affected by the tumor.

Among these, tumors that preferentially affect the speech structures of the dominant hemisphere can lead to disorders of the *language*, including aphasia, dysarthria, and other communication difficulties (such as semantics or communicative pragmatics disorders).

Finally, patients with glioma may experience emotional, relational, and psychological disorders. Depression, anxiety, mood disturbances, and personality changes are very common in patients with glioma and may be symptoms of the diagnosis itself, of the side effects of treatment, or even of the loss of independence [19, 25, 26]. Personality changes are among the most difficult symptoms to manage in brain tumor patients and are a major concern for both patients and their families [27–29], with a significant negative impact on quality of life and caregiver distress [19, 27]. Carers of people with brain tumors also report feeling unprepared or unable to cope with changes in their relative's personality and behavior, resulting in lower overall mastery [19, 23, 30].

20.3 Duration of the Rehabilitation Programs

Several investigations and reviews addressed the crucial topic of the duration of a proper rehabilitation program. The duration of rehabilitation was less than 6 months for most of the participants included in studies [2, 4, 6]. Several authors reported that the intervention was delivered at the time of adjuvant treatments (either at the time of discharge post-surgery or when receiving radiation and chemotherapy) [1, 2, 31]: this timing of intervention aligns with the supportive care framework for the management of high-grade gliomas (HGG) recommendation to share information about expected personality and behavioral changes upon the completion of radiotherapy [32, 33].

The NICE guidelines [34] underline the variability and fluctuation of neurological symptoms and problems that can occur at different points in the history of such diseases, and there is no recommendation about a specific timing or duration of the neurorehabilitation program. Therefore, these guidelines emphasize that referral for a neurological rehabilitation program should be considered at every stage of the disease, including at diagnosis. The importance of screening throughout the illness trajectory for personality and behavior changes is also echoed in the "Optimal care pathway for people with HGG." [35].

Early and individually tailored physical training (within weeks after surgery) results in significant functional gains for HGG patients. Such patients differ from other cancer diagnoses because of progressive neurological deterioration resulting in changing and complex symptoms along the disease and treatment trajectory. Only a multidisciplinary approach can address the multiple needs arising from this life-threatening condition. However, cognitive deficits, personality changes, lack of intuition and loss of empathy may impair the ability of HGG patients to consciously and actively participate in adjuvant therapies and postoperative monitoring [12, 36, 37]. Therefore, it is important that the interventions are strictly tailored to the specific patient's complaints, feelings, and needs [14].

Indeed, the overall goal of glioma rehabilitation programs is to maximize patients' independence and improve their Quality of life (QoL). The rehabilitation team must identify all types of impairments comprehensively and specifically and intervene in each area. The achievement is made possible by a team of individuals that includes physician, neurologist, neuropsychologist, cognitive therapist, and physiotherapist, which allows:

1. **Restoration of Physical Function**: Physical therapy focuses on regaining strength, coordination, balance, and mobility to optimize the patient's ability to enhance overall physical endurance [2, 6, 15].
2. **Cognitive Rehabilitation**: Cognitive therapies are tailored to address specific deficits, such as memory, attention, and problem-solving disturbances, with the aim of improving cognitive performance and facilitating a prompt return to daily activities and work, when possible. Due to the behavior of the disease itself, perioperative factors (such as significant blood pressure fluctuations, cerebral ischemia, and hypoxia), and the impact of surgical trauma, approximately half of glioma patients experience variable degrees of postoperative cognitive impairment, seriously affecting their overall oncologic prognosis [25]. In this complex process, the neuropsychologist identifies areas of impairment through a detailed assessment of cognitive function and guides the rehabilitation process based on patient-specific recovery goals. These goals vary according to the severity and specificity of the disorder and the residual resources [12, 38].
3. **Speech and Language Rehabilitation**: For patients with speech impairments and aphasia, therapy aims to restore communication abilities, not only including verbal production, but also comprehension, articulation, lexical and phonological, orthographical abilities, and fluency [14, 20]. It is also important to keep in mind the significant impact on QoL the swallowing disorders that tend to be greatly underestimated [36].
4. **Emotional and Psychosocial Support**: Psychological support and counseling are integral to rehabilitation, addressing issues of depression, anxiety, and emotional adjustment to illness [39].

20.4 A Memory-Centered Program and the Self-Transcendence Approach

Reed proposed the *self-transcendence* approach, suggesting that the enhancement of an individual's physical well-being and health status is a continuous process of personal growth and advancement [10]. By persistently seeking and exploring life's meaning, value, and truth, individuals can unlock their full potential to adapt effectively to life challenges such as a glioma diagnosis.

Within this framework, memory therapy emerges as a psychological intervention necessity. Its proper functioning allows the recollection of past emotions, thoughts, and experiences, aiding patients in coping with loss and bolstering their ability to adjust to a new environment [10, 40]. Studies have shown that memory therapy proven beneficial for patients with Alzheimer's disease and stroke, offering relief from negative emotions and improving cognitive function [41, 42].

However, reports on its use during the perioperative period for glioma patients are still scarce [43]. A retrospective cohort study involving 168 brain glioma patients identified post-surgical impairments in executive function, mental state, and memory, with incidences of 26.5%, 23.2%, and 19.3%, respectively [37].

A seminal investigation has linked the postoperative cognitive status of glioma patients to their psychological well-being, daily living capabilities, and overall QoL [44]. These findings underline the substantial incidence of cognitive impairment following glioma surgery, highlighting the importance of enhancing cognitive functions to improve the QoL and alleviate the adverse psychological impact on patients. In this study, after a proper neurorehabilitation program, the average Neurobehavioral Cognitive Status Examination (NCSE) scores of the observation group was significantly higher than that of the control group, whereas the scores of Clinical Dementia Rating (CDR), and other hospital stress scale were lower in comparison to those of the control group [2, 4, 5]. These outcomes suggest that memory therapy can promote postoperative cognitive function recovery in glioma patients and diminish anxiety and stress responses.

This improvement may be attributed to several factors: (1) The plasticity of the nervous system allows patients to continuously activate their memory's language networks through self-narration and recall, thereby enhancing abilities such as delayed and immediate recall, learning, language organization, and expression. (2) Memory therapy aids patients in retrieving and reconstructing memories, safeguarding residual memory, and expediting the recovery of postoperative cognitive function. (3) The interaction between the intervener and the patient boosts patient self-esteem prevents a loss of initiative and improves social connections, reducing social withdrawal, negative emotions, and psychological stress, thus further ameliorating cognitive impairments.

Memory therapy was previously demonstrated to significantly improve QoL and cognitive and memory abilities and reduce depression levels among the elderly [11]. Echoing the findings of this investigation, a care model based on memory therapy has been shown to potentially reduce the frequency of cognitive impairment and boost cognitive function in patients experiencing acute ischemic stroke [5, 41]. The rate of adverse outcomes in the observation group was found to be lower than that in the control group. Additionally, subsequent multivariate logistic regression analysis further supports the efficacy of memory therapy in reducing the probability of unfavorable outcomes following glioma surgery, thereby improving patient's overall functional and oncologic results.

The most challenging aspect of rehabilitation programs is determining which functions are impaired and whether the impairment is due to the disease, surgery, or adjuvant treatments. For this reason, patient evaluation needs to involve multiple disciplines and be ongoing with closed follow-up. Rehabilitation Hospitals *must* maintain close communication with the treatment centers where the patient is being treated, and follow-up plans *should* be made jointly [7, 14, 16].

20.5 The Need of a Multidisciplinary Approach

Effective rehabilitation in glioma patients requires a multidisciplinary team of healthcare professionals, each contributing expertise to address the patient's complex needs:

1. **Physiatrists**: Lead the rehabilitation team and develop a comprehensive, individualized rehabilitation plan.
2. **Physical Therapists**: Specialize in mobility, balance, and strength training, using both active and passive exercises to restore motor function.
3. **Occupational Therapists**: Focus on improving the patient's ability to perform ADLs by addressing upper body strength, dexterity, and functional adaptations to compensate for deficits.
4. **Speech-Language Therapists**: Evaluate and treat communication and swallowing disorders, with interventions aimed at improving speech clarity and language comprehension.
5. **Neuropsychologists**: Provide cognitive assessments and design rehabilitation plans to address deficits in memory, attention, memory, praxis and executive functions.
6. **Psychiatrists and Clinical Psychologists**: Offer emotional support and therapy to help patients and their families cope with the psychological impacts of glioma diagnosis and treatment.
7. **Social Workers**: Assist in discharge planning, home care arrangements, and connect patients to community resources for ongoing support.

20.6 Rehabilitation Phases

The rehabilitation process for glioma patients is individualized and typically begins in the hospital after surgery. Once the patient is stable, they may be transferred to an inpatient rehabilitation facility or continue their rehabilitation on an outpatient basis.

The rehabilitation process typically includes:

- **Assessment:** The rehabilitation team will conduct a comprehensive assessment to evaluate the patient's physical, cognitive, and emotional impairments.
- **Goal setting:** The rehabilitation team will work with the patient to set personalized and realistic rehabilitation goals.
- **Treatment:** The patient will participate in a variety of therapies, such as physical therapy, occupational therapy, speech therapy, cognitive rehabilitation, and emotional support therapy.
- **Education:** The patient and their family will receive psychoeducation about the disease, treatment, and rehabilitation process.
- **Discharge planning:** The rehabilitation team will work with the patient to develop a plan for discharge from the hospital or rehabilitation facility. This plan will include recommendations for continued therapy, home modifications, and community resources.

Neurological function decline following intrinsic brain tumor surgery is a common occurrence [6, 9, 12]. In certain instances, this deterioration is anticipated due to factors such as perioperative ischemic damage, operations in eloquent brain regions causing specific deficits, or the development of supplementary motor area (SMA) syndrome after procedures involving the supplementary motor complex [20]. However, the cause of postoperative neurological decline is not always clear-cut, and predicting the progression of the impaired function can be challenging. Up to 40% of patients may experience postoperative neurological deterioration, with a higher incidence of new deficits observed in patients with tumors in presumed eloquent areas compared to those in non-eloquent regions. These new deficits typically manifest immediately after surgery, with delayed neurological deterioration being less common, although seizures may lead to transient deficits. Tumors in eloquent locations are considered a strong predictor of postoperative neurological decline, and in high-grade glioma (HGG) surgery, pre-existing neurological deficits are likely to persist or worsen following surgical intervention [25].

Most studies report a 30–40% incidence of neurological deterioration after craniotomy for primary brain tumors [20]. However, this decline is often temporary, with 81% of patients experiencing complete or near-complete symptom resolution, and 66% achieving full recovery. Consequently, several authors report a lower incidence of permanent postoperative neurological deficits, around 6% for the entire patient group, with an additional 6% experiencing minor residual deficits that do not significantly impair function. A meta-analysis of glioma surgery outcomes revealed that early deficits occurred in 30% of patients [9]. In a study conducted by Gempt et al. [45], transient postoperative neurological deficits were observed in 17% of newly diagnosed gliomas and 32% of recurrent cases, while permanent neurological deficits were found in 7% and 16% of these cases, respectively.

20.7 Rehabilitation Phases for Patients with Glioma

The rehabilitation process for glioma patients consists of multiple stages that are determined by the time phase of pathology at which we will intervene.

1. **Acute Phase**: Rehabilitation begins during the acute phase of treatment, often immediately following surgery. Early mobilization, prevention of complications (e.g., deep vein thrombosis, pressure ulcers), and initial physical and cognitive therapy sessions are prioritized during this period.
2. **Post-Acute Phase**: Following discharge from the hospital, rehabilitation continues in either an inpatient rehabilitation facility or as outpatient therapy. The focus shifts toward more intensive therapy aimed at regaining lost functions and promoting independence.
3. **Long-Term Rehabilitation**: Glioma patients often require long-term rehabilitation due to the progressive nature of the disease and the cumulative effects of treatments. Maintenance therapies, including regular physical and cognitive exercises, are recommended to prevent further decline. Rehabilitation for glioma and glioblastoma is an ongoing process. Even after the patient has completed formal rehabilitation, they may need to continue with certain therapies or home exercises to maintain their gains. It is also important for patients to stay active and engaged in their community to help prevent further decline in function.

20.8 Specialized Rehabilitation Techniques

Several advanced rehabilitation techniques are particularly effective in glioma patients:

1. **Task-Specific Training**: Therapy that focuses on practicing specific tasks, such as walking or hand movements, has been shown to improve motor function through neuroplasticity, allowing the brain to rewire itself to compensate for damaged areas [16]. Very important in modern rehabilitation design is the use of dual-task tasks that allow motor recovery coupled with cognitive recovery.
2. **Constraint-Induced Movement Therapy (CIMT)**: This method is used to improve upper limb function in patients with hemiparesis by constraining the unaffected limb, thereby forcing the use of the affected limb [17]. However, this therapeutic method is less used today.
3. **Virtual Reality (VR) and Robotic-Assisted Therapy**: These technologies provide an immersive environment for rehabilitation exercises and have been shown to enhance motor recovery by providing real-time feedback and motivation.
4. **Cognitive Rehabilitation Therapy (CRT)**: This includes strategies such as memory exercises, attention drills, and problem-solving activities that are designed to improve cognitive functioning. Computer-based cognitive rehabilitation programs are increasingly being used for home-based therapy [15].
5. **Psychological Interventions**: Mindfulness-based stress reduction (MBSR), cognitive-behavioral therapy (CBT), and supportive psychotherapy are employed to help patients manage the emotional toll of glioma and its treatment.

20.9 Challenges in Glioma Rehabilitation

The rehabilitation of glioma patients presents numerous obstacles, with tumor recurrence and progression being the primary concern. Gliomas, especially HGGs, are notorious for their high likelihood of returning, which can lead to a swift deterioration in functional abilities and require modifications to rehabilitation objectives. Another significant challenge is fatigue related to cancer, a widespread and incapacitating symptom that often restricts patients' capacity to fully engage in rehabilitation programs. Additionally, cognitive deficits associated with gliomas may impede patients' ability to follow therapeutic instructions and adhere to exercises, particularly those aimed at rehabilitating cognitive functions. Psychological stressors, including anxiety, depression, and feelings of hopelessness, can undermine motivation and commitment to rehabilitation efforts. This necessitates the integration of psychological support throughout the rehabilitation process [19]. Although rehabilitation techniques have advanced, there remains a lack of high-quality research regarding the most effective rehabilitation protocols, resources, intensity, and duration for glioma patients. Further studies are necessary to enhance care models that consistently identify and address functional limitations in this patient group [46].

20.10 Latest Advances in Rehabilitating Glioma Patients

Recent advancements in glioma patient rehabilitation include monitor-augmented reality (MAR) supported exercises, which have demonstrated improvements in physical fitness, mental well-being, and quality of life for high-grade glioma patients undergoing radiotherapy [20]. The MAR system offers immediate feedback and guidance during exercises, enhancing awareness and self-perception of impaired or lost functions. Preliminary cognitive rehabilitation interventions, such as web-based working memory training and comprehensive mnemonic training, have shown promise and feasibility in enhancing cognitive function among glioma patients [21]. A study reported a 69% adherence rate and moderate to substantial effects on working memory assessments after a 5-week online training program [21]. Comprehensive inpatient and outpatient rehabilitation programs involving physiotherapists, occupational therapists, neuropsychologists, and other specialists aim to prevent disability and maximize function in glioma patients [21]. Tailored exercise prescriptions and individualized training programs are designed to address the specific needs and capabilities of glioma patients, leading to improvements in physical fitness, mental health, and quality of life [3, 20]. Emerging neuromodulation techniques in rehabilitation focus on enhancing functional prognosis and quality of life for glioma patients by leveraging brain plasticity and promoting cortical reorganization. These techniques can be invasive or non-invasive and include:

- Neuromodulation-Induced Cortical Prehabilitation (NICP): This approach seeks to minimize the risk of neurologic sequelae following surgery by inducing cortical reorganization through non-invasive and invasive methods such as Repetitive Transcranial Magnetic Stimulation (rTMS-NICP) and extra operative Direct Cortical Stimulation (eDCS-NICP) [3, 4].
- Non-Invasive Neuromodulation: This method employs techniques like rTMS to modulate brain activity and facilitate cortical reorganization. It has demonstrated effectiveness in reducing the risk of neurologic sequelae and improving functional outcomes in glioma patients [3, 4].

Despite these advancements, additional high-quality research is required to establish optimal rehabilitation protocols, resources, dosage, and duration specifically for glioma patients [18–21]. Larger clinical trials are essential to further evaluate the efficacy of these emerging rehabilitation techniques.

20.11 Role of Family in Rehabilitation

Family members play a crucial role in the rehabilitation of glioma patients. Their involvement in care can include helping with AAD, encouraging participation in rehabilitation activities, and providing emotional support [47]. Family and friends can play a vital role in supporting people with glioma and glioblastoma during the rehabilitation process [29]. They can provide emotional and practical support in attending therapies and help with ADLs. Therefore, families must be included and involved in the process at all stages to educate them about the goals of rehabilitation, the disorders encountered, and the specific needs of the patient [17, 19, 27]. This is essential to promote a supportive and motivating environment for the rehabilitation process itself.

20.11.1 The Role in Performance Status

A recent study by our research team [43] highlighted a key finding regarding patient recovery following surgical intervention during the pandemic: individuals exhibited a notably reduced performance status (measured using the Karnofsky performance scale, KPS) in the lockdown era compared to the pre-pandemic period. This decline was likely attributed to limited access to neurorehabilitation facilities, decreased caregiver availability, fewer centers offering chemo- and radiotherapy services, and an increased risk of medical care disruption. Interestingly, while patients diagnosed with GBM during the pandemic tended to have later detection of disease recurrence, their overall performance status was lower, characterized by diminished KPS and quality of life. This indirectly suggests that GBM patients at our center during lockdown experienced not only a decrease in rehabilitation activities but also a probable reduction in clinical and radiological follow-ups, thereby postponing the diagnosis of recurrence and subsequent treatment.

The pandemic's impact on various aspects of neuro-oncological care has led to modifications in clinical practices, including significant changes in pre-, peri-, and postoperative care [48]. Typically, most GBM patients undergo daily radiotherapy for 6 weeks, which ideally should not be interrupted. Maintaining this treatment regimen can be challenging during pandemics, leading to increased interest in hypofractionation for all tumor types. Moreover, radiation oncology departments are susceptible to unit closures or substantial service reductions due to staff shortages, while adhering to radiation protection regulations remains crucial. Consequently, hypofractionated programs should be employed to minimize exposure and infection risk from SARS-CoV-2 and to enhance the likelihood of completing a course of radiotherapy [48].

Currently, there is a lack of evidence on how to mitigate GBM-specific treatment interruptions and their impact on survival. Our series revealed an increase in the number of patients who had to discontinue radiotherapy for medical reasons, including COVID-19 positivity. During the pandemic, the risk of virus exposure escalated with each day of treatment, as patients required transportation to radiotherapy facilities, either alone, with family, or via transport services [49]. Occasionally, hospital admissions were necessary, involving hospital transfers, which were generally discouraged. Furthermore, most centers restricted visitors, causing additional stress and safety concerns for GBM patients, who often experienced cognitive impairment [43].

20.12 Conclusion

Glioma patient rehabilitation is a complex and evolving process that demands a holistic, individualized approach. By targeting the specific physical, mental, and psychological challenges associated with glioma, rehabilitation can substantially enhance patient outcomes and QoL. The adoption of cutting-edge rehabilitation technologies and tailored treatment strategies shows potential for future improvements in glioma patient care. Rehabilitation plays a crucial role in the overall treatment plan for glioma and glioblastoma patients. A team-based approach, with support from loved ones, can assist patients in regaining functionality, enhancing their QoL, and fostering greater self-sufficiency. Despite the considerable advantages of rehabilitation, there is a scarcity of robust research on ideal protocols, resource distribution, and treatment intensity and duration specifically for glioma patients. Additional studies are necessary to create improved care models that consistently recognize and address functional limitations in this group.

References

1. Sun Y, Xiong ZY, Yan PF, Jiang LL, Nie CS, Wang X. Characteristics and prognostic factors of age-stratified high-grade intracranial glioma patients: a population-based analysis. Bosn J Basic Med Sci. 2019;19(4):375–83. https://doi.org/10.17305/bjbms.2019.4213.
2. Zhao K, et al. Rehabilitation therapy for patients with glioma. Medicine. 2020;99(45):e23087. https://doi.org/10.1097/md.0000000000023087.
3. Weyer-Jamora C, Brie MS, Luks TL, Smith EM, Braunstein SE, Villanueva-Meyer JE, Bracci PM, Chang S, Hervey-Jumper SL, Taylor JW. Cognitive impact of lower-grade gliomas and strategies for rehabilitation. Neurooncol Pract. 2020;8(2):117–28. https://doi.org/10.1093/nop/npaa072.
4. Bergo E, Lombardi G, Pambuku A, Della Puppa A, Bellu L, D'Avella D, Zagonel V. Cognitive rehabilitation in patients with gliomas and other brain tumors: state of the art. Biomed Res Int. 2016;2016:3041824. https://doi.org/10.1155/2016/3041824.
5. Geler-Kulcu D, Gulsen G, Buyukbaba E, Ozkan D. Functional recovery of patients with brain tumor or acute stroke after rehabilitation: a comparative study. J Clin Neurosci. 2009;16(1):74–8. https://doi.org/10.1016/j.jocn.2008.04.014.
6. Kushner DS, Amidei C. Rehabilitation of motor dysfunction in primary brain tumor patients†. Neurooncol Pract. 2015;2(4):185–91. https://doi.org/10.1093/nop/npv019.
7. Piil K, Jakobsen J, Christensen KB, Juhler M, Guetterman TC, Fetters MD, Jarden M. Needs and preferences among patients with high-grade glioma and their caregivers—a longitudinal mixed methods study. Eur J Cancer Care (Engl). 2018;27(2):e12806. https://doi.org/10.1111/ecc.12806.
8. Pace A, Metro G, Fabi A. Supportive care in neurooncology. Curr Opin Oncol. 2010;22(6):621–6. https://doi.org/10.1097/CCO.0b013e32833e078c.
9. Spina S, Facciorusso S, Cinone N, Pellegrino R, Fiore P, Santamato A. Rehabilitation interventions for glioma patients: a mini-review. Front Surg. 2023;10:1137516.
10. Reed PG. Self-transcendence and mental health in oldest-old adults. Nurs Res. 1991;40:5–11.
11. Bazrafshan MR, Faramarzian Z, Soufi O, Delam H. The effect of group reminiscence therapy on death anxiety and adaptation of the elderly to old age. Arch Psychiatr Nurs. 2022;41:312–6.
12. Schei S, Solheim O, Salvesen Ø, Hansen TI, Sagberg LM. Patient-reported cognitive function before and after glioma surgery. Acta Neurochir. 2022;164:2009–19.
13. Hallford DJ, Hardgrove S, Sanam M, Oliveira S, Pilon M, Duran T. Remembering for resilience: brief cognitive-reminiscence therapy improves psychological resources and mental well-being in young adults. Appl Psychol Health Well Being. 2022;14:1004–21.
14. Hansen A, Pedersen CB, Jarden JO, Beier D, Minet LR, Søgaard K. Effectiveness of physical therapy–and occupational therapy–based rehabilitation in people who have glioma and are undergoing active anticancer treatment: single-blind, randomized controlled trial. Phys Ther. 2020;100(3):564–74.
15. Zhao K, Yu C, Gan Z, Huang M, Wu T, Zhao N. Rehabilitation therapy for patients with glioma: a PRISMA-compliant systematic review and meta-analysis. Medicine. 2020;99(45):e23087.
16. Vargo M, Henriksson R, Salander P. Rehabilitation of patients with glioma. Handb Clin Neurol. 2016;134:287–304.
17. Boele FW, Butler S, Nicklin E, Bulbeck H, Pointon L, Short SC, Murray L. Communication in the context of glioblastoma treatment: a qualitative study of what matters most to patients, caregivers and health care professionals. Palliat Med. 2023;37(06):834–43.
18. Mesti T, Ocvirk J. Malignant gliomas: old and new systemic treatment approaches. Radiol Oncol. 2016;50(2):129–38. https://doi.org/10.1515/raon-2015-0003.
19. Gregg N, Arber A, Ashkan K, et al. Neurobehavioural changes in patients following brain tumour: patients and relatives perspective. Support Care Cancer. 2014;22(11):2965–72.
20. Salvati M, Armocida D, Pesce A, Palmieri M, Venditti E, D'Andrea G, Frati A, Santoro A. No prognostic differences between GBM-patients presenting with postoperative SMA-syndrome and GBM-patients involving cortico-spinal tract and primary motor cortex. J Neurol Sci. 2020;419:117188. https://doi.org/10.1016/j.jns.2020.117188.
21. Mukand JA, Blackinton DD, Crincoli MG, Lee JJ, Santos BB. Incidence of neurologic deficits and rehabilitation of patients with brain tumors. Am J Phys Med Rehabil. 2001;80:346–50.
22. Duffau H. Lessons from brain mapping in surgery for low-grade glioma: insights into associations between tumour and brain plasticity. Lancet Neurol. 2005;4(8):476–86.
23. Thakur D, Dhandapani M, Ghai S, Mohanty M. Assessment of behavioral symptoms of postoperative patients with intracranial tumor and dis-

tress among their caregivers. Nurs Midwifery Res J. 2020;16(2):84–94.
24. Gehrke AK, Baisley MC, Sonck AL, Wronski SL, Feuerstein M. Neurocognitive deficits following primary brain tumor treatment: systematic review of a decade of comparative studies. J Neuro-Oncol. 2013;115(2):135–42. https://doi.org/10.1007/s11060-013-1215-2.
25. Long A, Halkett GK, Lobb EA, et al. Carers of patients with high-grade glioma report high levels of distress, unmet needs, and psychological morbidity during patient chemoradiotherapy. Neurooncol Pract. 2016;3(2):105–12.
26. Lök N, Bademli K, Selçuk-Tosun A. The effect of reminiscence therapy on cognitive functions, depression, and quality of life in Alzheimer patients: randomized controlled trial. Int J Geriatr Psychiatry. 2019;34:47–53.
27. Cavers D, Hacking B, Erridge SE, et al. Social, psychological and existential well-being in patients with glioma and their caregivers: a qualitative study. CMAJ. 2012;184(7):E373–82.
28. Halkett G, Lobb E, Shaw T, et al. Do carer's levels of unmet needs change over time when caring for patients diagnosed with high-grade glioma and how are these needs correlated with distress? Support Care Cancer. 2018;26(1):275–86.
29. Schmer C, Ward-Smith P, Latham S, Salacz M. When a family member has a malignant brain tumor: the caregiver perspective. J Neurosci Nurs. 2008;40(2):78–84.
30. Wright KM, Simpson GK, Koh E-S, et al. Development and evaluation of information resources for patients, families, and healthcare providers addressing behavioral and cognitive sequelae among adults with a primary brain tumor. J Neurosci Nurs. 2015;47(3):135–45.
31. Cramer CK, Cummings TL, Andrews RN, Strowd R, Rapp SR, Shaw EG, Chan MD, Lesser GJ. Treatment of radiation-induced cognitive decline in adult brain tumor patients. Curr Treat Options in Oncol. 2019;20(5):42. https://doi.org/10.1007/s11864-019-0641-6.
32. Philip J, Collins A, Brand C, et al. A proposed framework of supportive and palliative care for people with high-grade glioma. Neurooncology. 2018;20(3):391–9.
33. Victoria CCVaDoH. Optimal care pathway for people with high-grade glioma. 2nd ed. Melbourne: Cancer Council Victoria; 2021.
34. (UK). NGA. Evidence reviews for supporting people living with a brain tumour: brain tumours (primary) and brain metastases in adults: evidence report D. London: National Institute for Health and Care Excellence (NICE); 2018.
35. Schiffbauer H, Ferrari P, Rowley HA, Berger MS, Roberts TP. Functional activity within brain tumours: a magnetic source imaging study. Neurosurgery. 2001;49:1313–20.
36. van Loon EM, Heijenbrok-Kal MH, van Loon WS, van den Bent MJ, Vincent AJ, de Koning I, Ribbers GM. Assessment methods and prevalence of cognitive dysfunction in patients with low-grade glioma: a systematic review. J Rehabil Med. 2015;47:481–8.
37. van Kessel E, Emons MAC, Wajer IH, van Baarsen KM, Broekman ML, Robe PA, Snijders TJ, Van Zandvoort MJE. Tumor-related neurocognitive dysfunction in patients with diffuse glioma: a retrospective cohort study prior to antitumor treatment. Neurooncol Pract. 2019;6:463–72.
38. Gil I, Santos-Costa P, Bobrowicz-Campos E, Silva R, de Lurdes AM, Apóstolo J. Effectiveness of reminiscence therapy versus cognitive stimulation therapy in older adults with cognitive decline: a quasi-experimental pilot study. Nurs Rep. 2022;12:339–47.
39. Sherwood PR, Given BA, Given CW, et al. The influence of caregiver mastery on depressive symptoms. J Nurs Scholarsh. 2007;39(3):249–55.
40. Piil K, Juhler M, Jakobsen J, Jarden M. Controlled rehabilitative and supportive care intervention trials in patients with high-grade gliomas and their caregivers: a systematic review. BMJ Support Palliat Care. 2016;6(1):27–34. https://doi.org/10.1136/bmjspcare-2013-000593.
41. Cheng C, Fan W, Liu C, Liu Y, Liu X. Reminiscence therapy-based care program relieves post-stroke cognitive impairment, anxiety, and depression in acute ischemic stroke patients: a randomized, controlled study. Ir J Med Sci. 2021;190:345–55.
42. Thomas JM, Sezgin D. Effectiveness of reminiscence therapy in reducing agitation and depression and improving quality of life and cognition in long-term care residents with dementia: a systematic review and meta-analysis. Geriatr Nurs. 2021;42:1497–506.
43. Armocida D, D'Angelo L, Pietro R, Chiarello G, Jiang T, Rizzo F, Garbossa D, Frati A, Marampon F, Santoro A. The impact of the COVID-19 pandemic and lockdown on the outcome of glioblastoma. J Neurol Surg A Cent Eur Neurosurg. 2024; https://doi.org/10.1055/s-0044-1779262.
44. Zanotto A, Glover RN, Zanotto T, Boele FW. Rehabilitation in people living with glioblastoma: a narrative review of the literature. Cancers. 2024;16(9):1699.
45. Gempt J, Lange N, Bette S, Foreman SC, Cammardella JH, Albertshauser J, Gradtke C, Buchmann N, Ryang YM, Schmidt-Graf F, Meyer B, Ringel F. Factors influencing neurocognitive function in patients with neuroepithelial tumors. Sci Rep. 2017;7(1):17764. https://doi.org/10.1038/s41598-017-17833-w. Erratum in: Sci Rep. 2018 Mar 6;8(1):4274. https://doi.org/10.1038/s41598-018-21908-7.
46. Arber A, Hutson N, de Vries K, Guerrero D. Finding the right kind of support: a study of carers of those with a primary malignant brain tumour. Eur J Oncol Nurs. 2013;17(1):52–8.
47. Dhandapani M, Gupta S, Dhandapani S, et al. Study of factors determining caregiver burden among

primary caregivers of patients with intracranial tumors. Surg Neurol Int. 2015;6:160. https://doi.org/10.4103/2152-7806.167084.

48. Lozano-Sanchez F, Ursu R, Di-Stefano AL, et al. Descriptive and retrospective analysis of diffuse glioma patients with symptomatic SARS-CoV2 infection during the first wave of the pandemic. Neurooncol Adv. 2021;3(01):vdab078.

49. Pesce A, Palmieri M, Armocida D, Frati A, Santoro A. Letter: neurosurgery and coronavirus (COVID-19) epidemic: doing our part. Neurosurgery. 2020;87(01):E48–9.

21 Artificial Intelligence (AI) in Neuro-Oncology: A Never Updated Introductive Guide to AI Algorithms and Potential Applications

Leonardo Tariciotti, Youssef Zohdy, Marco Riva, Riccardo Levi, Federico Pessina, and Gustavo Pradilla

21.1 Introduction

Despite continuous advancements in the classification and management of CNS tumours, many of these entities are still associated with a barely unchanged poor prognosis [1, 2], posing tremendous responsibilities on researchers' and clinicians' shoulders for the future. To investigate these vacant challenges, the employment of cutting-edge medical technologies and research methodologies followed over the last decades. However, much work is still needed to improve neurooncological patients' quality of life and survival. The evolution and recent large-scale spread of artificial intelligence (AI) algorithms has been proposed as an innovative and—optimistically—revolutionising technology to change the medical research landscape and eventually empower physicians with new tools and capabilities to deliver better healthcare worldwide. An enormous growing list of publications (academic articles, policy reports, media coverage) has been produced as a translation of the spreading use of AI algorithms in the industrial field. However, the widely applied medical AI is still an embryonal concept, and successful employment is present but limited. Hence, the public attention attracted is somewhat unjustified by the compelling results demonstrated to solve real medical problems.

It is out of the question that AI will be impactful and beneficial in healthcare, especially in an evolving multidisciplinary field like neuro-oncology. However, validation, reliability, and generalisability are the pillars of public trust in AI for a significant adoption. To do so, a joint commitment of physicians, government, policy-makers, and AI experts is mandatory to identify

L. Tariciotti (✉)
Department of Neurosurgery, Emory University School of Medicine, Atlanta, GA, USA

Department of Oncology and Hemato-Oncology, University of Milan, Milan, Italy
e-mail: leonardotariciottimd@gmail.com

Y. Zohdy · G. Pradilla
Department of Neurosurgery, Emory University School of Medicine, Atlanta, GA, USA

M. Riva · F. Pessina
Department of Biomedical Sciences, Humanitas University, Pieve Emanuele (MI), Italy

Department of Neurosurgery, IRCCS Humanitas Research Hospital, Rozzano (MI), Italy

R. Levi
Unit of Neuroradiology, IRCCS Humanitas Research Hospital, Rozzano (MI), Italy

D. Armocida et al. (eds.), *Neurosurgery's Frontline Role in Gliomas Treatment*,
https://doi.org/10.1007/978-3-031-81850-9_21

the appropriate strategies for investigation and the case uses for such technology [3, 4].

However, a joint effort requires a shared background and a common language: to obtain that, medical professionals and researchers must become proficient in understanding the basic principles of AI models, critically reviewing their applications reported in the literature, and evaluating opportunities for future uses.

Two final key points deserve to be pointed out: first, an extensive approach to reviewing the whole available body of literature was not intentionally pursued in producing this chapter. This is due to the already extensive availability of systematic reviews on the topic, which would nullify our efforts and scarce longevity as updated documents [5–8]. The release of new algorithms and the extreme scientific hype on the subject produce exponential growth in published articles, whose quality is seldom easy to measure. Second, a neglected point of view in medical AI is the inadequate background of the medical curriculum in providing any spendable insight into understanding these advanced methodologies (i.e., computing literacy). We then focused on educative content, providing the essential notions for navigating this topic with caution and judice. To better integrate with this evolving landscape and grasp any potential benefit from it to apply to our patient's care, the question "Should medical professionals and researchers be trained to understand, code, optimise, and critically analyse (especially from an ethical standpoint) AI algorithms and tools" has already been postulated. Familiarity with programming languages and data repositories is becoming increasingly relevant, especially in research [9–13].

This chapter aims to provide an introductory repository of information for readers with a medical background to understand the basic principles of artificial intelligence through a structured description of the principal methods available, providing references for accessing these resources, understanding their potential use in research, and by reviewing the major field of current investigation in neuro-oncology.

21.2 Principles for Understanding Artificial Intelligence

AI comprises a broad spectrum of disciplines encompassing neuroscience, psychology, linguistics, philosophy, statistics, computer science, and computer engineering. AI can be defined as the ability of machines to perform tasks that typically require human intelligence, such as learning, problem-solving, information retrieval, and adaptation to external inputs.

AI is currently at the artificial narrow intelligence (ANI) stage. ANI excels at handling vast amounts of data, learning through pattern recognition, and performing tasks such as complex text generation, image classification, voice recognition, data clustering, and advanced programming. Its capabilities depend on the training dataset, often achieving expert-level performance in specific tasks, sometimes surpassing human abilities [14]. "Artificial General Intelligence (AGI)", which would think, reason, and recall information like a human, remains a distant goal, with ongoing research attempting to develop such algorithms. "Artificial Superintelligence (ASI)", a theoretical concept, posits that AI could surpass human intelligence in all aspects, raising ethical and philosophical questions about its potential impact [14].

The foundation of AI relies on the application of advanced statistical methods for modelling input data, which are part of machine learning (ML). ML is an ensemble of methods where algorithms are trained to learn patterns from pre-collected data using pre-compiled programming functions [6]. In neuro-oncology, ML models can be trained to identify and segment tumours in MRI scans by analysing large human annotated datasets. The quality and quantity of these annotations directly influence model performance. DL, a subset of ML, employs neural networks that iteratively create complex recognition patterns, often achieving superior results in respect of previous medical imaging algorithms. However, the interpretability of these models can be challenging, necessitating additional steps to ensure their predictions are understandable and critically reviewed, particularly in medical applications. ML models can be categorised by their learning methods, characteristics, and tasks they perform, which will be explored further in the chapter.

21.2.1 Supervised ML

The previous example of identifying tumours within an MRI scan using a labelled database is an instance of supervised ML. In supervised learning, a structured training database provides the algorithm with information about the meaning of the input data. This enables the machine to learn how to make accurate predictions by optimising the learning process and minimising errors. The performance of these models is tested on both the training set and on unseen (hold-out) data, which must share the same data structure. Supervised ML models are commonly used with pre-labelled image, textual, and numeric datasets or for building predictive models based on various medical data sources [15]. Additional resources on supervised ML models are available in Table 21.1.

21.2.2 Unsupervised ML

In contrast to supervised learning, unsupervised ML works with unlabeled input data and identifies intrinsic patterns within the data without knowing the specific attributes of each data set [16, 17]. These methods are instrumental in grouping (i.e., clustering) data based on their similarities. Several clustering algorithms in unsupervised ML follow different rules, such as exclusive, overlapping, hierarchical, and probabilistic clustering.

Other models analyse unlabeled datasets to identify and exclude variables that do not alter the integrity of the data batch, a process known as "dimensionality reduction". This simplifies large datasets, making them more manageable. A helpful example in clinical medicine is principal component analysis (PCA), which applies a linear transformation to generate a new dataset with principal components [18, 19]. The first component intersects the dataset, maximising the variance of the sample; the second does the same but intersects the multidimensional plane of data orthogonally with the first principal component. This process can be repeated multiple times depending on the dimensionality of the input data, allowing for the labelling of patients into novel clusters using only significant variables.

A more modern example of unsupervised learning is the autoencoder, an architecture famous in many DL models today [20–22]. It compresses the dimensionality of data through inner layers, storing information from the input data in smaller nodes (encoding). It then reconstructs this data (decoding) to perform any trained task. A significant portion of modern computer vision relies on this principle. Additional resources on unsupervised ML models are available in Table 21.2.

21.2.3 Reinforcement Learning (RL)

Reinforcement learning (RL) is based on an unsupervised trial-and-error training process, where the model executes predictions and receives feedback from human interaction at the output level. After a series of trials, positive or negative feedback is provided, allowing the model to learn association patterns and adjust its performance according to the operator's feedback (reinforcement). Essentially, the model iterates to find a balance between exploring new patterns in the data, which carries the risk of negative feedback, and exploiting existing knowledge, which has a higher chance of positive reinforcement. This maximises long-term positive outcomes. The environment for such iterations is usually designed as a Markov decision process (MDP), as many RL processes incorporate dynamic programming features. The main difference is that RL does not assume any fixed knowledge of the mathematical model of the MDP [23, 24]. An example of RL in neuro-oncology is determining medication dosing in clinical trials, where models can learn the optimal dosing to reduce tumour volume based on previous data. The same approach can be applied to radiation therapy [25]. Additional resources on RL models are available in Table 21.3.

Table 21.1 Overview of supervised LM models

Year	Model	Python Package	R Package	Description	Open Source	Potential Use	Reference (Python)	Reference (R)
1957	Linear discriminant analysis	Scikit-learn	MASS::Lda	A method used to find a linear combination of features that separates two or more classes of objects or events.	Yes	Tumor classification and predicting patient outcomes.	https://scikit-learn.org/stable/modules/lda_qda.html	https://cran.r-project.org/web/packages/MASS/index.html
1963	Support vector machine	Scikit-learn	e1071::Svm	A classifier that finds the hyperplane which best separates different classes of data.	Yes	Classifying tumor types based on imaging data.	https://scikit-learn.org/stable/modules/svm.html	https://cran.r-project.org/web/packages/e1071/index.html
1972	Ridge regression	Scikit-learn	Glmnet	A method used to analyze multiple regression data that suffer from multicollinearity.	Yes	Predicting patient survival rates based on multiple correlated features.	https://scikit-learn.org/stable/modules/linear_model.html	https://cran.r-project.org/web/packages/glmnet/index.html
1973	Decision trees	Scikit-learn	Rpart	A non-parametric supervised learning method used for classification and regression.	Yes	Creating decision models for treatment planning.	https://scikit-learn.org/stable/modules/tree.html	https://cran.r-project.org/web/packages/rpart/index.html
1974	Naive Bayes classifier	Scikit-learn	e1071::naiveBayes	A classifier based on applying Bayes' theorem with strong independence assumptions between the features.	Yes	Classifying tumor types from radiographic features.	https://scikit-learn.org/stable/modules/naive_bayes.html	https://cran.r-project.org/web/packages/e1071/index.html
1984	Artificial neural network	Tensorflow, keras, pytorch	Neuralnet, keras	A computing system inspired by biological neural networks, designed to recognize patterns.	Yes	Image recognition for tumor detection and segmentation.	https://www.tensorflow.org/, https://keras.io/	https://cran.r-project.org/web/packages/neuralnet/index.html, https://cran.r-project.org/web/packages/keras/index.html
1986	Multi-layer perceptron	Scikit-learn	Nnet	A class of feedforward artificial neural network.	Yes	Deep learning for complex pattern recognition in medical images.	https://scikit-learn.org/stable/modules/neural_networks.html	https://cran.r-project.org/web/packages/nnet/index.html
1989	Stochastic gradient descent	Scikit-learn	Sgd	An iterative method for optimizing an objective function with suitable smoothness properties.	Yes	Training large-scale machine learning models for imaging data.	https://scikit-learn.org/stable/modules/sgd.html	https://cran.r-project.org/web/packages/sgd/index.html
1992	Logistic regression	Scikit-learn	Stats::Glm	A statistical model that in its basic form uses a logistic function to model a binary dependent variable.	Yes	Predicting binary outcomes such as survival or recurrence.	https://scikit-learn.org/stable/modules/linear_model.html	https://cran.r-project.org/web/packages/stats/index.html
1995	Random forest	Scikit-learn	random-Forest	An ensemble learning method for classification and regression that operates by constructing multiple decision trees.	Yes	Predicting patient outcomes and treatment responses.	https://scikit-learn.org/stable/modules/ensemble.html	https://cran.r-project.org/web/packages/randomForest/index.html
1996	AdaBoost	Scikit-learn	Adabag	An ensemble learning method that combines the performance of many weak classifiers to improve classification results.	Yes	Enhancing the accuracy of tumor classification algorithms.	https://scikit-learn.org/stable/modules/ensemble.html#adaboost	https://cran.r-project.org/web/packages/adabag/index.html

1997	Gradient boosting machines	Xgboost, lightgbm	Xgboost, lightgbm	A machine learning technique for regression and classification problems, which produces a prediction model in the form of an ensemble of weak prediction models.	Yes	Improving the performance of predictive models for patient outcomes.	https://xgboost.readthedocs.io/, https://lightgbm.readthedocs.io/	https://cran.r-project.org/web/packages/xgboost/index.html, https://cran.r-project.org/web/packages/lightgbm/index.html
1998	K-nearest neighbors	Scikit-learn	Class::Knn	A simple, instance-based learning algorithm used for classification and regression.	Yes	Classifying patients into different risk categories based on similar cases.	https://scikit-learn.org/stable/modules/neighbors.html	https://cran.r-project.org/web/packages/class/index.html
1999	Extra trees	Scikit-learn	extraTrees	An ensemble method that fits a number of randomized decision trees on various sub-samples of the dataset.	Yes	Robust prediction models for treatment outcomes.	https://scikit-learn.org/stable/modules/ensemble.html#extra-trees	https://cran.r-project.org/web/packages/extraTrees/index.html
2002	Bagging	Scikit-learn	Ipred::Bagging	An ensemble method designed to improve the stability and accuracy of machine learning algorithms.	Yes	Combining multiple models to improve prediction accuracy.	https://scikit-learn.org/stable/modules/ensemble.html#bagging	https://cran.r-project.org/web/packages/ipred/index.html
2002	Elastic net	Scikit-learn	Glmnet	A regularized regression method that linearly combines the L1 and L2 penalties of the lasso and ridge methods.	Yes	Handling multicollinearity in prediction models for patient outcomes.	https://scikit-learn.org/stable/modules/linear_model.html#elastic-net	https://cran.r-project.org/web/packages/glmnet/index.html
2005	Bayesian network	Pgmpy	Bnlearn	A probabilistic graphical model that represents a set of variables and their conditional dependencies via a directed acyclic graph.	Yes	Modeling the probabilistic relationships between patient data and outcomes.	https://pgmpy.org/	https://cran.r-project.org/web/packages/bnlearn/index.html
2006	Gradient boosted decision trees	Xgboost, lightgbm	Gbm	An ensemble technique that builds trees sequentially, with each tree correcting the errors of the previous one.	Yes	Enhancing prediction accuracy for complex patient data.	https://xgboost.readthedocs.io/, https://lightgbm.readthedocs.io/	https://cran.r-project.org/web/packages/gbm/index.html
2006	AdaBoost	Scikit-learn	Adabag	An ensemble learning method that combines the performance of many weak classifiers to improve classification results.	Yes	Enhancing the accuracy of tumor classification algorithms.	https://scikit-learn.org/stable/modules/ensemble.html#adaboost	https://cran.r-project.org/web/packages/adabag/index.html
2009	LightGBM	Lightgbm	Lightgbm	A gradient boosting framework that uses tree-based learning algorithms, designed to be distributed and efficient.	Yes	Fast and efficient modeling of large-scale patient data.	https://lightgbm.readthedocs.io/	https://cran.r-project.org/web/packages/lightgbm/index.html
2012	Extreme gradient boosting	Xgboost	Xgboost	An optimized distributed gradient boosting library designed to be highly efficient, flexible, and portable.	Yes	Advanced predictive modeling for patient outcomes and treatment responses.	https://xgboost.readthedocs.io/	https://cran.r-project.org/web/packages/xgboost/index.html
2014	CatBoost	Catboost	Catboost	A gradient boosting library that handles categorical features automatically.	Yes	Building accurate models for categorical patient data.	https://catboost.ai/	https://cran.r-project.org/web/packages/catboost/index.html

Table 21.2 Overview of unsupervised ML models

Year	Model	Python Package	R Package	Description	Open Source	Potential use	Reference (Python)	Reference (R)
1965	K-means clustering	Scikit-learn	Stats::Kmeans	A method that partitions data into K distinct clusters based on similarity.	Yes	Segmenting MRI images to identify different tissue types.	https://scikit-learn.org/stable/modules/clustering.html#k-means	https://cran.r-project.org/web/packages/stats/index.html
1974	Hierarchical clustering	Scipy.Cluster.Hierarchy	Stats::Hclust(dist())	A method of cluster analysis which seeks to build a hierarchy of clusters.	Yes	Grouping similar patient cases for personalized treatment.	https://docs.scipy.org/doc/scipy/reference/cluster.hierarchy.html	https://cran.r-project.org/web/packages/stats/index.html
1980	Principal component analysis (PCA)	Scikit-learn	Stats::Prcomp	A technique for reducing the dimensionality of datasets, increasing interpretability while minimizing information loss.	Yes	Reducing dimensionality of imaging data for visualization and analysis.	https://scikit-learn.org/stable/modules/decomposition.html#pca	https://cran.r-project.org/web/packages/stats/index.html
2000	Independent component analysis (ICA)	Scikit-learn	fastICA	A computational method for separating a multivariate signal into additive, independent components.	Yes	Analyzing complex biomedical signals for insights.	https://scikit-learn.org/stable/modules/decomposition.html#ica	https://cran.r-project.org/web/packages/fastICA/index.html
2000	Mean-shift clustering	Scikit-learn	meanShiftR::knn_meanShift	A clustering algorithm that assigns each data point to the nearest cluster.	Yes	Segmenting regions of interest in MRI images.	https://scikit-learn.org/stable/modules/clustering.html#mean-shift	https://cran.r-project.org/web/packages/meanShiftR/index.html
2000	Latent Dirichlet allocation (LDA)	Scikit-learn	Topicmodels	A generative statistical model that explains a set of observations through unobserved groups.	Yes	Identifying hidden patterns in patient data.	https://scikit-learn.org/stable/modules/decomposition.html#lda	https://cran.r-project.org/web/packages/topicmodels/index.html
2002	DBSCAN clustering	Scikit-learn	Dbscan	A density-based clustering algorithm that can discover clusters of varying shapes and sizes.	Yes	Identifying regions of interest in radiology images.	https://scikit-learn.org/stable/modules/clustering.html#dbscan	https://cran.r-project.org/web/packages/dbscan/index.html
2002	Gaussian mixture	Scikit-learn	Mclust::Mclust	A probabilistic model that assumes all the data points are generated from a mixture of several Gaussian distributions.	Yes	Modeling the distribution of tumor characteristics.	https://scikit-learn.org/stable/modules/mixture.html	https://cran.r-project.org/web/packages/mclust/index.html
2003	Affinity propagation	Scikit-learn	Apcluster	A clustering algorithm that identifies exemplars among data points and forms clusters based on their similarities.	Yes	Grouping similar patients based on treatment response.	https://scikit-learn.org/stable/modules/clustering.html#affinity-propagation	https://cran.r-project.org/web/packages/apcluster/index.html
2003	Spectral clustering	Scikit-learn	Kernlab	A technique which uses the eigenvalues of a similarity matrix to reduce dimensionality before clustering in fewer dimensions.	Yes	Identifying complex structures in medical imaging data.	https://scikit-learn.org/stable/modules/clustering.html#spectral-clustering	https://cran.r-project.org/web/packages/kernlab/index.html

2006	Non-negative matrix factorization (NMF)	Scikit-learn	NMF	A group of algorithms in multivariate analysis and linear algebra where a matrix is factorized into (usually) two matrices.	Yes	Extracting underlying features from imaging data.	https://scikit-learn.org/stable/modules/decomposition.html#nmf	https://cran.r-project.org/web/packages/NMF/index.html
2007	Self-organizing map	MiniSom	Kohonen	A type of artificial neural network trained using unsupervised learning to produce a low-dimensional representation of input.	Yes	Visualizing and interpreting high-dimensional patient data.	https://github.com/JustGlowing/minisom	https://cran.r-project.org/web/packages/kohonen/index.html
2008	BIRCH	Scikit-learn	Birch	An efficient data clustering method for very large databases.	Yes	Efficiently clustering large patient datasets for analysis.	https://scikit-learn.org/stable/modules/clustering.html#birch	https://cran.r-project.org/web/packages/birch/index.html
2008	Feature agglomeration	Scikit-learn	Base::Cutree	A method that merges features together to form a smaller number of aggregated features.	Yes	Reducing the dimensionality of features in large imaging datasets.	https://scikit-learn.org/stable/modules/clustering.html#feature-agglomeration	https://cran.r-project.org/web/packages/base/index.html
2009	t-distributed stochastic neighbor embedding (t-SNE)	Scikit-learn	Rtsne	A machine learning algorithm for visualization by reducing the number of dimensions while preserving similarities.	Yes	Visualizing high-dimensional imaging data for exploratory analysis.	https://scikit-learn.org/stable/modules/manifold.html#t-sne	https://cran.r-project.org/web/packages/Rtsne/index.html
2011	OPTICS	Scikit-learn	Dbscan::Optics	An algorithm for identifying density-based clusters in spatial data.	Yes	Discovering patterns in spatial distributions of tumors.	https://scikit-learn.org/stable/modules/clustering.html#optics	https://cran.r-project.org/web/packages/dbscan/index.html
2014	Uniform manifold approximation and projection (UMAP)	Umap-learn	Umap	A dimension reduction technique that is similar to t-SNE but faster and more scalable.	Yes	Visualizing and interpreting high-dimensional patient data.	https://umap-learn.readthedocs.io/en/latest/	https://cran.r-project.org/web/packages/umap/index.html
2014	Deep embedded clustering (DEC)	Keras, tensorflow	deepCluster	An unsupervised learning method that simultaneously learns feature representations and cluster assignments.	Yes	Automatically learning and clustering features from complex imaging data.	https://keras.io/, https://www.tensorflow.org/	https://cran.r-project.org/web/packages/deepCluster/index.html
2016	Generative adversarial networks (GAN)	Tensorflow, torch	Keras	A class of machine learning frameworks designed by training two neural networks, one generates candidates and the other tries to recognize true and generated data.	Yes	Generating synthetic medical images for training and research.	https://www.tensorflow.org/, https://pytorch.org/	https://cran.r-project.org/web/packages/keras/index.html
2022	Latent Dirichlet allocation (LDA)	Scikit-learn	Topicmodels	A generative statistical model that explains a set of observations through unobserved groups.	Yes	Identifying hidden patterns in patient data.	https://scikit-learn.org/stable/modules/decomposition.html#lda	https://cran.r-project.org/web/packages/topicmodels/index.html

Table 21.3 Overview of RL models

Year	Model	Python Package	R Package	Description	Open Source	Potential use	Reference (Python)	Reference (R)
1989	Q-learning	Gym, tensorflow	Reinforcement	A model-free reinforcement learning algorithm that learns a policy to maximize cumulative reward.	Yes	Optimizing treatment plans by learning the best action strategies over time.	https://gym.openai.com/, https://www.tensorflow.org/	https://cran.r-project.org/web/packages/reinforcement/index.html
1992	SARSA	Gym, tensorflow	Reinforcement	An on-policy temporal difference learning algorithm that updates the action-value function based on the action taken.	Yes	Adaptive radiotherapy scheduling based on patient responses.	https://gym.openai.com/, https://www.tensorflow.org/	https://cran.r-project.org/web/packages/reinforcement/index.html
2013	Deep Q-network (DQN)	Keras-rl, tensorflow	Reinforcement	Combines Q-learning with deep neural networks to learn policies from high-dimensional sensory inputs.	Yes	Developing adaptive protocols for neurosurgery simulations.	https://github.com/keras-rl/keras-rl, https://www.tensorflow.org/	https://cran.r-project.org/web/packages/reinforcement/index.html
2015	Double DQN	Keras-rl, tensorflow	Reinforcement	An improvement over DQN that reduces the overestimation bias by using a separate network to select actions.	Yes	Enhancing decision-making processes in robotic surgery systems.	https://github.com/keras-rl/keras-rl, https://www.tensorflow.org/	https://cran.r-project.org/web/packages/reinforcement/index.html
2016	Dueling DQN	Keras-rl, tensorflow	Reinforcement	Separates the estimation of state value and advantage to improve learning stability and performance.	Yes	Optimizing neurosurgical robotic control systems for better precision.	https://github.com/keras-rl/keras-rl, https://www.tensorflow.org/	https://cran.r-project.org/web/packages/reinforcement/index.html
2016	A3C (asynchronous advantage actor-critic)	Stable-baselines3, torch	Reinforcement	Uses parallel actor-learners to stabilize training and improve performance.	Yes	Real-time adaptation in brain-computer interfaces.	https://github.com/DLR-RM/stable-baselines3, https://pytorch.org/	https://cran.r-project.org/web/packages/reinforcement/index.html
2017	PPO (proximal policy optimization)	Stable-baselines3, torch	Reinforcement	Simplifies and improves the efficiency of policy gradient methods.	Yes	Developing personalized treatment strategies in neurooncology.	https://github.com/DLR-RM/stable-baselines3, https://pytorch.org/	https://cran.r-project.org/web/packages/reinforcement/index.html
2017	DDPG (deep deterministic policy gradient)	Stable-baselines3, torch	Reinforcement	Extends DQN to continuous action spaces using actor-critic architecture.	Yes	Enhancing control algorithms for surgical robots.	https://github.com/DLR-RM/stable-baselines3, https://pytorch.org/	https://cran.r-project.org/web/packages/reinforcement/index.html

2018	SAC (soft actor-critic)	Stable-baselines3, torch	Reinforcement	Combines maximum entropy reinforcement learning with actor-critic methods to improve exploration and stability.	Yes	Improving adaptive radiation therapy protocols.	https://github.com/DLR-RM/stable-baselines3, https://pytorch.org/	https://cran.r-project.org/web/packages/reinforcement/index.html
2018	TD3 (twin delayed DDPG)	Stable-baselines3, torch	Reinforcement	Builds on DDPG with improvements like the use of two critic networks to reduce overestimation bias.	Yes	Optimizing treatment schedules and drug dosing in neurooncology.	https://github.com/DLR-RM/stable-baselines3, https://pytorch.org/	https://cran.r-project.org/web/packages/reinforcement/index.html
2019	Rainbow DQN	Keras-rl, tensorflow	Reinforcement	Combines several improvements to DQN into a single algorithm, including double DQN, dueling DQN, and prioritized experience replay.	Yes	Enhancing precision in robotic-assisted surgeries.	https://github.com/keras-rl/keras-rl, https://www.tensorflow.org/	https://cran.r-project.org/web/packages/reinforcement/index.html
2020	TQC (truncated quantile critics)	Stable-baselines3, torch	Reinforcement	An extension of SAC that improves performance by using quantile regression.	Yes	Personalized adaptive therapies in neurooncology.	https://github.com/DLR-RM/stable-baselines3, https://pytorch.org/	https://cran.r-project.org/web/packages/reinforcement/index.html

21.2.4 Deep Learning (DL)

DL is a subset of AI and ML that utilises an architecture of data nodes and connections inspired by the structure of human neural networks, termed "artificial neural networks (ANNs)". Each node (neuron) represents a data point from the input, and each connection (synapse) represents a weighted value that transfers information to the next node using an activation function. This architecture comprises an input layer, an output layer, and multiple hidden layers, which is why it is termed "deep". Optimising this structure is a central research area; generally, the deeper the network, with more hidden layers and nodes, the more complex tasks it can perform. Consequently, larger datasets are required to train these architectures, leading to high computational costs and time.

DL is versatile and capable of being trained on various data modalities (text, images, audio, etc.) and dimensionalities, making it a powerful tool for clinicians and researchers handling large-scale data. The synergy between AI research and neuroscience is evident when tracing the advancements in DL network architecture over the past decade. Though simplified, the structure of these models resembles the network and interneuron connectivity of the human brain. Recent advancements in DL research continue to draw inspiration from neuroscientific methods and discoveries [26–28].

For instance, recent models have surpassed previous convolutional neural networks (CNNs) in image recognition by incorporating a visual attention mechanism that filters out irrelevant components, enhancing performance and reducing time and costs [29]. Advances in reinforcement learning include optimising episodic-like memory computations, enabling models to learn complex tasks with fewer trials [30]. Similarly, long-short-term memory (LSTM) networks maintain information in a fixed activity state until required for a different output, mimicking aspects of human working memory [31].

Continual learning studies in humans have also influenced AI research. Mechanisms like elastic weight consolidation (EWC) anchor weights to previously identified outputs, slowing new learning when relevant tasks are present and preventing the erasure of prior knowledge during new iterations. This allows learning multiple related tasks with relatively low computational costs, supporting continual learning [32]. Progressive networks, another human-inspired model, enable the transfer of previous knowledge to new tasks through analogies, significantly reducing computational time and costs for various applications [33]. Transfer learning, commonly used in medical AI, employs pre-trained neural networks for new tasks. Additional resources on DL models are available in Table 21.4. A pictorial representation of an ANN is available in Fig. 21.1.

21.2.5 Natural Language Processing (NLP) and Large Language Models (LLMs)

NLP is a subfield of AI that has significantly evolved in recent years. It is a multidisciplinary domain involving computer science, AI, and theoretical linguistics. It includes a broad range of models and techniques designed to process human language in various forms, from rule-based methods to advanced ML and DL approaches. Key applications of NLP include speech tagging, semantic labelling, text generation, and recognition [34, 35].

LLMs represent an advanced subgroup within the NLP domain. These models are based on DL architectures capable of analysing and generating human-like text. LLMs predict the likelihood of a word (token) or sentence based on the preceding text, generating contextually relevant output. They are an evolution of earlier NLP techniques, made possible by advances in hardware, data mining, and ML model structures. LLMs are

Table 21.4 Overview of DL models

Year	Model	Python Package	R Package	Description	Open Source	Potential use	Reference (Python)	Reference (R)
1986	Multilayer perceptron (MLP)	Tensorflow, keras, torch	Nnet, keras	A class of feedforward artificial neural network used for general pattern recognition tasks.	Yes	General pattern recognition tasks, including diagnosis and prognosis.	https://www.tensorflow.org/, https://keras.io/, https://pytorch.org/	https://cran.r-project.org/web/packages/nnet/index.html, https://cran.r-project.org/web/packages/keras/index.html
1998	Convolutional neural network (CNN)	Tensorflow, keras, torch	Keras	A class of deep neural networks, commonly applied to analyzing visual imagery.	Yes	Image recognition and classification in medical imaging, such as MRI and CT scans for tumor detection.	https://www.tensorflow.org/, https://keras.io/, https://pytorch.org/	https://cran.r-project.org/web/packages/keras/index.html
2012	AlexNet	Tensorflow, keras, torch	Keras	A convolutional neural network architecture that won the ImageNet competition in 2012, known for its deep structure.	Yes	Advanced image classification tasks, potentially improving tumor detection accuracy in complex imaging datasets.	https://www.tensorflow.org/, https://keras.io/, https://pytorch.org/	https://cran.r-project.org/web/packages/keras/index.html
2012	Deep belief network (DBN)	Tensorflow, keras, torch	Deepnet	A generative graphical model composed of multiple layers of latent variables, used for unsupervised learning.	Yes	Feature extraction and dimensionality reduction in medical imaging.	https://www.tensorflow.org/, https://keras.io/, https://pytorch.org/	https://cran.r-project.org/web/packages/deepnet/index.html
2013	RNN (recurrent neural network)	Tensorflow, keras, torch	Keras	A class of neural networks where connections between nodes form a directed graph along a temporal sequence, used for time-series data.	Yes	Time-series analysis of patient health data, predicting disease progression.	https://www.tensorflow.org/, https://keras.io/, https://pytorch.org/	https://cran.r-project.org/web/packages/keras/index.html
2014	LSTM (long short-term memory)	Tensorflow, keras, torch	Keras	A type of RNN that can learn long-term dependencies, widely used for time-series data.	Yes	Analyzing sequences of patient data over time, such as EEG signals or patient monitoring data.	https://www.tensorflow.org/, https://keras.io/, https://pytorch.org/	https://cran.r-project.org/web/packages/keras/index.html
2014	GRU (gated recurrent unit)	Tensorflow, keras, torch	Keras	A variant of the LSTM that uses gating units to manage the flow of information without needing separate memory cells.	Yes	Similar to LSTM, used for analyzing time-series data and sequential patient records.	https://www.tensorflow.org/, https://keras.io/, https://pytorch.org/	https://cran.r-project.org/web/packages/keras/index.html
2014	Generative adversarial network (GAN)	Tensorflow, keras, torch	Keras	A class of machine learning frameworks designed by training two neural networks to generate synthetic data.	Yes	Generating synthetic medical images for training and research, enhancing the diversity of training datasets.	https://www.tensorflow.org/, https://keras.io/, https://pytorch.org/	https://cran.r-project.org/web/packages/keras/index.html
2014	VGGNet	Tensorflow, keras, torch	Keras	A convolutional neural network model known for its depth and small convolution filters.	Yes	Fine-tuning for specific medical imaging tasks to enhance accuracy in identifying and classifying tumors.	https://www.tensorflow.org/, https://keras.io/, https://pytorch.org/	https://cran.r-project.org/web/packages/keras/index.html

(continued)

Table 21.4 (continued)

Year	Model	Python Package	R Package	Description	Open Source	Potential use	Reference (Python)	Reference (R)
2015	ResNet	Tensorflow, keras, torch	Keras	A convolutional neural network that introduces the concept of residual learning to solve the vanishing gradient problem.	Yes	Image recognition tasks requiring deeper architectures to identify subtle patterns in medical images for diagnosis.	https://www.tensorflow.org/, https://keras.io/, https://pytorch.org/	https://cran.r-project.org/web/packages/keras/index.html
2015	U-net	Tensorflow, keras, torch	Keras	A convolutional network architecture designed for biomedical image segmentation.	Yes	Segmenting tumors and other structures in medical images, aiding in precise treatment planning and assessment.	https://www.tensorflow.org/, https://keras.io/, https://pytorch.org/	https://cran.r-project.org/web/packages/keras/index.html
2015	Deep Q-network (DQN)	Tensorflow, keras, torch	NA	A reinforcement learning algorithm that combines Q-learning with deep neural networks.	Yes	Optimizing treatment strategies and personalized medicine using reinforcement learning techniques.	https://www.tensorflow.org/, https://keras.io/, https://pytorch.org/	NA
2016	DenseNet	Tensorflow, keras, torch	Keras	A convolutional neural network architecture where each layer is connected to every other layer, promoting feature reuse.	Yes	Enhanced feature extraction for complex medical imaging tasks, improving accuracy in tumor identification and segmentation.	https://www.tensorflow.org/, https://keras.io/, https://pytorch.org/	https://cran.r-project.org/web/packages/keras/index.html
2017	Transformer	Transformers, torch, keras	Keras	A model architecture that eschews recurrence and instead relies entirely on self-attention mechanisms to draw global dependencies between input and output.	Yes	Natural language processing for medical records, aiding in automated annotation and information extraction relevant to patient treatment.	https://huggingface.co/transformers/, https://pytorch.org/, https://keras.io/	https://cran.r-project.org/web/packages/keras/index.html
2017	SE-ResNet	Tensorflow, keras, torch	Keras	A combination of the ResNet architecture with squeeze-and-excitation blocks to improve model performance.	Yes	Enhanced image classification and recognition in medical imaging, providing better diagnostic accuracy.	https://www.tensorflow.org/, https://keras.io/, https://pytorch.org/	https://cran.r-project.org/web/packages/keras/index.html
2018	BERT	Transformers, torch, keras	Keras	A transformer-based model designed to understand the context of words in a text by looking at the words that come before and after it.	Yes	Processing and analyzing medical texts, aiding in research, and extracting relevant information from patient records.	https://huggingface.co/transformers/, https://pytorch.org/, https://keras.io/	https://cran.r-project.org/web/packages/keras/index.html
2018	EfficientNet	Tensorflow, keras, torch	Keras	A model that scales up various dimensions (depth, width, resolution) of convolutional neural networks to achieve better performance.	Yes	Efficiently scaling models for medical imaging tasks, allowing for accurate and resource-efficient tumor detection and classification.	https://www.tensorflow.org/, https://keras.io/, https://pytorch.org/	https://cran.r-project.org/web/packages/keras/index.html
2018	GPT	Transformers, torch, keras	Keras	A transformer-based model designed for natural language generation tasks.	Yes	Generating synthetic medical texts for training purposes, enhancing automated report generation for medical imaging findings.	https://huggingface.co/transformers/, https://pytorch.org/, https://keras.io/	https://cran.r-project.org/web/packages/keras/index.html

2018	Attention mechanism	Tensorflow, keras, torch	Keras	A technique in neural networks that allows the model to focus on different parts of the input sequence when predicting outputs.	Yes	Improving the interpretability and accuracy of models analyzing complex medical sequences.	https://www.tensorflow.org/, https://keras.io/, https://pytorch.org/	https://cran.r-project.org/web/packages/keras/index.html
2018	DeepLab	Tensorflow, keras, torch	Keras	A semantic image segmentation model that uses atrous convolution to capture fine details in medical images.	Yes	High-precision tumor segmentation in medical images.	https://www.tensorflow.org/, https://keras.io/, https://pytorch.org/	https://cran.r-project.org/web/packages/keras/index.html
2019	BigGAN	Tensorflow, torch	Keras	An improvement over the original GANs, capable of generating highly detailed synthetic images.	Yes	Creating high-quality synthetic medical images to augment training datasets and improve the robustness of deep learning models.	https://www.tensorflow.org/, https://pytorch.org/	https://cran.r-project.org/web/packages/keras/index.html
2019	YOLO (You only look once)	Torch, tensorflow	NA	A real-time object detection system that processes images in one go, improving speed and accuracy.	Yes	Real-time tumor detection and tracking in medical imaging.	https://pytorch.org/, https://www.tensorflow.org/	NA
2020	Vision transformer (ViT)	Tensorflow, torch	NA	A model that applies the transformer architecture to images by splitting them into patches and treating them as a sequence.	Yes	State-of-the-art performance in medical image classification, enhancing diagnostic accuracy and reliability.	https://www.tensorflow.org/, https://pytorch.org/	NA
2020	CLIP	Torch	NA	A model that learns to associate images and text by training on a large dataset of images paired with captions.	Yes	Improving multi-modal data analysis, allowing for better integration of image, text, and clinical data for comprehensive diagnosis and treatment planning.	https://pytorch.org/	NA
2020	Swin transformer	Torch	NA	A hierarchical transformer whose representations are computed with shifted windows, improving efficiency and accuracy.	Yes	State-of-the-art performance in medical image classification, enhancing diagnostic accuracy and reliability.	https://pytorch.org/	NA
2021	Perceiver	Torch, tensorflow	NA	A model designed to handle data from multiple modalities, including imaging, text, and clinical data, enhancing multi-modal learning capabilities.	Yes	Integrating multi-modal patient data for comprehensive diagnosis and treatment planning.	https://pytorch.org/, https://www.tensorflow.org/	NA
2022	SAM (segment anything model)	Torch, tensorflow	NA	A model designed for segmentation tasks that can handle various types of data and outputs detailed segmentation masks.	Yes	Segmenting tumors and other structures in medical images, aiding in precise treatment planning and assessment.	https://pytorch.org/, https://www.tensorflow.org/	NA

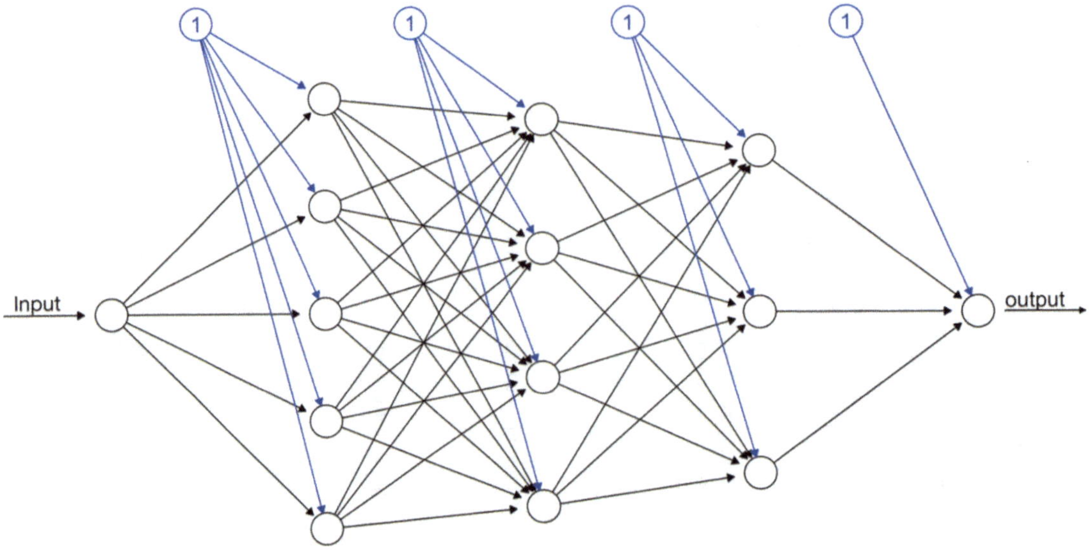

Fig. 21.1 A representation of an artificial neural network (ANN)

built on a DL model called the "Transformer", which uses a self-attention mechanism to evaluate the importance of different tokens (words) in an input sequence to understand context and produce output [36, 37].

LLMs have been employed for text generation in numerous commercial applications and research projects to process vast amounts of textual data. The development of multimodal models capable of processing various forms of information could further expand their potential applications in research. Despite their rapid adoption in the commercial world and significant public interest, the performance of LLMs remains a topic of debate. They can generate reliable outputs only when trained on massive datasets, which requires extensive computational power and energy. Additionally, LLMs are prone to errors and inaccuracies (often termed "hallucinations") and may produce biased content depending on the quality of the training data [38–41]. Traditional NLP models can still outperform LLMs at a lower computational cost despite being less flexible when presented with new tasks in specific subfields and applications. While the output of LLMs may resemble human reasoning, their performance is based on probabilistic modelling (learning statistical patterns from the input data), and it is clear that this does not represent an artificial form of "thinking" or "reasoning" [42]. Additional resources on LLMs are available in Table 21.5.

Table 21.5 Overview of LLMs

Year	Model	Python Package	R Package	Description	Number of Parameters	Open Source	Potential use	Reference (Python)	Reference (R)
2018	BERT	Transformers	Bert	A transformer-based model designed to understand the context of a word in search queries and improve performance on NLP tasks.	110 million (base)	Yes	Extracting relevant information from medical literature and patient records.	https://huggingface.co/transformers/model_doc/bert.html	https://cran.r-project.org/web/packages/bert/index.html
2018	GPT	Openai	NA	The original generative pre-trained transformer model, designed for various NLP tasks.	117 million	No	Generating medical documentation and performing language understanding tasks.	https://beta.openai.com/docs/	NA
2019	GPT-2	Transformers	NA	A transformer-based model designed for natural language generation tasks, capable of producing coherent and contextually relevant text.	1.5 billion	Yes	Generating patient reports and summarizing medical texts.	https://huggingface.co/transformers/model_doc/gpt2.html	NA
2019	XLNet	Transformers	NA	An auto-regressive pre-trained model that outperforms BERT on several benchmarks.	340 million	Yes	Improving accuracy in medical document analysis and interpretation.	https://huggingface.co/transformers/model_doc/xlnet.html	NA
2019	RoBERTa	Transformers	NA	A robustly optimized BERT approach that achieves better performance through longer training with more data.	355 million	Yes	Enhanced extraction of clinical insights from unstructured text.	https://huggingface.co/transformers/model_doc/roberta.html	NA
2020	T5 (text-to-text transfer transformer)	Transformers	NA	A model that treats every NLP problem as a text-to-text problem, providing a unified approach to various NLP tasks.	11 billion	Yes	Unified framework for handling diverse medical text processing tasks.	https://huggingface.co/transformers/model_doc/t5.html	NA
2020	GPT-3	Openai	NA	A language generation model that can produce human-like text and perform a variety of NLP tasks with few-shot learning.	175 billion	No	Generating detailed and coherent medical documentation.	https://beta.openai.com/docs/	NA
2020	Megatron-LM	Megatron-lm	NA	A large, powerful transformer model designed for NLP tasks, developed by NVIDIA.	8.3 billion	Yes	Large-scale data analysis and synthesis for research purposes.	https://github.com/NVIDIA/Megatron-LM	NA
2021	GPT-neo	Transformers	NA	An open-source model similar to GPT-3, designed to provide a large-scale language model accessible to the public.	2.7 billion	Yes	Accessible tool for research and development in medical NLP.	https://huggingface.co/transformers/model_doc/gpt_neo.html	NA

(continued)

Table 21.5 (continued)

Year	Model	Python Package	R Package	Description	Number of Parameters	Open Source	Potential use	Reference (Python)	Reference (R)
2021	Jurassic-1	NA	NA	A language model designed to perform a wide range of NLP tasks with high accuracy, developed by AI21 labs.	178 billion	No	High-accuracy processing of complex medical texts.	NA	NA
2021	Gopher	NA	NA	A model developed by DeepMind with a focus on improving performance across various language tasks.	280 billion	No	Advanced language understanding for detailed medical text interpretation.	NA	NA
2022	OPT (open pre-trained transformer)	Transformers	NA	A model designed to provide a transparent and reproducible approach to training large language models, developed by meta AI.	175 billion	Yes	Transparent and reproducible medical text processing.	https://huggingface.co/docs/transformers/model_doc/opt	NA
2022	PaLM (pathways language model)	NA	NA	A large-scale language model designed to advance natural language understanding and generation, developed by Google.	540 billion	No	Advanced language generation for complex medical documentation.	NA	NA
2022	LaMDA	NA	NA	A model by Google designed for dialogue applications, capable of engaging in open-ended conversations.	137 billion	No	Interactive systems for patient consultation and support.	NA	NA
2022	Bloom	Transformers	NA	A multilingual model developed by the BigScience project, aimed at providing an open-source alternative to GPT-3.	176 billion	Yes	Multilingual medical documentation and research.	https://huggingface.co/bigscience/bloom	NA
2022	Chinchilla	NA	NA	A model developed by DeepMind that focuses on achieving better performance with fewer resources.	70 billion	No	Efficient processing of medical text with fewer computational resources.	NA	NA
2023	GPT-4	OpenAI	NA	The latest iteration of OpenAI's language model, designed to be even more capable in understanding and generating text.	Unknown	No	Enhanced capabilities for medical text generation and analysis.	https://beta.openai.com/docs/	NA
2023	Claude	NA	NA	A model developed by anthropic focusing on AI safety and large-scale language understanding.	52 billion	No	Safe and robust NLP applications in clinical settings.	NA	NA
2023	Ernie 4.0	NA	NA	A model by Baidu focusing on language understanding and generation, optimized for Chinese.	260 billion	No	Chinese language processing for medical research and documentation.	NA	NA

2023	LLaMA (large language model meta AI)	Transformers	NA	A set of foundation language models ranging from 7B to 65B parameters, developed by meta AI.	7–65 billion	Yes	Flexible and scalable language model for diverse medical NLP tasks.	https://huggingface.co/docs/transformers/model_doc/llama	NA
2023	LLaMA 2	Transformers	NA	The second iteration of LLaMA models with improved performance and scalability.	7–70 billion	Yes	Enhanced NLP tasks in medical documentation and analysis.	https://huggingface.co/meta-llama/Llama-2-7b-hf	NA
2024	LLaMA 3	Transformers	NA	The latest iteration of LLaMA models with state-of-the-art performance.	8–70 billion	Yes	Cutting-edge NLP applications for comprehensive medical data analysis.	https://huggingface.co/meta-llama/Llama-3-8b-hf	NA
2023	Falcon LLM	Transformers	NA	A model developed by the technology innovation Institute in Abu Dhabi, aiming to advance state-of-the-art language understanding.	40 billion	Yes	Advanced NLP applications for medical data analysis and research.	https://huggingface.co/tiiuae/falcon-40b	NA
2023	MiniGPT-4	NA	NA	Enhancing vision-language understanding with advanced large language models.	Unknown	Yes	Multimodal understanding for interpreting medical images and related text.	NA	NA
2023	GLaM	NA	NA	Google's generalist language model designed to handle a wide variety of tasks.	1.2 trillion	No	General-purpose model for complex medical documentation and data analysis.	NA	NA
2024	Orca-2	NA	NA	A large language model focusing on conversational AI developed by meta AI.	200 billion	No	Enhanced interactive applications for patient engagement and support.	NA	NA
2024	DeepSeek-coder	NA	NA	Focused on coding and software development, enhancing AI capabilities in programming task	33 billion	Yes	Assisting in the development of medical software and tools.	NA	NA

21.3 How to Interpret AI Research Findings

The publication of new articles investigating AI models applied to medical problems has increased rapidly, and many experts in the medical field are now asked to review AI manuscripts without sufficient computer science literacy to analyse these reports critically. Here are some key points to consider:

The most relevant factor in reviewing the performance of an AI algorithm is the analysis of the training dataset in terms of quality and quantity. Authors should specify the exact source of data and detail how they were processed before training the model. Large DL models require extensive data to converge towards an accurate output. Moreover, the absence of a validation dataset (either internal or external) that the model has never encountered during training is a significant methodological red flag. AI models can perform surprisingly well on biased data but can be highly inaccurate on real-world data when tested prospectively [43, 44]. Consequently, most AI models published remain "proof-of-concepts", with only a tiny proportion ever validated.

Another red flag is a vague description of the model used or referring to "AI" in general. It is well-known in data science and medical implementation that different subsets of models perform better on specific tasks than others [45]. Therefore, a careful evaluation of the technical methodology should include a detailed explanation of the choice of the algorithm and their training parameters. Additional concerns involve evaluating the hypothesis being tested, ensuring the potential clinical use is relevant rather than purely speculative, explaining the model, and ensuring the dataset's and model code's availability in public repositories for reproduction by other research teams [46]. Several scientific societies have started publishing guides and recommendations for authors and reviewers to better evaluate the quality of this growing body of literature [47].

21.4 Applications in Neuro-Oncology

21.4.1 Neuropathology and Molecular Biology

As an explicative example, a database search of the terms "ML", "artificial intelligence", and "neuropathology" returned 2841 publications (1980–2024), confirming the vast investigation of this technology for improving the histopathological and molecular identification of CNS tumours despite being less represented than other fields.

The performance in correctly diagnosing a CNS tumour sample is based on the neuropathologists' experience and expertise, with adjunct employment of molecular signature, which further aids the diagnostic process and sub-classifies tumours for patients to the most suitable course of care. Even though molecular markers are becoming predominant in diagnosing CNS tumours, morphological analysis is paramount to triage the available sample, evaluate tumour heterogeneity, select the most appropriate region of interest to further test with molecular methods, and ultimately review potential anomalies and artefacts [2]. Since the wide adoption of Whole-Slide Imaging (WSI), namely "virtual microscopy", the availability of large amounts of digital data helps the field of automated computer vision flourish on the research ground [48–50]. AI and ML algorithms have been widely implemented to improve diagnostic accuracy, identify new prognostic and predictive labels, and reduce processing time and costs. Some examples of glioma grading using AI models are available in the literature. A large spectrum of databases is used for training such algorithms, achieving a fair accuracy in identifying the most common glioma subtypes according to the WHO CNS classification. More recent studies proposed automated models trained on the digitalised and open-source database "The Cancer Genome Atlas (TCGA)", achieving a 96% accuracy in differentiating glioblastomas from other models [51, 52]. However, this performance metric was carried out on a minimal validation sample, hampering the robustness of the findings. For similar reasons and scarce interstudy comparability, the discussion of AI studies in terms of classification performances without a careful analysis of their methodologies is meaningless and was limited in this chapter. In addition, recent findings confirmed that the kind of model adopted and the region of interest selected in the dataset can also dramatically influence the performance of these algorithms [53].

The histopathological workflow remains central in diagnosing CNS tumours and neurooncological research, even though the growing evidence on immunohistochemical and genetic analyses, which are already approved for clinical use, require a multiscale approach to the diagnostic or research process [2, 54–59]. DL models might help optimise laboratory pipelines by automatically triaging bioptic samples and predicting the presence of histological and molecular features, targeting those specimens more likely to benefit from more advanced analyses. However, several limitations are still in place. First, the digitalisation of all samples is a mandatory requirement. Since the introduction of WSI in 2014 and the later demonstration of non-inferiority in diagnosing performance compared to standard glass slides, virtual microscopy has widely spread in most high-income countries [60]. However, several regions still cannot afford to digitalize pathological slides nor store them for later use. Second, WSI requires large data storage capacity as single slides might reach several GB and require extensive and expensive post-processing. Finally, no consensus exists on a standardised paradigm for segmenting and selecting regions to be analysed. All these elements might drastically reduce the generalisability of any ML or DL model [61, 62].

21.4.2 Neuroradiology

Neuroimaging represents the perfect input source for evaluating artificial intelligence performance for several reasons. First, the extensive amount of data produced every day for clinical reasons and the harmless modality, summated to the growing availability worldwide of advanced imaging devices capable of producing multimodal imaging data in a shorter amount of time, incubate an ideal workplace for AI to flourish (published resources in neuroradiology accounts for more than 6000 indexed manuscripts, out of a total of 30.000 in radiology).

For obvious reasons, brain anatomy segmentation was the first and most relevant task enhanced with AI algorithms. It is a time-consuming task, but it gives access to quantitative morphological data otherwise only qualitatively assessed during routine radiological exams. It is impactful for diagnosing diseases, detecting subtle abnormalities, and classifying normal and pathological anatomical findings [63–65]. Besides oncological interest, brain tissue segmentation is a highly relevant function with a translational impact on any area of brain imaging healthcare and research.

CNNs mainly, but also ANNs, have been trained with neuroimages as input and supervised through human-made manual segmentation of sample cases to learn and replicate segmentation tasks on different imaging modalities. On the contrary, generative AI algorithms [including generative adversarial networks (GANs)] have been used to synthetically generate 7 T MRI-like scans from standard 3 Tesla MRI inputs or generate synthetic post-contrast T1 scans from volumetric T1, T2 or FLAIR sequences only. No statistically significant difference was encountered when evaluating patients' response to oncological treatments with the two modalities (control vs synthetically processed images). None of these techniques have yet reached clinical approval [66, 67].

An ideal and simplistic problem would be automatically identifying isocitrate dehydrogenase (IDH) mutations in gliomas through non-invasive imaging. IDH is the primary feature for classifying radiologically and even histologically-like tumours in segregated types. Its early identification might help tailor prognosis estimation, patient counselling, and optimal treatment planning. For example, lower-grade gliomas (IDH mutated) require a tailored approach and advanced intraoperative mapping strategy in most cases to preserve long-term neurological functions and quality of life, given the slow growth rate and potential neuroplasticity into play. In addition, the recent introduction of an IDH1 and IDH2 inhibitor, Vorasidenib (INDIGO trial), added another option for long-term treatment for these patients [68]. On the contrary, IDH wildtype gliomas without high-grade radiological or histopathological features still behave as highly aggressive tumours, and a maximal safe resection and fastest access to adjuvant treatments is the gold standard, with no room for morbid mid-term temporary deficits or staged surgeries. Knowing IDH status through AI algorithms in advance would provide valuable information to surgeons and oncologists so they can plan the best treatment. Several CNN models can achieve a 90% accuracy in this task evaluating preoperative MRI scans. At the same time, other algorithms were trained to identify O6-Methylguanine-DNA-Methyltransiferase (MGMT) methylation status, 1p19q collection or EGFR amplification, while no data is available on BRAF status [69–73].

Using a similar approach, WHO grade in CNS tumours can also be predicted with variable accuracy using batches of different MRI modalities. Multiple modalities combined in multidimensional input arrays also show higher performance (up to 96–97%) in paediatric cohorts [74–76].

A third relevant topic under extensive investigation is the differentiation of progression and pseudo-progression after treatment. The first is defined as identifying a contrast increase or T2/FLAIR area of intensity increase after 12 weeks of any radiation or combined radio-chemotherapy protocol. Pseudo-progression is usually paucisymptomatic, related to the mass effect on imaging scans, and does not evolve or resolve spontaneously in more than 15–30% of patients, with a lower proportion of unmethylated higher-grade gliomas [77]. Some pilot studies performed promisingly differentiating using ANN-based computer vision analyses pseudo-progression from true early progression in gliomas [72, 78–81].

Similarly to lower-grade gliomas in adults, accurate monitoring over time of tumour burden is paramount in paediatric populations with slow-growing tumours [75]. A study on 794 and 122 patient cohorts trained a 3D U-Net DL model to apply the Response Assessment in Paediatric Neuro-Oncology criteria (RAPNO) automatically on a sample of paediatric high-grade gliomas, medulloblastomas and other leptomeningeal spreading tumours obtained high reliability with human operators but higher performance in longitudinal assessments [75]. However, the study lacks an external validation, hampering the generalisability of these findings.

Not limited to gliomas, several groups applied DL algorithms to a variety of tumour histotypes, discriminating glioblastomas from primary CNS lymphoma or secondary tumours, pituitary adenomas from craniopharyngiomas, predicting the extent of resection or complication occurrence in complex skull base procedures, meningiomas grading and likelihood of recurrence regardless of the WHO grade assigned with promising performance metrics. However, a common limitation of the majority of these studies is the pilot design, with limited sample size, poor generalisability and external validation [76, 82].

21.4.3 Neurosurgery

Several of the previous applications apply to some extent to neurosurgical planning. However, specific paradigms for pre- and intraoperative applications are less represented. PubMed accounts for 2000 published manuscripts (2006–2024, with a real ML application in 2010) involving ML and AI applications in general to neurosurgery.

In the preoperative stage, the potential implementation of AI can be imagined, at a speculative level, as a perioperative management assistant and predictive tool. The large-scale and multidimensionality of electronic medical records (EMRs) offer a likeable candidate for training ML and DL algorithms to improve pre-and post-operative patient management by predicting—and, when possible—reducing preventable complications through physicians' intervention during the treatment timeline. Several models performing similar tasks have already been discussed in the previous sections. Other algorithms, on the contrary, reached high accuracy in identifying patients most likely to experience postoperative complications and unexpected morbidity resulting in non-home discharge, raising red flags for medical optimisations [83]. Similarly, an XGBoost model recently outperformed human operators in predicting 30-day mortality in brain metastases based on EMR data in a prospective cohort of about 3000 patients after being trained on over 28.000 patients [84].

The recent advancements in the field of NLP models and the introduction of LLMs might present new insight into how we analyse EMRs. NLP algorithms are, in fact, able to automatically process relatively unorganised and human unprocessed EMRs—which represents the main advantage of such algorithms—and label information for further use, summarising comorbidities, risk factors, and relevant prognostic factors, with the ability to stratify patients facing complications, non-home discharge and predict survival [85–87]. The exponential research evolution in the field of LLM can help organise EMRs for clinical and scientific use, minimising human effort and time consumption, and provide objective assessments of diagnosis likelihood and prognostication; moreover, LLM might help compare and combine data sources from different institutions and environment for creating large-scale datasets for further AI training, orienting AI research towards the harvesting of high-quality shared data across research teams [88, 89]. The availability of open-source LLMs from several sources might favour this kind of investigation.

AI applications in surgical planning rely mostly on neuroradiological assessments: the likelihood of a gross total resection is relevant surgical information that can be predicted on preoperative raw imaging data through computer vision algorithms or indirectly through extracting radiomics features from preoperative tumours or more from perioperative clinical and surgical datatypes. The latter models have been proposed for a vast proportion of CNS tumours for predicting several conditions, and several models implemented interpretation paradigms able to return to the operator the features driving the prediction (i.e., tumour location, the use of specific intraoperative tools like intraoperative monitoring, 5-aminolevulinic acid, ultrasound or MRI) [83, 84, 90]. Nevertheless, solid trials evaluating the impact on surgeons' decisions based on AI model predictions are missing, and most of these studies remain promising pilot investigations.

A previous section described the automatic classification (through AI) of tumour type by means of histological and molecular examination; however, several attempts have been made in the last 30 years to translate this application to real-time intraoperative diagnosis for adapting surgical goals [91]. Since the description by Orringer and colleagues of the stimulated Raman histology (SHR)—an advanced microscopy visualisation technique providing a digital image resembling haematoxylin and Eosin stained slides without requiring any staining processing—several approaches have been proposed to bring this technology into the operating theatre. Combining SHR with a DL model in an automatised pipeline, an expert pathologist-level response can be obtained in an almost real-time fashion, providing new valuable information to the surgical team [92–94].

Similarly, Raman spectroscopy analyses photon inelastic scattering to characterise the sample's chemical composition. Supervised and unsupervised ML and most DL models have recently been employed to build a classification model based on real-time acquired Raman spectra to predict tumour type and molecular labels [95]. However, the application of this technique is still in its infancy, and several limitations have been acknowledged. First, the input data heterogeneity across different laboratories nullifies any effort in comparing performances across trials. For this reason, a collection of high-quality spectra through an international consortium with standardised experimental conditions, standardisation of processing and normalisation of datasets is urgently needed to train reliable and generalisable AI models for this use. Finally, regardless of the application of ML and DL models, these analyses are computationally heavy, and time reduction must be addressed to provide a potential intraoperative tool. Additional information on Raman spectroscopy and related techniques are available elsewhere (see [96]). Alternative methods have been proposed for identifying MGMT methylation status and IDH mutation during surgery through DL models [97].

Intraoperative tools empowered by AI predicting tools have emerged in the scientific landscape, proposing intraoperative pipelines to guide surgeons' decisions. However, these applications are as sensitive as human examiners to tissue quality and quantity during tumour harvesting [92, 97, 98]. Moreover, non-standard computational resources are usually necessary for a fast and reliable result. This technique might stand in the future as user-friendly intraoperative predictive tools to tailor surgical decisions to tumour biology weeks before the final pathological report is drafted or in settings where a neuropathologist is not readily available.

The proposed uses of AI in neurological surgeries go beyond those reviewed here. Evaluation of surgeon's performance through recording of surgical videos, augmented reality headsets or motion analysis of instruments, synthetic simulations, and surgeons' hands might, in the future, quantify properties of our expertise, which are now indirectly measured; the latter might be beneficial in evaluating the training of junior neurosurgeons. Automatic segmentation of anatomical landmarks, automatic identification of surgical phases and surgical report redaction are additional examples [99–102].

The landscape of neurosurgical applications will probably change rapidly, and some new uses might still be incubated or translated from other fields. In the future, we might be called to investigate the use of AI-empowered robots for intraoperative use or operate with the assistance of semi- or autonomous robotic arms able to interpret and understand the surgical field. A pictorial example of such speculative but potential uses is a robotic arm guided by an AI algorithm capable of identifying fluorescent tumours through a filtered camera and manoeuvre a laser to automatically perform a tumour resection in a laboratory study on a tumour sample [103]. Considering the highly speculative timeframe we have experienced in these years and the need for a critical opinion on how AI is implemented in neuro-oncology, several clues suggest that artificial intelligence will be—to some extent—employed with success in our fields.

21.4.4 Radiation Oncology

As an explicative example, a database search of the terms "ML", "artificial intelligence", and "radiotherapy" or "radiosurgery" returned 4299 publications (1961–2024), with a notable trend since 2014. This confirms the scientific community's interest in applying these novel methods to radiation therapy planning, volume and dose tailoring, patient selection, and complication prediction, as much as outcome prediction.

Similar to the applications reviewed in the neuroradiology section, AI has been investigated for automating complex and time-demanding pipelines without sacrificing accuracy, quality, and standardisation during the treatment plan and execution [104–106]. Proposed applications comprehend imaging scan registration, target segmentation, radiation treatment planning, synthetic simulation of dose delivery, patient monitoring, and predictive models to assist physicians in multidisciplinary decision-making [106]. In several attempts, ML models aid in delineating and planning treatment delivery to improve the overall accuracy of therapeutic strategies [107]. In a small investigation with ground truth segmentation of stereotactic targets by experienced physicians, implementing an AI algorithm reduced inter-rater variability in target contouring and reduced processing time by 30% [107]. Similarly, this approach might be helpful in automatically detecting and segmenting brain metastases to candidates for radiosurgery with promising results in a pilot study [108].

Another field of application is the employment of GAN models to generate synthetic imaging scans. MRI is, in fact, the modality of choice to evaluate target volumes and trace high-risk structures to be spared, given the high resolution and contrast. Nevertheless, CT imaging is the warhorse of the radiotherapy apparatus for dose calculations through the planning systems [109, 110]. To reduce costs and time to treatment, several successful algorithms able to synthesise CT scans from MRI data based on DL algorithms are available, with a difference dose in dose delivery between synthetic-CT-based workflows and controls inferior to 2% [111].

Similarly, tumour response prediction or complication occurrence has been evaluated through different AI algorithms, returning in selected datasets an accuracy of 75% (above operators' performance) in identifying early responders to radiosurgery in a randomised clinical trial on over 200 brain primary and secondary tumours (SHIELD-RT), an XGBoost supervised model was able to identify those patients more likely to require acute care during radiation and chemotherapy regimen. The ML model classification was used to allocate these patients to a more stringent outpatient evaluation arm, reducing overall the rates of acute care in the investigation [104].

Several pilot studies have been reported for many applications in radiation therapy for CNS malignancies. Regardless of the high accuracies disclosed in internal or small validation datasets, to our knowledge, none of these methodologies has reached any clearance for clinical use. However, AI will likely be formally evaluated for clinical uses shortly, and the standard of care might be reshaped, to some extent, by implementing AI algorithms.

21.4.5 Clinical Oncology

Interestingly, querying the PubMed database for AI-related terms and "Neuro-Oncology" returns only 441 articles ever published (1991–2024), suggesting a more limited scientific interest in applying ML and AI algorithms to systemic treatments for CNS tumours. However, by combining different Booleans for oncological and brain-related keywords, we found up to 3000 manuscripts, which is still a relatively lower number than reported in other fields. Among the uses evaluated, potential employment might be using DL architectures for identifying novel drugs for pre-clinical tests. A pictorial example is a study by Neves BJ and colleagues, who published the performance of a supervised random forest model in assessing the blood-brain barrier penetration and efficacy against glioma cells in vitro of experimental molecules, identifying out of a rigorous pipeline two potential molecules just through an ML-based synthetic analysis [112] Among therapeutic agents already in use, AI algorithms can help tailor medication protocols (ex, temozolomide) for use in heterogeneous populations, reducing biases. Through an in silico simulation using a Monte Carlo tree search model, lower side effects and more significant tumour reduction were observed [113].

Similarly, other centres applied AI algorithms to genomic sequencing, helping to identify glioblastoma cell phenotypes that correlate better than standard classification labels with survival as a consequence of better treatment response. They also pointed out subgroups that might benefit from immune checkpoint inhibitors, whose indication is highly debated after the publication of unsuccessful clinical trials [114, 115].

21.5 Conclusions

CNS tumours present significant clinical challenges due to their complexity and poor prognosis. This chapter examined artificial intelligence's (AI) potential in neuro-oncology, acknowledging the need for cautious optimism. AI technologies, including ML, DL, and NLP, could enhance imaging techniques and tumuor detection in neuroradiology, assist in surgical planning and decision-making in neurosurgery, and optimise treatment protocols in radiotherapy. However, the complexity of this evolving research field requires rigorous validation before clinical deployment. Multidisciplinary collaboration and ethical considerations are essential to integrate AI into neurooncological practise effectively.

References

1. Miller KD, Ostrom QT, Kruchko C, et al. Brain and other central nervous system tumor statistics, 2021. CA Cancer J Clin. 2021;71:381–406.
2. Louis DN, Perry A, Wesseling P, et al. The 2021 WHO classification of tumors of the central ner-

vous system: a summary. Neuro-Oncology. 2021;23:1231–51.
3. Khosravi M, Zare Z, Mojtabaeian SM, Izadi R. Artificial intelligence and decision-making in healthcare: a thematic analysis of a systematic review of reviews. Heal Serv Res Manag Epidemiol. 2024;11:23333928241234863. https://doi.org/10.1177/23333928241234863.
4. Ramezani M, Takian A, Bakhtiari A, Rabiee HR, Ghazanfari S, Sazgarnejad S. Research agenda for using artificial intelligence in health governance: interpretive scoping review and framework. BioData Min. 2023;16:31.
5. Khalighi S, Reddy K, Midya A, Pandav KB, Madabhushi A, Abedalthagafi M. Artificial intelligence in neuro-oncology: advances and challenges in brain tumor diagnosis, prognosis, and precision treatment. NPJ Precis Oncol. 2024;8:80.
6. Baker CR, Pease M, Sexton DP, Abumoussa A, Chambless LB. Artificial intelligence innovations in neurosurgical oncology: a narrative review. J Neuro-Oncol. 2024;169:489. https://doi.org/10.1007/s11060-024-04757-5.
7. Shan G, Yu S, Lai Z, Xuan Z, Zhang J, Wang B, Ge Y. A review of artificial intelligence application for radiotherapy. Dose-Response. 2024;22:15593258241263687. https://doi.org/10.1177/15593258241263687.
8. Moassefi M, Faghani S, Erickson B. Artificial intelligence in neuro-oncology: predicting molecular markers and response to therapy. Med Res Arch. 2024;12:5523. https://doi.org/10.18103/mra.v12i6.5523.
9. Weidener L, Fischer M. Artificial intelligence teaching as part of medical education: qualitative analysis of expert interviews. JMIR Med Educ. 2023;9:e46428.
10. Weidener L, Fischer M. Teaching AI ethics in medical education: a scoping review of current literature and practices. Perspect Med Educ. 2023;12:399–410.
11. Weidener L, Fischer M. Proposing a principle-based approach for teaching AI ethics in medical education. JMIR Med Educ. 2024;10:e55368.
12. Morton CE, Smith SF, Lwin T, George M, Williams M. Computer programming: should medical students be learning it? JMIR Med Educ. 2019;5:e11940.
13. Law M, Veinot P, Campbell J, Craig M, Mylopoulos M. Computing for medicine: can we prepare medical students for the future? Acad Med. 2019;94:353–7.
14. Meskó B, Görög M. A short guide for medical professionals in the era of artificial intelligence. npj Digit Med. 2020;3:126.
15. Gupta V, Mishra VK, Singhal P, Kumar A (2022) An overview of supervised machine learning algorithm. In 2022 11th international conference on System Modeling & Advancement in Research Trends (SMART). IEEE, pp. 87–92.
16. Ghahramani Z. Unsupervised learning. In: Advanced lectures on machine learning. Berlin, Heidelberg: Springer; 2004. p. 72–112.
17. Montavon G, Kauffmann J, Samek W, Müller K-R. Explaining the predictions of unsupervised learning models. In: Holzinger A, Goebel R, Fong R, Moon T, Müller KR, Samek W, editors. Beyond explainable AI. Cham: Springer; 2022. p. 117–38.
18. Groth D, Hartmann S, Klie S, Selbig J. Principal components analysis. Methods Mol Biol. 2013;930:527–47.
19. Björklund M. Be careful with your principal components. Evolution (NY). 2019;73:2151–8.
20. Sandfort V, Yan K, Graffy PM, Pickhardt PJ, Summers RM. Use of Variational autoencoders with unsupervised learning to detect incorrect organ segmentations at CT. Radiol Artif Intell. 2021;3:e200218.
21. Singh A, Ogunfunmi T. An overview of Variational autoencoders for source separation, finance, and biosignal applications. Entropy. 2021;24:55.
22. Ullah I, Ali F, Shah B, El-Sappagh S, Abuhmed T, Park SH. A deep learning based dual encoder–decoder framework for anatomical structure segmentation in chest X-ray images. Sci Rep. 2023;13:791.
23. Leon V, Etesami SR. Online reinforcement learning in Markov decision process using linear programming. In 2023 62nd IEEE Conference on Decision and Control (CDC). IEEE. 2023: 1973–1978.
24. van Otterlo M, Wiering M. Reinforcement learning and Markov decision processes. In: Wiering M, van Otterlo M, editors. Reinforcement learning. adaptation, learning, and optimization, vol. 12. Berlin, Heidelberg: Springer; 2012. p. 3–42.
25. Hu M, Zhang J, Matkovic L, Liu T, Yang X. Reinforcement learning in medical image analysis: concepts, applications, challenges, and future directions. J Appl Clin Med Phys. 2023;24:e13898. https://doi.org/10.1002/acm2.13898.
26. Hassabis D, Kumaran D, Summerfield C, Botvinick M. Neuroscience-Inspired Artificial Intelligence. Neuron. 2017;95:245–58.
27. Brooks R, et al. Is the brain a good model for machine intelligence? Nature. 2012;482:462–3.
28. Anderson JR, Bothell D, Byrne MD, Douglass S, Lebiere C, Qin Y. An integrated theory of the mind. Psychol Rev. 2004;111:1036–60.
29. Mnih V, Kavukcuoglu K, Silver D, et al. Human-level control through deep reinforcement learning. Nature. 2015;518:529–33.
30. Hochreiter S, Schmidhuber J. Long short-term memory. Neural Comput. 1997;9:1735–80.
31. Graves A, Wayne G, Reynolds M, et al. Hybrid computing using a neural network with dynamic external memory. Nature. 2016;538:471–6.
32. Kirkpatrick J, Pascanu R, Rabinowitz N, et al. Overcoming catastrophic forgetting in neural networks. Proc Natl Acad Sci. 2017;114:3521–6.
33. Hong S, Oh J, Lee H, Han B. Learning transferrable knowledge for semantic segmentation with deep convolutional neural network. In 2016 IEEE conference on Computer Vision and Pattern Recognition Workshops (CVPRW). IEEE. 2016: 3204–3212.

34. Khurana D, Koli A, Khatter K, Singh S. Natural language processing: state of the art, current trends and challenges. Multimed Tools Appl. 2023;82:3713–44.
35. Yim W, Yetisgen M, Harris WP, Kwan SW. Natural language processing in oncology. JAMA Oncol. 2016;2:797.
36. XQ. Explained: tokens and embeddings in LLMs. Medium. 2023. https://medium.com/illuminations-mirror/on-tokenization-in-llms-34309273f238.
37. Menon P. Introduction to large language models and the transformer architecture. Medium. 2023. https://rpradeepmenon.medium.com/introduction-to-large-language-models-and-the-transformer-architecture-534408ed7e61.
38. Mugaanyi J, Cai L, Cheng S, Lu C, Huang J. Evaluation of large language model performance and reliability for citations and references in scholarly writing: cross-disciplinary study. J Med Internet Res. 2024;26:e52935.
39. Peng C, Yang X, Chen A, et al. A study of generative large language model for medical research and healthcare. npj Digit Med. 2023;6:210.
40. Filippova K. Controlled hallucinations: learning to generate faithfully from noisy data. In Findings of the Association for Computational Linguistics, EMNLP 2020. Association for Computational Linguistics, Stroudsburg, PA. 2020: 864–870.
41. Farquhar S, Kossen J, Kuhn L, Gal Y. Detecting hallucinations in large language models using semantic entropy. Nature. 2024;630:625–30.
42. Sejnowski TJ. Large language models and the reverse turing test. Neural Comput. 2023;35:309–42.
43. Estevez M, Benedum CM, Jiang C, Cohen AB, Phadke S, Sarkar S, Bozkurt S. Considerations for the use of machine learning extracted real-world data to support evidence generation: a research-centric evaluation framework. Cancers (Basel). 2022;14:3063.
44. Baxter JSH, Jannin P. Validation in the age of machine learning: a framework for describing validation with examples in transcranial magnetic stimulation and deep brain stimulation. Intell Med. 2023;7:100090.
45. Jayakumar S, Sounderajah V, Normahani P, Harling L, Markar SR, Ashrafian H, Darzi A. Quality assessment standards in artificial intelligence diagnostic accuracy systematic reviews: a meta-research study. npj Digit Med. 2022;5:11.
46. Rodgers CM, Ellingson SR, Chatterjee P. Open data and transparency in artificial intelligence and machine learning: a new era of research. F1000Research. 2023;12:387.
47. Karpov OE, Pitsik EN, Kurkin SA, Maksimenko VA, Gusev AV, Shusharina NN, Hramov AE. Analysis of publication activity and research trends in the field of AI medical applications: network approach. Int J Environ Res Public Health. 2023;20:5335.
48. Ker J, Bai Y, Lee HY, Rao J, Wang L. Automated brain histology classification using machine learning. J Clin Neurosci. 2019;66:239–45.
49. Klitzman R. Consenting for molecular diagnostics. Clin Chem. 2015;61:139–41.
50. Shafique A, Babaie M, Sajadi M, Batten A, Skdar S, Tizhoosh HR. Automatic multi-stain registration of whole slide images in histopathology. In 2021 43rd annual international conference of the IEEE Engineering in Medicine and Biology Society (EMBC), IEEE. 2021: 3622–5.
51. Ertosun MG, Rubin DL. Automated grading of gliomas using deep learning in digital pathology images: a modular approach with ensemble of convolutional neural networks. In AMIA annual symposium proceedings (AMIA Symp 2015). 2015: 1899–908.
52. Jin L, Shi F, Chun Q, et al. Artificial intelligence neuropathologist for glioma classification using deep learning on hematoxylin and eosin stained slide images and molecular markers. Neuro-Oncology. 2021;23:44–52.
53. Pei L, Jones KA, Shboul ZA, Chen JY, Iftekharuddin KM. Deep neural network analysis of pathology images with integrated molecular data for enhanced glioma classification and grading. Front Oncol. 2021;11:668694. https://doi.org/10.3389/fonc.2021.668694.
54. Di Nunno V, Franceschi E, Tosoni A, Gatto L, Maggio I, Lodi R, Angelini D, Bartolini S, Brandes AA. Clinical and molecular features of patients with gliomas harboring IDH1 non-canonical mutations: a systematic review and meta-analysis. Adv Ther. 2022;39:165–77.
55. Gatto L, Franceschi E, Tosoni A, Di Nunno V, Maggio I, Lodi R, Brandes AA. IDH inhibitors and beyond: the cornerstone of targeted glioma treatment. Mol Diagn Ther. 2021;25:457–73.
56. Gatto L, Franceschi E, Tosoni A, Di Nunno V, Bartolini S, Brandes AA. Molecular targeted therapies: time for a paradigm shift in Medulloblastoma treatment? Cancers (Basel). 2022;14:333.
57. Bush NAO, Chang SM, Berger MS. Current and future strategies for treatment of glioma. Neurosurg Rev. 2017;40:1. https://doi.org/10.1007/s10143-016-0709-8.
58. Touat M, Li YY, Boynton AN, et al. Mechanisms and therapeutic implications of hypermutation in gliomas. Nature. 2020;580:517–23.
59. Wen PY, Stein A, van den Bent M, et al. Dabrafenib plus trametinib in patients with BRAFV600E-mutant low-grade and high-grade glioma (ROAR): a multicentre, open-label, single-arm, phase 2, basket trial. Lancet Oncol. 2022;23:53–64.
60. Têtu B, Evans A. Canadian licensure for the use of digital pathology for routine diagnoses: one more step toward a new era of pathology practice without borders. Arch Pathol Lab Med. 2014;138:302–4.

61. Kurc T, Bakas S, Ren X, et al. Segmentation and classification in digital pathology for glioma research: challenges and deep learning approaches. Front Neurosci. 2020;14:27. https://doi.org/10.3389/fnins.2020.00027.
62. Levine AB, Schlosser C, Grewal J, Coope R, Jones SJM, Yip S. Rise of the machines: advances in deep learning for cancer diagnosis. Trends in Cancer. 2019;5:157–69.
63. Dora L, Agrawal S, Panda R, Abraham A. State-of-the-art methods for brain tissue segmentation: a review. IEEE Rev Biomed Eng. 2017;10:235–49.
64. Chen L, Bentley P, Rueckert D. Fully automatic acute ischemic lesion segmentation in DWI using convolutional neural networks. NeuroImage Clin. 2017;15:633–43.
65. Chu R, Kim G, Tauhid S, Khalid F, Healy BC, Bakshi R. Whole brain and deep gray matter atrophy detection over 5 years with 3T MRI in multiple sclerosis using a variety of automated segmentation pipelines. PLoS One. 2018;13:e0206939.
66. Qu L, Zhang Y, Wang S, Yap P-T, Shen D. Synthesized 7T MRI from 3T MRI via deep learning in spatial and wavelet domains. Med Image Anal. 2020;62:101663.
67. Jayachandran Preetha C, Meredig H, Brugnara G, et al. Deep-learning-based synthesis of post-contrast T1-weighted MRI for tumour response assessment in neuro-oncology: a multicentre, retrospective cohort study. Lancet Digit Heal. 2021;3:e784–94.
68. Mellinghoff IK, van den Bent MJ, Blumenthal DT, et al. Vorasidenib in IDH1- or IDH2-mutant low-grade glioma. N Engl J Med. 2023;389:589–601.
69. Choi YS, Bae S, Chang JH, Kang S-G, Kim SH, Kim J, Rim TH, Choi SH, Jain R, Lee S-K. Fully automated hybrid approach to predict the IDH mutation status of gliomas via deep learning and radiomics. Neuro-Oncology. 2021;23:304–13.
70. Chang P, Grinband J, Weinberg BD, et al. Deep-learning convolutional neural networks accurately classify genetic mutations in gliomas. Am J Neuroradiol. 2018;39:1201–7.
71. Kickingereder P, Bonekamp D, Nowosielski M, et al. Radiogenomics of glioblastoma: machine learning–based classification of molecular characteristics by using multiparametric and multiregional MR imaging features. Radiology. 2016;281:907–18.
72. Lu C-F, Hsu F-T, Hsieh KL-C, et al. Machine Learning–Based Radiomics for Molecular Subtyping of Gliomas. Clin Cancer Res. 2018;24:4429–36.
73. Akbari H, Bakas S, Pisapia JM, Nasrallah MP, Rozycki M, Martinez-Lage M, Morrissette JJD, Dahmane N, O'Rourke DM, Davatzikos C. In vivo evaluation of EGFRvIII mutation in primary glioblastoma patients via complex multiparametric MRI signature. Neuro-Oncology. 2018;20:1068–79.
74. Gates EDH, Lin JS, Weinberg JS, Prabhu SS, Hamilton J, Hazle JD, Fuller GN, Baladandayuthapani V, Fuentes DT, Schellingerhout D. Imaging-based algorithm for the local grading of glioma. Am J Neuroradiol. 2020;41:400–7.
75. Peng J, Kim DD, Patel JB, et al. Deep learning-based automatic tumor burden assessment of pediatric high-grade gliomas, medulloblastomas, and other leptomeningeal seeding tumors. Neuro-Oncology. 2022;24:289–99.
76. Maggio I, Franceschi E, Tosoni A, Di NV, Gatto L, Lodi R, Brandes AA. Meningioma: not always a benign tumor. A review of advances in the treatment of meningiomas. CNS. Oncologia. 2021;10:CNS72. https://doi.org/10.2217/cns-2021-0003.
77. Brandes AA, Franceschi E, Tosoni A, et al. MGMT promoter methylation status can predict the incidence and outcome of Pseudoprogression after concomitant Radiochemotherapy in newly diagnosed glioblastoma patients. J Clin Oncol. 2008;26:2192–7.
78. Kim JY, Park JE, Jo Y, Shim WH, Nam SJ, Kim JH, Yoo R-E, Choi SH, Kim HS. Incorporating diffusion- and perfusion-weighted MRI into a radiomics model improves diagnostic performance for pseudoprogression in glioblastoma patients. Neuro-Oncology. 2019;21:404–14.
79. Kniep HC, Madesta F, Schneider T, Hanning U, Schönfeld MH, Schön G, Fiehler J, Gauer T, Werner R, Gellissen S. Radiomics of brain MRI: utility in prediction of metastatic tumor type. Radiology. 2019;290:479–87.
80. Xia W, Hu B, Li H, et al. Deep learning for automatic differential diagnosis of primary central nervous system lymphoma and glioblastoma: multi-parametric magnetic resonance imaging based convolutional neural network model. J Magn Reson Imaging. 2021;54:880–7.
81. Park YW, Oh J, You SC, Han K, Ahn SS, Choi YS, Chang JH, Kim SH, Lee S-K. Radiomics and machine learning may accurately predict the grade and histological subtype in meningiomas using conventional and diffusion tensor imaging. Eur Radiol. 2019;29:4068–76.
82. Tariciotti L, Fiore G, Carrabba G, et al. A supervised machine learning algorithm predicts intraoperative CSF leak in endoscopic transsphenoidal surgery for pituitary adenomas: model development and prospective validation. J Neurosurg Sci. 2021;67:393. https://doi.org/10.23736/S0390-5616.21.05295-4.
83. Suter-Crazzolara C. Better patient outcomes through mining of biomedical big data. Front ICT. 2018;5:54434873. https://doi.org/10.3389/fict.2018.00030.
84. Zachariah FJ, Rossi LA, Roberts LM, Bosserman LD. Prospective comparison of medical oncologists and a machine learning model to predict 3-month mortality in patients with metastatic solid tumors. JAMA Netw Open. 2022;5:e2214514.
85. Jiang LY, Liu XC, Nejatian NP, et al. Health system-scale language models are all-purpose prediction engines. Nature. 2023;619:357–62.

86. Nunez J-J, Leung B, Ho C, Bates AT, Ng RT. Predicting the survival of patients with cancer from their initial oncology consultation document using natural language processing. JAMA Netw Open. 2023;6:e230813.
87. Muhlestein WE, Monsour MA, Friedman GN, Zinzuwadia A, Zachariah MA, Coumans J-V, Carter BS, Chambless LB. Predicting discharge disposition following meningioma resection using a multi-institutional natural language processing model. Neurosurgery. 2021;88:838–45.
88. Pease M, Gersey ZC, Ak M, et al. Pre-operative MRI radiomics model non-invasively predicts key genomic markers and survival in glioblastoma patients. J Neuro-Oncol. 2022;160:253–63.
89. Oh W, Nadkarni GN. Federated learning in health care using structured medical data. Adv Kidney Dis Heal. 2023;30:4–16.
90. Park D, Kim I. Application of machine learning in the field of intraoperative neurophysiological monitoring: a narrative review. Appl Sci. 2022;12:7943.
91. Sieben G, Praet M, Roels H, Otte G, Boullart L, Calliauw L. The development of a decision support system for the pathological diagnosis of human cerebral tumours based on a neural network classifier. Acta Neurochir. 1994;129:193–7.
92. Orringer DA, Pandian B, Niknafs YS, et al. Rapid intraoperative histology of unprocessed surgical specimens via fibre-laser-based stimulated Raman scattering microscopy. Nat Biomed Eng. 2017;1:0027. https://doi.org/10.1038/s41551-016-0027.
93. Ji M, Lewis S, Camelo-Piragua S, et al. Detection of human brain tumor infiltration with quantitative stimulated Raman scattering microscopy. Sci Transl Med. 2015;7:309ra163. https://doi.org/10.1126/scitranslmed.aab0195.
94. Hollon TC, Lewis S, Pandian B, et al. Rapid intraoperative diagnosis of pediatric brain tumors using stimulated raman histology. Cancer Res. 2018;78:278. https://doi.org/10.1158/0008-5472.CAN-17-1974.
95. Luo R, Popp J, Bocklitz T. Deep learning for raman spectroscopy: a review. Analytica. 2022;3:287–301.
96. Jones RR, Hooper DC, Zhang L, Wolverson D, Valev VK. Raman Techniques: Fundamentals and Frontiers. Nanoscale Res Lett. 2019;14:231.
97. Vermeulen C, Pagès-Gallego M, Kester L, et al. Ultra-fast deep-learned CNS tumour classification during surgery. Nature. 2023;622:842–9.
98. Hollon TC, Pandian B, Adapa AR, et al. Near real-time intraoperative brain tumor diagnosis using stimulated Raman histology and deep neural networks. Nat Med. 2020;26:52. https://doi.org/10.1038/s41591-019-0715-9.
99. Farquharson AL, Cresswell AC, Beard JD, Chan P. Randomized trial of the effect of video feedback on the acquisition of surgical skills. Br J Surg. 2013;100:1448–53.
100. Chan J, Pangal DJ, Cardinal T, et al. A systematic review of virtual reality for the assessment of technical skills in neurosurgery. Neurosurg Focus. 2021;51:E15.
101. Pangal DJ, Kugener G, Shahrestani S, Attenello F, Zada G, Donoho DA. A guide to annotation of neurosurgical intraoperative video for machine learning analysis and computer vision. World Neurosurg. 2021;150:26–30.
102. Kiyasseh D, Ma R, Haque TF, Miles BJ, Wagner C, Donoho DA, Anandkumar A, Hung AJ. A vision transformer for decoding surgeon activity from surgical videos. Nat Biomed Eng. 2023;7:780–96.
103. Tucker M, Ma G, Ross W, Buckland DM, Codd PJ. Creation of an automated fluorescence guided tumor ablation system. IEEE J Transl Eng Heal Med. 2021;9:1–9.
104. Hong JC, Eclov NCW, Dalal NH, et al. System for High-Intensity Evaluation During Radiation Therapy (SHIELD-RT): A Prospective Randomized Study of Machine Learning–Directed Clinical Evaluations During Radiation and Chemoradiation. J Clin Oncol. 2020;38:3652–61.
105. Cusumano D, Boldrini L, Dhont J, et al. Artificial intelligence in magnetic resonance guided radiotherapy: medical and physical considerations on state of art and future perspectives. Phys Med. 2021;85:175–91.
106. Gutsche R, Lohmann P, Hoevels M, Ruess D, Galldiks N, Visser-Vandewalle V, Treuer H, Ruge MI, Kocher M. PL01.6.A Radiomics outperforms semantic features for prediction of response to stereotactic radiosurgery in brain metastases. Neuro-Oncology. 2022;24:ii1–2.
107. Tsang DS, Tsui G, McIntosh C, et al. A pilot study of machine-learning based automated planning for primary brain tumours. Radiat Oncol. 2022;17:3.
108. Xue J, Wang B, Ming Y, et al. Deep learning–based detection and segmentation-assisted management of brain metastases. Neuro-Oncology. 2020;22:505–14.
109. Rai R, Kumar S, Batumalai V, et al. The integration of MRI in radiation therapy: collaboration of radiographers and radiation therapists. J Med Radiat Sci. 2017;64:61–8.
110. Hyun CM, Kim HP, Lee SM, Lee S, Seo JK. Deep learning for undersampled MRI reconstruction. Phys Med Biol. 2018;63:135007.
111. Isaksson LJ, Pepa M, Zaffaroni M, et al. Machine learning-based models for prediction of toxicity outcomes in radiotherapy. Front Oncol. 2020;10:790. https://doi.org/10.3389/fonc.2020.00790.
112. Neves BJ, Agnes JP, do Nascimento Gomes M, et al. Efficient identification of novel anti-glioma lead compounds by machine learning models. Eur J Med Chem. 2020;189:111981.
113. Houy N, Le Grand F. Personalized oncology with artificial intelligence: the case of temozolomide. Artif Intell Med. 2019;99:101693.

114. Wang Z, Wang Y, Yang T, Xing H, Wang Y, Gao L, Guo X, Xing B, Wang Y, Ma W. Machine learning revealed stemness features and a novel stemness-based classification with appealing implications in discriminating the prognosis, immunotherapy and temozolomide responses of 906 glioblastoma patients. Brief Bioinform. 2021;22(5):bbab032. https://doi.org/10.1093/bib/bbab032.
115. Arrieta VA, Dmello C, McGrail DJ, Brat DJ, Lee-Chang C, Heimberger AB, Chand D, Stupp R, Sonabend AM. Immune checkpoint blockade in glioblastoma: from tumor heterogeneity to personalized treatment. J Clin Invest. 2023;133(2):e163447. https://doi.org/10.1172/JCI163447.

MIX
Papier aus verantwortungsvollen Quellen
Paper from responsible sources
FSC® C105338

If you have any concerns about our products,
you can contact us on
ProductSafety@springernature.com

In case Publisher is established outside the EU,
the EU authorized representative is:
Springer Nature Customer Service Center GmbH
Europaplatz 3, 69115 Heidelberg, Germany

Printed by Libri Plureos GmbH
in Hamburg, Germany